The Nervous System

The Nervous System

BASIC SCIENCE AND CLINICAL CONDITIONS

THIRD EDITION

Adina T. Michael-Titus

Professor of Neuroscience
Centre for Neuroscience, Surgery and Trauma
Blizard Institute
Barts and The London School of Medicine and Dentistry
Queen Mary University of London
London, UK

Peter J. Shortland

Discipline Lead for Medical Science
Associate Professor of Human Anatomy
Western Sydney University
School of Science,
Penrith, New South Wales, Australia

Series Editor
Stephen Hughes BSc, MSc, MBBS, FRCSEd, FRCEM, FHEA

Consultant in Emergency Medicine, Broomfield Hospital
Senior Lecturer in Medicine, School of Medicine,
Anglia Ruskin University
Chelmsford, UK

For additional online content visit ExpertConsult.com

ELSEVIER

First edition 2003
Second edition 2010

ISBN: 978-0-7020-8340-2

Publisher: Jeremy Bowes
Content Project Manager: Fariha Nadeem
Design: Margaret Reid
Illustration Manager: Anitha Rajarathnam
Marketing Manager: Deborah Watkins

Copyedited by Editage, a unit of Cactus Communications Services Pte. Ltd.
Typeset by TNQ Technologies Pvt. Ltd.
Printed in Scotland

Last digit is the print number: 9 8 7 6 5 4 3 2 1

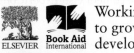

We would like to express our thanks to the various people who have supported us throughout the writing of this book, in particular during the production of the third edition.

Michael Parkinson encouraged us to write this volume. Very special thanks go to Fariha Nadeem and Jeremy Bowes who helped us, cajoled us and kept us on track, so that the work could be completed. Special thanks are due to our clinical colleague, Dr Stephen Hughes, who reviewed all the updated material and provided important comments on each chapter.

Most students now study medicine through a form of integrated curriculum. These courses blend basic science with exposure to clinical medicine from an early stage. These students have the good fortune to be left in no doubt, from the outset, why they are studying medicine. I teach in a medical school that delivers a fully integrated curriculum and I can compare it with the traditional model according to which I received my early medical education. That comparison is very favourable.

Unlike many other texts, the *Systems of the Body* series has been designed very specifically to support an integrated approach to learning medicine. Our carefully selected panel of authors drawn from across the English-speaking world have combined basic science with clinical application. Links to clinical skills, clinical investigation and therapeutics are made clear throughout.

The aim is to offer highly accessible guidance for all student types and stages. It will be invaluable to those who are approaching the subject for the first time or who may have found a topic challenging when using other more traditionally configured resources – as well as greatly assist all students wishing to excel as their course progresses. The clear layout and writing style, together with detail that informs without overwhelming, go a long way to supporting students. It may also provide welcome reminders to postgraduates facing their own examinations.

Whatever curriculum you follow, wherever you are in the world, and whichever stage you are at, we know that the *Systems of the Body* volumes will serve as great places to start when learning something new and enable you to effectively piece together the essential components of each major body system, in a modern clinical context.

Good luck!

Stephen Hughes, MSc MBBS FRCSEd FRCEM FHEA
Senior Lecturer in Medicine
Anglia Ruskin University
Chelmsford, UK
and
Consultant, Emergency Medicine
Broomfield Hospital
Chelmsford, UK

The diseases of the nervous system represent one of the most important challenges in modern medicine. Medical schools worldwide have adopted various strategies in the teaching of neuroscience. One of the more recent approaches combines anatomy, physiology and pharmacology in order to achieve an integrated view of the various pathologies, through the integrated analysis of clinical cases. The problem-based learning method in medicine is based on this concept of integration.

This book is part of the Systems of the Body series, which has been designed to provide a teaching tool for medical curricula that use problem-based learning. The aim of our book is to cover the basic science required to understand the structure and function of the nervous system, and its major pathologies, at a level appropriate to medical students in the first years of training. The volume comprises two parts. The early chapters offer an introduction to the general organization of the nervous system and the cellular and molecular mechanisms that govern its function. A separate chapter is devoted to the clinical examination of the nervous system. The later chapters, which form the main body of the book, are built around clinical cases. The chapters start with clinical scenarios, which prompt an exploration of specific issues, thus allowing us to introduce and discuss the knowledge that is required for the diagnosis and treatment of the conditions presented. To reflect the rapid pace of research in neuroscience, the information in the third edition has been updated throughout the text, and figures modified as appropriate, compared to the second edition.

Our experience of teaching medical students guided us throughout the writing of this text and we tried to present complex concepts in an accessible and clear manner. Our wish was not only to present the facts but also to increase the students' awareness of the many unresolved issues in neuroscience. It is our hope, therefore, that this book will not only assist students in the learning process, but also stimulate their interest and enthusiasm for the fascinating field of neuroscience.

Since the second edition of this book, we have lost our dear colleague and co-author, Dr Patricia Revest. We would like to dedicate this third edition to her memory.

ORGANIZATION OF THE NERVOUS SYSTEM

Chapter summary

1. The nervous system comprises two parts: the central nervous system (CNS), consisting of the brain and spinal cord, and the peripheral nervous system (PNS), which is divided into somatic, autonomic and enteric divisions.

2. The brain consists of three structural parts: two cerebral hemispheres and the cerebellum. They are composed of a thin external layer of cortex, consisting of grey matter densely packed with neurons. Below this is white matter, consisting of pathways that connect the different grey matter areas. The white matter aspect is conferred by the presence of myelinated fibres. Embedded in the white matter are nuclei, which are grey matter clusters of neurons that perform a similar function.

3. The brain has three main divisions: (1) the forebrain, comprising the cerebral cortex, which performs cognitive, perceptual and motor functions, and the diencephalon that controls information flow to the cortex (through the thalamus) and regulates homeostasis (through the hypothalamus); (2) the midbrain, which is important in consciousness and sleep functions and (3) the hindbrain, comprising the cerebellum, pons and medulla, which is concerned with motor coordination (cerebellum), cranial nerve functions and maintenance of life support systems.

4. The spinal cord has a central grey matter core divided into a dorsal sensory half and a ventral motor half. Surrounding the grey matter is white matter, which comprises axons travelling to or from the brain to convey sensory information or motor commands to neurons in the grey matter.

5. The somatic nervous system consists of 31 pairs of spinal nerves and 12 pairs of cranial nerves that give rise to specific peripheral innervation of the skin and skeletal muscles. The vast majority of nerves are mixed, in that they contain both sensory and motor axons, while a few are purely sensory or motor.

6. The autonomic nervous system (ANS) is distinguished from the somatic system by its disynaptic motor output, which consists of preganglionic and postganglionic motoneurons. The ANS has a major role in the control of visceral organs. It comprises three subdivisions: the sympathetic nervous system, which is an alarm system, and the parasympathetic nervous system, which is a rest and recuperation system. Their primary function is the maintenance of homeostasis. The third subdivision is the enteric system, which regulates gut function and operates semiindependently of the other divisions.

Introduction

The nervous system consists of the brain, spinal cord and peripheral nerves and is a highly specialized and complex structure. It is an information-processing system that regulates all the physiological functions of the organism. In addition, the nervous system performs unique functions that operate independently of other systems in the body. These underlie consciousness, memory, rationality, language and the ability to project our mental images forwards or backwards in time. Representations of the external world are transmitted, transformed and manipulated by the nervous system to affect behaviour. It has four important functions:

1. sensory function (gathering of information from the external environment)

2. integration (integration of information from all sources for assessment)

3. effector function (production of a motor response)

4. internal regulation (homeostasis for optimum performance).

The net result is the creation of a sensory percept of the external world, a behavioural response and, importantly, the creation of knowledge that is used to guide future behaviour in response to changes in the surrounding environment and experience.

In order to appreciate how the nervous system produces behaviour, it is necessary to understand how it is organized functionally and anatomically. The experience of examining a brain is very similar to the experience of buying a car. Before buying a car, you inspect it, and then take it for a test drive to make sure that it operates normally and runs smoothly without faults. Then you open up the bonnet to look at the engine. Unless you happen to be a trained mechanic or have an interest in car engines, you might be able to name a few parts, for example, the radiator, the battery and the fan belt, but not the rest of the mass of wires, spark plugs and assorted boxes. Moreover, the name does not always indicate what the function is or how all the different parts combine to burn petrol to make the car run. It is the same with the nervous system; you may be able to name some of the parts, such as the cortex, cerebellum and brainstem, and have some idea of what a few of the different parts do but have little idea of how they accomplish a task, such as reading this sentence. Moreover, when the car breaks down, we call the automobile rescue services. When the nervous system breaks down or misfires, we call neurologists, neurosurgeons or psychiatrists.

Although the anatomy of the nervous system appears complex and daunting, its organization is governed by a set of relatively simple developmental, organizational and functional rules that bring order to it, as summarized in Table 1.1.

The aim of this chapter is to provide a functional overview of the neuroanatomy of the brain, spinal cord and nerves. To do this, it is necessary to consider the basic parts of the nervous system to identify what they do and how they are related. Finally, we can see how the different parts interact, using the principles outlined in Table 1.1, to produce behaviour.

The nervous system comprises two parts: the peripheral nervous system (PNS) and the central nervous system (CNS). These two systems are anatomically separate but functionally interconnected and integrated (Fig. 1.1).

The PNS consists of nerve fibres that transmit specific sensory and motor information to the CNS, which comprises the spinal cord, brainstem and brain. The CNS is housed within the bony structures of the vertebral canal and skull for protection. Additional mechanical buffering protection of the CNS is afforded by the surrounding meninges and the fluid in the ventricular system.

Overview of brain anatomy

Based on neural development, the nervous system is initially comprised of three anatomical regions: the forebrain, midbrain and hindbrain. As the brain further develops, the CNS becomes six anatomically distinct regions: the cerebral cortex and diencephalon (thalamus and hypothalamus), which together form the forebrain; the midbrain, pons, medulla and cerebellum, which together comprise the hindbrain; and the spinal cord (Fig. 1.2). The best way to understand the anatomy is to look at the external and internal topography to identify anatomical structures and their relationships, and then to define the functions of the identified structures.

Meninges

If the skull cap is removed, the first thing seen is the membranes that cover the brain, called meninges. These membranes surround and protect the CNS. There are three layers: the dura mater, arachnoid and pia mater. The dura mater forms folds that separate different brain regions from each other and demarcate anatomical boundaries within the skull cavity. These layers are described in more detail in Chapter 12.

Cortical lobes

When the meninges are removed, one can observe the gross anatomy of the CNS. Anatomically, the cortex is described according to lobes that are named in relation to skull bones. Four lobes are visible on its lateral surface: the occipital, temporal, parietal and frontal lobes. However, there is one lobe that is not visible: the limbic lobe. It comprises the medial portions of the frontal, parietal and temporal lobes, forming a rim around the corpus callosum (a fibre tract that connects the two cortical hemispheres). Another cortical area, the insula, lies buried in the medial wall of the lateral fissure, overlain by parts of the frontal, parietal and temporal lobes; it is functionally associated with the limbic lobe. The lobes are divided into regions that are associated with specific functions (see Table 1.2).

Table 1.1 Principles underlying the functioning of the nervous system
Behaviour is produced by processing information in a sequence of 'in → integrate → out'
Separate sensory and motor divisions exist throughout the nervous system
The nervous system has multiple levels of function
The nervous system is organized both in parallel and in series
Most neural pathways relaying information decussate from one side of the central nervous system to the other
The nervous system regulates activity through excitation and inhibition
There is both symmetry and asymmetry in brain anatomy and function
Some of the functions of the brain are located in specific regions of the brain, while others are distributed

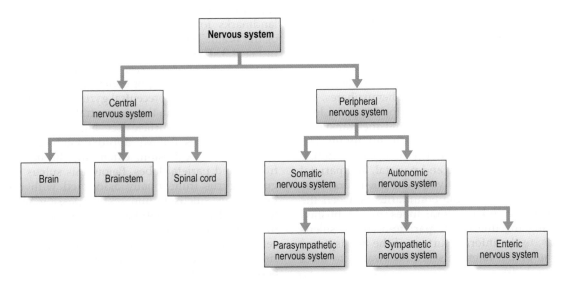

Fig. 1.1 Overview of the anatomical organization of the nervous system.

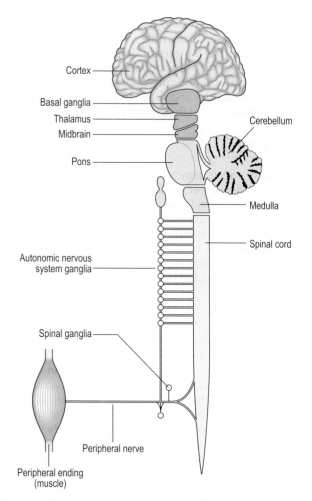

Cortex

Basal ganglia

Thalamus

Midbrain

Pons

Cerebellum

Medulla

Spinal cord

Autonomic nervous
system ganglia

Spinal ganglia

Peripheral nerve

Peripheral ending
(muscle)

Fig. 1.2 Schematic representation of the major parts of the nervous system. Light shading: structures of the supratentorial level. Dark shading: structures of the posterior fossa level. No shading: structures of the spinal level.

Table 1.2	Functions of brain lobes	
Lobe	**Important functional areas**	**Function**
Frontal	Primary motor cortex	Control of movement
	Broca's area	Expressive speech
	Motor association cortex	Intelligence, movement planning, intuition, rationalisation, object tracking
Parietal	Primary somatosensory cortex	Sensation
	Association cortex	Spatial awareness
	Taste cortex	Taste sensation
Temporal	Primary auditory cortex	Hearing
	Wernicke's area	Language comprehension
Occipital	Primary visual cortex	Vision
	Visual association cortex	Visual spatial awareness, colour processing
Limbic	Medial temporal lobe (uncus)	Emotions, memory
	Medial prefrontal cortex	Motivation, personality, emotional behaviour, risk-reward, working memory
	Cingulate cortex	Cognition, emotional affect
	Orbitofrontal	Olfaction, emotional behaviour

Surface features: sulci and gyri

The cortical surface is highly convoluted and is subdivided into fissures (deep grooves), gyri (elevated folds; singular = gyrus) and sulci (shallow grooves between folds; singular = sulcus). Gyri massively increase the surface area of the cortex. The longitudinal fissure separates the two cortical hemispheres, the lateral fissure (of Sylvius) separates the temporal lobe from the parietal and frontal lobes and the transverse fissure separates the forebrain from the hindbrain. The central sulcus and the parieto-occipital sulcus define the boundaries of the frontal and parietal, and parietal and occipital lobes, respectively. On the lateral surface of the hemispheres, the boundaries between the parietal, occipital and temporal lobes are established by continuing the line of the parieto-occipital sulcus downwards, to the inferior surface of the hemisphere, and the line of the lateral fissure backwards to meet this line (Fig. 1.3B).

The pattern of sulci and gyri is extremely variable, and defining even the major sulci and gyri is not always easy. In general, the surface of each lobe can be divided into three gyri by two sulci; this is easily seen in the frontal and temporal lobes, where the gyri are called superior, middle and inferior gyri. The sulci provide landmarks for identifying lobes and functional areas of the brain. The main lobes, gyri and sulci, are shown in Fig. 1.3. The central sulcus marks the position of two important functional areas: the primary somatosensory cortex and primary motor cortex. The latter lies anterior to this sulcus, in the precentral gyrus; the former lies posterior to the sulcus, in the postcentral gyrus.

On the medial surface (see Figs 1.3C and 1.5), the cingulate sulcus follows approximately the curvature of the corpus callosum, extending through both the frontal and parietal lobes. Below this sulcus is the cingulate gyrus (functionally associated with the limbic lobe). This sulcus terminates by passing upwards to form a sulcus that continues onto the lateral surface of the hemisphere as the postcentral sulcus (Fig. 1.3B). The central sulcus is usually the sulcus immediately anterior to this sulcus (on the lateral surface). The gyrus in between these two sulci is the postcentral gyrus, which

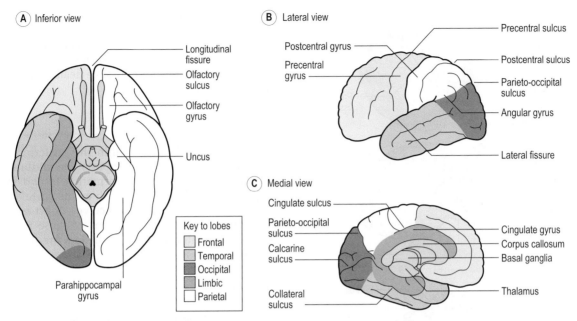

A Inferior view

Longitudinal fissure
Olfactory sulcus
Olfactory gyrus
Uncus

Parahippocampal gyrus

Key to lobes
- Frontal
- Temporal
- Occipital
- Limbic
- Parietal

B Lateral view

Postcentral gyrus
Precentral gyrus
Precentral sulcus
Postcentral sulcus
Parieto-occipital sulcus
Angular gyrus
Lateral fissure

C Medial view

Cingulate sulcus
Parieto-occipital sulcus
Calcarine sulcus
Collateral sulcus
Cingulate gyrus
Corpus callosum
Basal ganglia
Thalamus

Fig. 1.3 Main gyri, sulci, fissures and lobes of the brain.

contains the primary somatosensory cortex. Anterior to the point where the cingulate sulcus crosses (to the lateral surface of the brain) is the paracentral lobule, which contains the lower limb primary motor and somatosensory cortical function regions. The parieto-occipital and calcarine sulci are very prominent on the posteromedial part of the brain, to the extent that some consider them fissures rather than sulci. The lingual gyrus and cuneus region are located either side of the calcarine sulcus in the posterior part of the brain, and are associated with vision.

On the inferior surface (Fig. 1.3A) of the temporal lobe, the three gyri separated by two sulci are also obvious. The most medial gyrus is the parahippocampal gyrus, which expands at its anterior end to form the bulbous, hook-like uncus. These are evolutionarily old parts of the cerebral cortex and are concerned, in part, with the olfactory (smell) system and memory. It is separated from the middle gyrus, called the occipitotemporal (fusiform) gyrus, by the collateral sulcus, which becomes the rhinal sulcus at its anterior end, to separate it from the uncus. The most lateral sulcus is the inferior temporal gyrus (which is visible from the lateral and inferior surfaces). It is separated from the occipitotemporal gyrus by the occipitotemporal sulcus.

The orbitofrontal cortex (the part that sits above the orbit in the skull) is part of the inferior surface of the frontal lobe. Three gyri are also visible here: the gyrus rectus is the most medial and is the inferior continuation of the superior frontal gyrus. Adjacent to it are located two olfactory gyri, which are the inferior continuations of the middle and inferior frontal gyri from the lateral surface of the frontal lobe. The olfactory tract and bulb run over the surface of the olfactory sulcus between the gyrus rectus and olfactory sulcus. These cortical areas form part of the limbic system, which is involved in emotional processing and perception.

Cerebellum

Also visible on the inferior surface of the brain is the cerebellum. The cerebellum is the broccoli-like structure separated from the overlying occipital cortex by the transverse fissure. The function of the cerebellum is coordination of movements, including muscle tone, movement range, smoothness and equilibrium, as detailed in Chapter 9.

The cerebellum consists of a deeply convoluted cortex composed of numerous small gyri called folia and a core of white matter, within which are embedded the deep nuclei of the cerebellum (Fig. 1.4). The cerebellum has three lobes, the anterior, posterior and flocculonodular lobes (Fig. 1.4A, B), which are further subdivided into lobules. In the horizontal plane, there are three regions: the midline vermis separates the two lateral hemispheres. In the sagittal plane, the cerebellum forms the roof of the fourth ventricle (Fig. 1.4C), and it can be subdivided into three functional areas, the vestibulocerebellum, spinocerebellum and cerebrocerebellum (Fig. 1.4D), based on the source of afferent input. Each subdivision is associated with a pair of deep cerebellar nuclei. Input and output to the cerebellum are via three pairs of peduncles: the inferior, middle and superior cerebellar peduncles that attach to the different regions of the brainstem. The inferior cerebellar peduncle arises from the medulla and provides the predominant input to the anterior lobe from different body regions. The middle cerebellar peduncle is the largest and projects to the posterior lobe from the pontine

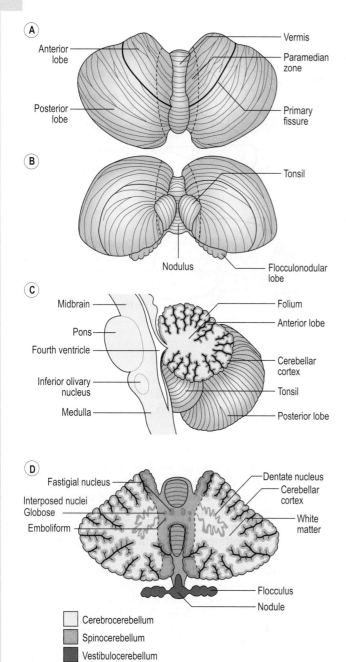

Fig. 1.4 Anatomy of the cerebellum: (A) superior view, (B) inferior view, (C) sagittal view and (D) horizontal view. (D) Shows the functional subdivisions and their associated deep cerebellar nuclei.

nuclei of the pons, carrying information from the motor cortex commissural fibres from one side of the cerebellum to the other. The superior cerebellar peduncle connects the posterior lobe to the midbrain and is predominantly an output pathway from the deep cerebellar nuclei, in particular, the dentate nucleus.

Also present on the inferior surface are the cerebellar tonsils, which lie lateral to the vermis of the cerebellum (Fig. 1.4B). They are easily identifiable, as their sulci are oriented at right angles to the general direction of the

other cerebellar sulci. They are anatomically important because they may herniate through the foramen magnum (in severe cases of raised intracranial pressure, see Chapter 11), resulting in compression on the respiratory centres of the medulla and possible death due to respiratory depression.

Brainstem

The brainstem is located within the posterior fossa of the skull and consists of three parts: the midbrain, pons and medulla. These relay information to and from the periphery to higher centres such as the cortex and cerebellum. The brainstem also receives direct input from the cranial nerves. The functions of these nerves and the internal anatomy of the brainstem are described in Chapter 6.

Medulla

On the ventral surface of the medulla are the pyramids (see Fig. 6.1) that contain descending motor fibres from the cerebral cortex that form the corticospinal (or pyramidal) tract (CST) of the spinal cord. The pyramidal decussation is where most of the CST fibres cross to the other side to become the lateral CST. The decussation marks the location of the spinomedullary junction, which is where the spinal cord ends and the brainstem begins. Lateral to the rostral part of the pyramids are two oval swellings that identify the inferior olivary nuclei (ION), which are functionally associated with the cerebellum. They provide a surface landmark for the emergence of cranial nerves IX–XII; nerve XII emerges between the ION and the pyramids (at the preolivary sulcus), whereas nerves IX–XI emerge laterally to the ION (from the postolivary sulcus).

On the dorsal surface of the brainstem, the medulla consists of two parts, the open and closed medulla, due to the emergence of the central canal from the spinal cord opening into the fourth ventricle. The point at which this occurs is called the obex. The closed part of the medulla shows a pair of gracile and cuneate tubercles that mark the positions of the gracile and cuneate nuclei (see Fig. 6.1), which transmit sensory information to higher brain centres.

Pons

The ventral pons has a transversely ridged appearance, with a shallow groove running along the midline, called the basilar sulcus, which contains the basilar artery. The ridged appearance is due to fibres entering the cerebellum from the nerve cells in the pons, which, in turn, are the recipients of a major input from the cerebral cortex (see Fig. 6.1). The trigeminal nerve is the only nerve to emerge from this ridged region, while cranial nerves VII and VIII exit at the cerebellopontomedullary angle. The position of cranial nerves VI–VIII identifies the pontomedullary junction on the ventral surface.

The pons is sharply demarcated both rostrally and caudally from the other parts of the brainstem. The open medulla and pons together form the floor of the fourth ventricle, which is diamond-shaped. The closure of the rostral part of the fourth ventricle to form the cerebral aqueduct and the cerebral peduncles demarcates the transition from the pons to the midbrain.

Midbrain

The midbrain (see Fig. 6.1) is short, and very little of it can be seen in the undissected brain. Ventrally, the cerebral peduncles are located lateral to two small, circumscribed mounds, which are the mammillary bodies (part of the hypothalamus). The peduncles are large bundles of fibres descending from the motor cortex to the brainstem and spinal cord and mainly comprise the pyramidal and corticopontine fibre systems. The dorsal surface of the midbrain is called the tectum and has two paired swellings, the inferior and superior colliculi, which are involved in auditory and visual reflexes. These are buried beneath the overlying cerebral hemispheres. Two cranial nerves exit the midbrain, cranial nerve III at the midbrain–pons junction and cranial nerve IV on the dorsal surface.

Spinal cord

The spinal cord connects the brain to the PNS. It is the part of the CNS located outside the skull, below the foramen magnum but within the vertebral column. The spinal level of the nervous system extends from the skull to the sacrum. The spinal cord receives input from the periphery, relays it to the brain and sends response signals back to the periphery. The spinal cord is not segmented; rather, the distribution of the peripheral nerve spinal roots gives it a functional segregation. The details of spinal cord function are described in Chapter 4. The spinal cord consists of grey matter and white matter, like the brain (except that in the spinal cord, the white matter is on the outside). The grey matter contains cells and is surrounded by white matter that mainly contains bundles of axons ascending and descending in the spinal cord.

Internal anatomy of the brain

The easiest way to see the various anatomical structures deep inside the brain is to cut it open. However, what is seen depends on the plane of section; the same structures look different in different planes (see Box 1.1). Many of these structures form the walls of the ventricular system.

Ventricular system

The ventricles are irregularly shaped cavities within the brain that contain cerebrospinal fluid (CSF). The main functions of the CSF are to provide buffering support

---

Box 1.1 Brain topography

Anatomical descriptions of images and tissue sections are based on four anatomical planes: sagittal, horizontal, transverse and median (Fig. 1.6). The horizontal (axial) plane is a plane across the brain that would be horizontal if the patient were standing up. The median plane is one that slices the brain vertically along the midline into two symmetrical halves; sagittal sections are vertical planes through the brain parallel to the median plane. The coronal (frontal) plane is one slicing the brain vertically across (e.g. from ear to ear).

In addition, structures towards the front of the brain are termed anterior (or rostral), and those towards the back are posterior (or caudal). Those towards the top of the brain are termed superior, and those towards the bottom are termed inferior. Structures located laterally are further away from the midline, and those located medially are nearer the midline.

---

during rapid head movements and to provide buoyancy to CNS structures, so that they are, in effect, weightless.

The ventricular system consists of two lateral ventricles, and the midline third and fourth ventricles, connected by the cerebral aqueduct (Fig. 1.5). The lateral ventricles are the largest cavities and are located deep within the brain. They are symmetrical structures. Each communicates with the third ventricle through the interventricular foramen (of Monro), and the latter is connected to the fourth ventricle via the cerebral aqueduct.

CSF drains from the fourth ventricle through a median and two lateral apertures in its floor (giving it a diamond-shaped appearance) into the subarachnoid space. These apertures are the only means by which the CSF can enter the subarachnoid space. The cerebellum forms the roof of the fourth ventricle, called the superior medullary velum.

All the ventricles contain variable amounts of choroid plexus, which is the main source for the production of CSF (see Chapter 12). If the flow of CSF becomes blocked (especially in the cerebral aqueduct), there is a rise in intracranial pressure. If this happens in infants, they may develop hydrocephalus and severe brain damage.

Sagittal sections

If the brain is sectioned at the midline, cutting along the longitudinal fissure, the cerebrum is divided into its two hemispheres, as shown in Fig. 1.7. In this plane, below the corpus callosum are the deep (diencephalic) structures of the brain: the thalamus, the hypothalamus and the ventricular system. Moving laterally in this plane, adjacent sections also reveal the appearance of the basal ganglia nuclei that are located on top of the thalamus and form part of the lateral walls of the ventricular system. The basal ganglia are better viewed in frontal and horizontal sections (see Figs 1.8 and 1.11). As shown in the upper part of Fig. 1.7, a thin membranous sheet—the septum pellucidum (which is torn in

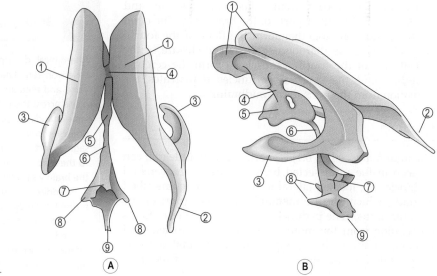

Fig. 1.5 Anatomy of the ventricular system from the (A) superior and (B) posterolateral aspects. 1, lateral ventricle; 2, posterior horn; 3, inferior horn; 4, interventricular foramen (of Monro); 5, third ventricle; 6, cerebral aqueduct; 7, fourth ventricle; 8, lateral aperture (of Luschka) and 9, median aperture (of Magendie).

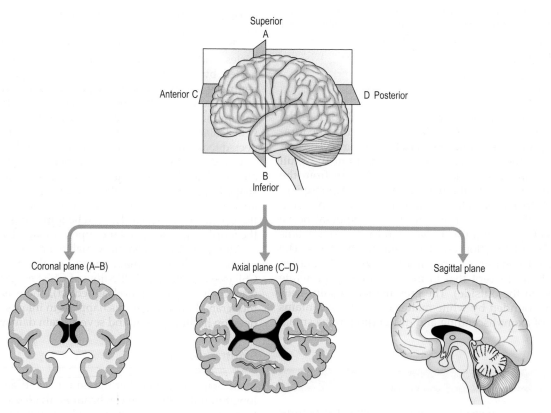

Fig. 1.6 Anatomical planes of sections. Shading: black, ventricles; grey, grey matter; yellow, white matter.

this specimen)—obscures them. Most of these structures are visible in the MRI image shown in the lower part of Fig. 1.7.

Coronal sections

Frontal (coronal) sections are the easiest to visualize because their orientation is such that viewing them is just like looking at another person face-on. When sectioning from front to back (Figs 1.8–1.11), the very first section in a coronal series would consist of just the tips of the frontal lobes, which are located right behind the forehead. The section shown in Fig. 1.8 is a little further caudal and is the first to show the internal structures. In these sections, the white matter (axons) appears white and the grey matter (cell bodies) appears grey. The first thing to notice is the corpus callosum. This major pathway

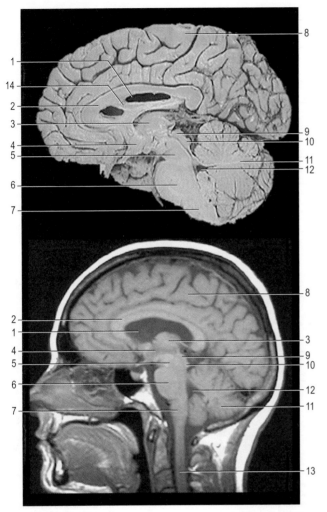

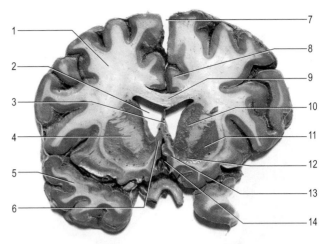

1. Frontal lobe
2. Lateral ventricle
3. Septum pellucidum
4. Anterior limb of internal capsule
5. Temporal lobe
6. Septal nuclei
7. Longitudinal fissure

8. Cingulate gyrus.
9. Corpus callosum
10. Caudate nucleus
11. Putamen
12. Nucleus accumbens
13. Hypothalamus
14. Third ventricle

Fig. 1.8 Coronal section of the brain.

1. Lateral ventricle
2. Corpus callosum
3. Thalamus
4. Hypothalamus
5. Midbrain
6. Pons
7. Medulla

8. Paracentral lobule
9. Superior colliculus
10. Inferior colliculus
11. Cerebellum
12. Fourth ventricle
13. Spinal cord
14. Septum pellucidum

Fig. 1.7 Midsagittal section of the brain shown in a gross specimen (top) and at the equivalent level on a magnetic resonance imaging scan (bottom).

connects the two hemispheres and serves as a useful landmark because it appears in all coronal sections in which deep structures are present.

Below the corpus callosum are the front ends of the two lateral ventricles, separated by the septum pellucidum. The masses of grey matter that form the lateral walls of the lateral ventricles are the caudate nuclei (part of the basal ganglia). The rule for identifying them is simple: if the lateral ventricles are visible, so is the caudate. This applies throughout the curved extent of the lateral ventricles, as the caudate follows them the whole way.

The caudate appears connected by threads of grey matter to another nucleus, the putamen. These two nuclei are almost always divided by a band of axons called the

internal capsule, which is a major pathway for connections between the thalamus and the cortex. In the rostral brain, these two nuclei are continuous at the base, so that in reality the caudate and the putamen are a single nucleus, divided in half by the internal capsule; hence, they are commonly called the striatum. Early anatomists did not realize this; therefore they were named separately, and the small ventral bridge below the internal capsule, which connects them, was named the nucleus accumbens. The nucleus accumbens and the septal nuclei are associated with conscious 'reward' and motivation and are part of the limbic system. These structures are involved in the mediation of the effects of addictive drugs, such as cocaine, heroin and amphetamines.

In the next most caudal section, shown in Fig. 1.9A, the nucleus accumbens has disappeared and the caudate and putamen are no longer connected. The caudate nucleus is decreased in size, and medial to the putamen, a new set of basal ganglia nuclei emerges—the globus pallidus external (GPe) and internal (GPi). The interventricular foramens—the diagonal openings that connect the lateral ventricles with the midline third ventricle—are clearly visible. The septum here is very small, and suspended from it are tracts called fornices (singular = fornix). The third ventricle is below the fornices. The fornix connects the mammillary body (part of the hypothalamus) to the hippocampus (in the temporal lobe). Below and lateral to the hypothalamus at the base of the brain is the optic tract. Below, between the putamen and GPe, and just above the temporal lobe is the anterior commissure, a white matter tract that connects the temporal lobes of each hemisphere. In the medial part of the temporal lobe is a circumscribed region of grey matter, the amygdala. The amygdala is a specialized part of the brain; it

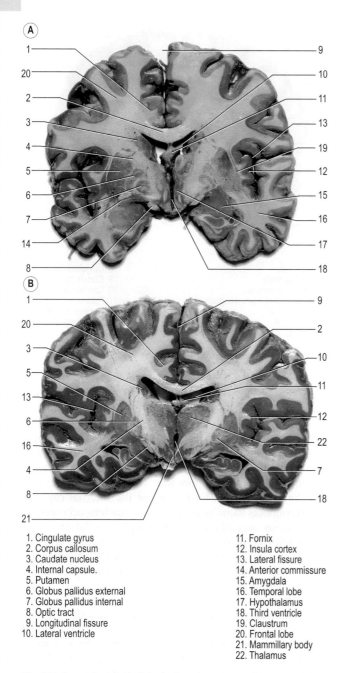

Fig. 1.9 Coronal section of the brain.

1. Cingulate gyrus
2. Corpus callosum
3. Caudate nucleus
4. Internal capsule.
5. Putamen
6. Globus pallidus external
7. Globus pallidus internal
8. Optic tract
9. Longitudinal fissure
10. Lateral ventricle
11. Fornix
12. Insula cortex
13. Lateral fissure
14. Anterior commissure
15. Amygdala
16. Temporal lobe
17. Hypothalamus
18. Third ventricle
19. Claustrum
20. Frontal lobe
21. Mammillary body
22. Thalamus

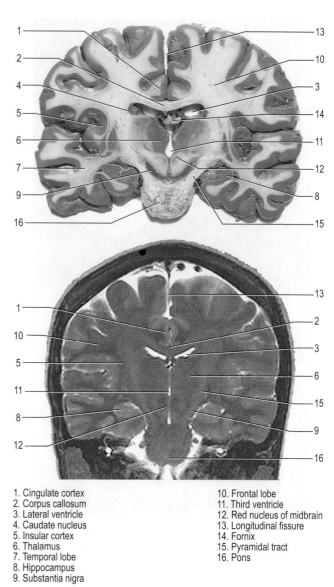

1. Cingulate cortex
2. Corpus callosum
3. Lateral ventricle
4. Caudate nucleus
5. Insular cortex
6. Thalamus
7. Temporal lobe
8. Hippocampus
9. Substantia nigra
10. Frontal lobe
11. Third ventricle
12. Red nucleus of midbrain
13. Longitudinal fissure
14. Fornix
15. Pyramidal tract
16. Pons

Fig. 1.10 Coronal section of the brain shown in a gross specimen (top) and at the equivalent level on a magnetic resonance imaging scan (bottom).

encompasses several nuclei and is part of the limbic system. It deals with the emotional significance of experiences. The insula cortex is also visible at this level, located medial to the lateral fissure. The insula is considered part of the limbic system and has a variety of roles including pain and taste perception, interoception, homeostasis and emotional and cognitive functions. It is a true integration hub where bodily sensations, emotional processing and autonomic functions converge. Between the insula and putamen is a nucleus called the claustrum. The claustrum has wide-ranging connections with the hippocampus, amygdala, caudate nucleus and premotor, prefrontal,

auditory and visual cortices. It seems to act as the conductor of cortical function to synchronise (bind) together the perceptual, cognitive and motor modalities relevant to consciousness and selective attention. The claustrum is separated from the insula by the extreme capsule and from the putamen by the external capsule.

Moving further caudally (Fig. 1.9B), another major nuclear structure, the diencephalon, appears, and it comprises the thalamus and hypothalamus. Both are a heterogeneous group of nuclei with specific functions: the thalami are the gatekeepers for any information passing to and from the cerebral cortex, while the hypothalamic nuclei regulate homeostasis and endocrine functions. The medial nuclei of the hypothalami and thalami form the lateral walls of the slit-like third ventricle. This provides another anatomical rule: if the third ventricle is

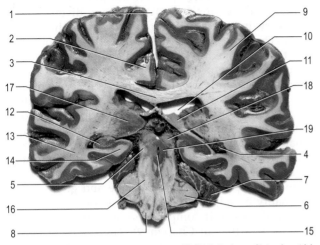

1. Longitudinal fissure
2. Cingulate cortex
3. Splenium of corpus callosum
4. Inferior horn of lateral ventricle
5. Midbrain
6. Middle cerebral peduncle
7. Cerebellum
8. Medulla
9. Parietal cortex
10. Posterior horn of lateral ventricle
11. Fornix
12. Hippocampus
13. Temporal lobe
14. Parahippocampal gyrus
15. Cerebral aqueduct
16. Pons

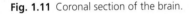

Fig. 1.11 Coronal section of the brain.

visible, so is the thalamus (or hypothalamus). The thalamus is located medial to the internal capsule (posterior limb), while the putamen and globus pallidus remain lateral to it; this relationship is always preserved and is easily seen in horizontal sections. The two swellings at the base of the midbrain are the mammillary bodies.

In Fig. 1.10, the globus pallidus and putamen have disappeared. The caudate nuclei are very small, and the thalami are larger. A new structure visible here in the medial temporal lobe, shaped like a sea-horse, is the hippocampus. At this level, more of the ventral surface of the brainstem has been sectioned. Medial to the hippocampus on either side are diagonally running white matter tracts that pass through the midbrain, pons and medulla. These are the pyramidal tracts. Also visible in the midbrain region is the substantia nigra, which has been cut obliquely, and the red nuclei. The ventral surface of the pons is also cut, showing the transverse cerebellopontine fibres.

Fig. 1.11 shows the last section of this series and much has changed. The posterior part of the left lateral ventricle is visible as a long diagonal slit comprising the posterior and inferior horns (and associated choroid plexus). The lateral ventricle, like many other structures in the brain, curves back and loops under itself like a big 'C'. The hippocampus, which is involved in memory formation, is clearly visible on the medial side of the lower part of the lateral ventricle, and is connected to the fornix, which runs inside the ventricles. This section is at the junction of the brainstem and cerebrum. The midbrain is identified by the cerebral aqueduct, which connects the third and fourth ventricles, and the paired superior

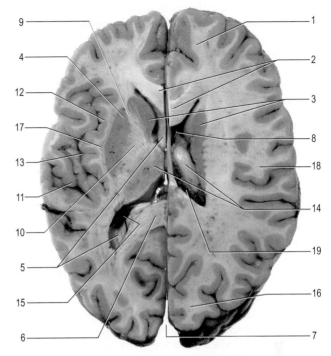

1. Frontal lobe
2. Genu of corpus callosum
3. Caudate nucleus
4. Putamen
5. Fornix
6. Splenium of corpus callosum
7. Longitudinal fissure
8. Anterior horn of lateral ventricle
9. Anterior limb of internal capsule
10. Posterior limb of internal capsule
11. Temporal lobe
12. Insular cortex
13. Lateral fissure
14. Thalamus
15. Posterior horn of lateral ventricle
16. Occipital lobe
17. Claustrum
18. Parietal lobe
19. Choroid plexus

Fig. 1.12 Horizontal section of the brain at the level of the lateral ventricles.

colliculi. Below the midbrain is the pons, with the two middle cerebellar peduncles (tracts of white matter) connecting the pons to the cerebellum.

Horizontal sections

In the horizontal plane, all the major subcortical nuclear structures are related to the positions of the ventricular system and internal capsule. Fig. 1.12 shows a brain cut at two different levels of the lateral ventricles—the right superior to the left. The caudate nuclei protrude into the anterior part of the lateral ventricles to form its lateral wall, and on the left, the putamen is separated from the caudate by the anterior limb of the internal capsule. The white matter tract immediately anterior and posterior to the ventricles is the corpus callosum, which crosses in and out of the plane of the page. Remember that, in the sagittal plane, it curves like a 'C' from front to back; in this horizontal section, it was cut through twice, at the front (genu) and back (splenium) end. At this level, on the left, the true shape of the internal capsule is apparent in the horizontal plane; it is V-shaped, with an anterior limb and a posterior limb. The third ventricle and the thalamic nuclei on either side are visible. The interventricular foramen between the lateral ventricles and the third ventricle is visible. Also visible in the left ventricle are the cut parts of the fornices.

Forebrain

This is the largest part of the brain (80% by volume) and comprises the cerebral cortex, limbic system and basal ganglia. The forebrain is involved with perception, cognition, motivation, memory, emotion and control of higher motor functions.

The architecture of the cortex differs between the cerebral cortex and limbic cortex. The limbic cortex is evolutionarily older and comprises only three (archi- or paleo-cortex) or four cell layers of grey matter, whereas the rest of the cortex, called the neocortex, is evolutionarily more recent and comprises six layers. The cortex consists mostly of pyramidal cells and granule cells; simplistically, granule cells (in layer 4) receive sensory input and pyramidal cells (layer 5) provide output. The other layers connect to other areas of the cortex on the same side of the brain via association fibres and to the contralateral side via commissural fibres.

The cortex is divided into areas that have a single function such as touch, vision, hearing, taste and smell or the production of movement. These are called primary areas (Table 1.2). Their function is to receive and start the initial processing of information. The rest of the cortex is association cortex, which provides higher-order processing of sensory and motor information. Some of these regions process complex aspects of a single sensory modality or information related to motor function, such as premotor cortex, or areas V2–V4 in the

visual system (Chapter 7). There are four main regions of association cortex, which carry out diverse types of sensory integration required for purposeful movements. They provide the link between sensations and (re)action by making connections with motor areas. These include the posterior parietal cortex, which integrates sensory and visual stimuli; it is associated with self- and spatial awareness, and is critical for attention to external events. The parietal–occipital–temporal association region coordinates somatosensation with visual and auditory cues to produce perceptual recognition or movements in response to visual or auditory stimuli. The frontal association cortex occupies most of the rostral part of the frontal lobe and gives us our personality by adjusting behaviour according to moral and social norms. It comprises several distinct regions (described further in Chapter 9). The premotor cortex is important in the planning of voluntary movements. The dorsolateral prefrontal region connects with the sensory and motor cortices and is associated with the attentional and cognitive consequences associated with movements. The ventromedial prefrontal cortex is interconnected with the limbic system to encode the emotional aspects of motor behaviour. The limbic association area is associated with the medial and inferior surfaces of the brain and is devoted mostly to memory, motivation and emotion. All the association areas feed into the higher-order motor areas, which then project to the primary motor cortex, which ultimately exerts control over the motor neurons (Fig. 1.13).

It is important to recognize the locations of the major functional areas of the cortex, particularly the primary somatosensory, visual, auditory and motor cortices (Figs 1.14 and 1.15). Selective damage to these regions leads to discrete neurological deficits.

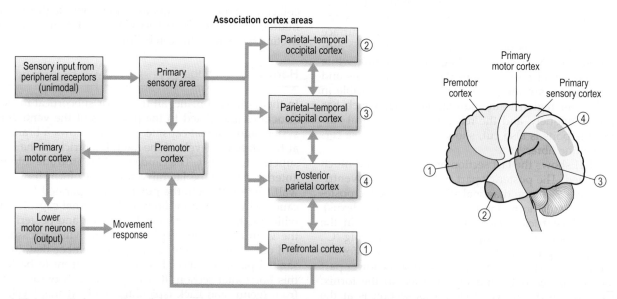

Fig. 1.13 Intercortical connections of primary, higher-order and association cortices used in processing a sensory stimulus to produce a behavioural response. Inset shows the location of the various association areas.

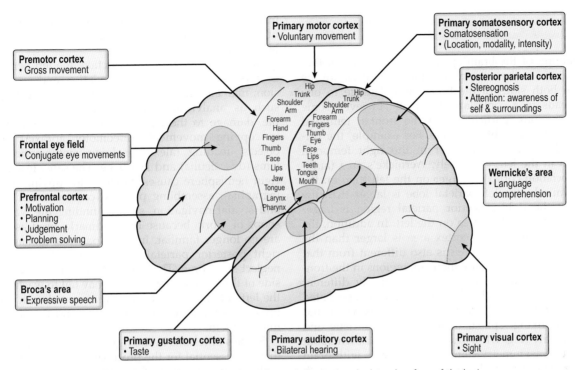

Premotor cortex
• Gross movement

Primary motor cortex
• Voluntary movement

Primary somatosensory cortex
• Somatosensation
• (Location, modality, intensity)

Posterior parietal cortex
• Stereognosis
• Attention: awareness of self & surroundings

Frontal eye field
• Conjugate eye movements

Prefrontal cortex
• Motivation
• Planning
• Judgement
• Problem solving

Wernicke's area
• Language comprehension

Broca's area
• Expressive speech

Hip
Trunk
Shoulder
Arm
Forearm
Hand
Fingers
Thumb
Face
Lips
Jaw
Tongue
Larynx
Pharynx

Hip
Trunk
Shoulder
Arm
Forearm
Fingers
Thumb
Eye
Face
Lips
Teeth
Tongue
Mouth

Primary gustatory cortex
• Taste

Primary auditory cortex
• Bilateral hearing

Primary visual cortex
• Sight

Fig. 1.14 Functional anatomy of specific cortical areas on the lateral surface of the brain.

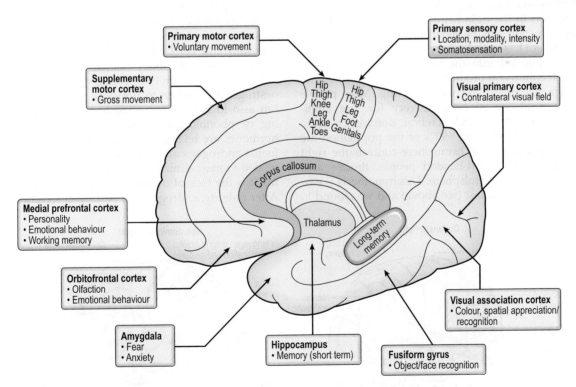

Primary motor cortex
• Voluntary movement

Primary sensory cortex
• Location, modality, intensity
• Somatosensation

Supplementary motor cortex
• Gross movement

Visual primary cortex
• Contralateral visual field

Hip
Thigh
Knee
Leg
Ankle
Toes

Hip
Thigh
Leg
Foot
Genitals

Corpus callosum

Thalamus

Long-term memory

Medial prefrontal cortex
• Personality
• Emotional behaviour
• Working memory

Orbitofrontal cortex
• Olfaction
• Emotional behaviour

Amygdala
• Fear
• Anxiety

Hippocampus
• Memory (short term)

Fusiform gyrus
• Object/face recognition

Visual association cortex
• Colour, spatial appreciation/recognition

Fig. 1.15 Functional anatomy of specific cortical areas on the medial side of the brain.

Hemisphere specialization

The anatomy of the brain appears symmetrical, in that most regions of the sensory and motor cortices are the same on both sides of the brain, and damage to one region leads to a contralateral deficit. However, some of these regions, particularly in the frontal, temporal and parietal lobes, differ in size. For example, the primary auditory cortex is larger in the right temporal lobe than in the left; conversely, Wernicke's area (auditory association cortex) is larger on the left than on the right. Similarly, the left parietal lobe is larger than the right, but the right posterior parietal region is larger than the corresponding area on the left. In addition, the left facial somatosensory cortex area is larger than the right. Broca's area on the left is also different from that on the right. This is because there are regions in the frontal and parietal lobes that have dramatically different functions in the left and right brain. These are associated with 'higher functions', such as language, analytical and intuitive thinking, spatial orientation and artistic and musical ability (Fig. 1.16). Much of what is known about hemispheric asymmetry comes from patients with brain lesions or who have had surgery to control diseases such as epilepsy or cancer.

The hemisphere that contains the centres for language production and comprehension is called the dominant hemisphere; in most people, this is the left hemisphere. Damage to the left hemisphere gives rise to difficulties in speech comprehension or production that do not occur if the lesion is in the right hemisphere. Lateralization of language function can be determined using the Wada test. If a patient has speech centres in the left hemisphere, anaesthetic injected into the left carotid artery blocks speech perception and production.

Another asymmetry occurs in writing. Most people are either right- or left-handed; very few are ambidextrous. Handedness and cerebral dominance were thought to be linked, since ~90% of the population are right-handed and the left hemisphere controls the right hand. Conversely, in left-handed people, Broca's area would be in the right hemisphere. This hypothesis is easily tested by the Wada test (see above) and was found to

be false; 97% of the population, including three-quarters of left-handers, have their language centres in the left hemisphere.

In addition to speech production, the left hemisphere is important in language articulation and comprehension, mathematical calculations and cognitive functions, such as analytical and rational thinking. For example, damage to the left parietal lobe causes difficulties in copying movements (ideomotor apraxia), naming objects, reading (alexia), solving mathematical problems (dyscalculia) and language. The same lesion in the right hemisphere causes difficulty in copying drawings (agraphia), assembling puzzles (constructional apraxia) and spatial navigation, such as finding the way to the shops or work, because the landmarks used as a guide are no longer familiar. In some patients, damage to the right posterior parietal cortex results in contralateral neglect syndrome. The patient fails to recognize the left side of the body as theirs. They may fail to wash or dress the left side of the body, and if presented with a stimulus such as pain, they may report it as hurting, but not as hurting them.

Studies of lesions in the right hemisphere have shown that it is essential for the processing of non-verbal sound patterns such as music; for example, patients with right-sided strokes can speak but often cannot sing properly. Lesions in the right hemisphere in regions corresponding to Wernicke's area produce deficits in music perception and the appreciation of tone and the emotional nuances of speech. Poetry, for example, may seem meaningless after a right area lesion.

Sex differences also exist in the CNS. Sexual dimorphism of the hypothalamic preoptic nucleus, corpus callosum and cerebral cortical regions has been documented. These are likely related to sex-specific behaviours associated with hormonal levels of testosterone and oestrogen that relate to not only reproductive function but also to non-reproductive (e.g. visuospatial processing or phonological language) functions. In addition, hormones are related to brain development. In the male foetus androgens are converted to oestrogen, and this is related to masculinization of the brain; in the female foetus it is the lack of oestrogen that leads to feminization. After puberty, androgen and oestrogen secretion leads to

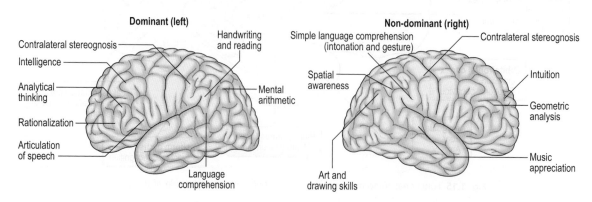

Fig. 1.16 Hemispheric specialization of function.

the development of secondary sexual characteristics, as well as sexually dimorphic behaviour.

Although these studies tell us that there are differences between the two hemispheres, it is unclear what this means. Cortical areas are more similar than they are different. However, if the hemispheres process information differently, this implies that they 'think' differently. There are various speculative theories as to why the brain evolved like this. One is that the left hemisphere is important in the control of fine movements, and this is important in controlling the production of speech, which involves fine control of the muscles of the larynx, tongue and oral cavity. The left hemisphere is also involved in the production of actions; damage leads to an inability to copy movements. Finally, another link between language and movement occurs in the representation of language areas. Verbs are 'doing' words that describe actions or states, whereas nouns are names of things. Verbs appear to be processed only in the left hemisphere, while nouns are processed in both hemispheres. Thus, the left hemisphere has a role in the production of both actions and mental representations of actions in the form of words.

If the left hemisphere is involved in fine motor control, what about the right hemisphere? One idea is that the right hemisphere is specialized for spatial movement relative to the surroundings, so that at a higher level, it can produce mental images of such movements. Damage to this lobe would impair such abilities. This is indeed the case.

One last controversial idea about asymmetry is that the left hemisphere is critical for language interpretation, and this is what sets humans apart from other animals. Evidence for this comes from 'split-brain' studies (Box 1.2), in which the corpus callosum was surgically cut in order to reduce the severity of seizures in patients with severe epilepsy. This meant that the two hemispheres could no longer communicate with each other. Patients undergoing this procedure were shown two pictures of related objects, to both hemispheres. Then several more pictures were shown, and patients were asked to select a picture that had an inferred relationship with the first two objects. For example, if the first two pictures were of rain and clouds, the third might be an umbrella. The right brain cannot make the connection, but the left can.

Box 1.2 'Split brain' syndrome

The brain houses two minds, not one, but they only orchestrate into a single personality if the two cerebral hemispheres communicate. Under normal conditions, both halves receive nearly identical information on the world, and life proceeds as though nothing is different about perception. Both hemispheres share the same knowledge base and reactive inclinations. Thus consciousness is controlled by both hemispheres, and there is a crossing over of functions so that one never normally experiences a dissociation of information. However, 'splitting' the brain by sectioning the corpus callosum and thereby disconnecting the hemispheres reveals separate functions. In the early 1960s, researchers showed that when a cat had its optic chiasm and corpus callosum severed, two independent learning centres were established, one in each hemisphere. The same effect was seen in humans. It was concluded that the brain had 'two separate realms of conscious awareness; two sensing, perceiving, thinking and remembering systems'.

Severing the corpus callosum was used by surgeons to treat chronic intractable forms of epilepsy. To the casual observer, split-brain patients appeared normal, and their seizures disappeared. However, psychological testing revealed that if the patient held up an object like a comb in the left hand, they could not say what it was. When it was transferred to the right hand, the patient had no trouble at all in communicating its identity. The same happened with words. If a card with a printed word like 'ring' was visible only in the patient's left visual field, they could not read it, yet vision in the left eye was fine. When the word

was in the right field, the patient immediately recognized it. In order to explain these observations, it was necessary to understand certain basic rules of perception. Right and left worlds of touch and sight project to opposite cerebral hemispheres. Sounds project to both hemispheres simultaneously, so the patient could be cued by the doctor's voice. Many things that people learn and think about are non-verbal: music, art, spatial relationships and geometry. To test the functions of the right hemisphere of split-brain patients, psychologists constructed a screen with a slot under which a patient could reach and touch objects, but not see them. Then they focused a picture of one object in the patient's left field of view (signalling the right hemisphere) and asked them to match the picture to the objects that they could feel behind the screen with the left hand. The patients passed the matching test, with scores similar to those of any normal person. However, when the same task was performed with the right hand, the patient failed to choose the objects correctly because the right hand is controlled by the left hemisphere, with which the patient cannot see the object, as it is not in the right visual field.

It is now recognized that cutting only the anterior three-quarters of the corpus callosum and the anterior commissure and leaving the splenium (posterior part) intact is sufficient to stop seizures completely or render them responsive to drugs. At the same time, psychological tests show results identical to those of normal subjects, suggesting that the cerebral hemispheres totally integrate if just a small fraction of the corpus callosum remains intact.

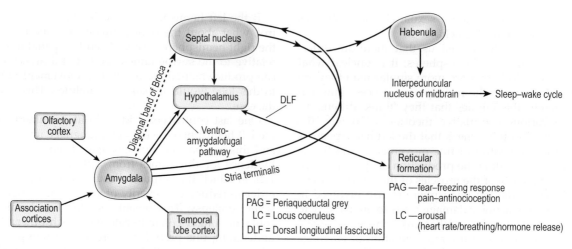

Fig. 1.17 The limbic system: neuroanatomical connections of the amygdala.

The same is true if words, rather than pictures, are used. The ability to infer leads to the ability to believe, and this sets humans apart from other animals. Parrots can be trained to talk, but they cannot infer or believe things.

Limbic system

The limbic lobe, situated on the medial side of the brain, surrounds the rim of the ventricles (see Figs 1.3C and 1.15). The cingulate and parahippocampal gyri, together with their associated nuclei—the hippocampus, amygdala, septal nucleus and insula—comprise the limbic system. The limbic system is evolutionarily old; it is found in fish, amphibians, reptiles and mammals. It controls emotional behaviour and the internal factors that motivate animals and people to adapt to a constantly changing external environment.

Emotions have three components: a visceral sensory component caused by endocrine and autonomic stimuli (a 'gut feeling'), a motor component involving the facial muscles to communicate the pleasantness or unpleasantness of the situation to others, and a cognitive–evaluative component to assess the situation. Pathology involving damage to the limbic system can elicit inappropriate behavioural patterns. These patterns include motivational behaviour relating to nutrition and fluid balance, sexual courtship behaviours and expressions of mood and affect. Memory is an important component of these patterns, and lesions within several limbic areas affect memory.

Input to the limbic system comes from the association cortex areas, olfactory cortex and medial temporal lobe regions, and is ultimately passed on to the hypothalamus, which controls the endocrine system and autonomic nervous system. The connections of the limbic system and the functions of the various nuclei are detailed in Figs 1.17 and 1.18 and Table 1.3.

The uncus of the medial temporal lobe houses the hippocampus and amygdala. The amygdala is a collection

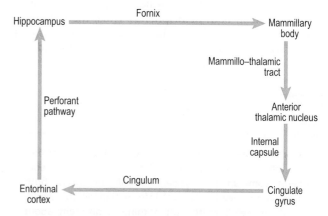

Fig. 1.18 The limbic system: the Papez circuit for emotions. Neuroanatomist James Papez demonstrated that emotions are not a function of any specific brain centre but involve a circuit comprising the hypothalamic mammillary bodies, thalamus, cingulate gyrus and hippocampus. Damage to any of these structures affects emotions and the ability to create memories.

Table 1.3 Functions of limbic system structures

Structure	Function
Hippocampus	Memory acquisition, consolidation and recall
Amygdala	Emotional content of stimuli; fear, anxiety and danger
Septal nucleus	Pleasure and reward
Cingulate cortex	Affective significance

of subnuclei and necessary for self-preservation. Clinical studies have shown that when stimulated, it gives rise to fear and anxiety or euphoria, depending on which part is stimulated. This structure is responsible for the feelings of fear or dread when you are walking home late at night and hear footsteps behind you. Another important

Klüver–Bucy syndrome

In the 1930s, Heinrich Klüver and Paul Bucy found that bilateral temporal lobectomy in monkeys produced a dramatic effect on the animals' responses to fearful situations. The bizarre behavioural abnormalities could be placed into five categories: visual agnosia, oral exploration of all objects, hyper-metamorphosis (a compulsion to touch everything, and place each found object into the mouth), altered and increased sexual behaviour and emotional changes, including fearlessness and decreased facial expressions usually associated with emotion. This constellation of symptoms is called Klüver–Bucy syndrome. Nearly all the symptoms of Klüver–Bucy syndrome reported in monkeys have also been found in humans with temporal lobe lesions. In addition to visual recognition problems, oral tendencies and hypersexuality, people appear to have 'flattened' emotions.

role is in recognizing the emotions indicated by other peoples' facial expressions. The amygdala receives input from the hippocampus, olfactory cortex and temporal lobe association cortex, and aminergic input from septal and brainstem nuclei. Its main outputs are to the septal nucleus and hypothalamus, via the stria terminalis and diagonal band of Broca (septal nucleus only), temporal cortex and other autonomic and brainstem reticular formation centres, and the nucleus accumbens (via the ventral amygdalofugal pathways). Damage to the amygdala is rare, but experimental studies show that bilateral damage may produce an inability to perceive situations as dangerous, which can have disastrous consequences for people and animals. Such lesions produce the Klüver–Bucy syndrome (Box 1.3).

The hippocampus is involved in memories and the recall of such information. It stamps the place, time and date on the memory and, in conjunction with other regions of the medial temporal lobe, medial thalamic nuclei and medial prefrontal cortex, is involved in the consolidation of information. Consolidation is sometimes termed 'long-term memory', and is stored as a modification of activity-dependent connections between neurons, and is analogous to information stored on the hard drive of a computer. The hippocampus allows humans to compare the conditions of a present situation, such as danger, with similar past experiences in order to decide what the best option is to guarantee survival. The hippocampus is part of the hippocampal formation, which includes the dentate gyrus and subiculum. The dentate gyrus is at the tip of the hippocampus, and the subiculum is at the base and is continuous with the entorhinal cortex of the parahippocampal gyrus. There is a one-way flow of information through the hippocampus. Information arrives via the perforant pathway from the entorhinal cortex to the dentate gyrus, which passes information to the CA3 region (CA stands for cornu Ammonis or 'ram's

horn' because of its shape). From CA3, it goes to the CA1 region and on to the subiculum, which is responsible for the output projection to either the nuclei of the mammillary bodies (part of the hypothalamus) via the fornix, or back to the sensory cortex via the entorhinal cortex. Somewhere along these pathways, memories are created. Bilateral damage to the hippocampi impairs the formation of new memories; nothing is retained, and information is soon forgotten. The hippocampus is also damaged in disease states such as dementia and epilepsy (see Chapters 13 and 14) and rabies.

The septal nuclei are the anterior thickenings of the septum pellucidum and are located immediately anterior to the anterior commissure. This area is a sexually dimorphic nucleus, and its stimulation evokes pleasurable sensations, particularly sexual sensations. It has been suggested that this is the location of the orgasm centre, and that women have four centres, while men only have one! Inputs are from the amygdala, hippocampus, mesolimbic dopaminergic system and olfactory tract. Outputs are to the hypothalamus (via the medial forebrain bundle), hippocampus and habenula (via the stria terminalis) and reticular formation.

The cingulate cortex evaluates the affective significance of events, that is, whether they are harmful or beneficial. Anatomical studies have revealed prominent afferent input to the cingulate motor areas from the limbic structures and the prefrontal cortex, which can send information about motivation and the internal state of subjects, as well as cognitive evaluation of the environment. The anterior cingulate cortex is also involved in pain perception, receiving input from the posterior insula cortex. Other important inputs are from the anterior thalamic nucleus, which receives its input from the mammillary bodies, forming the Papez circuit, involved in the cortical control of emotion (see Fig. 1.18). The anterior cingulate gyrus communicates between the prefrontal cortex and subcortical areas of the limbic system. Bilateral destruction releases the 'rage centres' of the amygdala and hypothalamus from any prefrontal inhibitory influence.

The limbic system is tightly connected to the prefrontal cortex, and together, they funnel emotional input to the hypothalamus. Frontal lobe asymmetry exists in regard to emotional processing. Activation in the left prefrontal regions may be part of a mechanism that inhibits 'negative' affects (e.g. sadness and disgust); conversely, the right prefrontal regions may inhibit positive emotions (e.g. happiness). People with increased left prefrontal activity are described as more 'optimistic' and more adept at minimizing negative emotions. Lesions of the left prefrontal neocortex are more likely to be associated with depression than lesions in the homologous location in the right hemisphere. During the Wada test, when the left hemisphere is temporarily anaesthetized, patients report negative changes in mood (e.g. sadness). Positron emission tomography (PET) studies have indicated increased left-side orbitofrontal blood flow during self-generated sadness.

Orbitofrontal cortex

The orbitofrontal cortex is part of the prefrontal cortex and anatomically linked with the limbic system and anterior temporal lobe cortex. It mediates the conscious perception of smell. The orbitofrontal cortex interacts with the limbic system in support of higher-order functions such as association, integration and regulation of central autonomic processes, mood and affect, and those motor patterns that are under limbic control. Orbitofrontal lesions interfere with motivation and arousal. Prefrontal leucotomy patients are typically unmotivated and lethargic. Orbitofrontal lesions reduce the sensation of chronic and intractable pain and sometimes reduce the expression of anger and frustration when expected rewards are not received. In the past, such findings gave impetus to the use of prefrontal leucotomy as a treatment for intractable emotional problems and psychosis. Orbitofrontal lesions interfere with the prediction of reward. Humans with orbitofrontal lesions are unable to anticipate the future positive or negative consequences of their actions, although immediately available rewards and punishments do influence their behaviour. A classic case of damage to the prefrontal and orbitofrontal lobes is that of Phineas Gage (see Box 15.7).

Basal ganglia

The basal ganglia are a group of large subcortical nuclei found in the forebrain. They are located above and anterior to the thalamus (see Figs 1.8, 1.9 and 1.12). They comprise the caudate nucleus, putamen and globus pallidus. The caudate nucleus fuses at its anterior end with the putamen to form the corpus striatum, which is named after the strands of grey matter that can be seen connecting the two structures as they become anatomically separated by the anterior limb of the internal capsule (see Fig. 1.8). At the bottom of the anterior part of the striatum is the nucleus accumbens. This structure, although anatomically part of the basal ganglia, is considered part of the limbic system and is involved in the reward systems of addiction mechanisms, as mentioned above. The body of the caudate runs over the thalamus, and then curves to pass into the temporal lobe, where it becomes the caudate tail and ends at the amygdala, which is another nucleus that is functionally part of the limbic system. The subthalamic nucleus and substantia nigra (in the midbrain) are functionally associated with the striatum and the globus pallidum. The basal ganglia are concerned with the initiation and maintenance of actions and are involved in decision-making about what the body is going to do next. The basal ganglia work via four circuit loops that start and end in the cortex:

- a motor loop, concerned with learned movements and involved in the correct sequencing of actions for the execution of learned motor programmes

- a cognitive loop, concerned with motor intentions and advanced planning for later movements

- a limbic loop, concerned with the emotive aspects of movement

- an oculomotor loop, concerned with voluntary saccadic eye movements.

Damage to basal ganglia structures results in movement disorders (see Chapter 10).

Diencephalon

The diencephalon connects the midbrain to the forebrain. It is located deep within the brain and comprises the epithalamus, thalamus, subthalamus and hypothalamus. The epithalamus forms the roof of the diencephalon and consists of the pineal gland (an endocrine gland involved in circadian rhythms and the onset of puberty) and the habenular nuclei, whose functions are associated with the limbic system, as they connect to the septal nuclei via a tract called the stria terminalis thalami. The subthalamus is located dorsolateral to the hypothalamus and has two notable cell groups: the subthalamic nucleus and the zona incerta. The former is part of the basal ganglia circuitry (see Chapter 10), while the latter is a rostral extension of the brainstem reticular formation.

Thalamus

This bullet-shaped structure is the largest nuclear mass in the body and, together with the hypothalamus, forms the lateral wall of the third ventricle. The two thalami face each other medially across the third ventricle and touch at the inter-thalamic adhesion. The thalamus comprises 12 subnuclei that have reciprocal connections with the cortex (except for the inhibitory reticular nucleus) via four thalamic peduncles that are incorporated into the corona radiata, which is a white matter tract in the brain. The thalamic input to the cerebral cortex is the first step in generating sensory perception. The thalamus is the gateway to the cortex and functions to coordinate and integrate sensory, motor and autonomic information to initiate appropriate responses.

The thalamus contains a sheet of fibres called the internal medullary lamina that divides the thalamus into three nuclear groups: the anterior, medial and lateral groups. The anterior and medial groups are associated with the limbic system. The lateral part of the thalamus receives restricted sensory or motor input, and is further subdivided into dorsal and ventral nuclei, based on function and projection.

Additionally, thalamic nuclei are classified into three functional relay groups: specific, association and diffuse (Table 1.4). Specific nuclei process either a single sensory modality or input from a motor region, and project to a specific (primary) cortical region. Each receives

Table 1.4 Functional organization of the thalamus

Nucleus	Functional group	Inputs	Outputs	Proposed functions
Anterior	Association nucleus	Hippocampus Mammillary body	Cingulate cortex	Limbic pathways
Medial dorsal	Association nucleus	Amygdala Olfactory cortex Hippocampus	Prefrontal cortex Hippocampus	Limbic pathways with major relay to the prefrontal cortex
Lateral dorsal	Association nucleus	Amygdala Olfactory cortex Hippocampus	Cingulate cortex Other limbic regions	Functions with the anterior nucleus to connect to limbic regions
Lateral posterior	Association nucleus	Superior colliculus Midbrain reticular formation	Occipital, parietal, temporal association cortex	Functions with the pulvinar to maintain a conscious alert state
Pulvinar	Association nucleus	Superior colliculus	Parieto-temporo-occipital association cortex	Behavioural orientation towards relevant peripheral stimuli
Medial geniculate	Specific nucleus	Inferior colliculus	Primary auditory cortex	Relays bilateral inputs to the auditory cortex
Lateral geniculate	Specific nucleus	Retinae of both eyes	Primary visual cortex	Relays bilateral inputs to the visual cortex
Ventral posterior Ventroposteromedial	Specific nucleus	Trigeminothalamic tract	Primary somatosensory cortex Primary taste cortex	Relays somatosensory and taste cranial nerve inputs to the cortex
Ventroposterolateral Posterior		Medial lemniscus Spinothalamic tract	Primary somatosensory cortex	Relays inputs to the primary somatosensory cortex
Ventral lateral	Specific nucleus	Globus pallidus internal Substantia nigra (pars reticulata) Deep cerebellar nuclei	Primary motor cortex Premotor cortex Supplemental motor cortex	Relays basal ganglia and cerebellar input to the motor cortex
Ventral anterior	Specific nucleus	Globus pallidus internal Substantia nigra (pars reticulata) Deep cerebellar nuclei	Frontal association (prefrontal, premotor and supplementary) cortex	Relays basal ganglia and cerebellar input to the motor cortex
Intralaminar	Diffuse nucleus	Spinal cord (spinothalamic tract) Reticular formation Cerebellar nuclei Globus pallidus Superior colliculus (deep layers)	Cerebral cortex Striatum	Conscious awareness Motor relay from the cerebellum and basal ganglia
Reticular thalamic	Diffuse nucleus	Reticular formation Corticothalamic efferents Thalamocortical afferents	Thalamic relay and intralaminar nuclei (GABAergic)	Regulates activity in other thalamic nuclei

reciprocal input from the region to which it projects. The association nuclei are reciprocally connected to association cortex areas of the brain and are predominantly involved in sensory integration, control of the emotional aspects of behaviour and the memory of stimuli. The diffuse nuclei have widespread projections to all functional divisions of the cortex and other thalamic nuclei. They are involved in arousal and regulate the level of cortical excitability. The intralaminar nuclei are housed in the internal medullary lamina and are considered a rostral extension of the reticular formation. The reticular nucleus is the only nucleus that does not directly project to the thalamus. It receives collateral input from the cor-

tex and thalamus. It is physically separate from the other thalamic nuclei, and its role is to modulate the activity of other thalamic nuclei, via activation of GABAergic synapses. If the thalamus is the gateway to the cortex, the thalamic reticular nucleus is the gatekeeper. It is active during sleep to inhibit information passing to the cortex.

Hypothalamus

This is the most ventral part of the diencephalon, lying anterior and inferior to the thalamus (separated by the hypothalamic sulcus), and extending from the optic

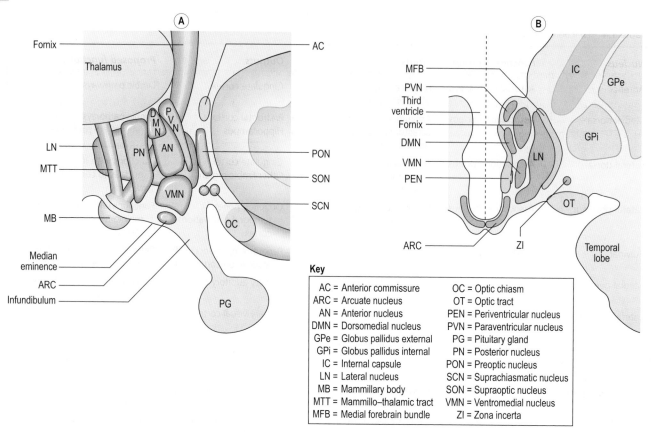

Fig. 1.19 Anatomical organization of the hypothalamus. (A) Lateral view. (B) Midline view.

Key

AC = Anterior commissure	OC = Optic chiasm
ARC = Arcuate nucleus	OT = Optic tract
AN = Anterior nucleus	PEN = Periventricular nucleus
DMN = Dorsomedial nucleus	PVN = Paraventricular nucleus
GPe = Globus pallidus external	PG = Pituitary gland
GPi = Globus pallidus internal	PN = Posterior nucleus
IC = Internal capsule	PON = Preoptic nucleus
LN = Lateral nucleus	SCN = Suprachiasmatic nucleus
MB = Mammillary body	SON = Supraoptic nucleus
MTT = Mammillo–thalamic tract	VMN = Ventromedial nucleus
MFB = Medial forebrain bundle	ZI = Zona incerta

chiasm to the caudal border of the mammillary bodies. The pituitary gland is connected to the hypothalamus by the infundibulum and is functionally related, as the posterior pituitary gland is a direct outgrowth of the hypothalamus. The hypothalamus forms the link between the neural and endocrine systems.

The hypothalamus is composed of 11 pairs of nuclei that form the major control centre of the visceral system. Its functions can be remembered using the mnemonic HEAL—homeostasis, endocrine control, autonomic control and limbic mechanisms—as it integrates activity from the limbic, autonomic and endocrine systems. It regulates the basic survival systems: sleep–wake cycles, thermoregulation, fluid intake, growth, metabolic energy expenditure and reproduction. The hypothalamus receives input from neural and circulatory systems. The neural input is from autonomic structures such as baroreceptors, which relay information about blood pressure (via the solitary nucleus), and chemoreceptors, which provide information about the chemical constituents of the fluid cavities. In addition, the level of neural arousal is signalled by pathways arising in the brainstem reticular formation and medial forebrain. The hypothalamus also receives input from the limbic and olfactory systems. Circulatory input arrives in the form of blood borne information concerning temperature, osmolarity, blood glucose and pH levels, as well as hormonal levels

that regulate growth, reproduction and feeding behaviour. The hypothalamus has reciprocal connections with many parts of the brainstem and cortex, especially the basal, frontal and medial cortical areas, and the reticular formation. It is considered part of the limbic system. It also has an important role in regulating hormone secretion from the pituitary gland. It is a critical player in regulating body homeostasis and appropriate behaviour in physical and social environments. Its control of stress, sex, thirst and hunger is mediated by the release of hormones from the pituitary gland, which act on specific target organs to induce the release of other hormones that act on body tissues and feed back to the hypothalamus and pituitary gland to regulate their activities.

The locations of the hypothalamic nuclei can be divided into four major regions in the antero-posterior plane: preoptic, anterior (supraoptic), middle (tuberal) and posterior (mammillary) (Fig. 1.19) and into three functional regions in the lateral-to-medial plane and periventricular, which surround the third ventricle. The fornix demarcates the boundary of the lateral and medial divisions. Within the lateral division runs the medial forebrain bundle, which conveys axons to and from other forebrain regions. The nuclei of the periventricular zone participate in neuroendocrine control, autonomic responses and biological rhythms and response to stress (Box 1.4), while the lateral nuclei are concerned

Stress

Nearly 60% of medical complaints seen by doctors are thought to be stress-related. Stress is defined as any external stimulus, physical or psychological, that threatens homeostasis. Stress both helps and harms the body. The body goes through three stages in response to a sudden stressor. Initially, there is a degree of shock, and this is followed by a stage of resistance, in which the body fights back. This is via activation of the sympathetic autonomic nervous system and the release of adrenaline, whose effects occur almost immediately, for example, increased heart rate, and put the body in a state of alert to deal with the immediate situation. Adrenaline also stimulates the periventricular nucleus in the hypothalamus to induce release from the adrenal cortex of the stress hormone cortisol, whose functions are 2-fold. In the short term, some of its effects are to help cope with the stress response, for example, mobilizing energy reserves for delivery to muscles and enhancing feeding to replenish energy sources after mobilization and use. The longer-term effects are to counteract the stress response, by re-establishing homeostasis by feedback inhibition of the hypothalamus. However, if there is too much cortisol produced for too long, the third stage—exhaustion—ensues, and this has deleterious effects on the body as its defence systems begin to break down. For example, chronic stressful situations such as a high-pressure job or a messy divorce lead to elevated cortisol and adrenaline levels in the body. This may lead to impaired immune function, chronic hypertension, obesity and atherosclerosis.

Table 1.5 Location and functions of hypothalamic nuclei

Antero-posterior subregions	Mediolateral subregions		
	Lateral	*Medial*	*Periventricular*
Preoptic		Medial preoptic (regulates gonadotrophic hormone secretion—sexually dimorphic nucleus)	
Anterior	Supraoptic (produces oxytocin and antidiuretic hormone, thirst regulation)	Anterior (temperature regulation—cooling and parasympathetic nervous system stimulation)	Suprachiasmatic (master clock for circadian rhythms)
	Lateral preoptic (role in sleep, thirst and reward behaviours)		Periventricular nucleus (regulates hormone release from anterior pituitary gland)
Middle	Lateral hypothalamic area (eating behaviour)	Ventromedial (satiety centre—inhibits eating)	Arcuate (produce dopamine- and gonadotrophin-releasing hormones to regulate hormonal release from the anterior pituitary gland via the tubero-infundibular tract)
		Dorsomedial (aggressive behaviour)	Paraventricular (synthesises oxytocin, antidiuretic and corticotrophin releasing hormones)
Posterior	Lateral hypothalamic area (eating behaviour)	Mammillary body (consolidation of memories)	Posterior hypothalamic (temperature regulation—warming and sympathetic NS stimulation)
	Mammillary body (consolidation of memories)		

with arousal mechanisms and motivational behaviour. The medial zone nuclei are involved in homeostasis and reproduction. Descending autonomic control arises from the paraventricular and dorsomedial nuclei, and their axons run in the dorsolateral funiculus through the brainstem to synapse with preganglionic neurons of the autonomic nervous system (ANS) in the brainstem and spinal cord. The organization and major functions of these nuclei are summarized in Table 1.5.

The suprachiasmatic nucleus contains intrinsic pacemaker cells that control the circadian rhythms of the body (body clock) via connections from specialized retinal ganglion cells and the pineal gland that are indirectly modulated by light. This may regulate sleep cycles. The medial preoptic nuclei and lateral hypothalamic area are also involved in sleep behaviour. Damage to these areas results in insomnia and hypersomnia.

Temperature is regulated by the preoptic and posterior nuclei. Cells act like miniature thermostats and are extremely sensitive to skin temperature changes. Correct body temperature is maintained by feedback circuits using behavioural or reflex mechanisms. For example, if one enters a room that is too cold, the heating is turned up, extra clothes are put on to warm the body or body heat is generated by shivering. If one is too hot, heat is lost by reflex measures, such as sweating, or by behavioural means, such as undressing.

The thirst centres reside in the supraoptic nucleus. Cells here are extremely sensitive to fluid volume and osmolarity. If the blood volume drops or the osmolarity is too high, water must be ingested. This is triggered by the release of vasopressin from the pituitary gland. Vasopressin acts on the kidney and leads to retention of water. The kidney signals back to the hypothalamus via the secretion of renin into the bloodstream, which leads to the formation of angiotensin II. This peptide feeds back to the hypothalamus by stimulating the subfornical organ in the lining of the lateral ventricles. This stimulates the thirst centres and ultimately leads to the intake of more water.

The hypothalamic control of eating and hunger is less well understood than other functions of the hypothalamus. Based on lesion studies, it was initially thought that there were two discrete centres for hunger and satiety in the lateral and ventromedial hypothalamic regions. Bilateral lesions of the former cause starvation behaviour, while damage to the latter causes overeating and obesity. This is an oversimplification, as lesions of the lateral hypothalamic region damage the medial forebrain bundle, leading to neglect syndrome; that is, there is no motivation to eat. Lesions of the ventromedial hypothalamus affect connections to the periventricular nucleus, disrupting satiety input signals from the digestive tract and giving the impression that the body is still hungry.

The hormones oxytocin and vasopressin are produced in the paraventricular and supraoptic nuclei of the hypothalamus, and are released at axon terminals that travel in the median eminence to the posterior lobe of the pituitary. Damage to these structures can result in diabetes inspidus and Cushing's disease. In contrast, the functional connection with the anterior lobe is vascular, and originates in the arcuate, preoptic, periventricular and ventromedial nuclei. These either promote or inhibit the release of various hormones from the anterior pituitary, such as adrenocorticotrophic hormone (ACTH), thyroid-stimulating hormone, growth hormone, prolactin, follicle-stimulating hormone and luteinizing hormone. Damage to the pituitary gland causes various clinical syndromes. Pituitary dysfunction results in hypothyroidism or hyperthyroidism (thyrotoxicosis) due to failure of thyroid regulation. Infertility is due to failure of gonadotrophic hormones, while growth hormone dysregulation results in acromegaly or dwarfism.

Table 1.6   Classification of peripheral receptors

Receptor type	Receptor end organ	Sensory modality
Mechanoreceptors	Hair follicles	Light touch
	Pacinian corpuscles	Vibration
	Ruffini endings	Skin stretch
	Merkel cells	Pressure
	Meissner corpuscles	Velocity
	Muscle spindles	Muscle length, joint position
	Golgi tendon organs	Muscle tension
	Free nerve endings	Nociception Pleasurable touch
	Auditory hair cells	Hearing
	Cupulae, maculae hair cells	Balance and motion
Chemoreceptors	Taste buds	Taste
	Olfactory receptor cells	Smell
	Visceral chemoreceptors	Pain
Photoreceptors	Rods	Vision
	Cones	Vision

Peripheral nervous system

The PNS includes all the nervous system structures outside the skull and vertebral column. It can be divided into the somatic nervous system, consisting of nerve fibres that transmit information from skeletal muscle, the skin and visceral organs and the ANS, which regulates automatic (involuntary) efferent control over visceral organs (see Fig. 1.1).

Somatic nervous system

The major structures of this section of the PNS are the peripheral receptors, neuromuscular junctions, peripheral nerves (trunks and plexuses) and their associated sensory ganglia.

Peripheral receptors

Receptors can be classified by sensory modality as mechanoreceptors, chemoreceptors or photoreceptors (Table 1.6 and Fig. 1.20). Each receptor is generally specialized to be sensitive to a specific type of stimulus.

The senses of smell, taste, vision and hearing have specialized receptors. Auditory and visual receptors are detailed in Chapters 7 and 8. Olfactory receptor cells have several hair-like cilia that are stimulated by odour molecules in the air. These generate action potentials that are transmitted to the mitral cells of the olfactory bulb, which

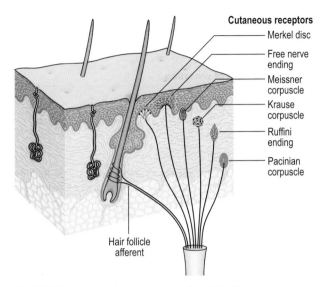

Cutaneous receptors
- Merkel disc
- Free nerve ending
- Meissner corpuscle
- Krause corpuscle
- Ruffini ending
- Pacinian corpuscle

Hair follicle afferent

Fig. 1.20 Types of peripheral receptor found in skin.

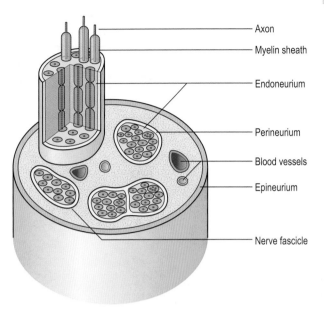

- Axon
- Myelin sheath
- Endoneurium
- Perineurium
- Blood vessels
- Epineurium
- Nerve fascicle

Fig. 1.21 Anatomical structure of a peripheral nerve.

then relay information to the primary olfactory cortex in the orbito-frontal and medial temporal lobe regions, where conscious appreciation of smell begins. Connections from this region to the limbic system and hypothalamus evoke emotional and memory responses to odours.

Taste buds on the tongue detect taste. Each taste bud has around 100 receptors that respond to sweet, sour, salt and bitter stimuli. A substance is tasted when the chemicals in food are dissolved in the saliva and enter the pores of the taste buds to stimulate the hair cells, which then relay signals to the gustatory cortex (in the parietal lobe) and the limbic cortex, for emotional labelling. Taste and smell are intimately linked to give the perception of flavour. Loss of smell leads to a reduction in taste sensation, manifested as a lack of flavour.

Sensory mechanoreceptors in the skin are either encapsulated or 'naked' (free nerve endings). Encapsulated endings 'tune' the axon to respond to a particular kind of stimulus. They are either rapidly adapting (RA), that is, they stop firing quickly in response to a constant stimulus, or slowly adapting (SA), that is, they do not stop firing. For example, if a pen is placed in the palm of your hand, the RA receptors fire on contact to let you know that something has landed in your hand. If the pen remains stationary, they will stop firing immediately, but the SA fibres (Merkel's and Ruffini's) keep firing to tell the brain that the pen is still there. Accurate manipulation of objects requires cooperation between all receptor types and the motor system. The ability to identify objects placed in the hand (without seeing them) is called stereognosis.

The receptors in skeletal muscle are the muscle spindles and the Golgi tendon organs. The muscle spindle is the major stretch receptor that monitors the length of the muscle, and, just like cutaneous afferents, it has RA and SA components. The Golgi tendon organs monitor the force exerted by a muscle during contraction and are found at the muscle–tendon interface. They are described in more detail in Chapter 9.

Pain and temperature sensory afferents do not have any specialized receptor organs; they use 'free nerve endings'. They are polymodal, that is, they respond to more than one kind of stimulus, for example, chemical, thermal or mechanical stimuli. Free nerve endings are found in all parts of the body except the interior of the bones and the interior of the brain itself. In the cornea of the eye, there are only free nerve endings; therefore abrasions of the cornea can be extremely painful. These are described in more detail in Chapter 5.

Peripheral nerves

Nerves are conduits for axons connecting the peripheral receptor to a neuron in the spinal cord or brainstem. The cell body of the sensory axon is housed in a specialized structure called a ganglion. Nerve fibres can be either myelinated or unmyelinated, and in the latter case, the nerve fibre covering is called a neurolemma. Nerve fibres are bound together by connective tissue called endoneurium, and gathered into bundles called fasciculi, which are enclosed in a connective tissue sheath called a perineurium. The whole nerve is encased in a tough coat called the epineurium (Fig. 1.21). This arrangement provides mechanical strength and support for the nerve. The epineurium is continuous with the dura mater, while the arachnoid and pia mater are continuous with the perineurium and endoneurium, respectively.

Nerve fibres are classified according to their diameter, and this is proportional to their conduction velocity, which is the speed at which impulses are transmitted. There are two commonly used systems. The Lloyd–Hunt system is used for afferents only and divides them into groups I–IV, while the Erlanger–Gasser system is used for afferents and efferents and separates them by size into groups A, B and C. Table 1.7 summarizes the generally accepted view

Table 1.7 Classification of peripheral nerve fibres

Class (group)	Myelin	Diameter (μm)	Conduction velocity (m/s)	Function/type of sensation
Afferents				
Aα (I)	Yes	12–20	>72	Joint receptors
Ia				Muscle spindles
Ib				Golgi tendon organ
Aβ (II)	Yes	6–12	30–72	Low-threshold mechanoreceptors (Pacinian corpuscles, Ruffini endings, Merkel cells, Meissner corpuscles, hair follicles)
				Secondary 'flower-spray' endings in muscle
Aδ (III)	Yes	1–6	5–29	Mechanical pain
	Thin			Muscle flexor reflex afferents
				Autonomic afferents
C (IV)	No	<1	<2.5	Low-threshold mechanoreceptors for affective touch
C (IV)	No	<1	0.5–2	Temperature, muscle and visceral nociception
Efferents				
Aα	Yes	12–20	>72	Motor to skeletal muscle fibres
Aγ		5–8	30–48	Motor to muscle spindle (Ia) fibres
B	Yes, thin	<3	3–30	Autonomic preganglionic efferents
C	No	<1	0.5–2	Autonomic postganglionic efferents

concerning human nerve fibres and their characteristics. There are four main fibre groups/classes:

1. The fastest fibres, both sensory and motor, mediate postural reflexes (e.g. monosynaptic reflexes) and are group I or Aα

2. Sensory fibres from specialized encapsulated endings responsive to low-threshold stimulation are group II or Aβ

3. Sensory fibres from non-specialized endings responsive to higher-threshold stimuli are group III or Aδ

4. Sensory fibres from unmyelinated fibres are group IV or C.

The muscle spindles are unique among sensory endings in that they have their own motor supply (Aγ fibres).

The somatic nervous system consists of 31 pairs of spinal nerves and 12 pairs of cranial nerves. The spinal nerves innervate the body and neck. At the level of the cervical and lumbar enlargements, spinal nerve fibres intermingle with each other in the brachial and lumbosacral plexuses to form peripheral nerves that have multiple spinal nerve contributions. The organization shows bilateral symmetry. Spinal nerves are formed by the union of dorsal and ventral roots; thus most spinal nerves are mixed nerves containing both sensory and motor fibres. However, the first cervical spinal nerve does not have a sensory root, and the fifth sacral and coccygeal spinal nerves do not have ventral roots. Dorsal roots transmit sensory information from skin, muscle, joints and, in some cases, viscera, to cells in the grey matter of the spinal cord. The dorsal root contains a swelling called the dorsal root ganglion that houses the cell bodies of all the sensory neurons that send axons into the spinal cord. Ventral roots transmit motor and autonomic information to the periphery (Fig. 1.22).

Spinal nerves divide into dorsal and ventral rami. Each ramus contains both sensory and motor fibres, just like a spinal nerve. The dorsal rami serve sensorimotor functions of the posterior body, while the cervical, lumbar and sacral ventral rami do not project directly to body structures; they merge with adjacent rami to form four major plexuses that have important motor functions (Table 1.8). The thoracic ventral rami project directly to the ribcage and stomach muscles.

The cranial nerves that innervate the face and head originate from different parts of the brainstem. Three cranial nerves are purely sensory, five are motor only and four are mixed. Four contain autonomic (parasympathetic efferent) fibres (see Chapter 6).

Dermatomes

Each spinal nerve innervates a specific skin region called a dermatome (Fig. 1.23), and the muscles innervated by a single ventral root are called a myotome. Most muscles are innervated by axons from two spinal segments (although the intrinsic muscles of the hand are unisegmental). Muscles sharing a common primary action are supplied by the same segment, and opposing muscles by segments in sequence with the former.

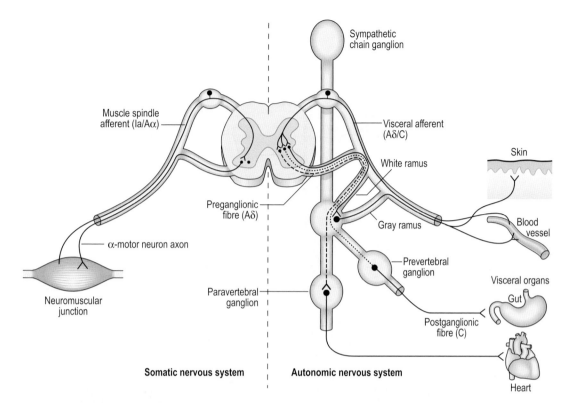

Fig. 1.22 Comparison of reflex circuitry in the somatic and autonomic nervous systems.

Plexus	Function	Main peripheral nerves	Clinical deficit
Cervical (C1–C5)	Respiration	Phrenic	Respiratory paralysis (see Box 1.5)
Brachial (C5–T1)	Movement of the hand	Radial	Wrist drop
		Median	Ape hand (unable to grasp objects)
		Ulnar	Claw hand (unable to spread fingers)
Lumbar (L1–L4)	Movement of the leg and foot	Femoral	Unable to extend knee and flex hip
Sacral (L4–S4)		Sciatic	Unable to flex knee and extend hip
		Peroneal	Foot drop

Table 1.8 Main functions of nerve plexuses

For example, in elbow movement, spinal cord segments C5 and C6 supply the biceps flexors and C7 and C8 innervate the triceps extensors. There is some functional overlap at the boundaries between adjacent dermatomes and myotomes. This acts as a sort of biological 'damage insurance', for if one spinal nerve is damaged, not all of the sensory information for that skin region will be lost, as some is carried in nerves of the adjacent spinal nerves. Thus, in reality, for a sensory or functional deficit to be seen, more than one spinal root must be damaged. Knowledge of the skin regions corresponding to particular dermatomes, therefore, plays an important role in the clinical diagnosis of peripheral nerve lesions (Table 1.9). Diseases that damage the nerves or muscles are called neuropathies and myopathies (Box 1.6).

Autonomic nervous system

The ANS consists of peripheral afferent and efferent neurons that regulate the body's internal environment and control exchanges between the internal and external environment. Together with the endocrine system, the ANS regulates homeostasis and controls a myriad of body functions and behaviours. As homeostasis is a prerequisite for survival, the ANS is an evolutionarily primitive neural system. Much of its normal function is accomplished involuntarily, without conscious intervention, through a series of reflexes that require input from viscera, smooth muscle, cardiac muscle and secretory glands.

It comprises three spatially segregated divisions:

1. the enteric system (ENS), which controls the smooth muscle functions of the gut, blood flow, mucosal transport and has immune and endocrine roles

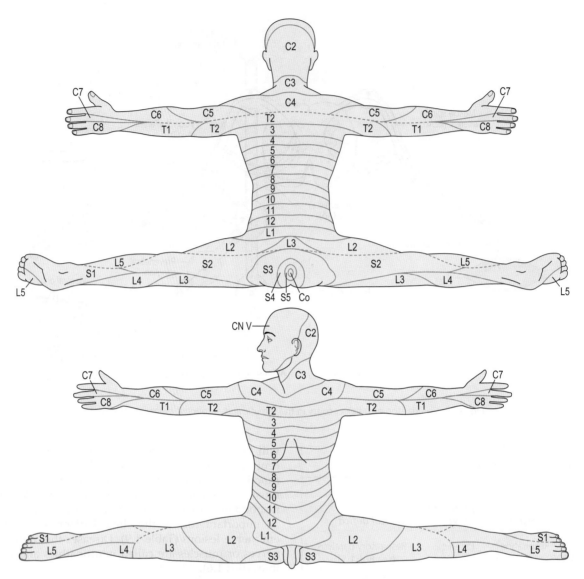

Fig. 1.23 Cutaneous dermatome distribution.

Phrenic nerve damage

The mnemonic 'C3, 4, 5, keeps you alive' refers to the function of the phrenic nerve. Each phrenic nerve innervates half the diaphragm, and paralysis of both, as can occur in spinal cord injury at high cervical levels, is often fatal. Unilateral damage does not affect the other side because of its separate nerve supply. Unilateral damage can be detected radiographically by observing asymmetry of the diaphragm position. Normally, during inspiration, the diaphragm dome is forced downwards by the muscle fibre contraction (and the action of the external intercostal muscles), but on the paralysed side, the dome rises as it is compressed by the displaced abdominal viscera, which are being compressed on the active side. During expiration, the dome returns to its original position in response to positive pressure in the lungs.

2. the parasympathetic division, which is involved in rest and recuperation
3. the sympathetic system, which acts as the body's alarm system for stress and danger and prepares the body for increased levels of activity; it is involved in flight, fright and fight reactions.

The basic organizational plan of the ANS is illustrated in Fig. 1.24. ANS fibres are found in peripheral and some cranial nerves. The afferents arise from visceral organs and blood vessel walls and have cell bodies located in spinal or cranial ganglia (Table 1.10). Their function is to initiate visceral reflexes.

Most visceral sensations do not reach the level of consciousness, and those that do, such as nausea and hunger, are poorly localized and are transmitted via sympathetic afferents. Parasympathetic afferents are more concerned with reflex activity control such as coughing or pupillary light reflexes. The afferents connect to neu-

Table 1.9 Functions of some specific dermatomes and myotomes

Root	Skin area	Motor function
C5	Lateral shoulder (over deltoid muscle)	Shoulder abduction (e.g. beer drinking!)
		Body rotation
C6	Lateral forearm, thumb and index finger	C5 and C6 forearm flexion (e.g. biceps)
C7	Middle finger	Finger (C7) and forearm extension (C7–C8)
C8	Ring and little finger	Digit abduction/adduction (C8–T1)
T1–T12	Skin overlying ribs	Breathing (external and internal intercostals)
T6–T12		Production of speech (stomach muscles)
L2	Anterior thigh skin	Hip, thigh and knee extension, thigh adduction
L3	Anterior knee skin	
L4	Medial lower leg skin	
L5	Lateral lower leg skin, toes 1–3	Ankle and toe dorsiflexion
S1	Toes 4 and 5, sole of foot	Ankle plantar flexion

Box 1.6 Neuropathies and myopathies

Peripheral neuropathy is a disease of the nerves and disrupts the flow of information between the central and peripheral nervous systems, producing sensorimotor deficits. Mononeuropathy affects a single nerve, whereas polyneuropathy affects several nerves. There are a variety of causes: direct trauma or entrapment (e.g. carpal tunnel syndrome), infection (e.g. HIV), toxicity (e.g. anticancer or anti-HIV drugs), genetic (e.g. Friedreich's ataxia), metabolic (e.g. diabetes), neoplasm or idiopathic (e.g. Guillain–Barré syndrome). The common symptoms are pain and paraesthesia of the affected area, with a temporal profile that is acute, chronic or relapsing.

The cardinal feature of myopathy is motor weakness, although the muscle reflexes may appear normal on examination. Myopathies can be caused by tissue degeneration, toxicity or inflammatory disease. Genetically inherited myopathies, called muscular dystrophies (e.g. Duchenne's dystrophy), involve progressive wasting and weakness of the muscles. Peripheral myopathies are non-painful.

rons of the spinal cord, brainstem reticular formation and solitary nucleus. This latter nucleus integrates sensory information from internal organs and coordinates motor output via interactions with parasympathetic brainstem nuclei and reticulospinal tracts. It also relays information to the hypothalamus, which is the main gatekeeper

of ANS preganglionic function. The hypothalamus and reticulospinal tracts have axons that converge on the common output neuron, the preganglionic neuron.

A key feature of the ANS is that the efferent output consists of two neurons: the preganglionic and postganglionic neurons. The cell bodies of the former are located within the CNS at either the craniosacral or thoraco-lumbar levels (see Fig. 1.24), while the latter are the true effector (motor) neurons but are located outside the CNS in peripheral ganglia. Preganglionic fibres leave the CNS in the ventral roots, while postganglionic fibres are only found in peripheral nerves or nerve plexuses. Thus visceral reflexes are disynaptic and thereby differ from the reflexes in the somatic nervous system, where monosynaptic reflexes occur. Other differences from the somatic nervous system include the speed of motor system action: somatic α-motor neurons rapidly excite skeletal muscle, whereas ANS actions are slower and more widespread in effect. The ANS balances excitatory and inhibitory effects to achieve coordinated and graded control. A good example of this is the male penile erection. Activation of the parasympathetic system is initially needed to erect the penis through engorgement with blood, while activation of the sympathetic system is needed to maintain the erection and achieve orgasm and ejaculation. The CNS coordinates the whole process. Any male will know the effects of increased anxiety or nervousness on 'performance'—impotence or premature ejaculation!

The effects of the two systems on target organs are largely antagonistic or reciprocal (see Fig. 1.24); they cannot act strongly at the same time, and the CNS inhibits activity in one division while the other is active, so that if levels of activity in the sympathetic system are high, activity in the parasympathetic system will be low. However, some targets—glands—only receive a single innervation. For example, sweat glands have only sympathetic innervation, while salivary and lacrimal glands have only parasympathetic innervation. Many other anatomical and functional differences exist between the two divisions (see Table 1.9); for example, sympathetic preganglionic fibres terminate in paravertebral or prevertebral ganglia, but not both, whereas parasympathetic preganglionic motor fibres terminate in terminal ganglia located in or near the effector organ. This difference in axon length results in parasympathetic activation producing localised effects, whilst sympathetic axons can produce widespread effects through their synapses within paravertebral chain ganglia (see Fig. 1.22). The paravertebral chain ganglia are also called sympathetic trunk ganglia and comprise 20–25 pairs that run along the vertebral column. The prevertebral ganglia are located along the abdominal aorta, particularly around the coeliac, superior and inferior mesenteric arteries, innervating the gut.

There are similarities and differences in their pharmacology: both divisions use acetylcholine (ACh) as a neurotransmitter in pre- and postganglionic motor fibres, just like the somatic motor system. ACh acts on nicotinic ACh

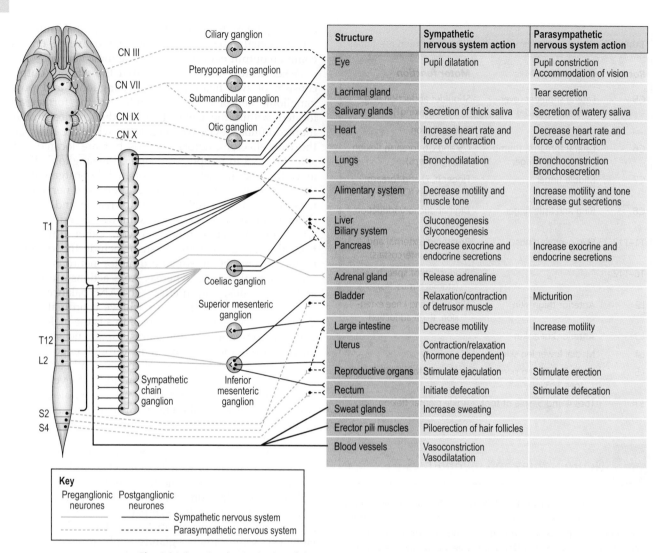

Structure	Sympathetic nervous system action	Parasympathetic nervous system action
Eye	Pupil dilatation	Pupil constriction Accommodation of vision
Lacrimal gland		Tear secretion
Salivary glands	Secretion of thick saliva	Secretion of watery saliva
Heart	Increase heart rate and force of contraction	Decrease heart rate and force of contraction
Lungs	Bronchodilatation	Bronchoconstriction Bronchosecretion
Alimentary system	Decrease motility and muscle tone	Increase motility and tone Increase gut secretions
Liver Biliary system	Gluconeogenesis Glyconeogenesis	
Pancreas	Decrease exocrine and endocrine secretions	Increase exocrine and endocrine secretions
Adrenal gland	Release adrenaline	
Bladder	Relaxation/contraction of detrusor muscle	Micturition
Large intestine	Decrease motility	Increase motility
Uterus	Contraction/relaxation (hormone dependent)	
Reproductive organs	Stimulate ejaculation	Stimulate erection
Rectum	Initiate defecation	Stimulate defecation
Sweat glands	Increase sweating	
Erector pili muscles	Piloerection of hair follicles	
Blood vessels	Vasoconstriction Vasodilatation	

Fig. 1.24 Functional organization of the autonomic nervous system. CN, cranial nerve.

(ionotropic) receptors of the preganglionic cells to evoke fast excitatory postsynaptic potentials that ultimately trigger action potentials, in the same way as occurs at the neuromuscular junction. However, ACh can also act on postganglionic muscarinic ACh (metabotropic) receptors that produce slower excitatory postsynaptic potentials, which do not produce action potentials unless repetitive activation occurs. Parasympathetic fibres release ACh, which has very localized effects on its targets. The sympathetic postganglionic fibres use mostly noradrenaline to activate their targets. Noradrenaline activates either α- or β-adrenergic receptors. The adrenal medulla, an endocrine gland, is essentially a modified sympathetic ganglion that secretes adrenaline (80%) and noradrenaline (20%) into the bloodstream and augments the localised effects of noradrenaline release at sympathetic targets. This accounts for the 'adrenaline rush' experienced when people encounter life-threatening or thrilling situations. The widespread action of blood-borne catecholamines, such as noradrenaline and adrenaline, and the high degree of neuronal divergence in the sympathetic system (see Table 1.10), lead to a whole-body action. This, together with the multiple release sites for neurotransmitters associated with the numerous varicosities along their terminal axons, contribute to the diffuse action of the sympathetic division.

Table 1.11 shows the effects of drugs that work on the different receptor systems associated with the sympathetic system. A drug that enhances the actions of noradrenaline is called a sympathomimetic drug, while drugs that are agonists at muscarinic ACh receptors have a parasympathomimetic profile. Sympathomimetics are primarily used to treat hypotension and cardiac arrest. They are also used to dilate bronchioles in asthma attacks or cases of anaphylactic shock. Adrenergic drugs are also used in local anaesthetic injections to constrict blood vessels, increasing the duration of effect of the anaesthetic drug by slowing down the rate of its washout. β-blocker drugs (sympathetic antagonists) are primarily used to treat hypertension, asthma and heart disease. Propranolol, a non-selective β-adrenergic antagonist, is used to slow the heart rate.

Table 1.10 Comparison of autonomic nervous system divisions

	Sympathetic	*Parasympathetic*
Afferent cell body location	T1–L2 spinal ganglia	Cranial nerve sensory ganglia (V, VII, IX, X)
		Spinal nerve ganglia S2–S4 (splanchnic nerves)
Peripheral innervation	Skin, blood vessels and viscera throughout body	Limited to head (lacrimal, salivary glands and eye muscles) and viscera of chest, abdomen and pelvis
Preganglionic cell body location	Intermediolateral horn of T1–L2 spinal cord	Brainstem and intermediolateral horn of S2–S4 spinal cord
Postganglionic cell body location	Paravertebral and prevertebral chain ganglia	Near or in peripheral target organ
Preganglionic/postganglionic fibre ratio	1:17—widespread effects	1:2—localized effects
Neurotransmitter	Acetylcholine Adrenaline	Acetylcholine
Neurotransmitter receptors		
Preganglionic	Nicotinic cholinergic	Nicotinic cholinergic
Postganglionic	Adrenergic (α1, α2, β1, β2, β3) (muscarinic, cholinergic at sweat glands)	Muscarinic cholinergic
Function	Alarm and arousal system (fight, flight and fright)	Homeostasis (rest and recuperation or growth, immunity, digestion and energy conservation)

Table 1.11 General effects of blocking cholinergic or adrenergic receptors

Site of action	*Effect of cholinergic receptor blockade*	*Effect of adrenergic receptor blockade*
Heart	Tachycardia	Bradycardia
Eye	Pupil dilatation, paralysis of accommodation	Pupil constriction
Gastrointestinal tract	Decreased tone, secretion and motility constipation	Decreased gluconeogenesis, increased tone and motility
Bladder	Urinary retention	Incontinence
Sweat glands	Decreased sweating and warm skin	Decreased sweating and warm skin
Salivary glands	Dry mouth	Dry mouth
Arterioles	Vasodilatation	Vasoconstriction
Veins	Venodilatation	Venoconstriction

Table 1.12 Signs of autonomic nervous system dysfunction

Sign	*Cause*
Postural hypotension	Postural hypotension reflects dysfunction of the baroreflex pathways, either the afferent limb in the vagus nerve or the efferent limb in the splanchnic nerves
Tachycardia	Defective sympathetic nervous system activity
Impotence Bladder/bowel dysfunction	Bladder and sexual dysfunction reflect demyelination of preganglionic fibres
Anhydrosis	Diminished or no sweating is most pronounced distally and reflects involvement of postganglionic sympathetic fibres to sweat glands

Parasympathomimetic drugs are also used to treat urinary incontinence or stimulate bowel function after surgery.

Clinical signs and symptoms of autonomic nervous system dysfunction

Autonomic dysfunction may occur due to a disease process that is selective for ANS cells and fibres, as seen in pure autonomic failure, multiple system atrophy (Shy–Drager syndrome) and genetically acquired syndromes such as familial dysautonomia (Riley–Day syndrome). It may also be secondary to other medical conditions, as in Parkinson's disease, diabetes, infectious peripheral neuropathy, alcoholism, multiple sclerosis and spinal cord damage. The cardinal signs of ANS dysfunction are detailed in Table 1.12.

In peripheral neuropathies such as Guillain–Barré syndrome (Box 2.2), these signs are accompanied by distinct signs of peripheral nerve damage. The initial signs are distal paraesthesia, numbness and muscle weakness, muscle wasting and decreased stretch reflexes, but no fasciculation. The autonomic signs develop more slowly and become prominent as the weakness advances proximally.

Diabetes is the most common cause of peripheral neuropathy with ANS involvement. The early compromise of small-diameter axons leads to distal loss of pain and temperature sensation, which precedes loss of vibration and position sense. Sweating is impaired and blood flow to the affected region is increased due to sympathetic denervation. The latter signs appear before the somatic sensory signs. Gustatory sweating—abnormal sweating of the face, scalp and neck that starts within a few minutes of starting to chew food—is common in diabetic peripheral neuropathies.

Multiple sclerosis and spinal cord lesions disrupt ANS function by disconnecting the preganglionic neurons from its supraspinal control. The effects depend on the level and severity of the lesion. Complete spinal cord transection is devastating to body temperature control, blood pressure regulation and bowel, bladder and sexual function.

The ENS is the largest division of the ANS, comprising hundreds of millions of neurons. It innervates the oesophagus, stomach, intestine, pancreas and gallbladder, and is composed of two plexuses, the myenteric and submucosal, which register changes in the tension of the gut wall and the chemical composition of the stomach and intestinal contents, to control the process of food digestion and transportation for excretion. It is a functionally separate system that works independently of the sympathetic and parasympathetic systems, but because of the large numbers of neurons, it acts as a 'second brain' to independently control gut functions, so that the cortex does not have to accommodate all these neurons and associated circuitry. Many neurotransmitters, anatomical connections and signalling pathways are common between the CNS and ENS, and there is a two-way communication process between the two systems. This has prompted the idea that, since they share neuronal and immune pathways, this can allow diseases to spread from the gut to the brain (e.g. along the vagus nerve); many CNS conditions also present with ENS deficits. Currently, much research is focused on the gut-brain axis and its roles in neurological conditions, such as autism, amyotrophic lateral sclerosis, Parkinson's disease and Alzheimer's disease.

Congenital abnormalities in the ENS system lead to Hirschsprung's disease (megacolon), characterized by an absence of ganglion cells in the myenteric plexus. Sufferers have an enlarged colon and the major symptom is constipation. Surgical intervention is required to remove the affected part of the colon.

Putting it all together: from anatomy to behaviour

To produce behaviour, external sensory inputs are relayed from the periphery to the brain, which then integrates and assesses the information to produce a motor response. This principle can be extended down to lower organizational levels, such as the nucleus (e.g. brainstem nuclei provide input to the thalamic nuclei that is then relayed to different cortical nuclei) and the individual neuron (where inputs from individual fibres converge onto a single neuron, which then integrates the information and passes it to other neurons).

Sensory and motor systems exist at all levels of the nervous system. Peripheral nerves have sensory and motor components, and these separate in the CNS to become specialized grey matter areas and nuclei associated with either sensory or motor functions. These specific functions are then relayed to separate areas in the cerebral cortex where they are separated in two ways: a specific primary area for discrete sensations within cortex lamina 4 always receives sensory input, while laminae 5 and 6 provide motor output (the other cortical layers are integrative in function).

An important but unexplained feature of the organization of the brain is that most pathways are bilaterally symmetrical, and they cross from one side of the nervous system to the other. Thus each cortex receives sensory input from the opposite side of the body and controls the movement of the contralateral side. Different pathways cross at different levels. For example, the pain pathway crosses in the spinal cord, whereas the pathway for voluntary control of movement crosses at the junction of the brainstem and spinal cord. Crossing in the visual system is more complicated (see Chapter 7). One problem posed by this organization is that information reaching one side of the body has to be integrated with information reaching the other side. This occurs via commissural pathways, which contain only axons crossing from one side of the brain to the other. The most prominent and largest of these is the corpus callosum, which connects the frontal, parietal and occipital lobes on each side; the anterior commissure connects the temporal lobes on either side.

Although the brain is anatomically symmetrical in some respects, in terms of some functions the brain is asymmetrical. This is certainly true of higher mental functions such as control of speech or spatial navigation.

In order to produce behaviour, neuronal circuits are regulated by coordinated excitation and inhibition. This principle applies to both single neurons and groups of neurons (nuclei). Neurons pass information to each other by being switched 'on' or 'off' by the appropriate neurotransmitter or combinations of neurotransmitters (neurons release mostly one neurotransmitter, but cases of co-release of different neurotransmitters do occur in the nervous system, and the implications of this phenomenon are still incompletely understood).

At the level of circuits, consider the role of the basal ganglia in movement. One of its functions is to scale the activity of the thalamic nuclei in regulating the size of the movement. Damage to the basal ganglia affects the activity of the thalamus and results in altered, abnormal movements; damage to one nucleus produces increased movement, while damage to another produces the opposite effect (see Chapter 10). This is analogous to the actions of the sympathetic and parasympathetic nervous systems; that is, one is excitatory, and the other is inhibitory for a given function (see Table 1.10).

The multiple levels of function seen in the nervous system are a product of evolution. As the brain evolved, new areas were added to the preexisting ones. Consider the evolution of movement: fish have no legs and use whole-body movements to swim, controlled by the spinal cord and hindbrain. Amphibians developed legs and control regions in the brainstem. Humans developed the ability to walk on two legs and independent control of limbs and digit movement, requiring further control areas, which are housed in the forebrain. For sensory areas, the newer regions are the association cortex regions, which provide higher mental processing of inputs such as shape, colour and size.

Sensory, motor and motivational (emotional or limbic) systems are organized both in parallel and in series to produce a unified conscious experience. Each has anatomically and functionally distinct subsystems that perform specialized tasks; for example, there are parallel systems for touch, smell, taste and hearing, and within each system, there are specialized subsystems for different aspects of the modality—sensation is broken down into parallel pathways for pain, proprioception, posture and balance. Motor systems likewise have parallel pathways, one to control voluntary fine movements, and others to control reflexes and body posture (see Chapter 9). The most striking feature of these pathways is that they are topographically organized so that there is a complete spatial map of the periphery in the brain for each modality. A key feature of the map is that it is distorted, so that, for example, regions that are important in sensory discrimination have the largest cortical representation. Another feature of the system is that there are interconnections between the different parallel streams.

An intuitive assumption based on the many different functions of the nervous system is that distinct brain functions are localized to specific areas of the brain, and indeed, this is true for many functions. Thus localized focal brain lesions lead to discrete neurological deficits. Other higher mental functions have a more widespread distribution throughout the cortex. For example, there is no one area that we can call primary pain cortex; different aspects of pain are processed in widely anatomically separated brain regions. Similarly, language ability (comprehension, production and appreciation) is widely separated across different lobes of the brain, and damage to focal regions may produce subtle deficits, whereas widespread injury, as occurs in stroke, often causes severe language deficits.

Thus knowing the names of the different parts of the nervous system is just the beginning of understanding how humans behave. It requires integration of the motivational, sensory and motor systems. Consider this the next time you are hungry and you go out to buy food. The decision to go to get food arises in the limbic system, which then instructs the somatic motor system to enact, causing you to walk to the shops and buy food. The processes of eating and tasting your favourite meal are provided by the sensory and motor systems. In addition, this influences the ANS, which feeds back to the hypothalamus to tell the brain that the hunger has been satiated (via increases in blood glucose levels).

There are more than 1000 disorders of the nervous system. Neurological disease and mental illness affect millions of people worldwide and cost billions to treat. The following chapters aim to shed light on how knowledge of the functional anatomy, physiology and pharmacology of the nervous system can be used to diagnose and treat some of the more important nervous system disorders.

ELEMENTS OF CELLULAR AND MOLECULAR NEUROSCIENCE

2

Chapter summary

1. The cellular components of the nervous system are neurons and glia. Neurons are the main communicators while glial cells play roles in support, immune surveillance and homeostasis.

2. The main components of a neuron are the soma, dendrites and axon. They display the fundamental property of excitability. The presence of an axon is the key characteristic that differentiates neurons from glial cells.

3. Glia comprise astrocytes, microglia and oligodendrocytes. Astrocytes provide structural support and play roles in trophism and homeostasis; they are also involved in the formation of the blood–brain barrier and the scar reaction of the nervous system to injury. Microglia are key players in immune surveillance, control of inflammatory responses in response to infection or trauma, and the stabilisation of neural circuits during development. Oligodendrocytes are specialised cells whose main role is the production of central nervous system (CNS) myelin—a lipid-rich sheath that covers certain axons. Schwann cells are the equivalent of oligodendrocytes in the peripheral nervous system (PNS).

4. The resting membrane potential (RMP) of neurons is determined by the intrinsic permeability of cells to potassium, sodium and chloride ions. A variety of stimuli can trigger changes in the membrane potential via depolarisation or hyperpolarisation of neurons. Summation of small amplitude depolarisations can reach the threshold required to trigger a larger scale depolarisation—the action potential. The potential propagates unidirectionally and non-decrementally in axons. Action potentials are all-or-none events; they are triggered, or not, in a neuron and their amplitude is always the same. In myelinated axons the propagation is saltatory, between the nodes of Ranvier in the myelin sheath, whereas in unmyelinated axons propagation is passive via sequential opening and closing of ion channels.

5. Neurons communicate through synapses, which are specialised zones of communication between cells. Synapses comprise a presynaptic component, a postsynaptic component and a synaptic cleft. The presynaptic side contains vesicles filled with neurotransmitters. Vesicles can release their content through an exocytosis process, following local depolarisation.

6. Neurotransmitters of the CNS and PNS are endogenous compounds that belong to a variety of families, for example, peptides, amino acids and monoamines. In most cases neurotransmitters are synthesised in the presynaptic terminal, through enzymatic reactions. Following synthesis, the neurotransmitters are packaged in vesicles. After release, the neurotransmitters can act on a variety of receptors that are located presynaptically or postsynaptically. Neurotransmitters can be taken back into the presynaptic terminal through specialised transporters and they can be inactivated by specific enzymes.

7. Neurotransmitter receptors can be divided into various classes. The two main classes are ionotropic and metabotropic receptors. Ionotropic receptors are multimeric ligand-gated ion channels that control the flow of various cations and anions and the subsequent change of excitability of neurons. Metabotropic receptors are G-protein coupled receptors; ligand binding leads to the activation of a G-protein response and various changes in intracellular signalling.

Introduction

The central nervous system (CNS) and peripheral nervous system (PNS) contain two main cell types: neurons and glia. A few other minor types of cell with specific functions, such as the choroid epithelial cells, are present in the brain, but these are described in other chapters.

Neurons

Neurons are the cells of the nervous system that receive signals, process them and transmit the appropriate response either to another neuron or to an effector such as a secretory cell or a muscle. The number of neurons in the human nervous system is estimated to be approximately 100 billion (1×10^{11}). The signals may be received directly from the environment, for example, light falling on the photoreceptor cells of the retina, in the form of chemicals released from other neurons at specialised junctions between them or as electrical signals directly transmitted through low-resistance gap junctions between adjacent neurons.

Neurons have a variety of sizes and morphologies, although they all have three elements:

1. A cell body (soma), which contains the nucleus and other intracellular organelles concerned particularly with protein synthesis, cellular housekeeping functions that are essential for cell survival and secretory processes. The large numbers of ribosomes, particularly those associated with the rough endoplasmic reticulum or polyribosomes, appear in tissue specimens as darkly stained 'Nissl bodies'. Cell body diameter ranges from 5–120 μm.

2. Highly branched processes extending from the cell body, called dendrites, which may be covered with protrusions (spines, hence the term 'spiny' neurons); cells without spines are called aspiny neurons. These form the dendritic tree, which receives most of the synaptic inputs from other cells.

3. A single axon extends from the cell body to the target cell. Axons may extend just a few millimetres to a nearby cell or, as in the case of the motor neurons supplying muscles distant from the spinal cord, for

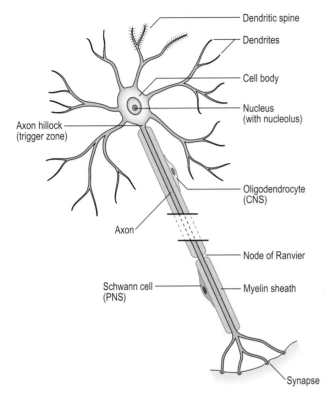

Fig. 2.1 A typical multipolar neuron. *CNS*, Central nervous system; *PNS*, peripheral nervous system.

several metres. The axon emerges from the soma at the axon hillock. Close to the axon hillock is the axon initial segment (also known as the trigger zone), where electrical signals called action potentials are generated. These are then propagated along the axon, which terminates at a synapse. Axon diameter varies from 0.2–20 μm.

The basic structure of a neuron is exemplified by the typical multipolar neuron shown in Fig. 2.1.

The cytoskeleton of the neuron, like that of all cells, consists of microtubules (composed of tubulin), microfilaments (made from actin) and intermediate filaments called neurofilaments, which form the core of the axon. Intracellular organelles, for example, mitochondria, are generated in the cell body and are physically transported along the axon by fast axonal transport along microtubules (anterograde transport) towards the axon terminal; materials for recycling are returned in the same way in the reverse direction (retrograde transport), using the motor proteins kinesin and dynein. Slower axonal transport, which transports proteins to the synapse, may also involve neurofilaments.

A single axon may give off occasional branches called axon collaterals before reaching its target. At the end of every axon there are a large number of branches, each ending within a specialized structure called a synapse. This is where signals are transmitted to other cells.

A typical synapse consists of a presynaptic terminal and a postsynaptic region. Axons may contain swellings along their length called varicosities, before forming the presynaptic terminals, which are at the end of the axonal branches. These contain secretory vesicles and large numbers of mitochondria. The presynaptic membrane is slightly thickened and presents inward projections called active zones. The postsynaptic region may also display a zone of increased density. In some axons there are synapses along the length of the axon without obvious contact zones, which appear as swellings. These vesiculated axons are common in autonomic nervous system (ANS) efferents. Both axons and dendrites are generically called 'neurites', but can be distinguished by their morphology, their organelles and the organization of their microtubules.

In general, neurons can be classified into one of three major types, depending largely on the position and number of dendrites and the position of the trigger zone.

Most neurons are multipolar neurons, like the one shown in Fig. 2.2A (and Fig. 2.1), and have many processes, which consist of one axon and many dendrites. The trigger zone is close to the cell body. These are the most common types of neurons and examples are the pyramidal cells of the cortex and the Purkinje (see Fig. 2.2A) cells (PCs) of the cerebellum.

Bipolar neurons (see Fig. 2.2B) have a single axon and a single dendrite, which only branches at its end. These are relatively rare and are almost all found in special sensory organs. An example is the bipolar cells found in the retina of the eye. The trigger zone is often found in the same location as in multipolar neurons.

Pseudo-unipolar neurons (see Fig. 2.2C) have only a single process extending from the cell body, which is situated part of the way along the axon. This divides the axon into central and peripheral processes. At the end of the peripheral process lies a sensory ending, which may be a bare axon, with the axon hillock and trigger zone very close to the sensory ending. Pseudo-unipolar neurons have no dendrites. The commonest pseudo-unipolar neurons are the sensory neurons found in the PNS, which convey signals from the periphery to the spinal cord in the CNS. Their cell bodies are found in the spinal (dorsal root) or cranial nerve ganglion of the PNS, and they synapse with neurons in the spinal cord or brainstem.

Owing to their very active nature, neurons in general have a very high metabolic rate and they need a continuous secure supply of oxygen and glucose. Any interruption of this supply is critical, as oxygen- and nutrient-deprived neurons will start to die very rapidly. This is particularly problematic because, under most conditions, mature neurons do not divide. During development, epithelial cells lining the neural tube give rise to neuroblasts. These cells divide mitotically to produce amitotic neurons, which then migrate to their final positions in the brain. As this occurs during foetal development and is completed in early childhood, the mature brain does not generally contain neurons that can divide. Therefore, the implication is that lost neurons cannot be replaced, not even in part. However, recent research has

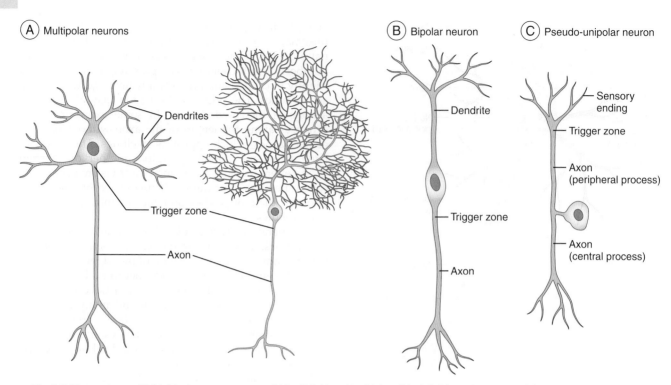

(A) Multipolar neurons

(B) Bipolar neuron

(C) Pseudo-unipolar neuron

Dendrites

Trigger zone

Axon

Dendrite

Trigger zone

Axon

Sensory ending

Trigger zone

Axon (peripheral process)

Axon (central process)

Fig. 2.2 Neuron types. (A) Multipolar neurons—pyramidal cell (left) and Purkinje cell (right). (B) Bipolar neuron. (C) Pseudo-unipolar neuron.

shown that some degree of neurogenesis (formation of new neurons) continues in the adult brain (Box 2.1).

One result of the predominant non-mitotic characteristic of neurons is that brain tumours derived from neurons are very rare and occur almost exclusively as neuroblastomas in children. Most primary malignant brain tumours (those derived from brain cells and not caused by metastases from elsewhere in the body) are gliomas, which are derived from glial cells (see below).

Glial cells

The other main category of cell in the nervous system is glial cells, of which there are several types. The term 'glia' derives from the German word for glue/putty, as proposed by the German physician Rudolph Virchow in the 19th century. These cells have several functions including structural and metabolic support, immune functions, electrical insulation of axons and support of impulse conduction. In the CNS astrocytes, oligodendrocytes and ependymal cells form the macroglia and are derived from the ectoderm. In contrast, microglia originate from the mesodermal/ myeloid tissue. In the PNS the macroglia include Schwann cells, satellite cells of sympathetic and sensory ganglia, and glia present in the enteric nervous system.

Astrocytes

In the CNS the most abundant glial cells are astrocytes (also called astroglia), characterised by their star-like appearance (Fig. 2.3). They are distinguished from neurons by the lack of Nissl substance and the presence of a specific structural protein—glial fibrillary acidic protein—which is a key component of glial filaments. The abundance of these glial filaments is not consistent. Astrocytes are very heterogenous; their functions and morphology differ by their location, developmental stage and subtype. Fibrous astrocytes contain large numbers of filaments and long unbranched processes; they are found in the white matter tracts of the brain. Protoplasmic astrocytes are the most prevalent, have fewer filaments and very branched tertiary processes and are found mainly in the grey matter in the proximity of synapses. In the human brain, a single protoplasmic astrocyte has within its domain as many as 2 million neuronal synapses. Astrocytes have a number of fine processes that surround neurons, capillaries and the ependymal cells lining the ventricles and the pia mater, forming the glial membrane. These astrocytic end-feet do not touch the capillaries, but release factors that induce blood–brain barrier characteristics in the capillary endothelial cells (see Chapter 12). Astrocytes are important in regulating K^+ levels in the extracellular medium around neurons, and in providing a store of glycogen to neurons, in the form of lactate, when required. Astrocytes surrounding neurons play an important role in controlling the distribution of neurotransmitters released by the neurons. They do this in two ways: first, by restricting diffusion, and second, by transporting neurotransmitters into the astrocyte, where they can be metabolized or recycled. Astrocytes can also produce neurotrophic factors, such

Box
2.1 ## Neural stem cells

During the development of the nervous system, cells in the neural tube become multipotent stem cells, which can divide into all the different cells of the brain. The mammalian brain contains resident precursor cell populations that contribute to neural development and persist into adulthood. These findings have led to the idea that activation of endogenous precursors may promote tissue repair. There is now clear evidence that neurogenesis and gliogenesis can continue throughout life. This is particularly valuable concerning the human brain, which displays limited self-repair after injury. Various terms are used to designate the cells that can potentially support neural repair: 'neural stem cells', 'neural progenitor cells' and 'neural precursor cells (NPCs)'. The first term defines cells that are multipotent and have very high self-renewal potential. They can give rise to a progeny which can differentiate into neuronal and non-neuronal cells. The second term defines cells with more limited self-renewal ability. Finally, the third term is often used to collectively designate both neural stem cells and neural progenitor cells. The brain contains distinct populations of NPCs. These include the cells in the subventricular zone (SVZ) and hippocampal NPCs that generate neurons and glia, as well as the more specialised oligodendrocyte precursor cells (OPCs) that generate oligodendrocytes throughout life.

In rodents, NPCs in the forebrain SVZ contribute to olfactory memory, while NPCs in the hippocampal dentate gyrus contribute to spatial learning and memory. Agents have been identified that can induce proliferation and differentiation of NPCs in vivo and can promote brain repair in experimental models. One of the most exciting developments in neurobiology in the last 15 years, rewarded by the Nobel prize in 2012 to John Gurdon and Shinya Yamanaka, is the ability to reprogramme adult differentiated cells (e.g. skin fibroblasts) into stem cells, through the technology of inducible pluripotent stem cells (iPSCs), using specific combinations of transcription factors. These cells can then be differentiated in vitro to produce various cell types, e.g. astrocytes, oligodendrocytes or neurons. Therefore, it has become possible to study the specific response of patient-derived neurons to various stimuli, thus providing a basis for a better understanding of physiopathology and also supporting the development of personalized therapeutics.

as glial-derived neurotrophic factor (GDNF), essential for the development and survival of dopaminergic neurons. Astrocytes play a critical role in the formation and maintenance of synapses, the control of blood flow and the regulation of blood–brain barrier function.

Astrocytes have recently been shown to play a potentially more active role in signalling. Gap junctions link adjacent astrocytes, through which small molecules can diffuse, thus forming a complex communication network. When stimulated by neurotransmitters they show changes in intracellular levels of Ca^{2+} ions, which spread between astrocytes as waves. Gap junctions also occur between astrocytes and neurons, possibly modulating the behaviour of the neurons by allowing the passage of Ca^{2+} between them (termed gliotransmission). After an injury, astrocytes can become activated and rapidly form a barrier around the affected area to contain the toxic processes triggered by injury. When persistent, this barrier becomes a glial scar, which prevents CNS regeneration (see Chapter 4 for further details).

The precursors of astrocytes are radial glial cells which, during early development, span the cerebral cortex, forming a scaffolding for the migration of new nerve cells to their destinations. In the adult brain they are present as Müller cells of the retina or Bergmann cells in the cerebellum, which perform the same repair functions in these regions as activated CNS astrocytes.

Microglial cells

Microglial cells were first characterised by Rio Hortega at the start of the 20th century. They are derived from the yolk sac during embryonic development and rapidly colonise the brain, where they ultimately represent 10%–15% of cells. They are maintained throughout life, through proliferation. These cells are relatively small and characterised by a stellate morphology under resting conditions (Fig. 2.4A). During the development and maturation of the CNS they release growth factors and also act as macrophages, removing debris produced by the programmed cell death which occurs on a large scale at this time, and assisting in the processes of dendritic pruning and synapse elimination, which refines neuronal circuits. In the adult they are normally relatively inactive, playing a local surveillance role in tissue, somewhat like a community police officer on patrol. However, in the presence of almost any type of injury or insult to the nervous system (e.g. stroke, infection or traumatic brain injury) they become activated. They multiply and change their morphology into an amoeboid, globular appearance (see Fig. 2.4B), move rapidly towards the site of the problem and revert to the role of phagocytotic macrophages; they change from friendly police officers into the riot squad! In this activated state microglia can adopt one of two major polarisation states: M1 or M2. The M1 phenotype is related to release of inflammatory cytokines, such as tumour necrosis factor (TNF)-α, interleukin (IL)-1β and also reactive oxygen species, whereas the M2 phenotype is anti-inflammatory, linked to the release of cytokines such as interleukin (IL)-10, and also participates in tissue remodelling after injury. M2 microglia possibly support oligodendrocyte differentiation towards remyelination (see below). It must be noted that this M1/M2 dichotomy is rather simplistic, and some perceive it as unhelpful and somewhat misleading, as there is ample evidence that microglia can exist in a variety of intermediate states between M1 and M2. Genome-wide expression profiling will no doubt contribute to a more thorough characterization of the extreme

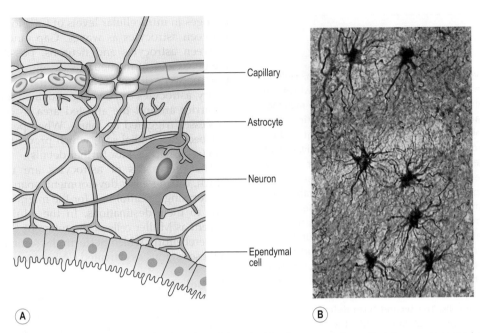

Fig. 2.3 (A) Drawing of an astrocyte. (B) Astrocytes that have been injected with a fluorescent dye so that the processes can be clearly seen. (From Young B, Heath JW. (2000) Wheater's functional histology, fourth ed, by permission of Harcourt Publishers.)

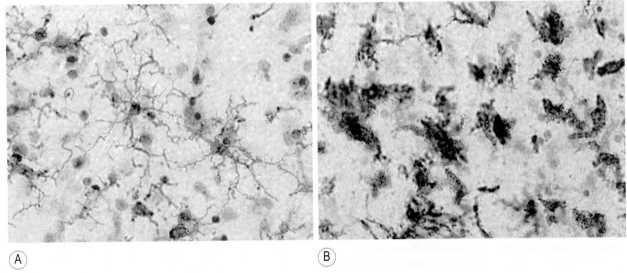

Fig. 2.4 Morphology of resting and activated microglia. (A) Ramified microglia exhibit highly branched processes with which they are in contact with the surrounding microenvironment. (B) Activated microglia retract processes and become enlarged due to organelle build-up and increased metabolic activity (from Lowe J. (2020). Stevens & Lowe's Human Histology. Oxford: Elsevier Ltd.).

complexity of microglia in the future. In neurodegenerative diseases, such as Alzheimer's disease or Parkinson's disease, the sustained state of activation of microglia may become responsible for exacerbated synaptic loss.

Oligodendrocytes and Schwann cells

Oligodendrocytes and Schwann cells are involved in electrically insulating axons in the CNS and PNS, respectively. They are large cells with few processes, which wrap around the axons forming multiple lipid bilayers, with their plasma membranes generating a myelin sheath. Damage to these cell types leads to demyelinating diseases (Box 2.2). These membranes have a high lipid/protein ratio, which makes them excellent insulators (see below). The myelination of nerve fibres is an important process and the number of myelin whorls around an axon is related to the conduction velocity of that axon. Oligodendrocytes can myelinate more than one axon and the cell body lies between them. Schwann cells

Demyelinating diseases

Multiple sclerosis is a progressive autoimmune disease, first named by the neurologist Jean Martin Charcot in 1838. It primarily affects young adults, occurring more often in females than in men. Areas of the myelin sheath, mainly in the brain, brainstem, cerebellum, spinal cord and optic nerve, are damaged, impairing nerve conduction. This is a chronic inflammatory process and there is evidence of both genetic susceptibility and environmental causes, which trigger an immune response. There are two main theories as to how the disease arises, termed the 'outside-in' theory and the 'inside-out' theory. In the former, dysregulation of the peripheral immune system leads to an autoimmune response against CNS myelin, while the latter proposes that damage to oligodendrocytes triggers an innate immune response and subsequently an autoimmune reaction. There are four major types of multiple sclerosis: primary progressive, secondary progressive, relapsing-remitting and clinically isolated syndrome. The relapsing-remitting form accounts for ~75% of multiple sclerosis cases. Areas of demyelination, called plaques, evolve into areas of scar tissue that may be partially remyelinated, restoring much of the function, so the disease shows periods of remission. However, other plaques form and eventually there is an accumulation of damage that causes permanent deficits. The loss of myelin in multiple sclerosis causes the failure of saltatory conduction, as there are no ion channels on the denuded axon. Major symptoms of multiple sclerosis include muscle weakness, lack of coordination, visual disturbances, spasticity and pain. These symptoms are due to a slowing or lack of nerve conduction. In many patients, the disease has phases of remission, which vary significantly in their duration. These are thought to be caused by temporary remyelination or by the insertion of new voltage-dependent Na^+ channels in the area lacking myelin. There is no cure for multiple sclerosis and treatment is symptomatic. Drugs aim to speed up the remission phases or slow the demyelination phases. This involves the use of disease-modifying immunomodulatory drugs such as beta interferon, glatiramer acetate, cladribine, natalizumab, alemtuzumab, ocrelizumab and siponimod.

Another type of demyelinating disease is the Guillain–Barré syndrome, in which infection by a variety of bacteria or viruses triggers an inflammatory demyelination of neurons in the peripheral nervous system. It classically presents with distal lower limb paraesthesia—proximal muscle weakness that rapidly affects the rest of the body. Facial weakness occurs in 50% of cases. Treatment consists of measures to shorten the course of the disease (plasmapheresis or immunoglobulin therapy to inhibit the autoantibodies) and most patients make a good recovery.

to regrow, the tip of the axon must make contact with a Schwann cell. This stimulates mitosis in the Schwann cell, which then extends processes towards the growth cone of the axon. The axon regrows at a rate of 2–5 mm per day along the Schwann cells, which remyelinate the new axon. Damaged neurons in the CNS do not regenerate successfully; one of the reasons is because CNS glial cells release a host of factors that specifically inhibit axon growth. Another major reason is that Schwann cells have a basement membrane along which the regenerating axon can grow, whereas oligodendrocytes do not.

Not all axons are myelinated. These are seen in the brain and spinal cord as grey matter, which consists of cell bodies and unmyelinated axons. In contrast, white matter consists of axons, most of which are myelinated. Dendrites are never myelinated. However, *all* axons have an oligodendrocyte or Schwann cell covering, although unmyelinated axons have only a single layer (Fig. 2.5), meaning that there are both myelinating and non-myelinating subtypes of Schwann cells and oligodendrocytes.

Neuron excitability

The basic function of a neuron is to receive signals, either directly from the environment or from other cells. The signals, which may be chemical or electrical, all produce graded electrical changes in the neuron. The input signals mainly occur in the dendrites and cell body of the neuron and may be excitatory or inhibitory. The graded electrical potentials produced are called excitatory postsynaptic potentials (EPSPs) or inhibitory postsynaptic potentials (IPSPs). These graded electrical potentials summate over time and space (temporal and spatial summation) and, if their total exceeds a threshold value, the trigger zone of the neuron initiates or 'fires' an electrical impulse called an action potential. This impulse is of a fixed size and is propagated unchanged along the nerve axon to the synapse, where the neuron makes contact with either another neuron or an effector. At the synapse endogenous compounds called neurotransmitters are released, which affect the postsynaptic target cell, making it more or less likely to produce a response. In specific cases, such as at the neuromuscular junction, a single action potential in the nerve is sufficient to produce muscle contraction.

Resting membrane potentials

All cells in the body have a voltage difference across the plasma membrane, called the resting membrane potential (RMP). In neurons, this is approximately –75 mV (the inside is negative relative to the outside). This is a consequence of the unequal distribution of ions across cell membranes and the different permeabilities of the neurons to these ions.

only myelinate a single axon and the cell body is closely apposed to the myelin sheath in the outermost layer.

Schwann cells play a role in the regeneration of peripheral axons following injury. In order for a peripheral nerve

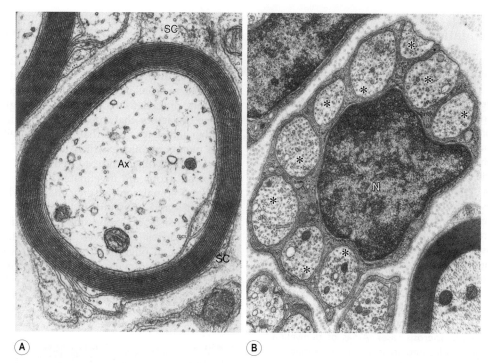

Fig. 2.5 Myelinated and unmyelinated axons. (A) Electron micrograph of myelinated axon in the peripheral nervous system (PNS) shown in cross section. The axon (Ax) is seen at the centre within a sheath consisting of multiple wrappings of the Schwann cell's cytoplasmic membrane. The Schwann cell soma (SC) is at the upper right. (B) Electron micrograph of unmyelinated axons in the PNS. Nine axons (*asterisks*) cut in cross section are seen embedded in a Schwann cell whose nucleus is at the centre (N). In the lower right area a portion of a myelinated axon is visible (from Lowe J. (2020). Stevens & Lowe's Human Histology. Oxford: Elsevier Ltd.).

Table 2.1 Ionic concentrations of intracellular fluid and extracellular fluid

Ions	Intracellular concentration (mM)	Extracellular concentration (mM)
Na^+	12	145
K^+	139	4
Cl^-	4	120
Large anions (A^-)	140	–
Ca^{2+}	<0.0002	1.8

The two most common cations found in total body water are sodium (Na^+) and potassium (K^+). Their distribution in intracellular and extracellular fluids are very different. Intracellular fluid (ICF) contains predominantly K^+, while extracellular fluid (ECF) contains predominantly Na^+ (Table 2.1). It is this difference in ionic concentration between ICF and ECF that allows the generation of the RMP and provides the energy that drives the action potential. The predominant extracellular anion is chloride (Cl^-), whereas the intracellular cations are balanced by the presence of large intracellular anions (A^-), mainly phosphates and the negatively charged side chains of proteins.

The concentration gradients for Na^+ and K^+ are established by the active transport of Na^+ and K^+ by an Na^+/K^+-ATPase known as the Na^+/K^+ pump (Fig. 2.6). This uses the energy derived from breaking down the high-energy phosphoanhydride bond of ATP to pump both Na^+ and K^+ against their concentration gradients. Because the ATPase pumps three Na^+ ions out for every two K^+ ions, this produces a small potential of approximately 5 mV. On the extracellular face of the Na^+/K^+ pump is a binding site for the glycoside ouabain, which inhibits the activity of the pump. The Na^+/K^+ pump is essential to all cells, not just excitable cells, as the ion gradients it establishes are used to power many transport processes.

For a voltage to be generated current must flow and this occurs due to the presence in the plasma membrane of protein channels that selectively allow ions to diffuse passively down their concentration gradients. At rest, the plasma membrane is slightly permeable to K^+ and almost impermeable to Na^+. This means that K^+ will tend to diffuse out of the cell, but this cannot be electrically balanced by the inward diffusion of Na^+. Therefore as K^+ diffuses out, down its concentration gradient, an electrical potential develops, with an excess of negative charge inside the neuron. The neuron also contains negatively charged ions, but these cannot leave the cell as they are too large to cross the plasma membrane. The negative charge inside the neuron creates an electrical gradient, which will tend to pull positively charged ions into the cell. As

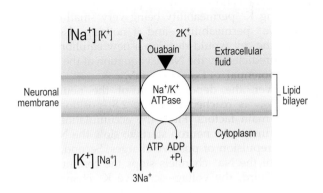

Fig. 2.6 Diagram of an Na⁺/K⁺ pump. The square brackets represent ionic concentrations, a large symbol indicates a high concentration, and a small symbol indicates a low concentration.

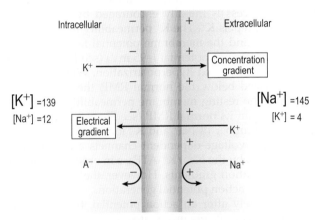

Fig. 2.7 Passive movements of ions across the plasma membrane at rest. Intracellular and extracellular concentration are shown in mmoles per litre.

the membrane at rest is virtually impermeable to Na⁺, the only ion that can be attracted into the cell is K⁺ (Fig. 2.7).

This means that there is an equilibrium position, whereby the amount of K⁺ leaving the cell down its concentration gradient is balanced by the amount being drawn into the cell by the electrical gradient, and there is no net movement of K⁺ across the cell membrane. However, at this equilibrium position, there is a small excess of negative charge inside the cell and this produces the RMP. Because this potential difference is generated across a very small distance—the width of the plasma membrane—the actual difference in the number of ions needed on both sides of the membrane to produce the voltage difference is very small and represents a concentration difference of approximately one part in 10^8. If the membrane is assumed to be permeable only to K⁺, the predicted RMP can be calculated using the Nernst equation.

At 37°C, the Nernst equation reduces to:

$$E_m = \frac{61.5}{Z} \, log_{10} \frac{[C_0]}{[C_1]}$$

where Z= valency of the ion; C_o= external concentration; C_i= internal concentration; and E_m= membrane potential.

| Box 2.3 | Goldman–Hodgkin–Katz equation |

$$V_m = RT \, log_e \frac{P_K[K^+{}_o] + P_{Na}[Na^+{}_o] + P_{Cl}[Cl^-{}_i]}{P_K[K^+{}_i] + P_{Na}[Na^+{}_i] + P_{Cl}[Cl^-{}_o]}$$

where P_K, P_{Na} and P_{Cl} are the relative permeabilities of the plasma membrane to K⁺, Na⁺ and Cl⁻. R, gas constant; T, absolute temperature (in Kelvins); V_m, voltage across membrane; Log_e, Log_{10}.

If the values for K⁺ (C_o = 4 mM, C_i = 139 mM, Z = + 1) are inserted in the equation, the value calculated is approximately –95 mV (negative inside). This is called the K⁺ equilibrium potential ($E_K{}^+$) and is slightly more negative than the measured RMP of approximately –75 mV. It is also called the reversal potential, as at values above and below this potential the current flowing through the channel goes in opposite directions. If the values for Na⁺ are used instead, the Na⁺ equilibrium potential ($E_{Na}{}^+$) is approximately +66 mV. Thus it is obvious that the movement of K⁺ is largely responsible for determining the RMP.

However, if the very slight permeability of the membrane to Na⁺ (~1/75th of that of K⁺) is taken into account, a more complicated equation, called the Goldman–Hodgkin–Katz equation (Box 2.3), is used to calculate the RMP. This allows the relative permeabilities of Na⁺, K⁺ and also Cl⁻ to be taken into account and is a better reflection of the roles of all these ions. At rest, the permeability (P) ratios are $P_K/P_{Na}/P_{Cl}$ = 1.0:0.04:0.45, which gives an RMP of –75 mV for the concentrations in Table 2.1.

The membrane permeability to K⁺ (and Na⁺) is due to the presence of integral transmembrane proteins that form ion channels. The channels are passive, leak channels, which do not seem to be regulated and are always open. These channels are ion-selective and the greater permeability of the plasma membrane to K⁺ is simply due to the fact that there are more K⁺ leak channels than Na⁺ channels.

However, present in the membranes of excitable cells, such as neurons and muscles that can fire action potentials, are also other types of ion channel that are voltage-activated and do not normally open in the resting state.

Action potentials

All cells have an RMP, but cells that can generate and conduct action potentials are said to be excitable—a principal characteristic of neurons. Action potentials are rapid changes in the potential difference across the axonal plasma membrane. During an action potential the membrane potential first depolarizes very rapidly from –75 mV to approximately +40 mV (positive inside). It then repolarizes to approximately –95 mV (a slight hyperpolarization) before returning relatively slowly to its RMP (Fig. 2.8, which shows a typical action poten-

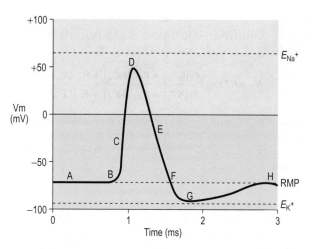

Fig. 2.8 A typical action potential. For events occurring at positions A–H, see text. *RMP*, Resting membrane potential.

tial as recorded from a neuron). The action potential is an all-or-nothing phenomenon, in that once initiated it has a fixed size. The ability of neurons to generate action potentials is due to the presence in their plasma membrane of ion channels that respond to changes in the membrane potential; they are voltage-sensitive. The different phases of the action potential are due to the opening of two types of voltage-sensitive channel, which are Na^+- and K^+-selective. The different properties of these two types of channel determine the characteristics of the action potential.

A neuron may be initially at rest (see Fig. 2.8, position A). The initial stimulus for the generation of an action potential is depolarization of the neuron at the trigger zone (how this is produced is explained later).

Voltage-sensitive Na^+ channels, which have a particularly high density in this part of the axon, will open almost instantaneously, within microseconds, in response to depolarization—a process called activation—and Na^+ ions will flow down their concentration gradient into the neuron. However, these channels will also close again within approximately 0.5–1 ms and be in a state in which they cannot be reopened; they are inactivated. If the depolarization of the trigger zone is small then only a few Na^+ channels will open. Unless the total Na^+ permeability (gNa^+) is greater than the resting K^+ permeability (gK^+), after they close nothing else will happen. This occurs when the graded input signals to the neuron are weak and the depolarization is subthreshold.

However, when the depolarization of the trigger zone is larger (see Fig. 2.8, position B), usually to approximately −55 mV, a greater number of Na^+ channels are activated. Once the Na^+ permeability exceeds the resting K^+ permeability, positive feedback occurs, by which depolarization of the membrane will open more Na^+ channels, depolarizing the membrane further until all local Na^+ channels are open, allowing Na^+ influx.

The voltage then changes rapidly (see Fig. 2.8, position C) to a value approaching + 40 mV. The local area

of membrane is now effectively permeable only to Na^+—the resting K^+ permeability being very small compared to the Na^+ permeability—and if nothing else were to happen the cell would develop a new equilibrium position, as predicted by the Nernst equation at the Na^+ equilibrium potential, of $E_{Na^+} = +66$ mV.

However, the depolarization of the neuron stops before E_{Na^+} is reached (see Fig. 2.8, position D), due to three main factors. First, the accumulation of positive ions inside the neuron starts to slow the Na^+ influx, through repulsion of positive charges. Second, the inactivation of the Na^+ channels stops the continued influx of Na^+. Third, the voltage-sensitive K^+ channels open. These channels are activated by the same depolarization that triggered the opening of the Na^+ channels, but they open more slowly. The axon now becomes highly permeable to K^+ ions, which can now leave the neuron down their concentration gradient (see Fig. 2.8, position E). This process is initially encouraged by the positive charge that repels K^+. The K^+ permeability is now higher than at rest and the membrane potential falls to close to the K^+ equilibrium potential (−95 mV) (see Fig. 2.8, position G). This is called hyperpolarization. When the axon is repolarized below the normal RMP, the K^+ channels close and the resting membrane permeability allows the axon to regain its normal RMP (see Fig. 2.8, position H). The small number of Na^+ and K^+ ions that have moved through the voltage-dependent channels are eventually redistributed by the Na^+/K^+-ATPase in order to maintain the concentration gradients. However, the pump has no active role in action potential generation.

Immediately after an action potential, the Na^+ channels remain completely inactivated for a short period and cannot be opened by depolarization, however large. The Na^+ channels only regain their normal resting state once the membrane has repolarized (see Fig. 2.8, position F). This is called the absolute refractory period (see Fig. 2.8, positions B–F) and ensures that action potentials occur separately and do not propagate in the reverse direction along an excited axon. However, for a short time after this, during the period when some K^+ channels are still open and when the membrane is hyperpolarized, it is possible to initiate another action potential if the stimulus is larger than normal—a suprathreshold stimulus—but the action potential remains a fixed size. This second period is called the relative refractory period (see Fig. 2.8, positions F–H). Table 2.2 lists a summary of the events during an action potential.

The all-or-nothing nature of the action potential, and the enforced time gap between action potentials, means that the action potential is a binary signal. Action potentials are clearly separated one from another, which ensures that the number of action potentials in a given period is clear. This is very important in a system where stimulus strength is coded by frequency. Binary-coded information can be transmitted with less degradation due to noise, an important consideration when the action potentials are transmitted across large distances.

Table 2.2 Sequence of events during an action potential (see Fig. 2.8)

Event	Channels	Ion movements	Notes
Initial depolarization to threshold (approximately −55 mV) (A)	Na⁺ channels open (B)	Na⁺ influx (C)	Absolute refractory period (B–F)
Depolarization to approximately +40 mV	Na⁺ channels close and	K⁺ efflux (E)	
	K⁺ channels open (D)		
Repolarization, then hyperpolarization (−95 mV)	K⁺ channels close (G)		Relative refractory period (F–H)
Return to resting membrane potential (H)		Movement of K⁺ through leak channels (G–H)	

Nerve conduction

So far we have considered only the activity at a given position on the axon, but it is the inactivation of Na⁺ channels that also enables the action potential to travel along the axon from the trigger zone to the synapse.

The depolarization caused by the opening of Na⁺ channels at any given point will spread passively along the axon equally in both directions. However, any Na⁺ channels in the direction from which the action potential has come will still be inactivated and only those Na⁺ channels further down the axon, which have not yet been opened, will be activated by the depolarization. In this way the wave of depolarization (like a Mexican wave) will propagate from the trigger zone to the synapse, with the depolarization being continually regenerated by newly opening Na⁺ channels.

In unmyelinated axons voltage-gated Na⁺ and K⁺ channels are located all along the axon and the action potential travels continuously along the axon. However, in myelinated axons there is a different mode of propagation. Owing to the tight insulation of the axon by oligodendrocytes (in the CNS) or Schwann cells (in the PNS) the axon is effectively separated from the ions that would flow in, except at tiny gaps where the myelin sheath does not cover the surface of the axon. Occurring at regular intervals, these gaps in the myelin are called nodes of Ranvier (see Fig. 2.1) and are zones where the Na⁺ and K⁺ channels are concentrated. Depolarization at the preceding node spreads passively along the interior of the axon but, as the myelinated axon cannot depolarize,

this spread is more rapid than in bare axons. The action potential does not decay as rapidly as in unmyelinated axons, because of the insulation, and at the next node the depolarization is sufficiently large to trigger the opening of large numbers of Na⁺ channels. This will regenerate the depolarization to its full voltage. In this way the action potential jumps rapidly from node to node, a process called saltatory conduction. Failure of saltatory conduction may underlie certain pathologies (see Box 2.2).

The advantage of myelination is an increase in the speed of conduction without a large increase in metabolic cost. Another way of increasing the speed of conduction is by increasing the size of the axon, which reduces the internal electrical resistance and increases the passive depolarization. This strategy is seen in its most exaggerated form in the giant axons of some invertebrates, particularly the giant squid. The large size of these axons means that they are easier to examine experimentally than smaller mammalian axons. Much of the early work on the action potential was done on these axons by Hodgkin and Huxley in the 1950s.

In humans the fastest axons are both large and myelinated. As detailed in Table 1.7, nerve fibres can be categorized based on conduction velocity according to their axon diameter. A difference in conduction velocity can be seen when a mechanical trauma is experienced. The sensory input from mechanical nociceptors travels along myelinated axons (Aδ fibres) and arrives before the signal carried by unmyelinated axons (C fibres). This gives rise to fast and slow pain. Although the C fibres are smaller, most of the difference in velocity is due to the myelin.

Because myelination allows rapid conduction with a smaller diameter, this allows more axons to be packed into a smaller volume, a significant advantage when wiring something as complex as a brain.

Although the electrical polarity of the membrane changes during an action potential the numbers of Na⁺ and K⁺ ions which flow into and out of the neuron in order to bring about this change are relatively small and do not significantly change the internal concentration of either ion. This is because the RMP is only a local charge separation, involving only a very small proportion of the positive charges present, and the main bulk of the intracellular ions is electrically balanced. This can be shown clearly when an axon is poisoned with ouabain (a plant derived toxin). Despite the inhibition of the Na⁺/K⁺-ATPase the axon is able to fire many thousands of action potentials, only stopping eventually when the ion gradients are dissipated.

Synaptic transmission

The specialised site where the axon terminal meets the target cell is the synapse. This is where the signal is transmitted either to another neuron or to an effector, such as a muscle or a gland. There are two types of synapses: electrical and chemical.

Electrical synapses are present throughout the CNS, for example, in the cortex, hippocampus, thalamus, locus

ELEMENTS OF CELLULAR AND MOLECULAR NEUROSCIENCE

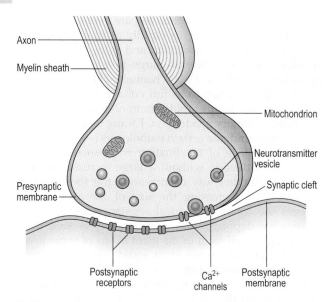

Fig. 2.9 Simplified diagram of a synapse. For clarity, only a few vesicles are shown.

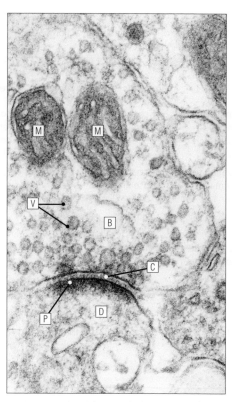

Fig. 2.10 Electron micrograph of a synapse. The synaptic bouton (B) is making contact with the dendrite (D). The bouton contains many small vesicles (V) and mitochondria (M). The synaptic cleft (C) contains faint granular material above the postsynaptic membrane (P) which presents an area of thickening (from Lowe J. (2020). Stevens & Lowe's Human Histology. Oxford: Elsevier Ltd.).

coeruleus and olfactory bulb. In an electrical synapse the two cellular elements are connected by gap junctions. At these junctions, cells interact through a cluster of integral membrane proteins around a pore called a connexon. Each connexon is formed from six connexin proteins and is aligned with a connexon in the opposing cell. This forms a channel between the cells that allows the free passage between them of water and small molecules (<1.2 nm in diameter) including some signalling molecules such as inositol trisphosphate (IP_3) and Ca^{2+}. The intercellular space is approximately 2–4 nm. Gap junctions play important roles in the electrical and metabolic coupling of cells. They are particularly important in coordinating electrical activity in smooth and cardiac muscle. They are also found between astrocytes and between neurons in the retina, where horizontal cells are electrically coupled. Electrical synapses are bidirectional—electrical signalling can flow both ways across the synapses.

In humans, most synapses are chemical synapses and are unidirectional—the presynaptic element releases chemicals called neurotransmitters into the small gap between the neuron and the subsequent cell (postsynaptic element). The gap measures approximately 15–25 nm and is called the synaptic cleft. A simplified image of the chemical synapse in shown in Fig. 2.9. There is evidence that the synaptic cleft is not devoid of molecules as it contains some proteinaceous material. There is also evidence of specific protein interactions that establish discrete molecular bridges across the cleft (e.g. between the cell-adhesion proteins, *neurexin* on the presynaptic side, and *neuroligin* on the postsynaptic side). These complexes stabilize synapses and maintain the perfect alignment of presynaptic and postsynaptic membranes.

At chemical synapses, when the propagated action potential reaches the axon terminal, release of neurotransmitters (one or several different transmitters)

occurs by a process called exocytosis. The neurotransmitter diffuses across the gap and interacts with receptor proteins in the postsynaptic membrane of the target cell.

The presynaptic terminal contains numerous membrane-bound organelles such as mitochondria and smooth endoplasmic reticulum. However, the most distinguishing feature is the presence of large numbers of storage vesicles, which contain neurotransmitters. These can be easily visualized on electron micrographs (Fig. 2.10). Vesicles have a variety of morphological characteristics corresponding to the type of neurotransmitter that they contain.

While many of the vesicles are distributed throughout the presynaptic terminal, there are some that are anchored close to the synaptic cleft at the presynaptic membrane, ready to be released in areas known as active zones. When an action potential invades the presynaptic terminal the depolarization opens voltage-sensitive Ca^{2+} channels, which allow Ca^{2+} to flow into the synapse (the concentration of Ca^{2+} is much higher in the ECF than in the ICF (see Table 2.1)). Ca^{2+} acts at a number of sites to facilitate exocytosis. During exocytosis, SNARE (from SNAP Receptor) proteins play an essential role in vesicle docking, priming, fusion with the plasma membrane and neurotransmitter release into the synaptic cleft. SNARE proteins can be divided into vesicle, or *v-SNAREs* (part

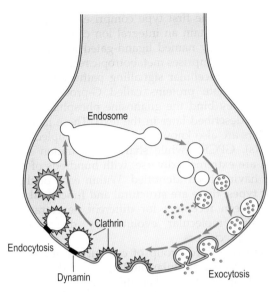

Fig. 2.11 Neurotransmitter is released by exocytosis. The vesicle membrane is coated with clathrin and the vesicle is retrieved by endocytosis. The vesicle then fuses with an endosome. New vesicles are budded from the endosome and filled with neurotransmitter, ready for release.

Table 2.3	Examples of neurotransmitters
Type	**Neurotransmitter**
Amino acids	Glutamate
	Aspartate
	γ-Aminobutyric acid (GABA)
	Glycine
Amines	Acetylcholine
	Dopamine
	Noradrenaline
	Adrenaline
	Serotonin (5-hydroxytryptamine, 5-HT)
Peptides	Endorphins
	Enkephalins
	Substance P

of the membranes of vesicles), and target, or *t-SNAREs* (associated with the presynaptic membrane), and these two classes interact during exocytosis. Synaptobrevin, syntaxin and synaptotagmin are examples of SNARE proteins involved in the process of exocytosis. First, the vesicle is released from the cytoskeleton. Second, it partially fuses with the presynaptic membrane with the help of SNARE proteins in the vesicle and presynaptic membranes. The active zone of the presynaptic membrane contains the primed vesicles and a high density of SNARE proteins. The influx of Ca^{2+} following depolarisation activates synaptotagmin, which allows the complete fusion and development of a pore through which the neurotransmitter can diffuse into the synaptic cleft.

Exocytosis incorporates vesicle membrane into the presynaptic membrane. If the vesicle membrane were to remain there the surface area of the neuron would increase and the plasma membrane would also contain vesicle membrane proteins. Therefore, in order to retrieve the vesicle for reuse, the vesicle membrane is recycled back into the synapse by a process called endocytosis (Fig. 2.11). The vesicle membrane is first coated with a protein called clathrin, which forms a 'cage' around the vesicle; this is then pulled back into the cell by the cytoskeleton, with the help of a 'collar' of dynamin. The retrieved vesicle is fused with an endosome, from which new vesicles can bud off. The empty vesicles can then be refilled with neurotransmitter and reused.

Patterns of vesicle release vary enormously across synapses. At many synapses in the CNS, not every action potential will release vesicles; the average probability of release is usually less than one. However, at the other extreme, in the PNS, at the synapses between motor

nerves and skeletal muscles, the skeletal neuromuscular junction, a single action potential releases approximately 30 vesicles containing neurotransmitter, which is sufficient to produce a twitch of the target muscle.

Neurotransmitters

The first endogenous compound to be identified as a neurotransmitter was acetylcholine (ACh), when its effects on the frog heart were described by Otto Loewi in 1926. Since then, a wide range of endogenous compounds have been identified which act as neurotransmitters, which are responsible for signalling at chemical synapses (Table 2.3). There are distinct patterns of distribution for various neurotransmitter systems and in some cases particular neurotransmitters are associated with specific functions in the brain.

Peripheral neurotransmitters

In the ANS the major neurotransmitters are noradrenaline and adrenaline, which are released onto target organs and tissues by the sympathetic nervous system, and ACh, which is released by the parasympathetic nervous system. ACh is also released at all skeletal neuromuscular junctions, although the receptor subtypes on the muscle are different from those in the ANS. ACh is also the neurotransmitter that acts at all autonomic ganglia, both sympathetic and parasympathetic.

Central neurotransmitters

In the CNS the major excitatory and inhibitory neurotransmitters are the amino acids glutamate and γ-aminobutyric acid (GABA), respectively. These are the main mediators of fast signalling in the brain and spinal cord. Other neurotransmitters include a number of monoamines, such as noradrenaline, 5-hydroxytryptamine

(5-HT, serotonin) and dopamine. These monoamine neurotransmitters mainly act in a slower manner than amino acids and are often described as 'neuromodulators', as their (excitatory or inhibitory) effects depend on the receptor type stimulated. Many neurons release more than one neurotransmitter, although the patterns of excitation required to stimulate their release may differ. One of the neurotransmitters may be, for example, glutamate, whereas the second neurotransmitter may be a peptide. Peptides are released at a higher firing frequency. The slow-acting neurotransmitters frequently have long-lasting modulatory effects on their target neurons.

Histamine, as well as acting as an important neurotransmitter in the brain, is also an inflammatory mediator, released from mast cells and basophils, and promotes vasodilatation and increased capillary permeability.

Following its discovery as a key molecule in the control of blood pressure, nitric oxide (NO), a short-lived gas, is a more recent addition to the list of neurotransmitters. It is produced from L-arginine, through the action of NO synthases. One of these synthases is expressed in neurons, and NO can be produced postsynaptically and act after diffusion on the presynaptic element as a retrograde signalling agent. While it fulfils the criteria for a neurotransmitter, it does not act on cell surface receptors but binds to the intracellular enzyme guanylate cyclase, causing changes in intracellular biochemistry. It has been suggested that one role for NO in the CNS may be in the hippocampus, in the formation of new memories. There are also lipid-derived neurotransmitters such as the endogenous cannabinoids (e.g. anandamide), which can be produced on demand by the postsynaptic element, and diffuse across the synapse to exert their effects on receptors located on the presynaptic terminal—another example of retrograde signalling.

Postsynaptic events and postsynaptic receptors

The neurotransmitter that is released into the synaptic cleft diffuses to the postsynaptic membrane, where it binds to specific receptors. Typically, this takes less than 5 μs, as the cleft is very narrow, measuring approximately 15–25 nm. Not all the released neurotransmitter reaches the receptors, as diffusion out of the cleft and specific inactivation mechanisms may reduce the amount available for receptor binding.

The action of a given neurotransmitter on a target neuron (or peripherally on a target organ) depends on the identity of the receptors present on the postsynaptic target. Almost all neurotransmitters identified and characterised so far have multiple receptor subtypes that they can activate. Receptors for most neurotransmitters (unlike those for some hormones and NO) are integral membrane proteins, which have their neurotransmitter binding sites in receptor structural domains located near the extracellular surface. There are two major types

of receptors. The first type comprises ionotropic receptors, which contain an integral ion channel; hence they are alternatively named ligand-gated ion channels. The second type comprises metabotropic receptors, which are linked to intracellular signalling pathways via a group of intermediate proteins called G-proteins (so called because they bind the guanosine phosphates, GTP and GDP, as described later in the text). These metabotropic receptors are also known as G-protein-coupled receptors (GPCRs). GPCRs, while sharing a common structural motif, are extremely diverse, with hundreds of different types having been identified. Within each of these two major types, there are structural and functional similarities between receptors for different neurotransmitters, suggesting molecular evolutionary divergence from common precursors.

There is a third group of cell surface receptors consisting of an extracellular binding site and an intracellular catalytic site that, when the receptor is activated by the ligand, phosphorylates tyrosine residues. These are receptor tyrosine kinases (RTKs). There are more than 20 subclasses of RTK (e.g. the epidermal growth factor family, the fibroblast growth factor family and the vascular endothelial growth factor family) and they are the targets for peptide growth factors (including neurotrophic factors such as nerve growth factor (NGF) and brain derived neurotrophic factor (BDNF)), cytokines and various hormones. They can exist as single subunit receptors and also as multiple subunit complexes. The catalytic domain responsible for the kinase activity of these receptors is located in the C-terminal domain of the subunits, which is intracellular. After activation, RTKs can undergo internalisation in a manner similar to metabotropic receptors (see later).

Some ligands, such as the steroid hormones, are lipophilic and can diffuse across the cell membrane. Others, such as thyroid hormone, are internalized by specialized transport mechanisms. These ligands bind to nuclear receptors which act as transcription factors, thus affecting the level of gene transcription.

Ionotropic receptors

Ionotropic receptors are integral membrane-spanning proteins with multiple subunits (hence the name 'multimeric') that group together to form an ion channel complex that has different ion selectivities and multiple associated ligand-binding sites. Receptors of this type (Table 2.4) can be divided into many subtypes. In some cases the distribution of the subtypes clearly varies over developmental time and by location (see later chapters for further details on specific receptors). Ionotropic receptors are anchored to the membrane through a complex scaffolding which consists of proteins with specific structural domains that enable them to couple both to receptor subunits and to the cytoskeleton or to intracellular signalling complexes. Ionotropic receptors are responsible for fast signalling such as on the millisecond scale.

Table 2.4 Ionotropic receptors

Neurotransmitter	Receptor type
Acetylcholine	Nicotinic acetylcholine
Glutamate	NMDA
	AMPA
	Kainate
GABA	GABA$_A$
Glycine	Glycine
Serotonin	5-HT$_3$

5-HT, 5-Hydroxytryptamine; AMPA, amino-3-hydroxy-5-methyl-4-isoxazole propionic acid; GABA, γ-aminobutyric acid; NMDA, N-methyl-D-aspartate.

An example of an ionotropic receptor is the nicotinic ACh receptor (nAChR) (Fig. 2.12; see also Chapter 17). It is formed of five subunits—α, β, γ, δ and ε—as a homomer (the same subunit) or a heteromer (different subunits). The open nAChR allows the flow of Na$^+$, Ca^{2+} and K$^+$ across the membrane. The subunit composition dictates the biophysical and pharmacological properties of this type of receptor. This is a general principle applicable across all ionotropic receptors.

Neurotransmitter binding to ionotropic receptors triggers a conformational change that allows ions to flow selectively through the channel. The subsequent current flow sets up a potential difference called a postsynaptic potential, which may be excitatory (EPSP) or inhibitory (IPSP), depending on the ion selectivity and the membrane potential, and makes the neuron more (EPSP) or less (IPSP) likely to fire an action potential. If the current flowing through each type of channel is measured at different membrane potentials, there is a voltage at which the net current is zero. For example, if the channel is only permeable to K$^+$, this will occur at the Nernst potential for K$^+$. This is because at this voltage—called the reversal potential—the numbers of ions moving in and out of the neuron are exactly balanced (see earlier). For any given channel, if the membrane potential is higher than the reversal potential, activation of the channel will produce an IPSP, and if it is lower, it will produce an EPSP.

If we consider the case of ACh receptors at the neuromuscular junction (also called the motor endplate), the RMP will be approximately –85 mV. On activation, current will flow through the ACh receptor, making the membrane potential more positive, and in skeletal muscle this depolarization is sufficient to activate voltage-sensitive Na$^+$ channels, producing an action potential, which, via the subsequent release of Ca^{2+} from the sarcoplasmic reticulum, causes the muscle to contract.

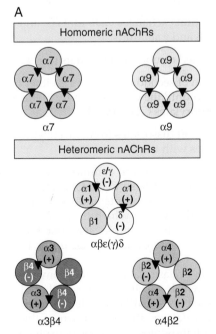

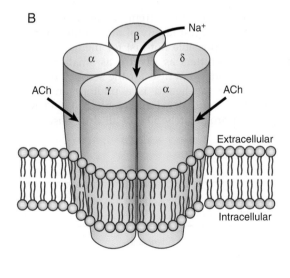

Fig. 2.12 The multimeric structure of the nicotinic neuronal and muscle acetylcholine (ACh) receptors. (A) Homomeric or heteromeric combinations of various subunits define the ion channel and form receptors with different properties. The ACh binding sites are illustrated as triangles. The different subunits are labelled α, β, δ/ε and γ. (B) Location of the muscle-type nACh receptor in the membrane showing its quaternary structure—the straight arrows indicate the binding sites for the neurotransmitter and the curved arrow indicates the flow of sodium though the channel. (A, From Ho Thao N.T., Abraham N., Lewis R.J. (2020). 'Structure-Function of Neuronal Nicotinic Acetylcholine Receptor Inhibitors Derived From Natural Toxins', *Frontiers in Neuroscience*, 14. http://doi:10.3389/fnins.2020.609005; B, From Karlin A. (2002). 'Emerging structure of the Nicotinic Acetylcholine receptors', *Nature Reviews Neuroscience*, 3:102-114.

In studies on the motor endplate, it was observed that small EPSPs called miniature endplate potentials (MEPPs) occurred spontaneously at a rate of approximately 1 per second. They were of similar size (~ 0.5 mV) and duration (rising rapidly and decaying more slowly in a total of ~5 ms), and all EPSPs were multiples of MEPPs. This is because neurotransmitter release occurs in distinct packets called quanta. Each MEPP represents the release of a single vesicle containing ACh, which is the minimum possible amount that can be released. The amount of ACh in each vesicle is approximately the same and the stimulated neurotransmitter release therefore consists of release from several vesicles, so the response will be multiples times the effect of a single vesicle.

This phenomenon has been more difficult to establish in the CNS, possibly due to the variable size and content of the vesicles and the smaller number of vesicles released by each action potential. The amount of neurotransmitter reaching the postsynaptic receptors may be affected by the high-affinity uptake of neurotransmitter into glia and surrounding neurons, through specialised transporters (see below). It is also important to note that the neurotransmitter released from the presynaptic terminal can also activate presynaptic receptors. These are called 'autoreceptors' and they often act through a negative feedback mechanism: if neurotransmitter in the synaptic cleft reaches too high a level, the activation of autoreceptors may limit further release or even ultimately lead to reduced neurotransmitter synthesis.

Metabotropic receptors

Metabotropic receptors, or GPCRs, while having a common mode of action, are extremely varied in their ligands. They are the largest family of membrane-bound receptors and are responsible not just for mediating the effects of neurotransmitters as diverse as small amino acids and large peptides, but also for the sensory reception of light (where the ligand is a photon) and for detecting some tastes and all odours (Table 2.5). GPCRs are the target of approximately 50% of all drugs used at present.

Table 2.5 A selection of endogenous ligands that have metabotropic receptors

Acetylcholine	Adenosine
Adrenaline	Serum calcium
Noradrenaline	Anandamide
Serotonin	Bradykinin
Dopamine	Oxytocin
Histamine	Somatostatin
Glutamate	Vasopressin
GABA	β-endorphin

The common structure of these receptors is that of a single protein with seven transmembrane segments, with an extracellular domain that often contains the ligand-binding site and an intracellular domain that is involved in the interaction with G-proteins (see Fig. 2.13). Some metabotropic receptors are anchored to specific postsynaptic proteins, in a manner similar to ionotropic receptors. G-proteins are trimers of membrane-associated proteins and consist of alpha (α), beta (β) and gamma (γ) subunits. The inactive α subunit has guanosine diphosphate (GDP) bound to it. This is exchanged for guanosine triphosphate (GTP; present in the cytoplasm) upon activation of the G-protein trimer by a receptor, resulting in the α subunit separating from the β and γ subunits. The activated α subunit then alters the activity of an enzyme involved in the synthesis of a second messenger. The α subunits come in different forms, which interact with different intracellular enzymes, and can either stimulate or inhibit these enzymes. A few seconds after the GDP/GTP interchange, the molecule of GTP is converted to GDP by the intrinsic GTPase activity of the α subunit, which renders the α subunit inactive, whereupon it recombines with the β and γ subunits. The β and γ subunits, which are also released from the receptor, remain bound to each other throughout, and have roles distinct from that of the α subunit. At its simplest, the sequence of events triggered by the binding of a ligand to a metabotropic receptor is as follows (see Fig. 2.13):

1. The ligand binds to the receptor.

2. The receptor binds the G-protein trimer.

3. The α subunit exchanges GDP for GTP and separates from the β and γ subunits.

4. The activated α subunit binds to its target enzyme.

5. Production of second messengers is either increased or reduced until the GTPase activity of the α subunit dephosphorylates GTP to GDP.

6. The α subunit dissociates from the enzyme and recombines with the βγ subunit.

The target enzymes are commonly either adenylate cyclase or phospholipase C (PLC) (Fig. 2.14). At least 17 genes code for α subunits and they can be grouped according to the way in which they modulate intracellular signalling, for example, whether they stimulate or inhibit adenylate cyclase (α_s or α_i) or they activate PLC (α_q).

Adenylate cyclase catalyses the conversion of ATP to cAMP, which itself activates other intracellular enzymes such as cAMP-dependent protein kinase A (PKA). PLC catalyses the breakdown of the membrane lipid phosphatidylinositol 4,5-bisphosphate into two second messengers, diacylglycerol (DAG) and inositol 1,4,5-trisphosphate (IP_3). DAG is an activator of protein kinases, in this case protein kinase C (PKC). IP_3 diffuses into the cytoplasm and binds to specific IP_3 receptors on intracellular organelles containing Ca^{2+} stores, causing

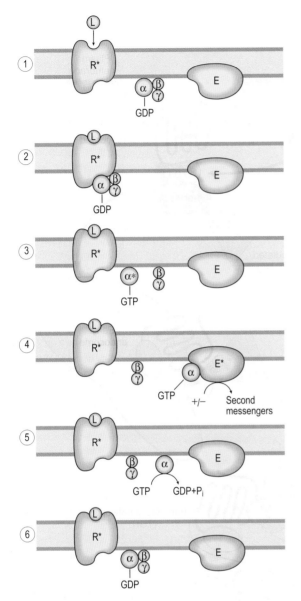

Fig. 2.13 Sequence of events associated with the activation of a G-protein-coupled receptor. *E*, Enzyme; *GDP*, guanosine diphosphate; *GTP*, guanosine triphosphate; *L*, ligand; *P_i*, phosphate; *R*, receptor; *α*, *β* and *γ*, G-protein subunits; *, activated state.

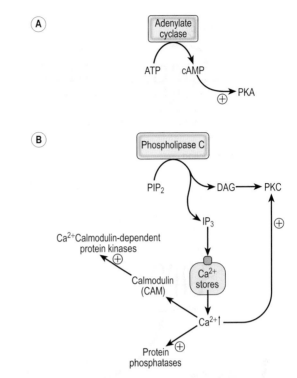

Fig. 2.14 Diagram of second messenger pathways. (A) Pathway generating cyclic AMP (cAMP). (B) Pathway generating diacylglycerol (DAG) and inositol 1,4,5-trisphosphate (IP_3). *PIP_2*, Phosphatidylinositol 4,5-bisphosphate; *PKA*, protein kinase A; *PKC*, protein kinase C.

the release of Ca^{2+} into the cytoplasm. Ca^{2+} can activate both protein kinases such as PKC and protein phosphatases (see Fig. 2.14). It can do this either directly or, in some cases, via a Ca^{2+}-binding protein called calmodulin; in this case, the resulting Ca^{2+}–calmodulin complex activates the target protein. cAMP, DAG, IP_3 and Ca^{2+} are called second messengers, as they act within the cell. In this context the neurotransmitter (ligand) is called the first messenger, although this term is very rarely used.

An important aspect of signalling via GPCRs is that an activated receptor may itself activate multiple G-proteins before the ligand is removed. Additionally, each α subunit can bind to a single enzyme molecule, although the enzyme activity is changed for the entire time that the α

subunit is bound, which can lead to a large change in the concentration of second messengers. This is especially true in the case of PLC-linked systems, as the second messenger IP_3 can itself release large amounts of Ca^{2+}. This amplification of the neurotransmitter signal can produce significant downstream biochemical changes in the neuron through the levels of protein phosphorylation by activated kinases and phosphatases.

After activation of the receptor, the response of the receptor to the ligand may be reduced. One mechanism that may be linked to this reduced response is the internalisation of the receptor. Internalisation occurs in several steps and may have different consequences. As described in Fig. 2.15, the first step is the phosphorylation of the receptor by a specialised kinase—GPCR-associated kinase (GRK). The phosphorylation can lead to fast desensitisation of the receptor. The phosphorylation can also be followed by the binding of a protein called β-arrestin, which will trigger internalisation of the receptor through clathrin-coated membrane pits. The β-arrestin-bound receptor-ligand complex can trigger intracellular signalling through enzymatic pathways such as those involving the mitogen-activated protein-kinase (MAPK) system of phosphorylation cascades. The complex can also be diverted towards the lysosomal compartment, where the receptor and ligand are degraded, or the receptor is dephosphorylated and recycled back to the plasma membrane. Signalling can be triggered by the internalized receptor through the endosome or the

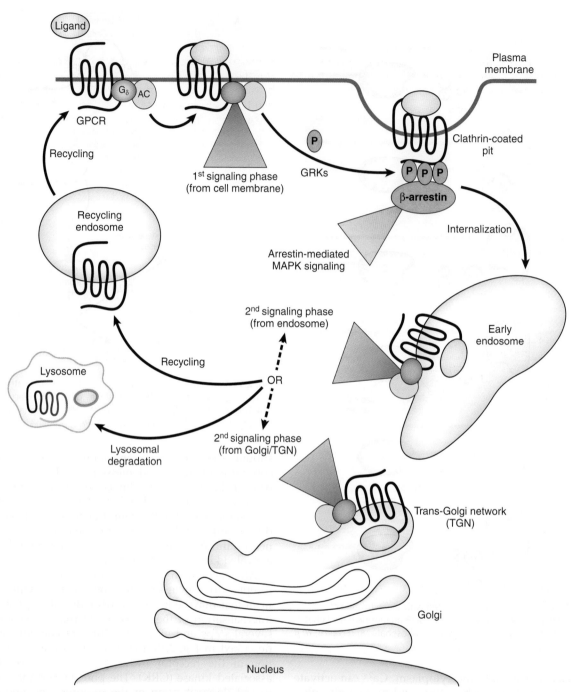

Fig. 2.15 The dynamics of GPCR internalization and intracellular signalling. The receptor can be rapidly phosphorylated by a GRK, and β-arrestin is rapidly recruited. The complex can then be internalized and directed towards the endosomal compartment and towards the trans-Golgi network. During this internalization, GPCR can continue to be involved in signalling processes. *GPCR,* G-protein coupled receptor; *GRK,* GPCR kinase; *MAPK,* mitogen-associated protein kinase; *TGN,* trans-Golgi network. (From Calebiro D, Godbole A. (2018) Internalization of G-protein-coupled receptors: implication in receptor function, physiology and diseases. Best Practice and Research: Clinical Endocrinology and Metabolism 32:83–91.)

trans-Golgi network—a major secretory complex which directs proteins to various subcellular locations.

One of the consequences of GPCR activation is the modulation of neuronal excitability. Many of the ion channels present in neuronal membranes can, like many intracellular proteins, have their properties changed by altering their state of phosphorylation. This can determine the conditions under which they open and for how long they open. GPCRs can lead to changes in the level of channel phosphorylation. Changes in the opening of ion channels then influences whether a neuron fires in response to the stimulus produced by ionotropic receptors and other metabotropic receptors. In this way, GPCRs affect the overall excitability of neurons and thus their firing patterns. In some cases, it has been shown that both α and βγ subunits can interact directly with ion channels to modulate their activity, without the intervention of an enzyme or second messenger.

Neurotransmitter synthesis

The small 'classical' neurotransmitters (amino acids and amines) are biosynthesized from precursors in reactions catalyzed by enzymes present in the presynaptic terminal. For example, in the case of glutamate, it is synthesized either from glucose provided by the Krebs cycle or from glutamine produced by glial cells. It is important to note that glutamate is present in large amounts in the cell and has different metabolic and neurotransmitter pools. After biosynthesis, neurotransmitters are concentrated in vesicles through an antiport system, for example, transporting H^+ out of the presynaptic storage vesicle in exchange for the neurotransmitter. The high concentration of H^+ in the vesicles is maintained by an H^+-ATPase in the vesicle membrane.

Peptide transmitters are manufactured in the cell body as larger precursors, by ribosomes in the rough endoplasmic reticulum, and are processed and packaged via the extensive Golgi system into vesicles that are transported down the axon via anterograde transport. They appear in the presynaptic terminal in large dense-core vesicles, which are found further away from the synaptic cleft than the small clear vesicles that contain neurotransmitters like the amino acids and amines. They are released from the synapse when the frequency of action potentials is high and the intracellular Ca^{2+} concentration reaches higher values than under lower-frequency stimulation.

It is possible to trace the neurotransmitter pathways in the brain by immunocytochemistry, using antibodies for the specific enzymes associated with a particular neurotransmitter. For example, ACh is made from acetyl coenzyme A (acetyl-CoA) and choline by the enzyme choline acetyltransferase (ChAT), and the presence of ChAT can be used to identify neurons that synthesize and release ACh.

Neurotransmitter inactivation

After release, enzymes present on the postsynaptic side can inactivate neurotransmitters. ACh is inactivated by enzymatic degradation within the synapse by acetylcholinesterase (AChE) at the neuromuscular junction or other cholinergic synapses. The enzyme is found in the folds of the postsynaptic membrane, located close to the receptors. The esterase activity cleaves ACh into its inactive components—choline and acetate. Choline is then transported back into the presynaptic neuron by an Na^+-dependent choline transporter, where it can be used to resynthesize ACh in combination with acetyl-

CoA derived from glycolysis. As well as the membrane-bound AChE, there are two soluble esterase enzymes. One of these is another type of AChE, found in the cerebrospinal fluid, and the other, called butyrylcholinesterase (BChE) or pseudocholinesterase, is found in plasma. It is less substrate-specific than the AChE and can hydrolyse a wide range of esters. Suxamethonium is a commonly used, short-acting neuromuscular blocking agent that is normally inactivated by BChE. However, approximately 1 in 3000 individuals have an inherited condition in which they have a modified form of BChE that fails to metabolize suxamethonium. These mutated forms are the consequence of various genetic mutations in the BChE gene that are associated with loss of function. These individuals show neuromuscular paralysis that lasts for several hours instead of a few minutes, and hence will need to be ventilated until the suxamethonium is degraded. These variations in BChE may also underlie increased susceptibility to the toxic effects of organophosphorus compounds such as nerve agents, which can be inactivated by non-mutated BChE.

Most classical neurotransmitters are *de facto* inactivated—their action at their receptors is terminated by their removal from the synaptic cleft by high-affinity Na^+-dependent uptake systems (also known as sodium symporters). These transporters are found on neurons and, in some cases, glial cells. The importance of these mechanisms is highlighted by the fact that drugs that inhibit neurotransmitter uptake can have profound effects on brain function. Cocaine inhibits dopamine uptake, which at least partly accounts for the euphoria and addiction associated with the drug. More usefully, tricyclic antidepressant drugs, which block the uptake of serotonin and adrenaline (and also in some cases dopamine) and selective serotonin uptake inhibitors such as fluoxetine (Prozac®) are widely used in the treatment of depression, although the link between reuptake blockade and the long-term therapeutic effect is rather complex. The signals mediated by glutamate or GABA can also be terminated by removal of these neurotransmitters through transporters such as the excitatory amino acid transporter (EAAT) family, and GAT-1, respectively. Simple diffusion away from the synaptic cleft may also be important in the inactivation of transported molecules, and is a mechanism of inactivation for peptide neurotransmitters, in parallel with the action of specific peptidases. As diffusion may be slow, this may explain why peptide actions are more long-lasting that the effects of transmitters such as ACh or monoamines. Finally, removal of ligand-bound receptors by internalisation, as discussed above, is another mechanism of termination of the synaptic signal.

Summation and neuronal integration

Each neuron in the brain establishes tens of thousands of synaptic contacts with other neurons. If a given input is closer to the trigger zone of the neuron, then it is more

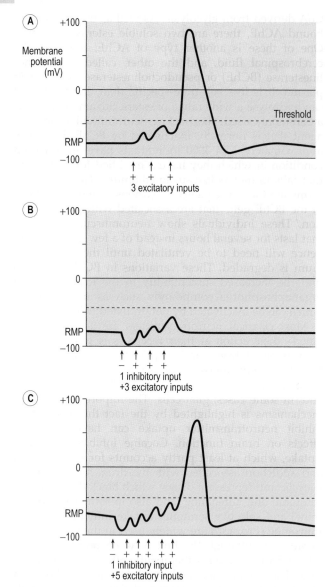

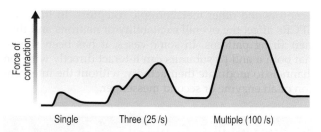

Fig. 2.17 Single twitch and summation of inputs produces tetanus in skeletal muscle. The force of contraction in a skeletal muscle depends on the frequency of firing of the motor nerve.

Fig. 2.16 Integration of excitatory and inhibitory inputs. (A) Three closely spaced excitatory inputs cause the neuron to exceed the threshold and fire an action potential. (B) A single inhibitory input prior to the three excitatory inputs prevents the neuron from firing. (C) Increasing the number of excitatory inputs enables the threshold to be reached and an action potential to fire.

likely to affect the firing of that neuron. This is often the case with inhibitory inputs. If the firing frequency of the input is high, then the EPSPs may summate to produce an action potential (Fig. 2.16A), a process known as tem-

poral summation. If another synapse also contributes, then the electrical potentials from all inputs summate in spatial summation. If there is an IPSP, then this may prevent the action potential (see Fig. 2.16B). The number of EPSPs would have to increase to overcome the inhibition (see Fig. 2.16C). The density of a given type of receptor at a given synapse will also affect the subsequent behaviour. This spatial and temporal summation, along with the current electrical status of the neuron (i.e. how depolarized or hyperpolarized the neuron is), will all determine whether it fires or not. In most cases neurons will require the simultaneous activation of a number of excitatory inputs in order to fire, thus ensuring integration of signals.

Sometimes, the sum of the inputs will ensure firing of the postsynaptic cell in all cases, but this seems to be relatively rare. At the neuromuscular junction, firing of the motor neuron releases so much neurotransmitter that muscle contraction is always activated, although for a large contraction it requires a high frequency of inputs, as single twitches summate to produce a tetanus (Fig. 2.17). In the cerebellum, inputs from a climbing fibre always cause the firing of the large PC that it innervates. The cerebellum is involved in the acquisition and refining of motor patterns, and this climbing fibre/PC signal is activated when an error of execution occurs.

Finally, beyond the temporal and spatial integration which is a fundamental characteristic of the function of local neuronal circuits, there is now awareness of a higher level of integration of signals between neuronal populations in different regions of the brain, based on the 'connectome'—the whole network of structural connections in the CNS. The present goal of the study of the connectome is to deepen the understanding of the dynamics of the cerebral networks that underlie normal function and neurodevelopment and analyse how these networks are disrupted very distinctly by pathological processes that characterize specific diseases.

CLINICAL ASSESSMENT

3

Chapter summary

1. The clinical examination consists of several parts: gaining the patient's consent, taking a history (presenting complaint and medical, drug, family and social histories) and then performing the relevant component parts—the neurological examination, mental state examination and clerking the observations.

2. Major common clinical laboratory techniques that can provide additional or confirmatory information relevant to the clinical examination include neurophysiological, medical imaging, biochemical, immunological, microbiological and haematological tests.

Introduction

A clinical examination has three components: the history, the examination and the explanation, where the doctor discusses the nature and implications of the clinical findings. A patient seeks medical help for three main reasons: diagnostic purposes, treatment or reassurance or a combination of these factors. The foundation of the patient–doctor relationship is based on establishing a good rapport during the history taking and the examination.

Although increasingly sophisticated tests are available to support the diagnostic process in neurology and psychiatry, the history and clinical examination remain the core of the assessment of a patient who suffers from some form of damage to, or dysfunction of, the nervous system. The important point is to be systematic. This chapter aims to provide a brief overview of the essential points of the clinical examination and to describe the main additional laboratory-based investigations that may help in the formulation of a diagnosis.

The clinical examination is preceded by obtaining the patient's consent to perform the assessment. This is best done by introducing oneself, explaining who you are and what you do and asking permission to talk with them and examine them. Additionally, clues as to the potential issues can be gained by general observation of the patient as they enter the consulting room or at the patient's bedside, for example, the use of aids such as hearing aids, crutches, walking sticks etc., whether they appear unwell and observation of any obvious physical signs, such as muscle atrophy, abnormal gait or scars. These may provide clues to the experienced clinician of a preliminary diagnosis.

Next comes the taking of the patient's history; this provides essential information about the possible aetiology of the disease. It is the most important part of the clinical assessment, during which, the following information is obtained about the patient: age, gender, race, occupation and handedness. It comprises several parts: history of the present complaint (e.g. onset, is it sudden or gradual; nature and distribution, is it uni- or bilateral; symptom onset/frequency), past medical history (including past and/or present drug treatment and associated conditions like diabetes, hypertension), family history and social history. For example, the temporal evolution of the problems that the patient is experiencing provides important clues as to their nature. An acute onset is characteristic of trauma or a major vascular accident. Development over days may suggest an inflammatory component. Neoplasms develop, in general, over months or years. Neurological problems resulting from an immune mechanism, such as multiple sclerosis, also have an evolution over months and years, with a pattern of relapse and remission. Neurodegenerative diseases, such as Parkinson's disease, motor neurone disease or Alzheimer's disease, develop inexorably over years. In some cases, if the patient presents with an impaired state of consciousness, either transient (e.g. seizures) or chronic (e.g. dementia), a complete history of the patient's problems will require involving others, such as relatives, carers or the general practitioner. Psychiatric histories are often more detailed, as more detail is needed about the patient's personal life, family and social background (e.g. siblings and 'family' illnesses, home circumstances, diet, smoking status, drug and alcohol history and sexual orientation and history).

A general physical examination is performed. This is important, as systemic disease may lead to neurological complications (e.g. links exist between atherosclerosis and stroke, cancer and cerebral metastases, diabetes and peripheral neuropathy and rheumatoid arthritis and cervical cord compression). The whole of the clinical examination is performed gently, tactfully and with consideration for the patient, who may be surprised or intimidated by some of the questions or procedures that are part of the examination, or may perceive them as completely unrelated to the complaint. Avoid using medical jargon, using instead simple explanations and common language, building the patient's trust and gaining their confidence, thus making the examination as participatory and interactive as possible.

There is no absolute 'gold standard' way to perform a neurological examination, and methods vary between clinicians, hospitals and countries. However, any basic neurological clinical examination includes an evaluation of the follwoing: (1) mental state, (2) sensory systems, (3) cranial nerves, (4) motor system and reflexes, (5) coordination, (6) gait and (7) cortical function.

A general practitioner of medicine could carry out a first assessment of this type before involving a specialist. For diseases in the field of psychiatry, such as depression or schizophrenia, more specialized tests and rating systems may be required, as mentioned in the corresponding case analyses discussed in this book. It is also important to note that the autonomic nervous system is not tested directly during the examination. However, the patient may present with complex indirect signs and symptoms of dysfunction in the sympathetic or parasympathetic systems (e.g. postural hypotension, constipation or faecal incontinence, urinary retention or incontinence, pupillary immobility, disturbances of sweating or erectile failure). If required, the Valsalva manoeuvre is the gold-standard test used to assess the integrity of the autonomic nervous system. It requires the patient to take a deep breath and, while pinching the nose and keeping the mouth closed, to try to exhale against a resistance of 40 mmHg for 15 seconds. During this test, the heart rate increases, and then returns to normal once the subject breaths normally.

After the clinical examination, a series of laboratory-based investigations may be required in order to obtain information that the clinical examination cannot reveal. Inconsistencies in the history or examination should make one think about the possibility of a functional non-organic disorder.

Mental state

The mental state examination is the psychiatric equivalent of the physical examination. It is a thorough and systematic evaluation of the emotional and mental state of a patient carried out as an interview. The following areas must be assessed:

- appearance and behaviour

- speech

- mood

- thought content

- abnormal experiences and beliefs

- cognitive state

The time devoted to each component depends on the patient's answers and the diagnostic possibilities; much of this information is gathered through observation and interaction with the patient during the history taking and the initial general physical examination.

The patient's appearance can often reveal much about an underlying psychiatric disorder. Important points to look for include dress, personal hygiene and general grooming. The general appearance and demeanour of the patient may suggest self-neglect, depression or anxiety. The latter may also be revealed by hyperventilation or sweating. The way in which a patient sits also gives important hints to a possible underlying pathology; are they relaxed and at ease or sitting tensely and fidgeting? The agitated depressive or the excited manic or schizophrenic may be so agitated that they get up from the seat and pace around the room. A demented or confused patient may leave the chair because they do not understand what is going on. The presence of delusions of persecution may lead the patient to feel threatened by the proceedings and to become angry or terminate the consultation. Alternatively, patients may appear to drift off to sleep repeatedly, suggesting either a confusional state, with fluctuating levels of consciousness or over-sedation due to existing medication.

The patient's behaviour during the interview may be disinhibited, as in the manic patient who strips; the patient may be manipulative or seductive and may threaten violence if their wishes are not met. Alternatively, the patient may appear unduly submissive or self-critical or make little or no eye contact with the interviewer. They may appear suspicious of questions due to an underlying personality disorder or paranoid illness. The patient may also appear inattentive to the interviewer or to be listening to someone else when there is no one else in the room; this suggests that they are experiencing auditory hallucinations. Undue terror without any obvious cause or attempts to touch or shoo away non-existing objects suggests that the patient is experiencing visual hallucinations.

Gradually, the clinician can also assess whether the patient is confused or, on the contrary, has good insight into their condition. Assessment of drug/alcohol use and social and family circumstances should also be considered. It must be remembered that bizarre behaviour or inability to relate to the interviewer may reflect subnormal intelligence.

Speech is a form of behaviour, and thus it is important to assess its production, form and content. Does the patient speak at all or are they mute, and if so, is this deliberate, organic or part of a depressive stupor? In a mute patient, it is important to assess all aspects of speech production, including the ability to produce sounds and communicate non-verbally. If the patient does speak, is this spontaneous or only in answer to questions, with monosyllabic or fuller and more elaborate replies, or is the patient vague and evasive? Is speech unduly slow, as in depressive illness, or so quick and continuous that it is impossible to interrupt, as in hypomania and mania? A sudden change in verbal style may indicate an emotionally sensitive subject requiring further questioning. Language production is related to handedness; dysphasia (difficulty in verbal communication) is a feature of dominant hemisphere dysfunction (see Chapter 1).

Mood has both a subjective component, which is reflected in the way the patient describes their emotional state, and an objective component, that is, what the interviewer sees. The subjective and objective components of mood are usually, but not always, congruent. Facial expression is one of the outward signs of the patient's mood. For example, tearfulness or poverty of expression in depression, elation in mania, tenseness in anxiety and perplexity in schizophrenia are observed. The emotional expression may be abnormally labile, as in mania or organic brain disease. A patient's mood can be probed using direct questions, for example, 'How have you been feeling lately?' Psychiatric symptoms (e.g. paranoid delusions or profound thought disorder) may become apparent during the conversation with the patient.

Abnormal moods most commonly include depression and anxiety; they also include elation, irritability, anger and perplexity. When the mood is abnormal, it should be evaluated in detail, in the same way as any other presenting symptom. Some severely depressed patients may see no future, feel despairing and hopeless and have suicidal thoughts. Suicidal ideation must always be sought for in depressed patients, and it is also appropriate to ask about suicidality in those with other disorders such as schizophrenia, alcohol dependence, hypomania and severe anxiety disorders. Not only is it incorrect to think that discussing suicide with patients encourages them to commit suicide, but failure to discuss it may lead to tragedies that could have been prevented. Intent to commit suicide can be probed with questions such as 'Is life worth living nowadays? Have you seriously contemplated ending it all?'

The patient should be asked what their main worries are and whether they are preoccupied by any thoughts, for example, morbid thoughts. Obsessional ruminations are stereotyped thoughts that the patient recognizes as their own and realizes are silly but unsuccessfully tries to resist. They occur in obsessive-compulsive neuroses and may be associated with obsessional rituals, that is, acts that the patient feels compelled to carry out, even though they recognize them as being absurd, for example, compulsive hand washing because they 'feel dirty'. For obsessional rituals, the patient realizes that the compulsion comes from within, unlike delusions of influence, in which the impulse is felt to come from outside forces.

Perceptual abnormalities most often take the form of hallucinations or delusions. Patients suffering delusions have a false and unshakeable belief that is out of keeping with the social milieu from which they come. Hallucinations are apparently normal perceptions that occur in the absence of an appropriate stimulus. In psychiatric illness, hallucinations occur in organic and functional psychoses, for example, in schizophrenia and affective illnesses, cases of severely raised levels of anxiety due to hyperventilation, grief reactions and hysterical illnesses. Illusions occur when the object is real but perception is disturbed. They are usually related, in the psychiatric sense, to disorders of the perceptual environment of the object, thereby leading to decreased visual clarity coupled with a state of high emotion in the perceiver. Illusions are common in psychiatric illness, particularly acute confusional states. In affective disorders, the content of any hallucinations or delusions is generally mood-congruent. Depressed patients may think that they are evil, while manic patients may believe that they are God.

Impaired concentration is a characteristic sign of depression; it also occurs in dementia and acute confusional states. Cognitive function can be assessed using the Mini Mental State Examination (see Table 14.3). It includes several components: the level of consciousness, the orientation in time and place, general appearance, mood, interaction with the examiner and attention and memory.

Cranial nerves

Abnormalities in cranial nerves may occur in isolation and involve one nerve only or may affect several nerves. Assessment aids lesion localisation and in an unconscious patient can give prognostic information.

Cranial nerve I (olfactory)

The olfactory nerve is tested by exposing the patient to a range of scents (e.g. cinnamon, cloves, vanilla, tobacco mint, oranges or coffee). With the patient's eyes closed, each nostril is alternately occluded, while the other nostril is tested. Odours that produce irritation are avoided (e.g. ammonia). It is also important to note that anosmia (loss of the sense of smell) may not have a neurological

cause but be simply due to a sinus inflammation (catarrh), which may be linked to an infection. Anosmia is an important symptom of SARS-CoV-2 viral infection (which causes COVID-19). Olfactory hallucinations may be associated with epilepsy. Testing of this nerve is not routinely performed but is carried out when patients report a decrease in their sense of taste or smell. It is also performed in patients with suspected dementia and in patients with tumours or fractures through the cribriform plate of the skull or damage to the nasal passages, where there may also be associated optic nerve or frontal lobe damage. Loss of the sense of smell may significantly affect the sense of taste.

Cranial nerve II (optic)

Testing of the optic nerve starts with an assessment of the patient's ability to read printed material with each eye separately, that is, visual acuity using a Snellen chart. Testing consists of a series of letters whose sizes are such that the biggest letter can be seen at a distance of 60 m, whereas the smallest can be seen with normal vision at 5 m. If the patient wears glasses, the type of lens worn is determined in order to differentiate between myopia and hypermetropia. Acuity at the normal reading distance is also assessed. The visual fields are then tested by moving an object (usually the examiner's finger) into the four visual quadrants. The left and right eyes can be tested together at first (binocular vision), and then monocular testing can be performed. Any subjective visual sensations are also noted, for example, visual hallucinations or white flashes in the visual field. Fundoscopic examination of the retina can detect the possible presence of papilloedema, suggesting raised intracranial pressure, and retinal haemorrhages, which may occur in diabetics or hypertensives. Colour blindness, although not regularly tested, is assessed using Ishihara plates, in which a series of coloured spots contain numerical shapes that the patient must identify.

Cranial nerves III (oculomotor), IV (trochlear) and VI (abducens)

The examination of these three nerves assesses eye movements and pupillary function. The examiner first notes the position of the eyes during gazing straight ahead (where a squint or strabismus could become evident), and then assesses any symmetrical or asymmetrical change in the movement of the eyes when performing specific tests. Visual tracking is tested by assessing the convergence response (depth of focussing), smooth pursuit is tested by observing the conjugate eye movements in response to drawing an imaginary letter 'H' and peripheral fields are tested by confrontation testing. Saccade responses (fast conjugate eye movements that shift the eyes between different targets) are assessed by asking the patient to rapidly and alternately fixate on the examiner's hands (e.g. thumb of one hand and finger of the other) several times in quick succession. The patient should be specifically asked for the presence of

Looking to the right

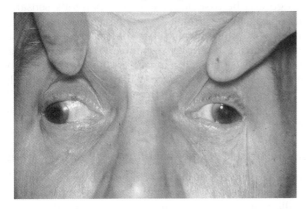

Looking to the left

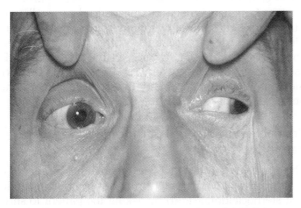

Fig. 3.1 Left oculomotor nerve lesion. Note the inability of the patient's left eye to adduct on command to look right. It deviates laterally due to the unopposed action of the lateral rectus muscle (innervated by cranial nerve six).

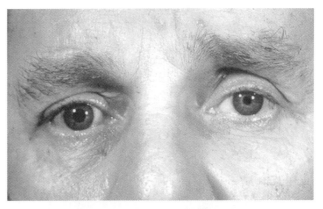

Fig. 3.2 Example of Horner's syndrome (left eye). Note the slight drooping of the patient's left eyelid and asymmetry of the pupils; the left is slightly smaller than the right.

any diplopia (double vision) on looking in particular directions. A lesion to cranial nerve III may lead to deficits of adduction (Fig. 3.1), depression or elevation of the eye and unilateral ptosis. A lesion of cranial nerve IV will result in deficient abduction and in the medial deviation of the eye. A lesion in cranial nerve VI leads to a deficit in the internal rotation of the eye and failure to abduct. Examination of the pupils involves assessment of the size, shape and mobility of the pupils, and the accommodation reflex response (see Chapter 6). Slight asymmetry between pupillary sizes occurs in up to 20% of people. The pupillary light response (direct and indirect) is also performed (see Chapter 6). Painful third nerve palsy can be a sign of an intracranial aneurysm (enlargement of an artery due to weakening of the arterial wall) pressing on the third nerve. Diabetic neuropathy and atherosclerosis can also cause pupillary dysfunction. A fixed, dilated pupil in a person with a mass lesion (e.g. tumour) can occur when the intracranial pressure has reached the point where the brain starts herniating to compress the third nerve. It is a sign of impending death in that situa-

tion. Drugs such as morphine and atropine can also alter pupillary size. A small pupil can be part of Horner's syndrome (Fig. 3.2), which may be due, for example, to a carcinoma impinging on the superior cervical ganglion or to damage to the sympathetic pathways anywhere along their cranio-cervical course.

Cranial nerve V (trigeminal)

Examination of this nerve involves assessment of the normal functioning of each of its three divisions: ophthalmic, maxillary and mandibular. Lesion of the whole nerve leads to a loss of sensation in the skin and mucous membranes of the face and nasopharynx. Sensory testing involves assessing the response to light touch and pinprick. The presence and symmetry of the corneal reflex (Chapter 6) are also tested. Motor function is assessed by asking the patient to clench their teeth (to check the masseter muscle), as well as testing the strength of the masticator muscles by asking the patient to open the mouth against resistance.

Damage to the motor division produces muscle wasting, which is most easily seen in the temporalis muscle (above the zygomatic arch). In addition, the mandible deviates to one side (indicating pterygoid muscle weakness on the side of nerve damage) rather than travelling vertically (normal) on opening and closing the mouth. The jaw-jerk stretch reflex (see Chapter 6) of the jaw-closing muscles (masseter and temporalis muscles) is weak or absent in normal subjects. Brisk or exaggerated jaw jerks often indicate bilateral lesions of upper motor neuron pathways.

Cranial nerve VII (facial)

The patient's face is inspected, looking for symmetry of movement—which is a key element in the testing of the facial nerve—when asked to perform specific movements, for example, eyebrow elevation, smile or show the upper teeth or blow out the cheeks. Several other manipulations can also reveal facial nerve dysfunction; for example, the patient may find it difficult to whistle.

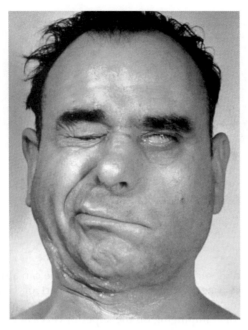

Fig. 3.3 Patient with left facial nerve palsy being asked to shut his eyes and grimace.

Lesions above the facial motor nucleus (located in the pons) cause supranuclear palsies, whereas lesions distal to the nucleus cause infranuclear (nerve) facial palsies. The ability to wrinkle the forehead is used to distinguish between upper and lower motor neuron damage to the facial nerve (Fig. 3.3), since the forehead muscles are bilaterally innervated by the corticobulbar tract, whereas the lower facial muscle motoneurons only receive a contralateral bulbar input (see Fig. 9.9). Supranuclear paralysis affects mainly the lower part of the face, whereas infranuclear palsies affect both parts of the face. The latter, but not the former, cause atrophy of the facial muscles. This is because the upper part of the face receives bilateral innervation from both facial nerves, unlike the lower part. The sensory component of this nerve is examined by assessing the response of the anterior two-thirds of the tongue to sweet, salty or sour solutions (on both sides).

Cranial nerve VIII (auditory and vestibular)

Hearing tests assess the auditory component of cranial nerve VIII. Hearing is tested by blocking one ear while testing the hearing in the other ear by whispering or varying the intensity of speech. This is followed, if necessary, by Weber's and Rinne's tests, which are tests of hearing involving the use of a tuning fork (see Chapter 8). The examiner also notes abnormal sensations (e.g. hyperacusis or tinnitus, although the former can indicate a lesion of the facial nerve). Vertigo (a sensation of spinning) and nystagmus (involuntary eye movements) reflect dysfunction in the vestibular component (although optokinetic nystagmus in response

to normal object tracking can occur physiologically). Vertigo can be associated with the patient's sensation that objects move around them. Nystagmus and vertigo can also be induced by sudden changes in head posture. Caloric testing, Hallpike's manoeuvre and Romberg's test may also be useful in aiding the investigation of vestibular dysfunction (see Chapter 8). A vestibular Schwannoma (acoustic neuroma) is a type of VIIIth nerve tumour that presents initially with only mild hearing loss.

Cranial nerves IX (glossopharyngeal) and X (vagus)

These nerves are tested functionally by observing the quality of speech and coughing, and monitoring taste, swallowing and the position of the palate at rest. The movement of the palate is also assessed during voluntary or reflex activity. Damage to the glossopharyngeal nerve is associated with loss of taste in the posterior part of the tongue. Lesions of the vagus nerve lead to swallowing (dysphagia) and voice (dysphonia) problems for example, a hoarse, deep voice, blurred and ineffectual speech and a displaced uvula. The last of these is assessed by asking the patient to say 'Ah', and observing the movement of the soft palate and uvula. Damage to either nerve results in loss of the gag reflex.

Cranial nerve XI (spinal part of the accessory nerve)

These nerves are tested by assessing the weakness or wasting of the innervated muscles (upper trapezius and sternocleidomastoid) by asking the patient to shrug their shoulders and turn their face to each side against resistance.

Cranial nerve XII (hypoglossal)

This nerve supplies the tongue muscles. If this nerve or its nucleus is damaged, a deviation of the tongue to the side of the lesion can be seen, as well as wasting and fasciculation of the tongue on the same side when the tongue is protruded (Fig. 3.4).

Motor function

Examination of motor function involves the assessment of the following:

- muscle bulk
- presence of involuntary movements
- muscle tone
- muscle power
- reflexes
- coordination
- gait

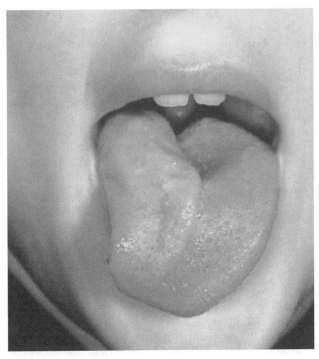

Fig. 3.4 Right hypoglossal nerve palsy; note the atrophy and fasciculation of the right side of the tongue.

Table 3.1	MRC scale for assessment of muscle power

0 = No muscle contraction visible (paralysis)

1 = Muscle contraction visible, but no movement of joint

2 = Joint movement when effects of gravity are eliminated

3 = Movement sufficient to work against gravity

4 = Movement overcomes gravity and resistance

5 = Normal power

Reflexes

Reflexes can be divided into the following types:

- stretch (deep tendon) reflexes

- superficial reflexes, such as the abdominal reflex and cremasteric reflex (not usually tested)

- brainstem reflexes: pupillary, corneal and gag reflexes (mentioned above)

- primitive reflexes: suck reflex, grasp reflex and palmomental reflex (their presence is often a sign of frontal lobe lesions)

Visual inspection to assess the bulk of muscles is commonly ignored, and this is an ill-advised omission, as wasting of muscles can occasionally give immediate clues to the pathology. Do not say there is no atrophy unless you have actually looked at all relevant muscle groups carefully! If necessary, ask the patient to remove or roll up clothing. Additionally, look for involuntary movements and fasciculations.

Muscle tone is tested by passively flexing and extending the elbows, the wrists and the hip, knee and ankle joints, and by pronating and supinating the wrists and assessing resistance to these movements. Muscles are hypertonic in Parkinson's disease, whereas hypotonia is seen in lower motor neuron or cerebellar damage. It is important to be able to assess the tone properly, as sometimes, it can be the only pointer to pathology in an otherwise normal clinical examination. Muscle tone is reflected in the intensity of the stretch reflexes.

Power is tested by assessing the strength of a muscle group across a joint and is graded against resistance applied by the examiner from 0 to 5 (Table 3.1). There are several tests for non-organic limb weakness. For example, if it is suspected that weakness of a leg is non-organic in origin, the hands of the examiner are placed below both the patient's knees, and the patient is asked to lift the allegedly weak leg. If there is genuine weakness, and the patient is really trying to lift that leg, the other leg will press down on the bed. If the weakness is not genuine (e.g. due to somatization of a psychological problem), the other leg will not move.

There are five deep tendon reflexes assessed in the neurological examination: the biceps, brachioradialis, triceps, knee and ankle reflexes. Their intensity can be graded from 0 to 5, where 0 is areflexia, 1 is sluggish, 2 is normal, 3 is hyperactive, 4 indicates the presence of non-sustained clonus and 5 is sustained clonus; 0, 4 or 5 are considered abnormal. There may also be a Hoffman's sign, which is increased rebound responses of the finger flexors in response to flicking the middle fingernail downwards (the thumb may also adduct and flex in response to this). The patient is examined in the seated or supine position, and the examiner uses a reflex tendon hammer to tap on the tendon of the muscle being tested. If reflexes cannot be elicited, reinforcement techniques, such as the Jendrassik manoeuvre (see Chapter 9), may be required. Asymmetrical decrease or loss of reflexes is due to peripheral nerve damage (radiculopathies, plexopathies or mononeuropathies). Hyperreflexia is a sign of upper motor neuron damage and is associated with spasticity and a positive Babinski sign. The latter is evaluated by the slow and firm scraping of the sole of the foot on the lateral side. This should elicit a flexor plantar response and adduction of the toes. The positive Babinski sign (see Chapter 9) consists of an extensor plantar response of the big toe and abduction of the other toes. A positive sign is normal in children aged up to 2 years (prior to independent walking). In adults, it is indicative of upper motor neuron damage. Occasionally, an equivocal response is obtained, when no movement of the big toe can be elicited at all. This can happen in some people naturally, as well as in some pathological conditions, as in the aftermath of spinal cord injury.

Superficial reflexes such as the abdominal reflex are normally elicited by lightly drawing a sharp object across the four abdominal quadrants supplying dermatomes T8–T12 to observe muscle contraction. This response is impaired if there is an upper motor neuron lesion above the spinal level tested. However, they are difficult to elicit in many patients (due to body fat obscuring muscle contraction) and so are less often tested.

Coordination and balance

Good coordination of movement reflects the cooperation of separate groups of muscles. Ataxia (poor coordination) can be sensory, caused by dysfunction of the afferent connections from muscles and joints within the nerve or spinal cord dorsal columns, or motor, caused by damage to the cerebellum. This can result in truncal ataxia of the proximal muscles when the midline cerebellum is affected or appendicular ataxia of the limbs when the cerebellar hemispheres are affected. The integrity of cerebellar function, and that of several other components of the motor system, is evaluated using coordination tests. For the upper limb, these include the finger-nose test (where the patient is asked to alternately touch their own nose and the examiner's fingertip as fast as possible) and rapid supination and pronation of the hand. The inability to execute rapid pronation/supination is termed dysdiadochokinesia and is a sign of cerebellar ataxia. For the lower limb, tests include the heel-knee-shin test (where the patient is asked to draw the heel of the contralateral leg up and down the lower limb of the ipsilateral leg), the heel-to-toe test (pigeon-toe walking in a straight line without losing balance) and Romberg's test. In this last test, the patient stands upright, feet together, hands by their side, with their eyes open and then closed. The clinician observes any signs of sway and loss of balance—termed a positive Romberg sign—which is worse with the eyes shut, indicating a sensory ataxia (and issues with the spinal cord dorsal columns). The test is based on the idea that a person needs two of the following three senses to maintain balance while standing: proprioception (the ability to know one's body position in space), vestibular function (the ability to know one's head position in space) and vision (used to monitor and adjust body position). A patient who has a problem with proprioception can still maintain balance by relying on vestibular function and vision. Romberg's test is used to differentiate between sensory and motor ataxia, the latter of which is caused by cerebellar dysfunction.

Gait

The examination of gait involves an assessment of the patient's ability to rise from a chair, posture and postural stability and ambulation. Difficulty in rising from a chair may reflect the weakness of muscles or basal ganglia disease. The posture of the patient is also pathognomonic for certain diseases. For example, Parkinson's disease patients have a stooped posture, whereas patients with progressive supranuclear palsy may have a rigid, hyper-erect posture.

During assessment of ambulation the examiner assesses speed, length of stride and ability to turn; leg circumduction (by abducting the hip and thigh in order to clear the foot above the ground during the swing phase of gait), stiffness, knee bending, arm swing and deviation from a straight line while walking are also noted. Patients with Parkinson's disease have a shuffling, festinating (i.e. rapid and increasingly accelerating) gait, experience difficulty in stopping at will and also have a decreased arm swing. Patients with progressive supranuclear palsy may present with a wide-based stride and slowing of ambulation. To detect subtle movement abnormalities, a forced gait test (walking on heels, tiptoes, inside/outside of the foot only, hopping or climbing stairs) can be performed.

For assessment of postural stability, the patient is asked to stand with the feet next to each other. Patients with cerebellar disease or labyrinthine problems may not be able to stand without separating the feet. The clinician may also perform the Romberg test, during which the patient is asked to stand still and close their eyes. Wide oscillations and a loss of equilibrium may reflect damage to the posterior columns. Truncal ataxia can also be assessed and is seen as an inability of the patient to walk in a straight line when asked to perform the heel-to-toe task, in which they must place the heel of one foot in direct contact with the toe of the other foot. The gait in cerebellar truncal ataxia is 'drunken'. A waddling gait (like that of a duck) is due to proximal muscular weakness and is seen in muscular dystrophies and myopathies. It is important to remember, however, that the commonest disorders of gait in the general population are due to local musculoskeletal pathology in the limbs, for example, arthritis of the hips, and it is important to exclude this.

Sensory examination

This part of the examination evaluates the response to painful stimuli, temperature and light touch, and also vibration and joint position sense. It is important to note that sensory changes may be milder and more difficult to detect than motor or reflex changes and depend on the patient's willingness or ability to express what they are feeling. Consequently, it can often be the hardest part of the examination to interpret with certainty. As in the cranial nerves and motor examination, it is important to compare both sides of the body (always with the patient's eyes closed) using each test before deciding whether the results are abnormal or normal. Nociception is tested through applying pinprick stimuli to the skin. Temperature perception is tested using a cold object (e.g. the side of a tuning fork) but is less often tested than the pinprick sensation. These are rarely tested together because if one is present, almost invariably so is the other. Vibration is tested by placing a vibrating tuning fork on the bony prominences of the various joints tested. Light touch is assessed by dabbing (static touch) or stroking (dynamic touch) a twist of cotton wool on the skin of the patient and asking them to say when and where they feel the stimulus.

During examination, comparisons of the two sides, and proximal to distal, are made in order to identify the site of the lesion. When a sensory deficit is suspected or identified, the examiner must determine its modality and map its distribution on a sensory examination chart to see if it matches that found with lesions of the peripheral nerve, spinal nerve, spinal cord, posterior fossa or supratentorial region. For example, decreased response to pinprick on one half of the body is due to a lesion in the contralateral ascending pathways or the cerebral hemisphere. If the deficit is mainly distal and bilateral (e.g. 'stocking' or 'glove' distribution of a deficit), the cause may be a peripheral neuropathy. It is also important to note that considerable individual variation occurs in the segmental or radicular (dermatome) innervation patterns and therefore also in the anatomical location of dysfunction.

Cortical function

Tests assessing sensory cortical function depend on the integrity of the pathways to the brain; if they are damaged, then these tests should not be performed. Certain sensory and higher mental functions require specific intact cortical lobes. Spatial awareness/perception (parietal lobe) can be assessed by examining sensory input and spatial limb position with a variety of tests. Stereognosis (the ability to identify objects using only tactile sensation) is assessed by asking the patient to identify common objects, such as a key or money, by touch alone. Graphesthesia (the ability to recognise any symbols drawn on the skin) loss is tested by using numbers or letters drawn on the skin, which the patient should identify by touch alone. Assessing the patient's ability to perform simple mathematical calculations, such as addition or subtraction, examines calculating skills, while asking a patient to copy a drawing of a symmetrical object, such as a clock, examines sensory neglect. All of these tests assess parietal lobe function. Damage to the parietal lobe (in particular, to the non-dominant parietal lobe) gives rise to various types of apraxia, that is, the inability to execute movements or tasks. Constructional apraxia—failure to build, draw or comprehend the spatial relationships of objects—can be identified by asking a patient to copy a construction made with building blocks, whereas ideomotor apraxia—failure to make movements upon a verbal command—can be identified by asking a patient to mimic getting dressed or copying arm movements made by the examiner.

Higher mental skills, such as reasoning, working memory, abstract thought and the organization and reorganization of information, are functions of the frontal lobes; damage to these results in characteristic deficits. These abilities can be assessed using the following tests. Reasoning and abstract thought can be assessed by asking the patient to explain the meaning of idioms in their own words, for example, 'people who live in glass houses shouldn't throw stones', or 'there's no smoke without fire' or identifying similarities between pairs of objects, for example, cats and dogs.

Working (short-term) memory is assessed by examining digit span recall. This involves paying attention to and verbally recalling the order of two series of numbers that are presented to the patient to view, and then removed. If all are correctly recalled, another (longer) series of numbers is used, and the test repeated. If these are all correctly recalled, the test is repeated until the subject makes an error on a trial at a given list length. Digit span corresponds to the length of the longest list for which the patient was correct in both trials. Normal short-term memory span is between five and nine items. People normally show greater recall of numbers at the beginning of the list, as they are rehearsed more often, and good recall of numbers at the end of the list, as they have the least time to decay from memory; numbers in the middle of the list are the ones most likely to be forgotten. Recent memory can also be tested by asking a patient to recall a list of items presented to them 3–5 minutes previously.

The Wisconsin card sorting test is a sensitive test of executive function, involved in processes such as rule changing or set shifting. The cards given to the patient have symbols on them that differ in number, shape and colour, and the examiner chooses a category for sorting the cards, such as by colour, shape or number. The patient must then sort the pack of cards by placing each card, in turn, under an appropriate stimulus card based upon a rule that the examiner has generated (colour, shape or number). After the patient places each card on top of an appropriate stimulus card, the examiner says 'correct' or 'incorrect', depending upon whether their rule is being obeyed. For example, if the rule is shape, for example, a circle, when the subject places a single cross on top of a single circle (working on a number rule), then they are wrong. The subject should continue placing the cards on top of the appropriate stimulus card until 10 successive correct placings have been scored. When this has been achieved, the sorting rule is changed. Scoring is performed in two ways: categories achieved within the number of cards given and perseverative errors. The former is the number of changes of criterion and the latter is the number of errors caused by the subject continuing to choose a discontinued criterion. Damage to the frontal cortex gives rise to errors of these types, and the effect is particularly severe if the dorsolateral frontal cortex is damaged.

Abnormalities of speech and language may interfere significantly with history taking and with the ability of the patient to perform parts of the rest of the examination; therefore the assessment of any impairments is often performed at the beginning of the clinical examination. The clinician may detect aphasia (i.e. disorders of understanding and expression), dysphonia (disturbance of voice production) or dysarthria (problems with the articulation of words). Damage to Broca's area produces difficulties with verbal output, but not with comprehension, whereas damage to Wernicke's area does not affect verbal output: the subject is normally fluent, but the comprehension of language is impaired, and they may talk rapidly, producing jumbled speech that resembles a 'word salad'.

People with diminished levels of consciousness are assessed using the Glasgow Coma Scale, which ranges from a minimum score of 3 to a maximum of 15 (see Table 11.7). The three parameters assessed are the verbal, eye-opening and motor responses. A score of 8 indicates coma, 8–12 indicates a severe head injury and 12 indicates a mild head injury.

The neurologist's approach to the examination of cortical function reflects the attempt to diagnose an organic (physical) disease of the brain that may disrupt mental functions, whereas in psychiatry, the clinician may be more interested in dysfunctional brain syndromes that may not be associated with organic disease.

Other investigations

In addition to the clinical examination, other diagnostic techniques may be employed to help identify or confirm the cause of the problem. These include haematological, microbiological, biochemical, immunological, neurophysiological and medical imaging. Some are outlined below.

Nervous system imaging

Radiography

X-ray contrast images are produced by the differential absorption of X-rays as they pass through air, water, fat and mineral components of the body. Structures such as the brain and spinal cord are mostly water and so are largely invisible on the image, whereas bone has a high calcium content and so absorbs much X-ray energy. Radiographic analysis can reveal bony fractures (skull or spine) or misalignment, tumours and metastatic processes, general alterations in the skull, inflammatory processes, vascular abnormalities (aneurysms or malformations) or degenerative processes (e.g. calcification of intervertebral discs).

Computed tomography

During computed tomography (CT), a beam of X-rays scans the head or spine in a series of successive planes, and the differential absorption of the rays by the tissue is reflected in an image of the structures scanned. Images are obtained in the coronal or axial plane. CT is used in the diagnosis of brain infarcts and haemorrhages, fractures, hydrocephalus, cerebral atrophy and tumours. For skull analysis, CT has superseded X-rays for most pur-

poses. It is relatively insensitive to spinal cord pathology, although it can detect herniated discs and bony fractures. An additional injection of contrast medium can help display the vascular system and identify aneurysms and arteriovenous malformations. CT or magnetic resonance imaging (MRI) can be used interchangeably in some indications. However, there are instances when one or the other technique is preferable. For example, CT is valuable in the evaluation of intracranial abnormalities in patients with craniocerebral trauma. Skull X-ray examination is more accurate for fractures of the cranial vault, whereas CT is preferable for fractures of the base of the skull. In particular, the acutely injured patient may not be amenable to a complex MRI scan. A CT scan (under 10 seconds) is also shorter than an MRI scan (5–10 minutes), which is an important factor. Acute haemorrhage is also better demonstrated by CT than by MRI analysis. In contrast, MRI is preferable for evaluation of patients in a subacute phase of injury or with chronic injury. For example, 48 hours after haemorrhage, even small collections of blood in subdural locations can be imaged by MRI, although they are not visible by CT. Herniation of discs, which ultimately results in compression of nerve roots, can also be rapidly imaged by CT.

Magnetic resonance imaging

MRI generates signals that are due to the interaction of hydrogen ions (essentially components of the water in the nervous tissue) with magnetic fields; it does not involve the use of X-rays. Initially, protons are oriented in a strong magnetic field, and they are subsequently excited using a lateral magnetic pulse. During relaxation they emit signals that can be decoded and transformed into an image that reflects anatomical structures as a function of their water content. Because grey matter contains more water than white matter, a clear difference between the two tissue types is readily seen. Two types of image are obtained: T1-weighted and T2-weighted images (Fig. 3.5). T1-weighted images show details of the anatomy, whereas T2-weighted images highlight areas of increased signal density or pathology. Table 3.2 summarises signal differences between T1- and T2-weighted images.

An easy way to differentiate between MRI and CT scans of the head is that bone appears white with CT and dark with MRI. Areas that are white or bright with CT are called high-density areas, whereas with MRI they are called high-signal areas. Gadolinium can be used as a contrast agent in MRI. Variations in MRI analysis include fluid-attenuated inversion recovery (FLAIR) and diffusion-weighted imaging (DWI); both are used for detecting areas of small lesions in acute ischaemic stroke. Although more cumbersome, MRI analysis has an advantage over the quicker CT scan. It is particularly good for seeing regions of demyelination in the central nervous system. For example, in multiple sclerosis, a normal CT scan may be obtained, whereas the MR image in the same patient will be

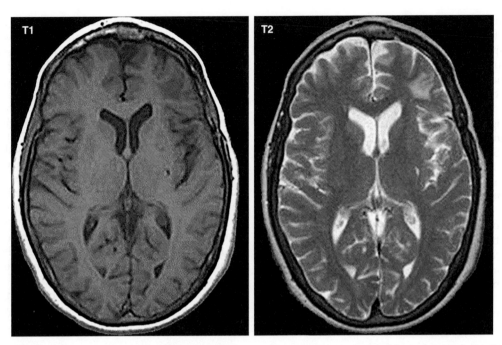

Fig. 3.5 Comparison of T1- and T2-weighted axial magnetic resonance images. The lipid component of the brain is bright in a T1-weighted image, so myelin gives a bright signal. Water (and hence cerebrospinal fluid-filled spaces) appears dark on T1-weighted images but bright on T2-weighted images.

Table 3.2 Differential signal characteristics of T1-weighted and T2 -weighted brain magnetic resonance images

	T1	*T2*
Cerebrospinal	Black	White
Fat	White	White
Cortical bone	Black	Black
White matter	Light grey	Dark grey
Grey matter	Dark grey	Light grey

grossly abnormal (e.g. T2-weighted images would show areas of increased signal intensity corresponding to plaques). MRI also gives better definition and sensitivity in tumour detection. MRI has become a procedure of choice for the evaluation of spinal abnormalities. MRI provides clear images of the spinal cord and roots and disc spaces and helps in the definitive diagnosis in cases of spinal cord compression, syringomyelia or tumours. A practical limitation of MRI is that, since its strong magnetic field tends to shift any ferromagnetic objects, it can only be used safely in the absence of metal implants (e.g. metal plates), defibrillators and pacemakers. In addition, since the MRI machine is like a tube in which the patient has to lie still for long periods for the scan, it is not suitable for claustrophobic patients or people who are not very cooperative, such as children or confused patients or people in a lot of pain.

Functional MRI (fMRI) is a variation of the technique that is predominantly used as an experimental research technique. It allows the correlation of anatomical location and function without injection of additional substances or tracers. In the brain, blood perfusion is related to neural activity; thus fMRI (like positron emission tomography [PET]) can be used to explore the activities of various brain regions when subjects perform specific tasks or are exposed to specific stimuli.

Diffusion tensor imaging (DTI) is a refinement of MRI based on mathematical algorithms that estimate water molecule diffusion in particular directions in the generated image. DTI provides a quantitative analysis of the magnitude and directionality of water molecules. It is now possible to use this to visualise, in three dimensions, specific white matter tracts in the brain, as axon bundles travelling in a particular direction constrain water molecule diffusion in a single direction; this is called tractography. It can identify major CNS tracts such as the corpus callosum or corticospinal tracts etc. and is used for presurgical operation planning, assessing white matter changes induced by tumours, microstructural alteration of white matter by diseases such as Alzheimer's disease (dysconnectivity and impact of plaque formation) or traumatic brain injury or investigating the anatomy of the developing brain.

Positron emission tomography and single photon emission tomography

PET is based on the use of compounds labelled with radioisotopes that emit positrons. There are 15O-labelled compounds that can be used to monitor cerebral blood flow and its fluctuations during cerebral activity. PET has a lower spatial and temporal resolution than fMRI. PET analysis using ^{18}F-fluorodeoxygluose can be used to gather information about cerebral glucose metabolism. PET analysis can also be used to follow the deposition of amyloid in the brain of individuals with Alzheimer's disease, using ligands such as ^{18}F-florbetapir or ^{18}F-florbetaben. Single photon emission computed tomography (SPECT) uses a similar principle to PET. The radioisotopes have a longer half-life than those used in PET and emit single photons. It is a less costly technique, but the resolution is significantly lower. Specific SPECT ligands could be used to detect, for example, neurode-generative processes. In Parkinson's disease, a disease characterised by loss of dopaminergic innervation, a DaT scan can be carried out for diagnostic purposes using SPECT and the tracer ioflupane (^{123}I), which is a marker of the dopamine transporter (uptake transporter) on dopaminergic fibres. Various PET or SPECT ligands for the translocator protein (TSPO), expressed by activated microglia, can be used to detect neuroinflammation.

Angiography

Angiography consists of the injection of contrast medium into the circulation, usually through a catheter placed in the femoral artery. It helps in the visualization of vascular abnormalities, aneurysms and the blood supply to tumours. This method has been superseded by magnetic resonance angiography, which provides detailed information on vascular anatomy and blood flow without need for the use of contrast medium, although this can be given intravenously if required.

Doppler/duplex scanning

This technique uses ultrasound imaging of the carotid arteries of the neck. It can reveal arterial stenosis and the characteristics of blood flow through arteries. This is a useful, non-invasive screening method in the investigation of cerebrovascular accidents or transient ischaemic attacks.

Electrical activity

Electroencephalography

Electroencephalography (EEG) recordings are used to globally characterize the electrical activity of the brain. The activity is recorded using scalp electrodes placed equidistantly on the head. A normal EEG recording is characterized by well-defined rhythms that have specific frequencies that vary with the level of patient alertness. Abnormal or asymmetric waveforms are indicative of pathology. EEG is used primarily in the diagnosis of epilepsy, as the analysis of the traces can help identify the seizure locus and, in some cases, the type of epilepsy. EEG is also useful in ventilated unconscious patients to detect seizures, as in these patients there may not be any external evidence of seizure activity. It is also occasionally used to confirm brain death, as it can show whether the electrical activity of the brain has ceased or not. EEG can be used in combination with MRI.

Event-related potentials

Changes in EEG recordings can occur in response to stimuli. These are called event-related potentials (ERPs). ERPs are evoked in the primary cortical regions that correspond to the type of stimuli used (e.g. cutaneous stimulation triggers ERPs in the somatosensory cortex). As an example, visual ERPs can be used to assess the integrity of the visual system and detect demyelination in the optic pathways. Auditory ERPs are less sensitive than visual ERPs but can detect the presence of acoustic neuromas. Somatosensory ERPs test the integrity of somatosensory pathways and are sensitive in detecting, for example, the demyelination associated with multiple sclerosis. Evoked potentials can be distinguished from background noise and spontaneous activity with the use of signal-averaging techniques.

Electromyography and nerve conduction tests

These procedures are used in the diagnosis of muscular and peripheral nerve disorders. In electromyography (EMG), spontaneous, voluntary and electrically stimulated muscle activity is recorded, using intramuscular needles or surface electrodes. This technique can detect fibrillations or fasciculations. The latter are due to spontaneous motor unit discharges in degenerating nerve fibres causing irregular flickering over the surface of the affected muscle. The former arise when muscle fibres are denervated and are due to the spontaneous and simultaneous discharges of muscle fibres in response to release of acetylcholine from degenerating motor fibres; they are not visible to the naked eye.

Nerve conduction velocity assessment is based on electrical stimulation of a nerve; the rate of action potential propagation along the nerve and the amplitude and time of the response are measured. Motor nerve, sensory nerve and mixed nerve conduction studies can be performed. Conduction studies are performed in patients with suspected peripheral nerve damage, such as carpal tunnel syndrome (where the median nerve is compressed in the carpal tunnel) or diabetic neuropathy.

Cerebrospinal fluid examination

Cerebrospinal (CSF) examination is a procedure commonly used for the diagnosis of infection in the nervous system, multiple sclerosis or other neuroimmunological disorders, as well as to identify bleeding into the subarachnoid space. The CSF is sampled using a lumbar puncture procedure (see Box 4.2). In general, a CT scan or fundoscopy should be performed before a lumbar puncture to rule out raised intracranial pressure. CSF pressure is measured, and fluid is withdrawn for analysis.

The normal volume of CSF is approximately 150 mL, and this is recycled approximately every 8 hours. Maximum lumbar CSF pressure is 180–190 mmH$_2$O. An increase indicates infection, increased CSF production or decreased resorption or the presence of a tumour. The normal concentration of glucose in the CSF is approximately 50–80 mg/dL (2.8–4.4 mmol/L). In conditions such as diabetes mellitus, it is greatly elevated (>200 mg/dL or 11.3 mmol/L). A low glucose concentration may reflect infection or meningeal inflammatory processes (see Table 12.5). The latter may also be suggested by the presence of polymorphonuclear leukocytes in the CSF. Numbers of mononuclear cells are increased in chronic inflammation. Analysis of the protein types present in the CSF can demonstrate the presence of specific antibodies in multiple sclerosis patients. The CSF can also be analysed serologically in the diagnosis of syphilis. The presence of red blood cells or xanthochromia (a yellow discolouration indicating the presence of bilirubin) in the CSF often indicates subarachnoid haemorrhage.

General comments

In order to make a diagnosis when a lesion or dysfunction in the nervous system occurs, clinicians use certain theoretical constructs. This is particularly the case in neurology and is reflected in this overview of how the clinical examination proceeds in a logical and orderly fashion through the complexities of the nervous system. Constructs and models are helpful, even if the constructs themselves are changed by the rapidly advancing pace of knowledge in neuroscience. The following are examples of such simple constructs: (1) the hierarchical organization of the nervous system (with higher functions represented rostrally and lower functions represented caudally), (2) the cerebral localization of function, (3) the topographical representation of body parts and (4) the dominance of one hemisphere. It is important to remember at all times that such constructs are only tools and the real world of neurology and psychiatry far exceeds any simple models of nervous system function. In practice, the neurological examination is rarely performed in its entirety. Importantly, impairment in one part of the examination may affect a patient's ability to perform other parts of the examination; this is especially true if there is cognitive impairment, as this will impair the motor and sensory examination. Thus the practitioner must appropriately modify the testing based on the patient's limitations. With experience, the practitioner learns to perform a screening examination of the most important elements, and then focuses on the most relevant in further detail.

THE SPINAL CORD

4

Chapter summary

1. The spinal cord is located between the cervical C1 and lumbar L1–2 vertebral levels; below this vertebral level only spinal roots are found, and they are known as the cauda equina.

2. The spinal cord is composed of white and grey matter. The white matter contains axons of ascending and descending pathways, to and from the brain, each of which has a specific location and carries specific information. Most of the pathways decussate at some point in the CNS, and it is important to know these decussation sites, as they are associated with particular neurological deficits.

3. The blood supply of the spinal cord is derived from two posterior and one anterior spinal arteries that originate from the vertebral artery circulation in the brainstem.

4. The three main sensory pathways that convey the sensory modalities of discriminative touch, pain, temperature, and balance (unconscious proprioception) are, the dorsal column medial lemniscus and the spinothalamic and spinocerebellar tracts, respectively. Each is associated with particular peripheral receptors and relay through specific brainstem, thalamic, and cerebellar nuclei to terminate in the cerebral or cerebellar cortex.

5. Damage to the spinal cord can cause loss of all functions below the lesion level, either immediately if the cord is completely transected, or within a few hours secondary to oedema, even if the lesion is incomplete. Following traumatic injury, there are two phases: spinal shock with complete areflexia, flaccid paralysis, atonic bowel and bladder function, and loss of vasomotor control, followed 1–2 weeks later (as the shock resolves) by hyperreflexia, hypertonia, limb spasticity, Babinski sign, autonomic hyperactivity (vascular and sweating) and impaired bladder and bowel functions (e.g. urge incontinence, automatic emptying). Certain symptoms are associated with distinct spinal cord syndromes.

Introduction

Spinal cord injury (SCI), whether through disease or trauma, can lead to a devastating loss of function below the level of injury and adversely affects several body systems. Moreover, because of the poor regenerative capacity of the central nervous system (CNS), patients suffer from lifelong disability that may range from partial loss of function to complete quadriplegia and artificial ventilation. In the UK there are more than 40,000 people suffering from traumatic SCI, with approximately 1200 new cases every year. Worldwide, 27 million people have SCI with 250,000 new cases each year. It is estimated that as a function of the severity of injury, each SCI case costs somewhere between £0.5 and 1.9 million in lifetime support and care. At least one-third to one-half of these patients are readmitted to hospital after the initial trauma.

Neurological assessment of patients with spinal cord damage requires an understanding of several concepts: the basic organization of the spinal cord, the relationships between the main nervous pathways that relay sensory and motor information to and from the brain, and the ability to correlate radiological evidence of injury to the vertebral column with different segmental levels of the spinal cord.

The aim of this chapter is to describe the organization of the spinal cord, the positions and functions of the various relay pathways that reside within it, and then to describe how these are affected in SCI.

Gross anatomy of the spinal cord and vertebral column

The spinal cord connects the brain to the peripheral nervous system (PNS). It is located within the vertebral canal, which provides structural protection, and is held in place by spinal roots and denticulate ligaments (Fig. 4.1). The adult spinal cord is approximately 18 inches (46 cm) long and extends from the foramen magnum to the level of the L2 vertebra. This is not so at birth, when it extends much lower (to the L3 vertebral level), but because the vertebral column grows faster than the cord, it leaves the cord positioned progressively higher up in the spinal canal. This means that different spinal cord levels can be related to specific vertebral levels (Table 4.1). The spinal cord tapers off at its caudal end to form the conus medullaris, and beyond this point, the spinal canal is filled only with spinal roots descending caudally to find their intervertebral foramen. In the sacral region these fan out, resembling a horse's tail, and this is termed the cauda equina (see Fig. 4.1).

The spinal cord and spinal roots are covered by the meninges and further protection is provided by the presence of cerebrospinal fluid (CSF), which surrounds the cord in the subarachnoid space. The pia mater is thin and

difficult to identify as a discrete membrane, except as the denticulate ligaments along the sides of the spinal cord. The denticulate ligaments attach the surface of the cord to the dura mater to stabilize the cord within the vertebral canal. The lowest level at which they are observed is the L1 lumbar root level. The filum terminale is an extension of the pia mater that is attached to the coccygeal segments, whose function is to suspend the cord in the CSF (like the denticulate ligaments). The arachnoid and dura mater extend beyond the L2 level to the level of the S2 vertebra. Thus, if a sample of CSF is needed, a lumbar puncture needle can be inserted below the level of the L2 vertebra without fear of damaging the spinal cord (Box 4.2). Spinal dorsal roots attach to the cord, and the posterolateral sulcus and ventral roots exit the cord at the anterolateral sulcus (Fig. 4.3).

The diameter of the spinal cord is not uniform along its length (Fig. 4.3). At the cervical and lumbar levels, the spinal cord locally enlarges to accommodate the increased sensorimotor connections involved with the limbs, via the cervical and lumbar enlargements. The cervical spinal cord is also largest because it carries tract fibres from lower body levels that are ascending to higher levels. The thoracic region is small because the input is only from

Box 4.1   Case history

Humpty Dumpty sat on a wall, and Humpty Dumpty had a great fall. He presents 2 weeks later, complaining of weak legs and unsteadiness of gait. He says that he was unable to walk the day after he fell, but progressively recovered movement later that week. Neurological examination reveals that he has muscle weakness and brisk reflexes in his right leg compared to the left leg, and there is a Babinski sign in the right foot. Abdominal and cremasteric reflexes are absent on the right side, and there is no voluntary movement of the right leg. There is loss of joint position sense in the right leg, as he has inability to sense movement of his toes either up or down, and there is loss of responses to light touch and vibration on the right leg, extending up as far as the belly button. In addition, there is a loss of temperature and pin-prick sensation in the left leg, which extends up the left side to his belly button. He is immediately sent for X-rays and further neurological tests at the local hospital.

This case gives rise to the following questions:

1. What is the location and organization of the sensory tracts in the spinal cord?
2. What is the location and organization of the motor tracts in the spinal cord?
3. What is the clinical significance of a Babinski sign?
4. Why are there dissociated sensory losses in both legs?
5. Where is the lesion?

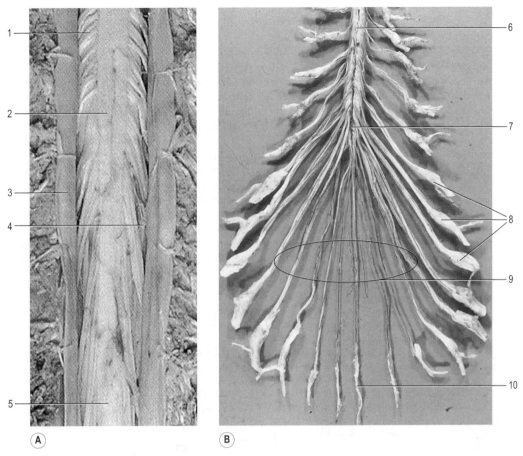

Fig. 4.1 Gross anatomy of the spinal cord. 1. Cervical dorsal roots, 2. posterior columns of cervical enlargement, 3. cut dura mater, 4. denticulate ligament, 5. thoracic cord, 6. spinal cord, 7. conus medullaris, 8. spinal ganglia, 9. cauda equina, 10. filum terminale. (A) Dorsal view of the cervicothoracic region showing spinal dorsal roots and meninges. (B) Caudal end of spinal cord showing the cauda equina, conus medullaris, filum terminale and spinal roots.

Table 4.1 Relationship between vertebral level and adult spinal cord segmental level

Vertebral level	Cord level
Cervical, e.g. C6	Add 1, e.g. C7
Upper thoracic, T1–T6	Add 2 segments
Lower thoracic, T7–T9	Add 3 segments
T10	L1–L2
T11	L3–L4
T12	L5
L1	Conus medullaris
L2–L5	Cauda equina

the ribcage area. Similarly, the size of the vertebral canal changes at different vertebral levels, being larger at the cervical and lumbar levels than at the thoracic levels. As the sacral bones are fused, the canal is reduced to tiny foramina that contain the nerve fibres of the cauda equina.

However, this has consequences, for if there is narrowing of the canal space, as in spinal stenosis or whiplash injuries that cause vertebral damage (fracture dislocation), subsequent compression of the spinal cord, either directly or indirectly due to oedema, may occur.

Functional organization of the spinal cord

The spinal cord receives sensory input from the periphery, relays it to the brain and sends motor response signals back to the periphery. The spinal cord is not segmented; rather, the distribution of the spinal roots gives it a functional segregation. The spinal cord comprises two distinct components: the grey matter and the white matter. The grey matter is reminiscent of the shape of butterfly wings (Fig. 4.3). The white matter surrounds the grey matter, and the amounts of grey and white matter vary at different levels of the spinal cord (Box 4.3).

The spinal cord has two main functions:

1. The grey matter specifies the characteristics of a stimulus in terms of its modality and location.

Lumbar puncture

Lumbar puncture is performed with the patient lying on their side or leaning forward with their lower back flexed so that the ligamentum flavum is stretched and the vertebral laminae and spinous processes are stretched apart. The skin overlying the lower lumbar vertebrae is anaesthetized with local anaesthetic, and the needle (fitted with a stylet) is inserted in the midline between the L3 and L4, or L4 and L5, vertebrae (Fig. 4.2). After penetrating 4–6 cm (more in obese patients), the needle punctures the dura and arachnoid mater to enter the lumbar cistern. This is the subarachnoid, or intrathecal, space. When the stylet is removed, cerebrospinal fluid (CSF) normally drips out at the rate of 1 drop/s. If the subarachnoid pressure is high, CSF may spurt out.

There are several reasons for performing lumbar puncture: retrieval of CSF is an important diagnostic tool for evaluat-

ing a variety of central nervous system diseases, as its cellular composition may change. Lumbar puncture can be used to introduce contrast media into the subarachnoid space to image the outline of the cord, and it can also be used to provide analgesic relief during childbirth by inserting the needle tip into the epidural (extradural) space between the dura mater and vertebral ligaments.

In certain pathological conditions, CSF pressure may be elevated. CSF pressure is normally approximately 180–200 mm H_2O. Lumbar puncture is not performed in patients if examination of the fundus of the interior of the eyeball with an ophthalmoscope reveals raised intracranial pressure. This is because the consequent release of pressure could cause a fatal herniation of the tonsils of the cerebellum through the foramen magnum onto the respiratory centres of the brainstem.

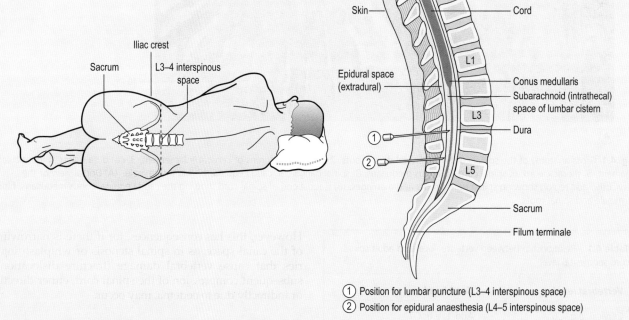

① Position for lumbar puncture (L3–4 interspinous space)
② Position for epidural anaesthesia (L4–5 interspinous space)

Fig. 4.2 Procedure for performing lumbar puncture. (Adapted from Moore KL, Dalley AF. (1999). Clinical Orientated Anatomy, 4th edn. LWW.)

2. The white matter serves as a relay conduit for impulse propagation to and from the brain. Sensorimotor information is relayed via the dorsal, lateral and ventral funiculi of the white matter.

The grey matter of the spinal cord contains cells and terminals of primary afferents from the periphery. It is subdivided into different functional regions: the dorsal (posterior) horn is associated with sensory perception and the ventral (anterior) horn is associated with motor functions such as reflex movements. The latter contains motor neurons whose axons exit the cord via the ventral root, on their

way to the muscles. At thoracic and sacral levels, these two regions are separated by the intermediate zone, which contains the lateral horn (see Fig. 4.3 arrows) that contains the cell bodies of the sympathetic and parasympathetic preganglionic fibres (the autonomic nervous system outflow).

The sensations of touch, pressure, pain, temperature and joint and muscle position sense (proprioception) are mediated by specific peripheral receptors. The primary afferents that carry these sensations terminate on cells in different regions (laminae) of the grey matter. The grey matter is subdivided into 10 laminae (Fig. 4.4A). The dorsal horn has six laminae based on cell size. Laminae

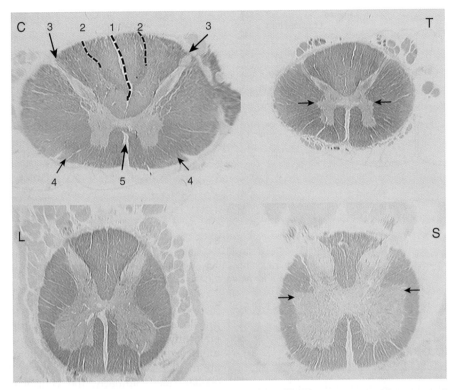

Fig. 4.3 Examples of transverse sections at different levels of the spinal cord showing relative differences in the amount of grey and white matter and the shape of the cord. 1. Posterior median sulcus, 2. posterior intermediate sulcus, 3. posterolateral sulcus (dorsal root attachment), 4. anterolateral sulcus (ventral root exit point), 5. anterior median fissure. Arrows point to the location of the intermediate horn, which houses autonomic preganglionic neurons. C, cervical; L, lumbar; T, thoracic; S, sacral.

I–II together constitute the superficial dorsal horn, which receives information from nociceptors (see Chapter 5). Lamina II—the substantia gelatinosa—is a pale-staining area through which a few myelinated fibres pass; it is also subdivided into two regions. The outer region—IIo—is involved in the processing of nociception from unmyelinated afferents, whilst the inner region—Iii—receives input from unmyelinated low threshold mechanoreceptors and thinly myelinated low threshold or itch responsive afferents. Laminae III–VI receive input from low-threshold cutaneous receptors. The ventral horn consists of laminae VII–IX and contains the cell bodies of motor neurons and interneurons and the terminals of primary afferents from muscle and joints. α-Motor neuron cell bodies are the most prominent cell structures visible in this region. Different muscles have their motor neurons located in discrete cell groups in the ventral horn. The motor neuron populations supplying different muscles are differentially organized within the ventral horn (Fig. 4.4B). Distal muscles are represented laterally, while proximal muscles are located more medially. Extensor muscle groups are located more ventrally within the ventral horn, compared to flexor muscle motor neurons. Visceral afferents, which primarily mediate unconscious sensory input from visceral organs and blood vessels, terminate in laminae I, IIo and V. They encode information in a way which is different from that of cutaneous and skeletal muscle afferents (see Chapter 5).

The grey matter is functionally organized by sensory modality in the dorsoventral plane. Proprioceptive afferents terminate in the ventral horn (to make connections with motor neurons to facilitate reflex activity), low-threshold cutaneous afferents terminate in the deep dorsal horn (laminae III–VI), and nociceptors terminate in the superficial dorsal horn (Fig. 4.4A). Within the grey matter at a given segmental level, there is also a topographical representation of the periphery in the mediolateral plane. Thus, contiguous skin areas occupy contiguous areas of the spinal cord, and each peripheral nerve has its own terminal area within the spinal cord. Therefore the site and nature of a peripheral stimulus is encoded by its rostrocaudal, mediolateral and dorsoventral position within the dorsal horn. This is called somatotopy, and this feature is faithfully replicated at all levels of the nervous system.

Likewise, the white matter is functionally and topographically organized. The dorsal funiculus contains only sensory axons travelling to the brainstem. At sacral, lumbar, and lower thoracic (below T6) regions, the white matter is termed the gracile fasciculus and contains sensory afferents innervating the lower half of the body. From C1–T6, the fasciculus is divided into two parts by the posterior intermediate sulcus (see Fig. 4.3). The white matter lateral to this sulcus is termed the cuneate fasciculus and receives input from the upper half of the body, whereas the white matter medial to it is the continuation of the

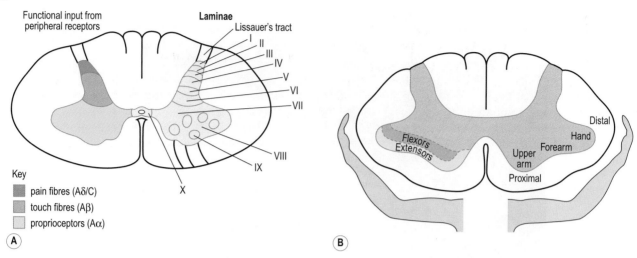

Fig. 4.4 (A) Schematic representation of the functional organization of sensory modalities into different laminae of the spinal cord (indicated by Roman numerals). (B) Schematic topographic organization of motor neurons in the cervical ventral horn.

Identifying segmental features of the spinal cord

From examination of the cross-sections of the spinal cords in Fig. 4.3, it is obvious that different levels of the cord are different in shape. It is important to be able to differentiate cervical from thoracic, lumbar, and sacral. Obvious things to look for:

1. Overall shape. Cervical sections tend to be wide and oval-shaped as compared to, for example, the lumbar section, which appears round.
2. Amount of white matter relative to grey matter. This decreases along the rostrocaudal length of the cord: the white matter of the cervical cord essentially contains all the axons going to or from the entire body. In the sacral cord, the white matter contains only those axons going to or from the last few dermatomes; all other axons have 'exited' at higher levels. This is why the sacral cord looks like it has so much grey matter; in reality, it has only lost most of the white matter fibres.
3. Ventral horn enlargement. At segments that control a limb, the motor neurons are large and numerous. This causes enlarged ventral horns at two levels: the lower cervical sections (C5–C8) and the lumbar/sacral sections. If an enlargement is seen, one needs to differentiate cervical from lumbar levels. This can be done by shape or by proportion of white matter.
4. Presence of pointed tips between the small dorsal and ventral horns. This region is the intermediate horn, or the intermediolateral cell column, and is the source of all of the sympathetic preganglionic neurons in the body. It occurs only in thoracic sections.

gracile fasciculus (see Box 4.6 for further details). The lateral funiculus contains both motor and sensory axons; motor axons of the descending lateral corticospinal tract are medial to the ascending axons of the dorsal spinocerebellar tract. Similarly, the ventrolateral funiculus also contains both ascending sensory (e.g. spinothalamic, spinoreticular) and descending (vestibulospinal and reticulospinal tract) axons (see Figs 4.10 and 9.8 for details).

Spinal cord cell types

Spinal cord cells are classified into two main types according to where their axons project:

- Interneurons represent approximately 97% of cells in the spinal cord. They are involved in modulating sensory input and motor output and make local connections with other cells in the spinal cord.

- Projection neurons represent the remaining cells. These are subdivided into cells that give rise to axons of the ascending pathways, comprising about 1% of the population, and motor neurons, representing the remaining 2% of spinal cord cells, whose axons innervate skeletal muscles.

Spinal cord interneurons are further classified into two main functional groups with respect to their action on other cells or sensory afferents:

1. Inhibitory neurons, which limit the receptive field (RF) size or activity of other neurons. They use inhibitory neurotransmitters such as γ-aminobutyric acid (GABA), glycine and enkephalin to regulate the activity of other neurons.

2. Excitatory neurons. These cells use glutamate and various neuropeptides as neurotransmitters, and their stimulation evokes action potentials in other cells.

The peripheral RF of excitatory neurons in the dorsal horn can be of three general types: those that are high threshold and respond only to noxious stimuli, those that are low threshold and respond only to innocuous stimuli, and wide dynamic range (multi-receptive) neurons, which respond to both noxious and innocuous stimuli.

Receptive fields

An afferent in a peripheral nerve may form several branches when it reaches its peripheral target, and each branch ends in the same type of receptor. The area of skin (or muscle/viscera) where a stimulus can excite the sensory fibre is its RF. Cutaneous RFs measure approximately 2 cm^2 on the arm but only 5 mm^2 on the fingertips. This gives rise to a differential sensory acuity between distal and proximal skin. For example, humans have better sensory acuity (ability to localize a stimulus) on the fingertips than on neck skin. The ability to distinguish between two separate simultaneous touches to the skin is called two-point discrimination.

The central branches of primary afferents converge onto cells in the spinal cord. Thus the RFs of spinal cord cells are larger than those of primary afferents. Consequently, because of convergence, the RFs of higher-order neurons in ascending relay pathways become larger. However, they do not lose the ability to localize stimuli because their RFs have a sensitivity gradient of excitation and inhibition; they are strongly excited in the middle of the RF and weakly excited at the edge due to a phenomenon called surround (lateral) inhibition (this also occurs in the auditory and visual systems). Stimulation of the peripheral area reduces neuronal firing and is brought about by activation of inhibitory interneurons. This process sharpens the spatial resolution to improve the contrast at boundaries between stimuli.

Somatosensory pathways

The somatosensory system includes many types of sensation from the body: touch, pressure, pain, itch, temperature, and joint and muscle position sense (proprioception). These modalities may or may not reach consciousness. They travel in different ascending pathways that are located in specific areas of the spinal cord white matter and terminate in specific areas of the brain. There are several ascending tracts, which travel to varying degrees in the spinal cord. Their names reflect where they originate and terminate in the nervous system (see Table 4.2).

There are three important pathways that run the entire length of the spinal cord, and it is essential to know the location and sensory modalities associated with these

Table 4.2 Main ascending spinal pathways

Pathway	Function
Dorsal column medial lemniscus	Tactile discrimination and conscious proprioception (limb position sense)
Spinothalamic tract	Pain and temperature sensation; crude touch, itch, tickle
Spinocerebellar tract	Unconscious proprioception; assessment and integration of motor performance
Spinoreticular tract	Affective components of pain
Spinotectal tract	Integration of spinal (head/neck) reflexes with visual and auditory stimuli
Spino-olivary tract	Motor learning and modifying motor actions

pathways, as damage to these pathways results in specific functional deficits.

1. The dorsal column medial lemniscus (DCML) pathway conveys information about discriminative touch. The perception of pressure, vibration and texture is mediated by Aα/β fibres and enables us to 'read' Braille letters or numbers (graphesthesia), or describe the shape and texture of an object without seeing it.

2. The pain and temperature system uses free nerve endings in skin, muscle, bone and connective tissue to perceive changes in temperature or tissue damage. This is mediated by Aδ/C fibres. These fibres also mediate the sensations of itch, tickle and crude touch. These modalities are conveyed by the spinothalamic tract (STT) pathway.

3. The third modality is called proprioception and is conveyed by Aα fibres, which include receptors for what happens below the body surface: muscle stretch, joint position and tendon tension. This pathway is the spinocerebellar tract (SCBT) pathway, and it terminates in the cerebellum, which needs continuous feedback regarding what the muscles are doing.

Each of these main pathways is described separately but they share important common features, for example, each pathway consists of four neurons. Another important feature for conscious sensations is that they decussate (cross-over) to the contralateral side. Whenever decussation occurs, it is always the second-order neuron that decussates. Conceptually, one can consider the transmission of sensory information to consciousness as a 400-m relay team. Runner 1—the peripheral receptor—transfers the information to runner 2 in the spinal cord or brainstem. It is this runner who runs round the bend or crosses over to the other side of the track (cord or brainstem) to take the information to runner 3, who usually resides in the thalamus (or cerebellum), depending on the pathway involved. This runner takes the information to its final destination in the cortex, where runner 4 receives the information. This relay is the most commonly used, but some afferent pathways, for example, the spinoreticular tract (SRT), use more neurons, which then activate other areas of the cortex. In other cases, neuron collateral branches contact motor neurons or interneurons, which then participate in reflex responses.

The discriminative touch system

The DCML system transmits mechanoreceptive sensations from the limbs, trunk, and posterior part of the head to the dorsal column nuclei in the medulla. An analogous trigeminal nerve pathway—the trigeminal lemniscus serving the face—transmits sensory information to the main sensory trigeminal nucleus in the pons. Receptors associated with these pathways have small RFs and do not show much convergence. Thus this system provides the capacity to accurately define the quality, place, intensity and pattern of a stimulus. The capabilities of this system are:

- Fine touch—the ability to recognize the exact location of light touch, and the ability to perform two-point discrimination

- Stereognosis—the ability to recognize an object by feeling it

- Conscious proprioception—the awareness of body position, and awareness of body movements (kinaesthesia)

- Weight discrimination

- Vibration detection

The pathway for this system is shown in Fig. 4.5. The primary afferents ascend to the medulla, on the same (ipsilateral) side of the cord as they entered, in the dorsal columns. A key feature of this pathway is that it is somatotopically organized such that afferents from the lower limbs and trunk travel more medially in the gracile funiculus, and afferents from the upper limb travel more laterally, in the cuneate fasciculus, to their respective nuclei in the medulla. Similarly, the trigeminal input from the head is positioned lateral to the input from the body in the medulla. After synapsing in the dorsal column (or the analogous trigeminal) nuclei, axons of the secondary neurons cross in the medulla and ascend as the medial lemniscus to the thalamus, where they synapse in the ventroposterior (VP) nucleus. In the VP nucleus, the head is represented medially and the rest of the body laterally. Finally, information ascends from the thalamus via the posterior limb of the internal capsule to the primary somatosensory cortex (SI) in the postcentral gyrus.

The SI is necessary for the conscious awareness that a stimulus has occurred and of its quality, location, intensity, and duration. The SI is not, however, the final station in the somatic sensory pathway. It sends information to other cortical areas. Further important analysis of somatosensory information occurs in the posterior parietal association cor-

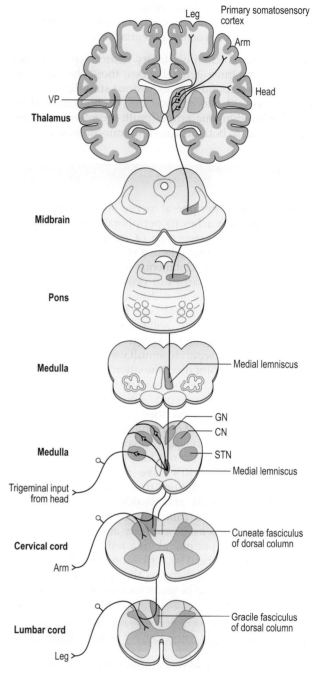

Fig. 4.5 The dorsal column medial lemniscus pathway. *CN*, Cuneate nucleus; *GN*, gracile nucleus; *STN*, spinal trigeminal nucleus; *VP*, ventroposterior nucleus.

tex. It is these areas that give meaning to the received stimulus. The SI is somatotopically organized (Box 4.4).

The SI is subdivided into four functionally different zones: Brodmann's areas 1, 2, 3a and 3b (see Fig. 4.6), named after the famous German anatomist. Areas 3a and 3b receive approximately 70% of the input from the VP thalamus, and the other 30% goes to areas 1 and 2. Each area receives input predominantly from one type of somatosensory receptor. Area 3b mostly receives cutaneous

Box 4.4 Somatotopic maps in the SI

The dorsal column medial lemniscus (DCML) system is very orderly, in that fibres and cells carrying information from one part of the peripheral receptive surface maintain their positions relative to fibres and cells representing neighbouring parts of the receptive surface. Thus different parts of the body are represented in an orderly sequence in the tracts and nuclei of the DCML system. This orderly arrangement of cells and fibres is called topographical organization. For the somatosensory system, it is usually called somatotopic organization (cf. retinotopic maps in the visual system and tonotopic maps in the auditory system). The somatotopic organization of the SI is shown in Fig. 4.6. The extent to which a body part is represented in the SI is related to its sensory acuity, not to its size.

The ability to perform point localization and two-point discrimination is best for the face (around the lips), hands (fingertips) and feet (toes). Somatosensory acuity—the ability to distinguish fine detail by touch—is directly related to the amount of neural tissue devoted to the representation of a body part, i.e. to the peripheral innervation density and to the volume of cortex representing the region. In general, the greater the peripheral innervation density, the smaller the receptive fields of the innervating neurons and the larger the volume of cortex representing that region. Surround (lateral) inhibition also enhances the ability to localize stimuli and perform spatial discriminations by sharpening the profiles of activity within the somatotopically organized neural system.

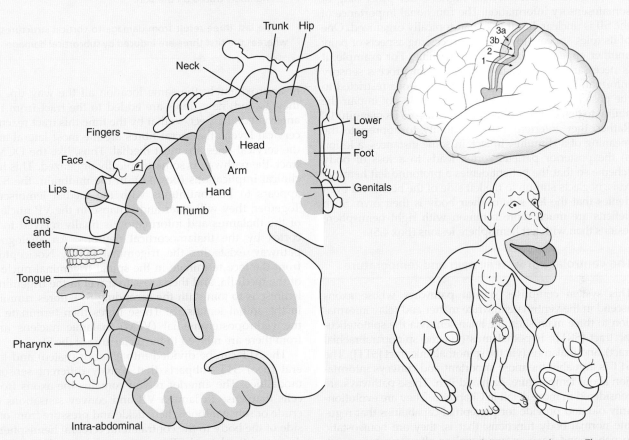

Fig. 4.6 Homuncular organization of the primary somatosensory cortex (SI) in a coronal section at the level of the postcentral gyrus. The body map is not scaled normally but looks like a caricature, with enlarged body parts correlating with areas of highest sensory acuity. The SI is subdivided into four Brodmann areas—1, 2, 3a and 3b—each of which process a different sensory modality (see text for further details). (Adapted from Penfield W, Rasmussen T. (1952) The Cerebral Cortex of Man. New York, Macmillan Press.)

input (from slowly and rapidly adapting receptors), and area 3a receives input from muscle proprioceptors. Area 2 mostly receives input from joints and deep tissues (thought to be important for stereognosis), and area 1 receives information from rapidly adapting cutaneous mechanoreceptors. This leads to multiple representations of the body in the SI and a rostrocaudal gradient of modality sensitivity in the order of muscle, skin and joint sensation. Within functional areas, cortical neurons are arranged in small vertical columns that have overlapping RFs, respond to the same submodality of stimulation, and have similar response latencies to synchronous afferent inputs.

Cells in the SI subregions also have different functions: area 3b is concerned with texture, shape and stimulus size; information about texture is transmitted to area 1; whilst information on size and shape is sent to area 2. Therefore discrete lesions in these areas produce predictable deficits. For example, lesions in area 3b cause deficits in texture and shape discrimination, area 1 lesions prevent texture discrimination, and area 2 lesions impair the ability to grasp objects and discriminate size and shape. This has been shown in experiments on monkeys, but in humans such lesions are rare and, in general, combination deficits occur.

These cortical areas have reciprocal connections with each other. Area 3a projects to areas 3b, 2 and the primary motor and premotor cortices, while area 3b projects to areas 1 and 2. All four areas send projections to an area called the secondary somatosensory cortex (SII) that is located in the parietal cortex immediately posterior to the SI. This area is necessary for higher-order processing of somatosensory information. The functional importance of the SII is unclear, but it is somatotopically organized. One of its roles appears to be in the processing aspects of pain; another appears to be in tactile learning. For example, it is necessary for stereognosis. SII cannot process sensory information independently of the SI. Lesions restricted to the posterior parietal association cortex do not impair the ability to detect a stimulus or even to assess its magnitude. Rather, they interfere with the ability to appreciate the meaning of a stimulus. In fact, in some instances, a lesion to the posterior parietal cortex leads to a loss of body scheme so that the patient denies a profound left hemiparesis, neglects stimuli to the left side of the body, and even denies that the left side of their body is their own. Such deficits are much more common with right hemisphere lesions than with left hemisphere lesions (Box 4.5).

The ventrolateral system: pain and temperature

This system comprises several pathways whose axons ascend in the ventrolateral white matter and relay information to three main sites: the brainstem (via the spinoreticular tract [SRT]), hypothalamus (via the spinoparabrachial tract), and thalamus (via the spinothalamic tract [STT]). The STT is arguably the most important and conveys information about temperature, pain and itch. These pathways are considered in more detail in Chapter 5. They are evolutionarily old and provide for perceptual capabilities that regulate normal body functions; that is, they are homeostatic in nature and have an emotional or affective component. The STT shares one major principle of organization with the discriminative touch system: primary afferents synapse ipsilaterally, and then the second-order neurons cross. The crossings occur at different levels; the STT crosses in the spinal cord (usually within one or two segments of entry), whereas the DCML crosses in the brainstem.

Nociceptive afferents enter the spinal cord and ascend one to two segments rostral or caudal in Lissauer's tract (Fig. 4.4A) before entering the grey matter to connect with cells of the STT. The STT ascends the entire length of the cord and brainstem, as shown in Fig. 4.7, staying

Box 4.5 Clinical features of dorsal column medial lemniscus system lesions

The following sensory deficits occur after lesions of the DCML system:

1. Decrease in two-point discrimination (increased threshold)
2. Decrease in vibratory sensibility
3. Decrease in position sense and kinaesthesia (patients have a positive Romberg sign, indicating sensory ataxia)
4. Astereognosis – inability to recognize objects by touch
5. Contralateral neglect – failure to perceive the stimulus on one side during double simultaneous stimulation
6. Agraphaesthesia – inability to recognize letters or numbers traced on the skin.

The last three result from damage to cortical structures, whereas the first three are induced by subcortical damage.

in approximately the same location all the way up. As they ascend, new fibres are added to the tract from the anteromedial aspect, so that by the time this tract reaches cervical levels, the sacral fibres are the most lateral and the cervical ones are most medial. Thus, like the DCML tract, the pathway is somatotopically organized. This has clinical implications (Box 4.6). In the midbrain, the STT appears to be continuous with the medial lemniscus. Together, they will enter and synapse in the VP nucleus of the thalamus and information is finally relayed to SI cortex by the thalamocortical neurons. An analogous pathway exists for the trigeminal nerve. Nociceptors from the face terminate in the spinal trigeminal nucleus of the medulla, and then cross to travel in the trigeminal lemniscus to join with the ascending STT fibres running in the spinal lemniscus. These fibres then terminate in the ventroposteromedial (VPM) thalamic nucleus and from there are relayed to the facial area of the SI.

The STT can be divided into anterior (paleo) and lateral (neo) STT subparts that convey different sensory modalities. The anterior region contains the axons from cells that arise in lamina VII and convey sensations of crude or sensual touch, itch, tickle and pressure from one side of the body to the contralateral cerebral hemisphere. Axons of the lateral STT are more concerned with 'fast pain' from one side of the body to the opposite cerebral hemisphere. This pathway encodes information about stimulus location, intensity and modality.

Other ventrolateral pathways

Spinoreticular tract

This is the oldest ascending pathway in evolutionary terms and mediates 'slow' pain. The cells originate in laminae V–VII and accompany the STT tract as far as

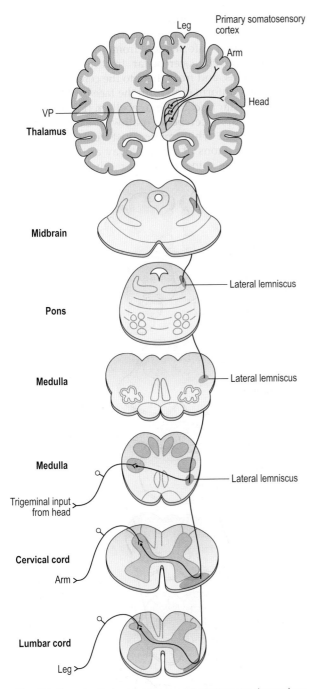

Fig. 4.7 The spinothalamic pathway. *VP*, Ventroposterior nucleus.

Box
4.6
Clinical relevance of topographical organization of neural pathways

All the main ascending and descending pathways are topographically organized with respect to the various segmental levels. For the DCML pathway, the sacral and lumbar segments are located medial to the thoracic segments, which are located medial to the cervical segmental input. In contrast, in the spinothalamic tract and corticospinal tract pathways cervical axons are most medial and sacral most lateral (Fig. 4.8). This is of clinical relevance when an injury or disease affects specific relay pathways. For example, if there is external pressure on the spinal cord, it can explain why there is first a loss of pain and temperature sensation in sacral dermatomes and, if the pressure increases, the loss progresses to lumbar and thoracic levels as higher dermatomes are affected. Similarly, if the problem occurs within the spinal cord, such as in syringomyelia or whiplash injury, the cervical dermatomes will be affected first and the lower body is less affected. Often, these patients show sacral sparing, with preservation of all sensations, reflexes and muscle tone in this region.

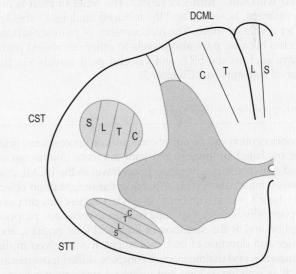

Fig. 4.8 Topographic organizations of the dorsal column medial lemniscus (DCML), spinothalamic (STT) and corticospinal (CST) tracts in a hemi-cross-section of the spinal cord. *C*, cervical; *T*, thoracic; *L*, lumbar; *S*, sacral.

the brainstem reticular formation to bilaterally activate the ascending reticular activating system and autonomic nuclei involved in pain responses (e.g. elevated blood pressure, increased heart and respiratory rates). Stimuli in this pathway are of a general and non-specific nature and act to participate in reflex activity or to relay information to the intralaminar thalamic nuclei, and from there to the prefrontal, anterior cingulate and limbic cortices (regions associated with cognitive and emotional aspects of pain). Ascending fibres of this tract are both crossed and uncrossed at segmental levels. Axons conveying visceral pain are also located in the midline of the dorsal columns (see Chapter 5).

Spinotectal tract

This pathway runs medially alongside the STT, from the cervical spinal cord to the superior colliculus in the midbrain. It is a crossed pathway that integrates visual input to mediate visuo-spinal reflexes in response to tactile stimuli by turning the eyes/head or body towards a tactile stimulus.

Spino-olivary tract

This crossed pathway runs laterally to the STT and ascends from the spinal cord to the inferior olivary nucleus (ION) in the medulla. The ION is associated with motor learning and relays information from proprioceptors to the contralateral cerebellum (see Chapter 9). It is thought that this tract may play a role in modifying movements when a moving body part encounters an unexpected obstacle.

Damage to the spinal ventrolateral pathways through injury or surgical intervention results in decreased pain and temperature sensitivity on the contralateral side below the level of the lesion. There is also reduced touch sensation. This is not the case if the lesion is in the brainstem because the fast pain fibres that ascend in the STT run laterally, whereas the slow pain fibres running in the SRT ascend more medially. Thus damage to the STT in the brainstem results in decreased sensitivity and localization of pain and temperature sensation but not the loss of the emotional quality of the sensation.

A surgical procedure called percutaneous chordotomy uses radiofrequency lesioning of the ventrolateral tracts at cervical levels to alleviate the intractable pain associated with some forms of cancer. The relief of pain is not permanent, however, and the induced analgesia subsides after a year or more. The reoccurrence of pain sensations occurs because pain also travels in other uncrossed pathways such as the SRT, and visceral pain travels via the dorsal columns (see Chapter 5).

The proprioceptive system

Proprioception can be either conscious or unconscious; both are mediated by muscle and joint afferents. Axons associated with conscious proprioception travel in the DCML and convey information such as judging the weight of an object or where a person's limbs are in space. Unconscious proprioception serves as an important backup to conscious proprioception and is the sensation of limb and joint position and range and direction of limb movement. It is involved in the acquisition and maintenance of complex, skilled movements, such as walking, talking and writing. Unconscious proprioception is mediated by the SCBT, whose primary function is to monitor and modify movements.

The proprioceptive system axons from muscle and joint receptors travel in the dorsal columns. Within a few segments, however, axon collaterals responsible for the proprioceptive information concerned with postural adjustments that occur unconsciously leave the white matter and synapse in Clarke's nucleus (nucleus dorsalis), which is located at the base of the medial dorsal horn from T1 to L1 of the spinal cord. The second-order neuron axons then enter the dorsal SCBT on the lateral edge of the cord and are somatotopically organized. This pathway ascends to the medulla without crossing to enter the cerebellum via the inferior cerebellar peduncle (ICP) to terminate on Purkinje cells. Purkinje cells relay the information to the deep cerebellar nuclei, and from there it is passed to other motor areas of the thalamus, brainstem,

and basal ganglia. Because Clarke's column only extends from T1 to L1, it only carries information from the lower body and trunk. Information from the upper body is relayed by the cuneocerebellar tract to the accessory cuneate nucleus, and from there to the cerebellum via the ICP. Similarly, information from the face travels in the trigeminocerebellar tract to the cerebellum (Fig. 4.9).

A second spinocerebellar pathway exists and travels in the lateral white matter, just ventral to the dorsal SCBT. The axons of this pathway arise from cells in lamina VII of the spinal cord that receive a diverse input

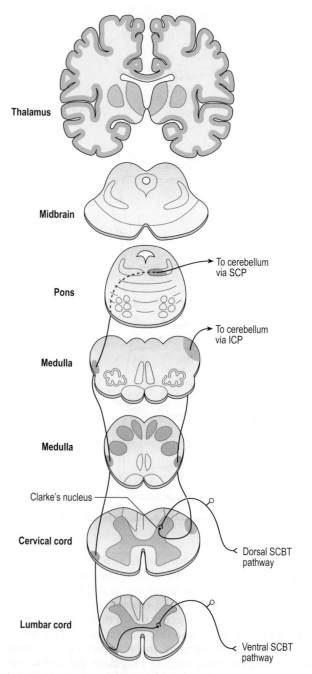

Fig. 4.9 The spinocerebellar tract pathway. *ICP,* Inferior cerebellar peduncle; *SCBT,* spinocerebellar tract; *SCP,* superior cerebellar peduncle.

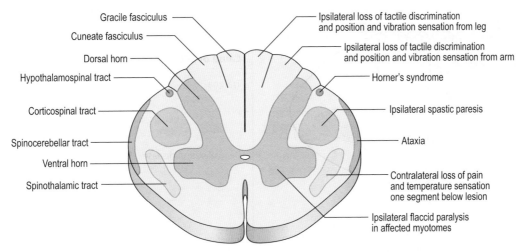

Gracile fasciculus

Cuneate fasciculus

Dorsal horn

Hypothalamospinal tract

Corticospinal tract

Spinocerebellar tract

Ventral horn

Spinothalamic tract

Ipsilateral loss of tactile discrimination and position and vibration sensation from leg

Ipsilateral loss of tactile discrimination and position and vibration sensation from arm

Horner's syndrome

Ipsilateral spastic paresis

Ataxia

Contralateral loss of pain and temperature sensation one segment below lesion

Ipsilateral flaccid paralysis in affected myotomes

Fig. 4.10 Clinical deficits associated with damage to the main ascending and descending pathways at the cervical spinal cord level. (Adapted from Fix JD. (1995). High Yield Neuroanatomy. Williams and Wilkins, Philadelphia.)

from proprioceptors, nociceptors and descending pathway tracts such as the vestibulospinal and reticulospinal tracts. The ventral SCBT seems to defy the ipsilaterality of the cerebellum because the fibres cross over in the cord. However, they cross back before entering the cerebellum via the superior cerebellar peduncle. Therefore, the cerebellum still receives information from the ipsilateral side of the body. Ventral SCBT cells have large RFs and appear to act as comparators of descending inputs and other inputs to motor neurons.

Summary of somatosensory pathways

Three main ascending somatosensory pathways each carry a specific modality of sensation associated with specific receptors. Each pathway is somatotopically organized so that a complete representation of the body is reproduced in each relay nucleus along the pathway. Any sensory system going to the cerebral cortex decussates at some point because the cerebral cortex operates on a contralateral basis. The discriminative touch system crosses in the medulla, and the pain system crosses in the spinal cord. The proprioceptive system ascends to the cerebellum and does not cross. There is some overlap of modalities between the ascending tracts: some light touch information travels in the STT so that lesioning the dorsal column does not completely abolish touch and pressure sensation; similarly, visceral pain fibres travel in the dorsal columns and not the STT. Discriminative proprioception also travels in the dorsal columns and follows the medial lemniscus all the way to the cortex, so there is conscious awareness of body position and movement. The pain and temperature system, although it does ascend to the somatosensory cortex, also has multiple targets in the brainstem and other areas. Knowledge of the pathways, point of decussation and cortical areas associated with conscious perception of sensation provides a framework for understanding sensory deficits after damage, as summarized in Fig. 4.10.

Table 4.3 Main descending spinal pathways

Pathway	Function
Corticospinal	Control of fine voluntary movement
Rubrospinal	Regulates muscle tone in anti-gravity (extensor) muscles
Vestibulospinal	Regulates neck muscles involved in head balance reflexes
Raphe spinal	Pain modulation
Coeruleospinal	Autonomic nervous system reflex modulation
Reticulospinal	Postural control via regulation of flexor and extensor reflexes
Tectospinal	Head and neck postural reflex responses to auditory and visual cues
Hypothalamospinal	Sympathetic nervous system control of visceral activity

As well as conveying sensory information to supraspinal levels, the spinal cord white matter contains many descending pathways (Table 4.3). The main descending pathway is the corticospinal tract (CST), which regulates the control of voluntary movement. Damage to this pathway produces hyperreflexia, hypertonia and a positive Babinski sign (extensor plantar response). These descending pathways and their dysfunction are more fully covered in Chapter 9.

The hypothalamospinal tract is clinically important, as damage to this pathway results in Horner's syndrome, which is characterized by miosis, ptosis and anhydrosis. Signs are always ipsilateral. The pathway runs directly from the hypothalamus to the ciliospinal centre, located in the intermediolateral cell column of the T1–T2 spinal cord. It descends through the lateral tegmentum of the brainstem to run in the dorsolateral quadrant of the dorsolateral funiculus.

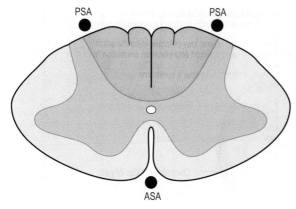

Fig. 4.11 Distribution of the main arterial supply to the spinal cord. The yellow area demarcates the distribution of the PSA; the remainder demarcates the ASA territory. *ASA,* Anterior spinal artery; *PSA,* posterior spinal artery.

Blood supply to the spinal cord

Two posterior spinal arteries and a single larger anterior spinal artery, which originate from the vertebral artery, supply the spinal cord. Each posterior artery supplies the ipsilateral posterior third of the cord, while the anterior spinal artery supplies the anterior two-thirds of the cord (Fig. 4.11). However, this is not enough to maintain an adequate blood supply to the spinal cord. At each spinal segment, these arteries are reinforced by segmental radiculospinal arteries, which are branches of the body wall arteries. In addition, the anterior spinal arteries give rise to smaller penetrating arteries, which anastomose with similar arteries from the posterior spinal arteries within the spinal cord tissue. Radicular arteries supply the dorsal and ventral roots. These do not connect to the anterior or posterior spinal arteries and only supply the roots. The venous drainage has a similar distribution to the arterial supply. Three anterior and posterior spinal veins drain along the nerve roots into the internal (epidural) and external vertebral venous plexus along the vertebral column, and from this plexus to ascending lumbar veins: the azygos vein and hemi-azygos veins.

Damage to the spinal cord

SCI commonly arises from trauma, degenerative diseases, ischemia or occlusion of spinal cord arteries, metastatic cancer, and infectious, toxic or metabolic disorders and should be treated as a medical emergency to limit any irreversible damage (Table 4.4). SCI can either be complete, meaning that there is no voluntary movement or sensation below the level of the lesion bilaterally, or incomplete, when there is a variable amount of function below the level of the lesion. The level of the lesion is helpful in predicting the deficits in body function that might occur and how much independence the patient might have after the injury (Table 4.5). The location of the lesion must be at, or

Table 4.4 Some common causes of spinal cord injury

Cause of SCI	Example
Trauma	Acts of violence
	Penetrating wounds
	Compression injury (e.g. prolapsed disc)
	Whiplash
	Sporting accidents (e.g. diving)
Demyelinating disease	Multiple sclerosis
	Spinal muscular atrophy
	Syringomyelia/Arnold-Chiari malformation
	Poliomyelitis
	Inflammatory (transverse) myelitis
	Spina bifida
Infection	AIDS
	Spinal meningitis
	Tuberculosis
	Syphilis
	Lyme's disease
	Abscess
Metabolic disorder	Subacute combined degeneration (vitamin B_{12} deficiency)
Vascular	Anterior spinal artery occlusion
	Spinal dural arteriovenous malformation
Tumour	Primary or secondary cancer

above, the level of the highest neurological sign. (For a better understanding of the impact of SCI, see the discussion on the descending pathways in Chapter 9). SCI is most often classified using the American Spinal Injury Association (ASIA) impairment scale based on neurological assessment of 28 dermatomes and 10 key muscles groups, 72 hours after injury. SCI is graded from category A to E (Table 4.6).

Cervical spondylotic myelopathy is the most common cause of spinal cord compression in people aged over 55 years, causing progressive loss of neurological function and may lead to tetraplegia if left untreated. Traumatic injuries are also common and can be caused directly by penetrating injuries such as gunshot or stab wounds, or indirectly as a result of compression or flexion/extension injuries of structures associated with the vertebral column. This can lead to sensory, motor or sphincter dysfunction or a combination of these, depending on whether the lesion is uni- or bilateral. One of the earliest signs of SCI is pain. Motor dysfunction also occurs early, resulting in hypotonia, muscle wasting and paralysis. Depending on the level of the lesion, there may be deficits in cardiovascular, respiratory and autonomic (bladder, sweating and sexual) function, as well as a loss of protective functions such as pain and temperature sensation (see Table 4.5). These lead to a number of secondary problems such as urinary infections and pressure sores, and a loss of unconscious control mechanisms such as regulation of CNS neuronal excitability.

Table 4.5 Effects of spinal cord injury at different segmental levels in humans

Segment	Consequence	Patient independence
C1–C2	Quadriplegia	None
	Requires ventilated respiration	Often die at scene of injury
	Acute sympathetic shock syndrome (bradycardia, hypotension, bilateral Horner's syndrome, and loss of thermoregulation)	
	Reflex bladder (damage to upper motor neuron control of micturition)	
C4–C5	Quadriplegia	None
	Impaired respiration	Requires constant care
	Reflex bladder (urinary retention and constipation)	
C6–C7	Quadriplegia with impaired arm control	Minimal
C8–T1	Impaired respiration	Requires personal care
	Reflex bladder	Can drive a car with special braces
	Paraplegia	
T2–T3	Impaired respiration	Complete
	Poor trunk control	
	Reflex bladder	
	Paraplegia	
T12–L1	Paraplegia	Complete
	Reflex bladder	
L4–L5	Paraplegia	Complete
	Reflex bladder	
S2–S3	Non-reflex bladder (damage to lower motor neurons leading to failure to void)	Complete

Imaging the spinal cord

In order to assess the possible causes of spinal cord damage, various imaging techniques are used. X-rays can detect vertebral damage due to trauma or cancer, and the radiographs are commonly viewed in the anteroposterior (longitudinal) and lateral directions. X-rays do not visualize the spinal cord but infer damage by changes in the alignment of the vertebral column or reduction in the size of the vertebral canal. Computed tomography (CT) can be used to visualize infarcts and tumours in neural tissue. Magnetic resonance imaging (MRI) can differentiate between grey matter and white matter, so this method is

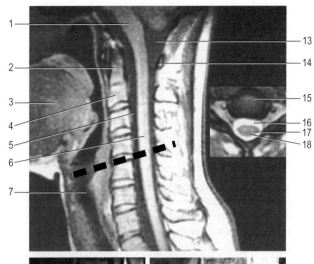

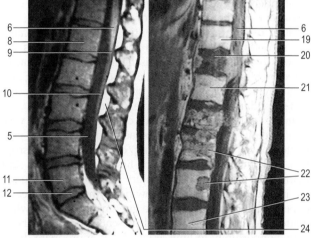

1. Medulla.
2. Dens of axis.
3. Tongue.
4. C2 vertebra.
5. Subarachnoid space.
6. Spinal cord.
7. Trachea.
8. L1 vertebra.
9. Conus medullaris.
10. Filum terminale.
11. L5 vertebra.
12. Intervertebral disc.
13. Foramen magnum.
14. Atlas.
15. Vertebral body.
16. Cerebrospinal fluid.
17. Grey matter.
18. White matter.
19. T11 vertebra.
20. Herniated cancerous disc.
21. T12 vertebra.
22. Degenerating vertebrae.
23. L4 vertebra.
24. Epidural fat.

Fig. 4.12 Magnetic resonance image of the spinal cord in the sagittal plane. Top: Cervical cord. Inset shows the cord imaged in the transverse plane at the level of the dashed lines. Here (in this T2-weighted image), the grey matter appears paler than the white matter and the cerebrospinal fluid is white. In the remaining images the cerebrospinal fluid appears black. Bottom left: A normal magnetic resonance image of the thoracolumbar vertebral region showing the end of the spinal cord. Bottom right: Magnetic resonance image showing metastatic intervertebral disc herniation into the spinal canal and compressing the spinal cord.

particularly sensitive for distinguishing CNS tissue. It is particularly sensitive for imaging areas of focal demyelination and spinal cord lesions. It can provide axial as well as longitudinal images of the entire spinal cord and is now the method of choice for study of the spinal cord, nerve roots, and disc spaces or signs of narrowing (stenosis) or damage (e.g. disc herniation, Fig. 4.12).

Pathophysiology of spinal cord injury

Spinal cord damage induced by a traumatic injury occurs in two phases:

1. Primary damage resulting from cord compression, contusion, laceration or haemorrhage, which occurs immediately on injury.

2. Secondary damage that is initiated by the trauma but occurs over a period of hours, days and months. This mainly involves physiological alterations due to trauma, hypoxia, ischemia and inflammation.

The cord is often swollen and congested after only mild focal indentation or severe haemorrhagic disruption, usually above and below the level of the lesion (Fig. 4.13). The swollen cord can occupy the entire vertebral canal, causing secondary ischemia when the swelling exceeds the venous blood pressure. This ischemia is further exacerbated by loss of autoregulation of blood flow, causing systemic hypotension, leading to spinal shock (see Box 4.7) and secondary damage through excitotoxicity.

In the acute phase of traumatic cord injury there are variable amounts of oedema, micro-haemorrhaging in the grey matter, axonal swelling, ascending/descending tract disruption, and foci of infarction. In the first 24 hours, axons start dying back from the point of injury and the area of the initial injury increases in size, growing further as the area of hypoperfusion spreads from the grey matter into the white matter. Clearly, this early period presents a period of therapeutic opportunity to limit lesion size if appropriate drugs can be used. Damaged cells, axons and blood vessels release

chemicals that cause reactive gliosis and damage neighbouring tissue. For example, the injury area is flooded with the neurotransmitter glutamate, which then overstimulates adjacent neurons and glial cells, leading to a massive Na^+ and Ca^{2+} influx into cells (neurons and glia) that cause them to swell and burst and release their cellular contents and free radicals into the extracellular space. This excitotoxic cascade also affects the oligodendrocyte cells that myelinate the CNS tracts. Vascular reperfusion of the damaged tissue also evokes excitotoxicity via the production of oxidative stress, excessive glutamate and ATP release. This leads to further demyelination of surviving fibres and more dysfunction.

Over the following days and weeks, there is macrophage infiltration and a gradual removal of degenerative debris (e.g. axons, myelin). At the site of injury, the grey matter becomes necrotic and may cavitate. As time progresses, there is hypertrophy of astrocytes and infiltration by fibroblasts forming scar tissue to spatially contain and isolate damaged tissue. However, reactive tissue repair mechanisms fail to occur, and the scar becomes a barrier to regeneration. Frequently, cavitation involves the ventral part of the dorsal columns, which is maximal at the site of injury but may extend a few segments rostral or caudal to the injury. Finally,

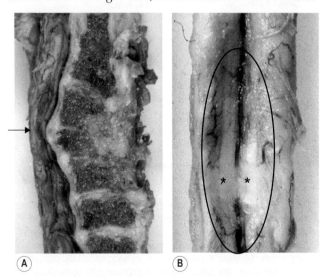

Fig. 4.13 Macroscopic anatomy of spinal cord injury. (A) Sagittal section of the spinal cord and vertebral column, showing focal indentation of the ventral spinal cord at the C4 level. (B) Gross anatomy of the cord following its removal from the vertebral column, showing compression of the ventral horn (oval).

> ### Box 4.7 Spinal cord shock and neurogenic shock
>
> Clinically, there is pain at the level of the injury and a variable amount of sensorimotor loss below the level of the lesion. Severe spinal cord injuries often initially produce spinal shock: a state of temporary loss of all of the functions, and muscle reflexes below the level of the lesion are depressed or absent, due to the removal of all descending motor pathways, giving the impression of flaccid paralysis of muscles and loss of sensation. If the lesion occurs above the T6 spinal level, the sympathetic nervous system is affected, and severe hypotension and thermodysregulation may occur as a result of loss of sympathetic vasomotor tone. This is neurogenic shock (autonomic dysreflexia) and is characterized by hemodynamic changes; spinal shock is not circulatory in nature, but symptoms can include neurogenic shock when the injury is at high thoracic or cervical levels. Spinal shock often lasts approximately 1 day but may persist for up to a month, after which the spinal cord neurons gradually regain their excitability and the flaccid paralysis gives way to spastic paresis. The first reflexes to reappear are the flexion reflexes. Even after these reappear, limbs are flaccid in the absence of tonic stretch reflex activation. After several months, a return of muscle tone and tendon reflexes may occur.
>
> The presence of spinal shock can be determined by testing the integrity of the anal sphincter reflex (checking for anal sphincter contraction after pulling of the glans penis or clitoris or by pulling on an inserted Foley catheter). However, a sacral cord lesion would nullify this test, as the S2–S4 nerve supply may be damaged.

days or weeks after the initial event, some cells undergo apoptosis, whilst Wallerian degeneration of damaged axons causes further gliosis and neuroinflammation that can result in another wave of death that may affect up to four spinal segments rostral or caudal to the injury site.

In almost all lesions, even in apparently complete SCI, not all ascending or descending axons are severed and a peripheral ring at the outer edge of the white matter remains intact (Fig. 4.14). For example, if as few as 10% of the descending CST fibres survive, the patient may be able to walk, whereas if less than 4% remain, they are unable to do so. However, surviving fibres often do not look normal; they are stripped of their insulation and so may not properly conduct nerve impulses.

The prognosis for SCI depends on whether the lesion is extrinsic, that is, outside the substance of the spinal cord (e.g. tumour, in which case, it can often be removed surgically, resulting in recovery of function) or intrinsic within the spinal cord. Research has shown that the most important predictor of improved spinal cord outcome is the retention of sacral sensation (S4–S5 dermatomes), especially pin-prick sensation, 3–7 days after injury. In general, most SCI patients may regain one level of motor function and most of the recovery, if it occurs at all, is seen within the first 6 months after injury. Ten to fifteen percent of ASIA grade A patients may progress to grade B–D, but very few regain functional strength below the level of the lesion, whereas half of grade B patients will regain functional strength below the lesion, and nearly 90% of grade C and D patients recover sufficient strength to walk again.

Spinal cord syndromes

Spinal cord compression is most often caused by extradural problems, such as spondylitis, disc herniation or primary or secondary vertebral tumours or abscesses (see Fig. 4.12). Tumours that arise outside the spinal cord, such as meningiomas or nerve fibromas, may compress the cord; those originating in the cord are rarer and include tumours such as gliomas (glial cell carcinomas). Pressure arising from any of these causes may interfere with the arterial or venous blood supply, causing ischemia or oedema and conduction blockage in fibres in the white matter, which, if prolonged, may cause focal demyelination. Compression may also cause blockage of CSF flow and changes in the composition of CSF below the level of the lesion. One of the earliest signs of compression injury is pain, which may be restricted to one or more spinal nerves and is made worse by exercise, coughing or sneezing, or lying down. Motor dysfunction occurs early, resulting in paralysis, spasticity and exaggerated reflexes below the level of the lesion. The degree of sensory loss will depend on the nerve tracts involved. Surgery to remove the extradural and extramedullary causes is usually successful at reversing the symptoms, provided that irreversible damage due to compromised blood flow has not occurred.

Fig. 4.15 details six distinct spinal cord syndromes caused by destructive lesions; the functional losses associated with these syndromes are predictable from knowledge of the anatomy of the spinal cord. The clinical symptoms associated with these syndromes are detailed below. In the first three, the characteristic symptoms appear after the initial period of spinal shock (see Box 4.7) has ended.

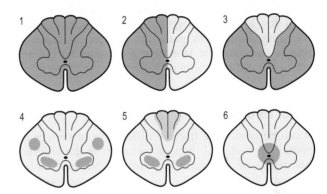

Fig. 4.15 Schematic representations of areas of damage in distinct spinal cord syndromes. *1*, Complete cord transection; *2*, spinal cord hemi-section; *3*, anterior cord syndrome; *4*, amyotrophic lateral sclerosis; *5*, infectious diseases; *6*, syringomelia.

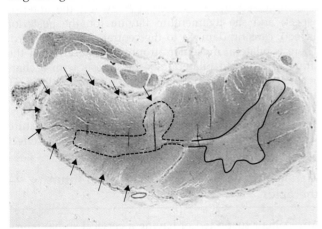

Fig. 4.14 Transverse section showing spinal cord compression. Note the distortion of the grey matter on the side of compression and demyelination at the lateral edge of the white matter of the cord on the injured side (arrows).

Table 4.6	ASIA impairment scale
Grade	**Description**
A	Complete SCI; no preservation of sensory or motor function in S4–S5 cord
B	Incomplete; sensory but not motor function below the neurological level and extending through to S4–S5 cord
C	Incomplete; motor function preserved below the lesion site; most key muscles have strength of <3 (Medical Research Council [MRC] grade score)
D	Incomplete; motor function preserved below the lesion site; most key muscles have strength of >3
E	Normal sensory and motor function

Complete cord transection

Here, there is complete loss of all sensory, voluntary movement and autonomic functions below the level of the lesion. Thus there is bilateral lower motor neuron paralysis and atrophy at the damaged level, bilateral spastic paresis and Babinski signs below the lesion, loss of bladder and bowel function, and bilateral loss of all sensation below the level of the lesion. If the injury is a vertebral fracture dislocation at L2–L3 or below, then no cord injury occurs; damage is confined to the cauda equina, and there are no upper motor neuron signs of damage, the only damage being to sensory, motor and autonomic nerve fibres.

Spinal cord hemisection (Brown–Séquard syndrome)

This can be caused by penetrating trauma injuries, for example, a stab or gunshot wound, or by vertebral damage. A pure hemisection results in ipsilateral loss of all sensations and voluntary muscle movement at the level of the lesion, ipsilateral spastic paresis below the level of the lesion, ipsilateral loss of discriminative (light) touch, vibration sensation and proprioception, and a contralateral loss of pain and temperature sensation below the level of the lesion. Damage to the hypothalamospinal (descending sympathetic pathway) tract at T1 or above produces an ipsilateral Horner's syndrome. Such pure lesions are rare and incomplete hemisections are more common.

Anterior cord syndrome

This can be caused by fracture dislocation of vertebrae, herniation of vertebral discs or occlusion of the anterior spinal artery by a tumour. It results in bilateral motor paralysis at the level of the lesion and bilateral spastic paresis below the level of the lesion. There is a dissociated sensory loss with bilateral loss of temperature and pain below the level of the lesion but no loss of light touch or vibration sensation (supplied by the posterior spinal arteries). Damage to the hypothalamospinal (descending sympathetic pathway) tract at T1 or above produces a bilateral Horner's syndrome, and damage to the parasympathetic centres at S2–S4 results in loss of voluntary control of bladder and bowel function.

Amyotrophic lateral sclerosis

This is a chronic progressive disease of which approximately 90% of cases are sporadic (unknown aetiology), whilst 10% have a genetic component (see Chapter 9, Box 9.7). Onset occurs in late middle age and is often fatal within 2–6 years of onset, although a small minority of people, such as Stephen Hawking, can survive well over 10 years from onset. It causes the death of both upper and lower motor neurons, resulting in symptoms such as muscle atrophy, weakness and fasciculation, spasticity and Babinski signs. There are no sensory deficits.

Infective diseases: poliomyelitis and syphilis

Polio is an acute viral infection that destroys the lower motor neurons of the spinal cord and brainstem, leading to progressive paralysis and muscle wasting. The lower limbs are more often affected than the upper limbs, and in severe cases, respiratory function may be threatened. The advent of immunization during the 1950s greatly reduced the incidence of this disease; however, post-polio syndrome can occur in those patients who have had the disease (see Chapter 9, Box 9.8). It is characterized by progressive weakness, fatigue and atrophy of previously affected muscles. In tabes dorsalis (neurosyphilis), the large-diameter myelinated fibres are affected. It results in chronic inflammation of the dorsal roots and spinal ganglia, causing pain and paraesthesia of affected dermatomes. The cells die, resulting in degeneration of the axons within the dorsal columns. The peak incidence of the disease occurs 15–20 years after the initial infection. It is a purely sensory disease and results in bilateral loss of discriminative sensation. If the gracile fasciculus is affected, a positive Romberg sign, indicating sensory ataxia, occurs.

Syringomyelia

This is a developmental abnormality that results in cavitation within the spinal cord around the central canal and is common in the cervical spinal cord. Thus it interrupts the STT bilaterally, resulting in loss of pain and temperature sensation below the level of the lesion, particularly in the hands. As the cavity enlarges, there is progressive bilateral flaccid paralysis as the lower motor neurons become affected. Horner's syndrome may become apparent if the descending sympathetic fibres that run in the lateral white matter are affected. Tactile discrimination, vibration and conscious proprioception remain intact.

A similar pattern of damage is seen in the central cord syndrome, which can be caused by whiplash injury (hyperextension of the cervical cord region). The cord is compressed by the vertebral body (on the anterior aspect) and the ligamentum flavum (on the posterior aspect), causing damage to the central part of the cord. There is bilateral muscular atrophy and paralysis at the site of injury and bilateral spastic paresis with a characteristic sacral sparing, as the sacral fibres of the CST are located furthest laterally and are thus least affected. The lower limbs are less affected than the upper limbs. Similarly, there is bilateral loss of pain and temperature sensation, again with sacral sparing, and a greater effect in the upper than in the lower limbs.

Management of spinal cord injury and future therapies

Any patient suspected of having a cervical spinal injury has their neck immobilized to prevent any potential bone fragments from penetrating or compressing the cord and causing further damage. Imaging of the cord and vertebral column is performed using X-rays, CT or MRI. The main aims of medical and surgical treatments in SCI patients are to prevent further damage and limit the area of secondary injury. Surgically, this can be achieved by removing fragments of damaged bone, discs and ligaments to decompress the cord. Pharmacologically, early administration of anti-inflammatory drugs appears beneficial by targeting the secondary effects of SCI (by reducing oedema, inflammation, glutamate release, and free radical accumulation). Clinical trials showed that high-dose steroids such as methylprednisolone were effective in preserving motor function if given within 8 hours of injury and continued for 48 hours, but their use remains controversial in some countries. Other promising pharmacological compounds that target immune cells that might be suitable for clinical trials are the tetracycline antibiotic minocycline, the omega-3 polyunsaturated fatty acid docosahexaenoic acid and peroxisome proliferator activated receptor gamma (PPARγ) agonists. Indeed, minocycline, when given within 12 hours and twice daily for a week, improved ASIA scores over 3–12 months. The other main treatment is rehabilitation medicine, which is used to help the patient make the most of what residual function they have left through functional retraining, and to prevent medical complications from occurring that often lead to re-hospitalization such as bladder infections, skin lesions and musculoskeletal problems.

Substantial progress has been made in understanding the cellular, genetic and molecular consequences of SCI, their spatial and temporal profile and how axons find their way to appropriate targets during normal development. Successful repair of SCI will involve overcoming (hierarchical) obstacles in four main areas: reducing cell death; promoting CNS axon regeneration or enhancing plasticity of residual, spared neural circuits; remyelination of damaged and regenerating fibres; and restoration of appropriate connectivity (Table 4.7). Consequently, researchers are now translating some of this knowledge to clinical trials. For example, the drug fampridine (4-aminopyridine)—a K⁺ channel blocker that restores action potential conduction in demyelinated fibres—reduced spasticity whilst increasing sensory and motor functions in some patients in phase 3 trials. Likewise, riluzole—a drug licenced for ALS—is in phase II and III trials. Giving riluzole orally twice a day for 2 weeks after SCI showed beneficial effects in terms of neurologic recovery, functional outcomes and quality of life outcomes.

The CNS environment, unlike the PNS, is hostile to regeneration because CNS neurons have a low intrinsic ability to regenerate and damage fails to stimulate growth-promoting molecules. More importantly, the damaged CNS is very inhibitory to axonal regeneration because it produces molecules that cause growth cones to collapse. One major source of the inhibition is myelin. At least three inhibitory proteins are known to exist: Nogo-A, myelin-associated glycoprotein and oligodendrocyte myelin glycoprotein. These molecules bind to a common receptor complex comprising the Nogo receptor (NgR1) and the p75 low-affinity neurotrophic factor

Table 4.7 Strategies for spinal cord repair

Level of difficulty	Objective	Technique
Low	Neuroprotection	Pharmacological, e.g. methylprednisolone, glutamate receptor antagonists, ion channel blockers
	Prevention of demyelination	Pharmacological, e.g. 4-aminopyridine
	Preventing scar formation	Targeting glial reaction, e.g. enzyme digestion
	Suppression of CNS inhibitory molecules	Neutralizing antibodies, vaccines, specific receptor antagonists
	Promoting axonal regeneration	Use of growth factors or stimulation of intrinsic growth potential
	Provision of permissive environment	Cellular bridges, e.g. nerve grafts, biodegradable conduits, Schwann cells, glial cell transplants
	Replacement of lost cells	Stem cells
High	Appropriate re-connectivity	Ensure specific target recognition

receptor, which activates the Rho signalling pathway to mediate growth cone collapse. Antibodies to Nogo-A have been shown in rodents to promote neuronal regeneration of the CST, both of injured and uninjured axons. Blocking the Nogo-A protein using antibodies or the NgR1 with drugs or decoy proteins (AXER 204) to trap myelin-associated inhibitors have all been tested in non-human primate models of SCI. Nogo-A antibodies and AXER 204 are now undergoing clinical trials for SCI.

Damage to the CNS produces a glial scar within a few weeks of injury that appears to have two opposing functions: to protect tissue and prevent repair. The scar is now recognized as a complex structure formed of several cell types with different functions. It is well known that the glial scar inhibits regeneration. Experimental therapeutic strategies use pharmacological, genetic, and surgical methods to reduce scar formation or block inhibitory extracellular matrix molecules like chondroitin sulphate proteoglycans (CSGPGs), which induces growth cone collapse. Enzymes that digest the CSPG side chains promote CNS regeneration. Alternatively, bridging of the scar region with biodegradable conduits that can be seeded with various trophic factors or cells, or nerve grafts, has provided limited regeneration across the injury site.

Another more controversial approach involves transplantation of Schwann cells, olfactory ensheathing cells (OECs), or neural progenitor or mesenchymal stem cells into humans. Cellular transplantation for SCI has been tried over the past 30 years, initially using embryonic tissue to bridge the lesion site and act as a relay between disconnected neurons. However, such approaches raised important ethical questions such as the source of the cells, delivery method, immunogenicity and control of growth that have largely precluded their incorporation into clinical practice. The early studies, especially with OECs, showed the feasibility of this methodology, as transplants were incorporated into the host tissue and produced some functional benefit in rodent models. OECs have been transplanted into human SCI patients in Portugal, Australia, China and Poland, with variable success in Poland and China, and it is unclear whether the transplants are directly responsible for the improvements. Inducible pluripotent stem cells (iPSCs) may circumvent the ethical issues associated with embryonic/foetal tissue use. Neural progenitor cells generated from iPSCs showed beneficial effects after transplantation in preclinical models of SCI, but it remains unclear whether meaningful differentiation into neurons occurs or if they only play a supportive role. A critical safety issue for the use of iPSCs is the risk of tumorigenicity.

It is highly unlikely that a single therapy will successfully treat SCI and lead to recovery of function. Multiple therapeutic approaches that target the different aspects detailed in Table 4.7 will be needed in a progressive and coordinated fashion to initiate, maintain, and guide appropriate regeneration from the injury site and to re-establish functional connections. Sadly, of 19 published clinical trials, none have translated into general clinical practice, aside from those countries that offer it as a form of medical tourism for non-validated therapies. However, an alternative strategy currently showing clinical promise is the use of functional electrical stimulation and brain computer interface (BCI) machines to recover function. Major advances (and failures) in neurosurgery, robotics, computational neuroscience and neuroengineering have populated SCI medicine with wearable and implantable neurotechnologies to enable and augment function, such as speaking or moving paralysed limbs via prosthetics. They share two common themes: to capitalize on the intrinsic capacity of spared circuits to produce movement, and their remarkable ability to reorganize with rehabilitation training to enhance recovery. The next generation BCIs aim to re-establish bidirectional communication between the brain and denervated body parts using wireless technology and implantable (miniature) CNS/PNS devices that will provide significant improvements in patient quality of life. SCI research has moved on from making people walk again, as for most SCI patients, walking is not at the top of their wish list for progress. It is the absence of bowel and bladder control and hand use, and the levels of neuropathic pain that emerge after injury, which control the quality of their lives. There are drugs that control incontinence and sexual dysfunction, pain and spasticity. For example, in rehabilitation medicine, oral or intrathecal baclofen—a $GABA_B$ receptor agonist—is used to reduce muscle spasticity by increasing general CNS inhibition via reduced neurotransmitter release and motor neuron activity. It also has effects on bladder function by decreasing hyperactive contracture of the external urethral sphincter. Next-generation implantable wireless technologies offer much hope for improving these adverse consequences post-injury.

Comments on the case history

Humpty Dumpty suffered spinal cord damage resulting in a Brown–Séquard syndrome. The level of the lesion is at T10—the highest level of neurological deficit on the right side. This syndrome results in dissociated sensory loss below the level of the lesion due to damage to the DCML and STT, and the Babinski sign is an indicator of damage to the CST. Humpty Dumpty's cord will not be put back together again!

Self-assessment case study

While on holiday, a 17-year-old boy playing with some friends dived off the rocks into the sea. He emerged motionless, face down in the water. His friends immediately rescued him, and on returning to shore, applied artificial resuscitation while the emergency services were called. The boy was put in a neck brace and flown by air ambulance to the nearest neurological trauma centre, where he underwent a complete neurological assessment and was sent for MRI. The MRI scan showed a complete fracture dislocation at C4, which had severed the spinal cord. The parents arrive and ask about his condition and what the prognosis is.

After studying this chapter, you should be able to answer the following questions:

1. Is it possible to give an accurate prognosis at this stage?

No, because after a major traumatic injury, an initial period of spinal shock sets in, whereby all physiological function of the cord is severely depressed, and this may last for up to 4 weeks after the initial injury. After this period has elapsed, signs associated with damage to various neuronal structures and pathways become evident. Depending on the exact nature of the injury, there may be some recovery of function.

2. What are the consequences of the lesion in terms of functional disability?

There is complete loss of all sensory, voluntary movement and autonomic functions below the level of the lesion. The patient is likely to be paraplegic with impaired respiration requiring artificial ventilation (due to damage to the phrenic nerve supplying the diaphragm). There is bilateral lower motoneuron paralysis and atrophy of the C4 dermatome innervating the posterior neck and shoulder muscles and bilateral spastic paresis and Babinski signs below the lesion, loss of bladder and bowel function and bilateral loss of all sensation below the level of the neck. A bilateral Horner's syndrome will also be present.

3. What are the medical complications associated with the scenario?

The patient will have no independence of life and will require constant care. Medical complications that can occur are: (1) bedsores over bony protuberances due to loss of sensation and inability to move; (2) bladder infections due to loss of bladder reflex control mechanisms; (3) muscle spasms due to loss of inhibitory control mechanisms leading to hyperactivity of gamma motoneurons that control the muscle spindles; (4) spontaneous neuropathic pain that is of a burning or shooting quality due to deafferentation of spinal cord neurons; and (5) nutritional deficiency due to the injury.

PAIN AND ANALGESIA

5

Chapter summary

Chapter summary

1. Pain is a multidimensional sensory modality. The perception and interpretation of pain involve the peripheral nervous system, and several subcortical and cortical areas in the central nervous system. This is commonly referred to as the pain matrix.

2. Pain has an essential protective function after acute injury, but under conditions of non-resolved inflammation or injury and following persistent damage to the nervous system, it can become profoundly maladaptive. Persistent neuropathic pain associated with injury in the central nervous system is linked to plastic adaptations of neural circuits, which involve peripheral and central sensitization that exacerbate pain.

3. Pain can be modulated through exogenous and endogenous mechanisms. Exogenous mechanisms often involve pharmacological or cognitive treatments, whereas endogenous mechanisms comprise two key processes: (a) a gating of nociceptive input at the first synapse in the spinal cord or brainstem and (b) by activation of descending pathways, which can modify the ascending nociceptive pathway transmission. This is done by presynaptic or postsynaptic inhibition.

4. The pain matrix circuitry involves multiple neurotransmitters, including peptides such as the enkephalins and substance P, purines such as ATP, and monoamines such as noradrenaline and serotonin, and glutamate. Management of pain is based on the use of non-opioid drugs and opioid drugs, whose use is titrated, so that therapy is based on a gradual escalation (known as the analgesic ladder), for example from non-steroidal anti-inflammatory drugs to low strength opioids and finally strong opioids. The mu opioid receptors are a major target for the modulation of pain, using agonists such as morphine or related compounds. However, long-term use of these agents is associated with a risk of tolerance and dependence. For chronic neuropathic pain, other drugs such as antidepressants, anticonvulsants, cannabinoid-based drugs or other interventional strategies are used.

Chapter summary—cont'd

5. Migraine is a distinct form of pain. It is a primary headache disorder whose pathophysiology is neurovascular. The trigeminovascular activation involved in migraine leads to release of vasodilatory agents, which trigger the specific pain that characterizes migraine attacks. Management involves treatment for the attacks and also prophylaxis, as needed. Drugs modulating 5-HT transmission (e.g. triptans) and calcitonin gene-related peptides (e.g. gepants) are specific therapies for the management of this condition.

6. Non-pharmacological approaches can also be used to control pain. They could involve surgical interventions (e.g. cordotomy) or various forms of neurostimulation such as transcutaneous electrical stimulation, vagus nerve stimulation, deep brain stimulation or remote electrical neuromodulation. Biofeedback, relaxation and distraction strategies can also help alleviate pain.

Box 5.1 **Case history**

A South-East Asian male was involved in an industrial accident when he was 18 years old; his shirtsleeve got caught in a machine, dragging his arm into the equipment. Surgeons tried to repair the arm but the blood supply was severely compromised and eventually the right arm was amputated above the elbow. Since the accident he has experienced phantom limb pain sensations that radiate up the right arm and appear to originate from the non-existent right hand. He describes the pain as shooting, burning and stabbing sensations, and it feels worse when it is cold. He rates it as 7 out of 10 on a visual analogue pain rating scale. Intermixed with these are sensations of hyperalgesia and allodynia when the skin over the stump is touched, and spontaneous pain that occurs sporadically and feels like electric shocks in the arm. When he is shaving he feels tingling sensations in the phantom hand. He describes the phantom hand as contorted, with the fist closed and the nails digging into the palm skin.

His GP initially prescribed mild analgesics to relieve the pain but these were largely ineffective. He sought alternative treatments such as transcutaneous electrical nerve stimulation (TENS) and acupuncture, but these have had mixed results; TENS made the pain worse and acupuncture only partially alleviated the pain. Likewise, anticonvulsant and tricyclic antidepressant drugs, such as carbamazepine and amitriptyline, had a limited effect, and stronger opiate drug treatment, such as morphine, was initially effective but now much higher doses are required to achieve the same effect.

He is referred to a pain clinic where the consultant tries a sympathetic nerve blockade that has limited effect. After unsuccessfully trying several new drug combinations, he prescribes the drug gabapentin. After a couple of months of treatment, the patient reports that suddenly the pain in his phantom limb has regressed to a point where he hardly notices it (pain rating, 1/10). The only side effect of this latest treatment was a mild dizziness that occurred during the first few days of treatment.

This case gives rise to the following questions:

1. What pathways transmit pain from the periphery to the brain?
2. Why were TENS and acupuncture ineffective?
3. How does morphine reduce pain and why did it become ineffective in this case?
4. What is the rationale for the other pharmacological and non-pharmacological treatments that were tried?
5. What are the mechanisms that may contribute to phantom limb pain?

Introduction

Pain is one of humanity's oldest and most dreaded fears. Pain is a sensation that evokes an emotional response and involves a complex interaction between the periphery, spinal cord, brainstem and higher cortical centres.

Intense pain is an extreme sensation that commands the person's attention and rapidly dominates the mind. To the neuroscientist, pain is a sensory phenomenon based on perception; to the psychologist, it may be a learned or conditioned behaviour, but to the doctor, it is a warning sign to be decoded for diagnosis and treatment. People go to see their doctors most often because they are in pain. Thus it is important that doctors have a sound knowledge of pain and its pathways, and of the treatments that are effective in alleviating pain. Pain is a learned experience, the perception of which depends on the emotional interpretation of pain, recall of past pain and social and genetic factors.

Pain is defined by the International Association for the Study of Pain (IASP) as 'an unpleasant sensory or emotional experience associated with, or resembling that associated with, actual or potential tissue damaging stimuli'. The definition includes the sensory-discriminative and motivational-affective components that make up the complex experience of pain. Among somatovisceral sensations, pain is arguably the most important. Although pain is used to define generically all sensations that hurt or are unpleasant, there are three distinct types of pain. The first two types of pain are examples of 'good' pain; the third is deemed 'bad' pain.

1. Nociceptive acute pain is elicited by a brief noxious stimulus such as a pinprick that induces a flexion withdrawal response to the stimulus. This type of pain is an adaptive sensation whose primary function is to protect the body from injury; it is an early warning alarm system. Loss of this type of pain through disease or injury can lead to life-threatening situations. People who have congenital insensitivity to pain with anhydrosis (CIPA)—a rare autosomal-recessive disorder— have recurrent episodes of unexplained fever, anhydrosis and absence of reaction to noxious stimuli, as well as mental retardation. Children with this condition often have to have their fingernails and teeth removed to stop self-mutilation (autotomy) behaviour, and many die young. Mutations in the sodium channel subunit $Na_V1.7$ also result in abnormal pain sensations; loss of the subunit results in analgesia, whereas increased expression results in conditions such as paroxysmal extreme pain disorder and erythromelalgia (Mitchell's disease). Pain also has a homeostatic function. A low level of pain is necessary to inform us when activities put excessive strain on the body, such as during certain movements or altered posture. Even when we sleep, nociceptors work to cause us to toss and turn during the night to prevent bedsores or musculoskeletal strain.

2. When pain is prolonged (e.g. sunburn), injury to the body has already occurred and the biological function of pain is to prevent further damage, assist healing and tissue repair. It does this by the development of areas of hypersensitivity in and around the injury site, which are the result of a decreased activation threshold of nociceptors—a phenomenon called peripheral sensitization. The pain recedes once healing has occurred.

3. Chronic pain is pain that has persisted for at least 2–3 months. Such pain is often neuropathic, due to damage of the nervous system. Chronic pain is defined by the IASP as 'pain resulting from disease or damage to the peripheral or central nervous systems, and from dysfunction of the nervous system'. Thus, it is a ubiquitous term covering a wide range of conditions such as pain in irritable bowel syndrome (a visceral pain disorder), through to muscle and joint pain disorders such as fibromyalgia and back pain, where there is no obvious nervous system damage, and to pain in diseases such as arthritis, diabetes, cancer and HIV/AIDS. The quality of pain sensations is distinct from that seen in acute pain (Table 5.1). In neuropathic pain, the pain persists in the absence of the initial injury. Chronic pain often results from abnormal sensitivity of nociceptors and non-nociceptors and pathological changes at multiple levels in the nervous system (Table 5.2). Pain, rather than the original injury, becomes of greatest concern and is often very difficult to treat.

Statistics suggest that the prevalence of chronic pain in the UK adult population is 35%–51%, with nearly two-thirds of those aged >75 years suffering from chronic pain. In 2018 in the United States, 50 million people were reported to suffer from chronic pain. The worldwide prevalence is about 30% of the population. Statistics from the United States suggest that the annual cost of chronic pain is $560–653 billion, with indirect costs (disability compensation and lost productivity) adding another $261–300 billion annually. These estimates do not include other costs such as legal fees, childcare, lost earning potential or personal suffering. Chronic pain costs more than heart disease ($309 billion), cancer ($243 billion) or diabetes ($188 billion). Chronic pain is expensive to diagnose, expensive to treat acutely, and expensive to live with long-term.

Table 5.1 Clinical features of neuropathic pain

Abnormal pain quality—burning, stabbing, gnawing and sickening

Sensory loss with associated hyperalgesia (increased painful response to a noxious stimulus), allodynia (pain in response to an innocuous stimulus) and hyperpathia (delayed perception, summation and painful after-sensations)

Paroxysmal pain (electric shock-like) episodes are common

Radiating dysaesthesia (non-painful abnormal sensations)

Pain is poorly localized and diffuse

Pain intensity is altered by emotion and fatigue

Onset of pain is immediate or delayed after injury

Sympathetic nervous system dysfunction may be present

Vasomotor (regulation of blood vessels) and sudomotor (stimulation of sweat glands) changes can occur

Table 5.2 Summary classification of some major characteristics of different types of pain

Type	Duration	Temporal features in relation to cause	Sensation	Nerve fibre class involved	Adaptive value	Example
Acute	Seconds	Instantaneous Simultaneous	Pain	C/Aδ	Preventive	Pinprick, muscle ache, visceral distension
Prolonged	Hours to days	Resolves on recovery	Hyperalgesia, allodynia	C/Aδ Aβ	Protective Recovery	Inflamed wound
Chronic	Months to years	Persistent; exceeds repair of injury	Hyperalgesia, allodynia, spontaneous pain	C/Aδ Aβ Aβ/δ/C CNS cells	None Maladaptive	Arthritis Neuropathy Central pain

Despite much research regarding the molecular and cellular aspects of nociception, pain therapy continues to be only partially effective and may be accompanied by distressing side effects or have abuse potential. For most acute pain conditions, non-steroidal anti-inflammatory drugs (NSAIDs) or opioids remain the first line of treatment, while these drugs are largely ineffective in neuropathic pain. Chronic pain can respond well to drugs whose primary use was not intended for pain, for example, antidepressants, anticonvulsants and local anaesthetics. It is becoming clear that no one class of drug is effective in treating all forms of pain. Moreover, different types of pain may involve common or dissimilar mechanisms. Therefore treatment, which traditionally was based on empirical measures such as symptom or temporal properties, may be improved by therapies targeting with more precision the underlying mechanisms. In the past 20 years, rapid progress has been made in uncovering new mechanisms, pathways, brain areas and drugs involved in pain perception, and modulation. However, we are still putting all the pieces of the pain puzzle together. This chapter aims to provide an overview of some of the pathways and mechanisms of nociception and pain, current therapies for pain management and new therapeutic concepts.

Nociceptors

Nociceptive afferents do not have specialized receptors; they use free nerve endings and most are polymodal, that is, they respond to more than one kind of stimulus such as chemical, thermal or mechanical stimuli. Free nerve endings are found in all parts of the body, except the interior of the bones and the brain itself. Acute pain is characterized by activation of nociceptors for a limited duration. Pain sensations can be broadly divided into bright, sharp, stabbing types of pain, and dull, throbbing, aching types. Aδ fibres mediate the former, or 'fast' pain, whereas C fibres signal the latter or 'slow pain'. Not all Aδ and C fibres are nociceptors. Some respond to low-threshold

Table 5.3 Comparison of pain characteristics from different target organs

Peripheral target	Sensation	Localization of pain
Skin	Pricking Stabbing Burning	Well localized
Muscle	Aching Soreness/tenderness Cramping	
Viscera	Dullness Vagueness Fullness Nausea	Poorly localized

stimuli such as sensual touching or brushing the skin; recent evidence suggests that these fibres contribute to pathological pain perceptions such as mechanical allodynia after injury. Many C fibres are thermoreceptors and respond to warm or cold, providing homeostatic responses via emotional tagging of sensations. For example, think how pleasant a cool shower feels after sunbathing for a while, and conversely, how unpleasant a cool shower feels first thing in the morning when the skin is cool! Additionally, there is a population of 'silent' nociceptors that reside in most tissues and are normally insensitive to mechanical and thermal stimuli. They become active under pathological conditions such as inflammation and nerve injury.

Interestingly, most of our knowledge about the neurophysiology of pain comes from the study of cutaneous nociceptors. Pain from each target organ has its own distinct perceptual quality, as shown in Table 5.3. However, cutaneous pain is clinically less common than muscle and visceral pain. Among the most common reasons for visiting the doctor are chest pain, neck pain, abdominal pain, headache and back pain. For example, back pain is extremely common, with up to 80% of the population suffering at some point in their life; it is the world number one chronic pain. Visceral pain represents a major clinical challenge, as its occurrence is not always correlated with disease severity. For example, bowel cancer produces little or no pain, whereas passing a kidney stone, or a stool in a patient with irritable bowel syndrome, can be excruciating.

There are several differences between cutaneous and muscle or visceral nociceptors. The first is that cutaneous sensation is well localized, and the pain is usually constant. Visceral and muscle pain is poorly localized due to the lower innervation densities of these tissues, and is often periodic. Secondly, visceral afferents are insensitive to direct trauma but very sensitive to distension (of hollow-walled muscular organs), whereas muscle and skin are not. In fact, early 20th century surgeons could perform abdominal surgery using only local anaesthesia of the body wall, as healthy organs are largely insensitive to direct mechanical trauma such as cutting or burning. All are sensitive to ischaemia and inflammation. Lastly, as most visceral organs have very few low-threshold myelinated fibres and comprise mostly of Aδ and C fibres, their stimulus response properties differ from cutaneous and muscle afferents, which have specialized receptors to detect innocuous stimuli. Visceral afferents encode a stimulus response in an intensity-dependent manner—the more painful the stimulus, the greater the number of action potentials and frequency of discharge.

Although acute pain results from damage to these free nerve endings; in reality, the pain is a result of substances released by damaged tissues such as prostaglandins, histamine, bradykinin, cytokines, peptides and H$^+$ ions. These activate specific receptors located on the free nerve endings. Nociceptors have more than 30 different ion channels or receptors and the list is functionally diverse and still growing! (see Table 5.4). Moreover, the molecular composition of the receptors and their relative ratios can change after injury.

Pain pathways

Cutaneous nociceptor afferents terminate mainly in laminae I, II and V of the spinal cord dorsal horn and synapse on second order neurons that carry the signal to either the brainstem or the thalamus. It is only when the nociceptive signal reaches the brainstem that it is translated into a conscious sensory percept. Three ascending pathways are concerned with pain transmission: the spinothalamic tract (STT), the spinoreticular tract (SRT) and the spinoparabrachial tract (SPBT). Each appears to be concerned with a particular aspect of pain processing. Simplistically, the sensory discriminative aspect is signalled by the STT, and the homeostatic and affective (emotional) qualities of pain by the SRT and SPBT (Fig. 5.1). Therefore fast and slow pain travel by different pathways to different areas of the brain. The fast pathway connects directly to the thalamus, which then relays the information to the primary sensorimotor cortices for analysis and response. Its function is

Table 5.4 Function of some of the receptor types and ion channels located on nociceptors

Receptor family	Function
P2X = purinergic ATP receptor ASIC = acid-sensing ion channel (chemical and mechanical stimuli) TRP = transient response potential receptors (temperature sensitive)	Involved in signal transduction
Voltage-gated Na$^+$ channels (tetrodotoxin resistant or tetrodotoxin sensitive) Voltage-gated Ca^{2+} channels α-amino-3-hydroxy-5-methyl-4-isoxazolepropionic acid + N-methyl-D-aspartate (AMPA + NMDA) = ionotropic glutamate receptors; mGluR = metabotropic glutamate receptors Voltage-gated K$^+$ channels γ-aminobutyric acid (GABA) receptors	Involved in membrane excitability
5-HT$_3$ = serotonin receptor CB$_1$ = cannabinoid receptor H$_1$ = histamine receptor EP = prostanoid receptors for prostaglandins IL-1R = receptor for interleukin 1 (cytokine) TrkA = tyrosine kinase A receptor for the neurotrophin nerve growth factor (NGF) BK$_2$ = bradykinin receptor	Involved in peripheral sensitization

to act as a warning system, by signalling the exact location and severity of the injury and duration of the nociceptive signal. Fast pain predominantly arises from the STT cells in laminae IV–V of the spinal cord. Slow pain is mediated by C fibres and signals the emotional aspects of pain. It reaches the thalamus indirectly via connections with the brainstem reticular formation. The slow pain axons innervate the non-specific intralaminar nuclei of the thalamus and the autonomic centres of the reticular formation in the brainstem. For example, axons of lamina I cells of both the STT and SPBT are more concerned with stimulus intensity than stimulus location. They form part of the forebrain pain pathways associated with the affective quality of pain (unpleasantness and fear of further injury) and involve the prefrontal cortex and amygdala. Slow pain may remind the brain that pain has occurred, that protective attention to the injury site is required, and that normal activity may need to be restricted while healing occurs.

The projections to the reticular formation underlie the arousal effects of painful stimuli, via activation of the ascending reticular activating system that projects to all areas of the brain. Activation of the reticular formation stimulates noradrenergic neurons in the locus coeruleus and thus decreases the pain transmission by activating the descending pain modulating systems (see below).

Thalamocortical axons transmit the information from the thalamus to the cortex. There is no one specific cortical region that is designated as 'pain cortex' (Box 5.2). Rather, functional brain-imaging studies have revealed

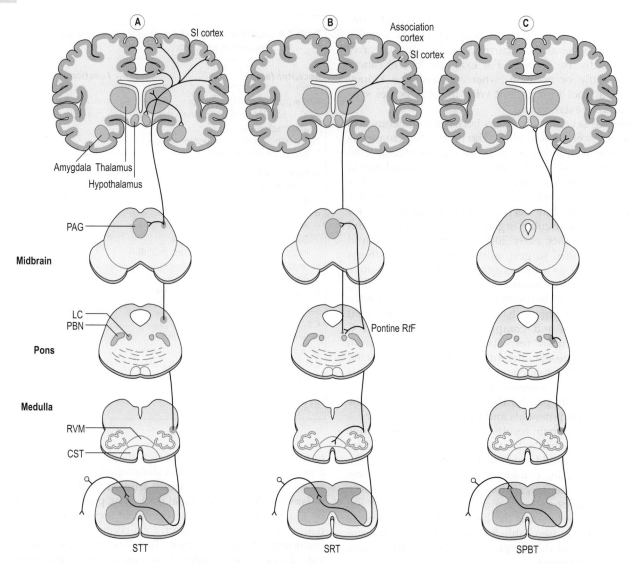

Fig. 5.1 Schematic representation of anterolateral pain pathways: (A) Spinothalamic tract (STT), (B) Spinoreticular tract (SRT), and (C) Spinoparabrachial tract (SPBT). Information is also transmitted to the amygdala and hypothalamic areas of the limbic system. *CST,* Corticospinal tract; *LC,* locus coeruleus; *PAG,* periaquductal grey; *PBN,* parabrachial nucleus; *RtF,* reticular formation; *RVM,* rostroventral medulla; *SI,* primary somatosensory cortex.

several regions that are active when a pain stimulus is sensed, and these are associated with different functional components of pain. The discriminative qualities (i.e. 'where and how much it hurts') involve the somatosensory cortex, whereas the affective-motivational aspects (e.g. 'I don't like it, or stop it!') are associated with the limbic regions (cingulate cortex, insula). Parts of the prefrontal motor cortex are also involved in cognitive evaluative processes, for example, attention to, anticipation of, memory of or escape from pain.

Visceral and muscular pain pathways

Considering that muscle and visceral pain evoke distinct sensations, it would be logical to expect to find cells in

the spinal cord that respond only to muscle or visceral stimulation. Interestingly, no such cells exist in the spinal cord. All cells that have either a visceral or muscle receptive field (RF) also have a separate cutaneous RF. This means that convergence occurs within the spinal cord. It provides an explanation for referred pain. Referred pain is a pain that is localized in one part of the body that is remote from its source. In contrast to cutaneous pain, which is well localized, visceral and muscle pains are poorly localized and are often sensed as somatic pain. This is because of afferent convergence onto spinal cord cells that have a cutaneous RF. The area of referral is related to the segmental dermatome and is often referred to skin or muscle. The classic example is angina in which ischaemic heart muscle causes pain over the skin and radiating down the left arm. Another example is stomach

Pain in the brain

The role of the cortex in pain has been debated for almost 100 years. Based on a careful study of patients with cortical or thalamic lesions, Dr. Henry Head showed that ablation of the thalamus eliminated all pain sensations, whereas cortical lesions did not. However, converging clinical, experimental and, more recently, functional imaging evidence, has now altered this view, to show that several brain regions are active, either directly or indirectly, in response to a painful stimulus but that they process different aspects of the stimulus (Table 5.5). These include the primary (SI) and secondary (SII) somatosensory cortex and the adjacent insula region, the anterior cingulate cortex and the ventromedial prefrontal cortex. Some regions, such as the anterior cingulate cortex and the ventromedial prefrontal cortex, directly feedback to the periaqueductal grey to stimulate anti-nociceptive pathways. Furthermore, pain perception modulation by hypnosis has been shown to alter activity in many of these brain areas.

Damage to the prefrontal cortex affects the evaluative cognitive responses to pain. For example, patients with frontal lobe damage which disconnects it from the thalamus rarely complain about the severity of pain. They acknowledge the presence of the pain but state that it does not bother them. Cingulotomy selectively decreases the emotional components of pain perception, although it fails to provide significant pain relief in approximately 25% of patients. It appears that the cingulate cortex may not

modulate some forms of chronic pain, for example, neuropathic pain. Patients with ischaemic damage to SI and SII areas show a loss of pain sensation with preservation of pain affect. Similarly, patients with damage to the insula and SII cortex have elevated pain thresholds to thermal stimuli. Table 5.5 summarizes the presumed functional roles of these cortical areas in pain perception.

Table 5.5 Presumed functional roles of cortical areas in pain perception

Cortical area	Presumed function
SI	Pain localization
SII	Pain intensity; spatially directed attention (touch, visual) to pain
Insula	Regulation of pain-related autonomic activity; pain intensity
Anterior cingulate	Response selection, attention, affect, motor suppression, anticipatory appraisal of pain; pain modulation
Prefrontal cortex	Affect, emotion, memory, anticipatory appraisal of pain; pain modulation

pain which can cause visceral organ spasm, muscle spasm, and a skin flare response due to autonomic activity. Referred pain is consistent enough to be of diagnostic value, for example, lower right quadrant abdominal pain can be used to diagnose appendicitis (Fig. 5.2). Another important feature is that the referral site may show signs of hyperalgesia due to a preexisting condition such as ischaemia, injury, disease or inflammation.

The central terminals of visceral and muscle nociceptors terminate in laminae I and V, but not lamina II, unlike skin nociceptor afferents. In lamina I, these fibres converge onto projection neurons of the STT and SPBT, which then project to the brainstem and thalamus, and from there to the somatosensory cortex. Visceral afferents also terminate on SRT neurons and onto cells that project to the dorsal column nuclei; recent research suggests that this latter pathway is exclusively involved in visceral pain, whereas the STT and SRT visceral pathways are more concerned with autonomic (visceral) reflex functions. Dorsal column lesions relieve chronic visceral pain and provide a new clinical treatment for managing visceral cancer pain.

Given that muscle, viscera and skin converge onto projection neurons that utilize common ascending tracts, how then does the brain know whether the pain is from skin, muscle or viscus? The answer is unknown but most likely involves differences in the temporal and spatial coding of inputs onto cells, inducing a differential processing of information by the brain.

How does the central nervous system interpret a stimulus as painful?

As lesion studies have confirmed the role of the STT in pain transmission, it might be expected that STT cells would be nociceptive specific (NS), that is, specifically responding to tissue-damaging stimuli. However, it is one of the paradoxes of pain that most of the cells of the STT are excited by non-noxious stimulation of the skin! Low-threshold sensory skin afferents synapse upon the proximal dendrites of the lamina IV and V neurons. These low-threshold inputs are the only inputs to lamina IV cells (i.e. they have no nociceptive inputs). The same low-threshold afferents also synapse on the dendrites of the lamina V cells. However, cells of lamina V extend some dendrites into laminae I–II where C/Aδ fibres contact the distal dendrites. Thus the lamina V cells receive convergent inputs from both nociceptor and non-nociceptor afferents (i.e. they are wide dynamic range cells). Therefore, the STT has axons of three different kinds of neurons: those that are nociceptor-specific (lamina I), those that are non-nociceptive (lamina IV) and those that have both nociceptive and nonnociceptive inputs (lamina V). The presence of this convergence of sensory modalities on the lamina V cells presents a problem. The forebrain can only know that action potentials are arriving in the axons of the STT. How can it tell which types of primary afferents are activating the lamina V cells, nociceptors (C/Aδ) or low-threshold Aβ afferents?

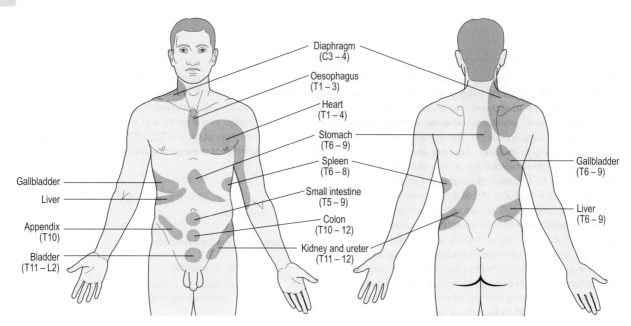

Fig. 5.2 Common cutaneous areas of referred pain from visceral organs; dermatomes of referred pain are in parentheses. *C*, Cervical; *L*, lumbar; *T*, thoracic. (Adapted from Moore KL, Agur AMR. (2002) Essentials of clinical anatomy, third ed. Lippincott Williams and Wilkins.)

One theory is that the lamina V cells make up the majority of the STT and have small RFs that signal the precise location of stimulus. However, because of the afferent input convergence in lamina V, they are non-specific in the type of stimulus that they register. The lamina I cells unequivocally signal that a noxious stimulus has occurred. However, these cells are fewer in number and have large RFs that cannot indicate the precise location of the painful stimulus. It is thought that the pain is signalled by the lamina I and V neurons acting together. If lamina I cells are not active, the detailed information about the type and location of a stimulus provided by the lamina V axons is interpreted as innocuous. If, however, a lamina I cell is active, the stimulation is recognized as painful. Thus, the lamina V cells provide the details about the location of a stimulus and the lamina I cells specify whether it is painful or not. This theory has been confirmed in recent animal studies where lamina I cells were selectively ablated using a neurotoxin, which led to a significant reduction in the behavioural hyperalgesia associated with tissue injury, without affecting the ability to locate the stimulus.

Physiology of pain modulation

The transmission of information from primary afferents to secondary neurons in the spinal cord is not simply a passive process but is dynamic, involving excitation, inhibition and modulation. The variable nature of pain responses also suggests that modulatory systems must exist in the CNS that regulate pain. Neurons in the superficial dorsal horn are subject to modulation that 'gates' the flow of information to the CNS. Nociceptive sensory information is gated in the substantia gelatinosa (lamina II of the spinal cord) where nociceptors synapse, by tonic or phasic inhibitory control mechanisms. Gating is of two kinds:

1. Local—'segmental antinociception' regulated by primary afferent inputs.

2. Widespread—'supraspinal antinociception', which utilizes descending pathways from the brainstem.

In attempting to explain various clinical pain phenomena such as allodynia, referred pain and the variable relationship between tissue injury and pain response, a theory about how pain is perceived—the 'gate control' theory—was proposed by Patrick Wall and Ronald Melzack in 1965 (Fig. 5.3, top). This theory states that pain is a function of the balance between the information traveling into the spinal cord through large (non-nociceptive) nerve fibres and information travelling into the spinal cord through small (nociceptive) nerve fibres. Without any stimulation, both sets of nerve fibres are inactive and the inhibitory neuron (I) blocks the signal in the projection neuron (P) that connects to the brain. The gate is 'closed' and therefore no pain is sensed. With non-painful stimulation, large nerve fibres are activated. This activates P but it also activates I, which then blocks the signal in P that connects to the brain. As the gate is 'closed', no stimulation is perceived by the brain. With noxious stimulation, nociceptive fibres become active. They activate P and according to the original theory, block I (it is now known that this does not occur). Since activity of the inhibitory neuron is blocked, it cannot block the output of the projection neuron that connects with the brain. Therefore if the relative amount of

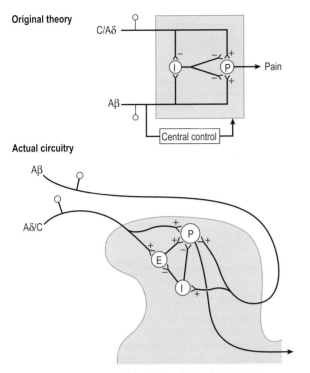

Original theory

C/Aδ

Aβ

Pain

Central control

Actual circuitry

Aβ

Aδ/C

Fig. 5.3 Gate control theory—original circuit shown on the top. The bottom part of the figure shows the actual circuitry involved. Nociceptors do not have an inhibitory effect on the inhibitory neuron as proposed in the original theory; they activate the P cell either directly or via an excitatory interneuron (E). The Aβ fibres have the connections as proposed in the original theory. *I*, Inhibitory neuron; *P*, projection neuron.

activity is greater in large nerve fibres, there should be little or no pain. However, if there is more activity in small nerve fibres, then pain ensues, because the gate is 'open'. Wall and Melzack also recognized that the brain could exert descending modulatory influences on the spinal cord. Their theory generated vigorous scientific debate; little was known about the neuroanatomy and neurochemistry of the dorsal horn back then. While the gate control theory can explain some observations seen in pain patients during therapy, it does not explain everything. Over the past 65 years, as new techniques such as transgenic models, genomics and, more recently, optogenetics, have explored and probed the functional neuroanatomy of the dorsal horn, the theory has undergone significant modification (see Fig. 5.3, bottom). For example, there is no evidence for an inhibitory connection to interneurons from small fibres, and the complexity and diversity of neuronal types and transmitters involved has exploded. Despite its limitations in the proposed circuitry, its most important contributions to pain research have been the appreciation that the CNS is intimately involved in pain modulation and that the brain has a dynamic role in pain processing. Psychological factors that had been previously thought of as reactions to pain are now considered integral to pain processing. Moreover, it offered new sites for pain modulation by

pharmacotherapy rather than surgery. Lastly, as a direct result, the theory has led to the production of counter-stimulation devices such as trans-cutaneous electrical nerve stimulators (TENS) and spinal cord stimulators, as well as other techniques that can alleviate pain.

Counter-stimulation analgesia

A bump on the head or kick in the shin by accident elicits acute pain. However, if the injury site is rubbed, the pain immediately subsides and it feels better. This reaction can be explained by the 'gate control' theory. Rubbing the head or shin stimulates the non-nociceptive afferents that send impulses into the spinal cord. According to the 'gate control' theory, lamina II inhibitory interneurons are activated either directly or indirectly by stimulation of these afferents from the skin that would then block the projection neuron and therefore block the pain. This may explain why 'counter-stimulation' techniques are sometimes effective at relieving pain. For example, this can be done simply by rubbing the skin over a sore muscle or may involve specially designed battery-powered devices designed to electrically stimulate nerves through the skin. The aim of these TENS machines is to stimulate the large (Aβ) sensory fibres in peripheral nerves in the hope that they will in turn activate the inhibitory neurons of lamina II and block pain transmission. Importantly, these devices work best when placed on/near the skin of the injured/painful region. They are commonly used by physiotherapists or midwives during labour and use high frequency, low intensity stimuli to activate the low-threshold fibres; recent evidence suggests that it is the Group 1 (Aα) afferents that are most effective at producing this effect. They are ineffective if they are positioned far away from the painful site. In practice, most counter-stimulation techniques require the use of 'near noxious' stimulation intensities (felt as a buzzing or tingling sensation), which recruit Aδ afferents to be maximally effective. From the spinal cord, the messages go directly to several places in the brain, including the thalamus, midbrain and reticular formation. It may be that Aδ fibres, rather than Aαβ fibres, are best at exciting lamina II inhibitory interneurons because the Aδ fibres are able to recruit the supraspinal control systems (described in next section). TENS is often used in the treatment of acute pain. It is not always useful in chronic pain, because some forms of chronic pain involve phenotypic changes in the properties of low-threshold afferents so that they behave more like nociceptors. In such cases, their activation may actually increase the pain rather than alleviate it.

Supraspinal (descending) analgesia

The 'gate control' theory introduced the concept that pain perception could be modulated in the spinal cord. It also became clear that pain could be modulated at each

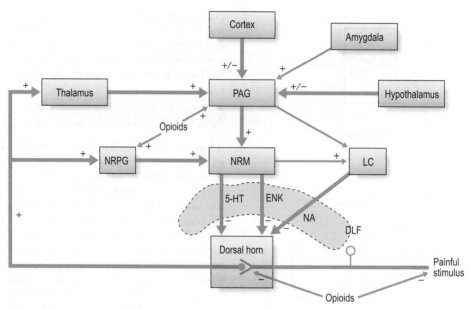

Fig. 5.4 Supraspinal control of pain and its pharmacological modulation by opioids. The periaqueductal grey (PAG) region can be stimulated by input from other regions. In turn, it causes activation of the nucleus raphe magnus (NRM) cells in the rostroventral medulla. Nucleus raphe magnus paragigantocellularis (NRPG) can also stimulate NRM. The NRM sends inhibitory enkephalinergic (ENK) and serotonergic (5-HT) axons via the dorsolateral funiculus (DLF) to the dorsal horn to inhibit substantia gelatinosa cells or nociceptors. Opioids excite cells of the PAG and NRM, as well as having a direct inhibitory effect in the dorsal horn on primary afferents and dorsal horn cells. The locus coeruleus (LC) sends separate noradrenergic (NA) inhibitory inputs to the dorsal horn via the DLF.

synapse along the pain pathways. Brain regions that are involved in pain perception and emotion project back to the brainstem and spinal cord, and these connections can change or modify information that is coming to the brain. This is one way that the brain can reduce pain by a mechanism known as supraspinal (descending) analgesia. It uses feedback loops that involve several different nuclei in the brainstem reticular formation (Fig. 5.4). There are now several lines of evidence to corroborate the involvement of brain mechanisms in analgesia, such as the fact that direct deep brain stimulation suppresses nociception, and the discovery of central endogenous opioid and cannabinoid transmission, which have modulatory roles.

Areas of the brainstem that are involved in reducing pain are the periaqueductal grey (PAG), nucleus raphe magnus (NRM), and locus coeruleus (LC). The PAG is very important in the control of pain. This region surrounds the cerebral aqueduct in the midbrain. Stimulation of parts of the PAG produces more pronounced analgesia than stimulation of either the NRM or LC. Neurosurgeons can implant stimulating electrodes near the PAG of intractable pain patients so that a small electrical shock can be delivered. The patient can control the level of self-stimulation and hence the level of analgesia. This is known as stimulus-induced analgesia. The PAG contains enkephalin-rich neurons that excite the NRM and/or LC neurons by inhibiting gamma-aminobutyric-acid or γ-aminobutyric acid (GABA) ergic interneurons in the PAG. This allows PAG (antinociceptor) neurons to excite amine-containing cells in the NRM and LC that in turn project to the spinal cord to block

pain transmission by dorsal horn cells. They can exert this inhibition by different mechanisms:

1. Direct presynaptic inhibition of neurotransmitter release from primary afferent terminals. This involves, for example, activation of G protein-linked receptors that cause calcium channels to close, thus reducing transmitter release (Fig. 5.5A).

2. Direct postsynaptic inhibition of projection cells causing hyperpolarization of the membrane, due to activation of G protein-linked receptors that cause potassium channels to open (see Fig. 5.5B).

3. Indirect inhibition via activation of local enkephalinergic and/or GABAergic inhibitory interneurons by the descending serotonergic and noradrenergic axons. These interneurons can act both postsynaptically on projection cells by opening potassium channels or presynaptically by closing calcium channels. Enkephalins bind to the same family of receptors as opiate drugs such as morphine and heroin. Therefore it seems likely that opiate drugs may act by mimicking the activity of the interneurons of lamina II.

Stimulation of the NRM causes activation of enkephalin- and 5-HT-containing neurons. Like noradrenaline-containing neurons, the majority of NRM axons synapse on lamina II cells. They also synapse on cells in laminae I and III. Stimulation of the raphe nuclei produces a powerful analgesia, and it is thought that the 5-HT released

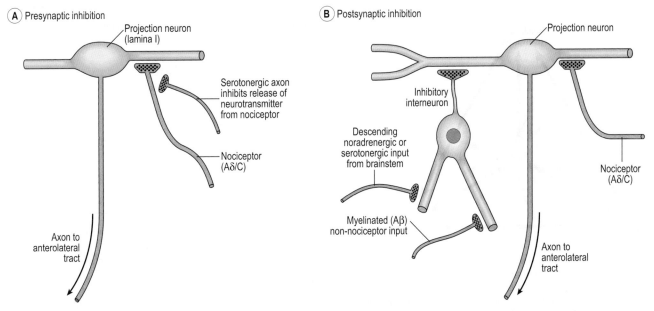

Fig. 5.5 Spinal cord mechanisms of descending inhibition. (A) Presynaptic inhibition; (B) Postsynaptic inhibition. See text for details.

by this stimulation activates the inhibitory interneurons even more powerfully than noradrenaline and so blocks pain transmission. However, 5-HT may not be specifically involved in the inhibition of pain transmission, as serotonergic agonists do not have significant analgesic effects. 5-HT neurons appear to inhibit all somatosensory transmission and may have a function in the initiation of sleep. A complicating factor is that 5-HT receptors are found in many locations in the dorsal horn, including on C fibres, and different 5-HT receptor subtypes mediate different effects of 5-HT.

Acupuncture analgesia

Acupuncture is a Traditional Chinese Medicine technique used to treat pain by inserting needles into specific points in the body (acupoints) and then either manually or electrically activating the deep tissue afferents to produce analgesia. There are several mechanisms by which analgesia is thought to occur. Electrical stimulation of the needles appears to work in a manner similar to TENS, by locally activating gate control. Increasing the intensity recruits the supraspinal descending pathways to produce analgesia via the release of endogenous opioid neurotransmitters. Some suggest that acupuncture is a form of distraction or diffuse noxious inhibitory control, whereby pain in another part of the body distracts the subject from the primary locus of pain. Electrical stimulation can also activate catecholamine nuclei within the brainstem to promote descending analgesia. Most recently, a subgroup of sensory afferents innervating deep tissues have been discovered by researchers at Harvard University that have the ability to selectively inhibit inflammation. They act on the vagal nerve to produce the release of noradrenaline and dopamine from the adrenal gland, to inhibit the activity of specific immune cells by activating their β_2 adrenergic or D_1 receptors. Additionally, by activating the splenic lymphocytes to induce release of acetylcholine, splenic macrophages can be inhibited. This raises the possibility that differential activation of selective neural circuits by electrical stimulation (by using a device akin to an electrical pacemaker) may provide a way to selectively inhibit local inflammatory responses without suppressing the entire immune system, thereby reducing adverse effects or infections.

Arousal analgesia

Recent work has clarified the mechanisms involved in the analgesia seen during intense excitement or arousal. During arousal the sympathetic nervous system is active in the body. Sympathetic fibres activate the slow pain pathways (STT and SRT) whose axons ascend to activate noradrenergic cells in the LC. Noradrenergic axons project back down to the spinal cord (via the dorsolateral funiculus) and synapse on the cells in laminae I–II, forming a feedback loop. Some lamina II cells contain the inhibitory transmitter GABA, and they in turn synapse on the cell bodies of large lamina I cells and on the distal dendrites of lamina V cells. Activation of the central noradrenaline system excites the inhibitory interneurons of lamina II and thus inhibits the lamina I STT cells, blocking pain transmission. Therefore, agents that increase noradrenergic transmission have analgesic potential.

Additionally, activity from autonomic-related brain areas such as the hypothalamus or the amygdala, stimulates the PAG to induce analgesia. This is involved in the 'fight-or-flight' reaction that produces hypoalgesia in life-threatening situations, for example, on the battlefield.

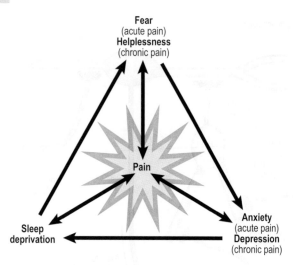

Fig. 5.6 The vicious psychological circle of pain. Untreated pain that persists for any length of time can cause fear and anxiety. If the pain fails to resolve, patients become depressed and lose confidence in themselves and their doctors. Sleeplessness may exacerbate the problem. (Adapted from Wall PD, Melzack R. (1994) Textbook of pain. Churchill.)

Psychology of pain

Emotions are central to the experience and expression of pain. Signs of emotional distress are the most frequently recognized evidence that a patient is in pain. The most common emotional aspects associated with pain are anxiety (that the pain will get worse), fear (that it may ultimately kill or severely impair them), and depression (that the pain may never go away or get better) that set up a vicious circle of pain that dominates the patient's life both in acute and chronic pain states (Fig. 5.6). Other emotions may be present such as aggression, anger, guilt or in some individuals, sexual arousal. Emotional distress is thus not only a component of pain but results from pain and can cause further pain; all these facets require the doctor's attention. In part, this helps to explain why drugs such as antidepressants are effective at relieving pain.

No two people's experience of pain is the same, and there are many psychological factors that affect pain. These are summarized in Table 5.6. There is evidence linking levels of pain perception with the opening or closing of the pain gate in the spinal cord. The gate can be opened or closed depending upon the messages received from the brain. This provides a psycho-physiological basis for factors that modulate chronic pain. This is summarized in Table 5.7.

While relatively little is known about the mechanisms involved, the limbic system and in particular, the hypothalamic–pituitary–adrenal axis that is involved in the stress response, have been implicated. Dysfunction of this pathway has been implicated in some chronic pain conditions such as arthritis and fibromyalgia.

Table 5.6 Psychological factors influencing pain responses

Prior experience

Cognitive appraisal (meaning of pain)

Mental attitude e.g. fear, anxiety, stress

Cultural beliefs

Personality (neuroticism or extroversion)

Coping strategies (attention, distraction, biofeedback)

Medication

Sex differences

Table 5.7 Factors that regulate spinal gate control

	Gate open	Gate closed
Physiological	C/Aδ fibres active	Aβ fibres active
Medical	Extent of injury Insufficient medication	Sufficient medication
Cognitive	Focus on pain	Distraction Reinterpretation of pain
Emotional state	Anxiety Fear Stress Depression	Happy, optimistic Relaxed Rested Prior experience of pain
Behavioural: personality	Introvert	Extrovert

Identification of factors that help reduce pain perception allows psychological management strategies to be employed in conjunction with pharmacotherapy. These include cognitive-behavioural therapies that change the patient's beliefs and perceptions of pain, educating the patient about their understanding of pain and addressing pain behaviour rather than the pain perception. One important psychological factor is the placebo effect or the expectation that the doctor will make the patient better (Box 5.3). Biofeedback (relaxation) techniques can be used to modify biological aspects of pain that produce changes in physiological parameters, for example, skin temperature and EMG activity have proven beneficial. Similarly, attention and/or distraction strategies that construct a separate image or reinterpret the pain can be very effective at reducing perceived pain levels.

Measuring pain

Several methods can be used to measure pain. The most common is a medical interview when patients are asked to use a rating scale. These scales range from verbal rating scores to visual analogue scales and box scales (Fig. 5.7) and the McGill Pain Questionnaire that consists of 78 adjectives organized into 20 groups based on similarities

Box 5.3 — The placebo effect

Placebo is Latin for 'I shall please'. Its main use is as a control to test the efficacy of new drugs in clinical conditions. Placebos can be pills, injections or even surgical procedures, and the patient who receives one believes that they have been given the 'good drug' that will alleviate their symptoms. In this regard, the placebo can be a powerful analgesic but there is great variability in patient responses. The biochemical basis and mechanism of action of placebos remain unclear. Several hypotheses have been suggested to account for its actions. Firstly, that it reduces pain perception by reducing anxiety levels. Secondly, that expectancy can account for the observed changes. Lastly, that the placebo effect is a case of Pavlovian conditioning, whereby association with the drug induces positive emotional responses. The placebo effect does have a physiological basis, as its analgesic effect can be antagonized by the opioid antagonist naloxone. Recent research suggests that the placebo effect can activate the dopaminergic reward system. Thus, the suggestion or belief that a treatment will work is enough to cause the release of endogenous opioids that may activate anti-nociceptive mechanisms and other neurotransmitters such as dopamine. The placebo response may also play a role in other alternative medical treatments such as hypnotherapy and acupuncture.

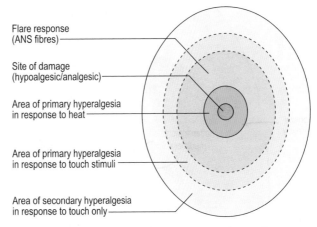

Fig. 5.8 Areas of analgesia flare, and primary and secondary hyperalgesia to different stimuli, after tissue injury. *ANS*, Autonomic nervous system.

response to pain such as grimacing, vocalization, limping etc. Lastly, there are physiological measures, such as changes in threshold for activation, autonomic activity changes (heart rate, skin temperature), or evoked potentials from reflex activity. Imaging techniques can also be used to measure changes in brain activity in patients in pain.

Pain mechanisms after tissue damage: peripheral and central sensitization

Normally, nociceptors require intense stimuli to activate them. However, pain sensation does not follow the firing pattern of nociceptors in a simple, predictable fashion. The central processing of this input in terms of summation of afferent input and inhibitory interactions is very important.

Peripheral tissue injury produces two types of change within the nervous system: *peripheral sensitization*, which is manifest as a reduction in the threshold for nociceptor activation, and *central sensitization*, an activity-dependent increase in the excitability of CNS neurons. Together they contribute to the post-injury hypersensitivity that is common in chronic pain syndromes.

Peripheral injury induces a decreased pain threshold at the site of injury, coupled with a variable loss of sensory input directly at the site of injury and in the surrounding tissue. The former is the area of primary hyperalgesia and is responsive to both thermal and mechanical stimuli, and is mediated by C fibres, while the latter is the area of secondary hyperalgesia that is only responsive to mechanical stimuli and is mediated by Aβ fibres. In addition, a flare response (reddening of the skin) due to activation of the sympathetic axons occurs, causing release of neuroactive substances that may potentiate the sensitization process (Fig. 5.8).

Much has been learned about the molecular mechanisms of peripheral sensitization after focal nerve or inflammatory injury. This is summarized in Fig. 5.9.

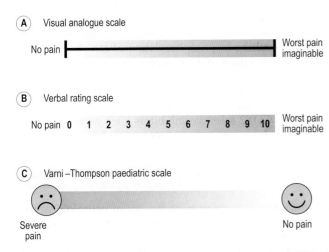

Fig. 5.7 Psychological evaluation of pain using rating scales. (A) Visual analogue scale where the patient marks a point along a line indicating their pain level. (B) Verbal rating scale where the patient rates the score on a scale of 0–10 where 0 is no pain and 10 is the worst pain imaginable. (C) Paediatric pain scale using smiley or sad faces to indicate the level of pain.

in pain quality. It offers the patient the opportunity to describe their pain using emotional and sensory descriptors. A pain rating is based on the scale value of the words, and the patient's personal interpretation of the pain is also considered. Non-verbal scales use behavioural assessments based on stereotypical behaviours in

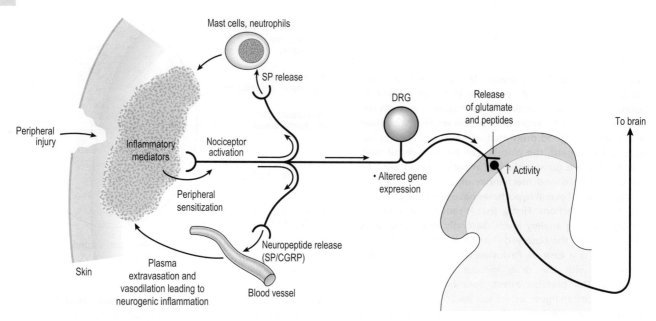

Fig. 5.9 Mechanisms of peripheral sensitization. Peripheral injury results in the creation of an acidic inflammatory 'soup' containing peptides, histamine, bradykinin, protons, adenosine, cytokines, serotonin and prostaglandins. These excite the appropriate receptors on the nociceptors causing activation of protein kinase A and C, leading to phosphorylation of various ion channels and receptors. This results in a lowering of the activation threshold and the excitability of the membrane increases. A secondary consequence of nociceptor activation is the induction of neurogenic inflammation, caused by the release of neuropeptides causing vasodilation and plasma extravasation of proteins from the blood stream, and activation of non-neuronal cells which in turn contribute substances to the inflammatory 'soup'. *CGRP,* Calcitonin gene-related peptide; *DRG,* dorsal root ganglion; *SP,* substance P.

Tissue damage leads to the production of an inflammatory 'chemical soup' that activates the various receptors on nociceptors (see Table 5.4). This leads to alterations in signal transduction sensitivity and also a change in the distribution of receptors, with down-regulation of some and upregulation of others. Primary hyperalgesia is mediated by a lowering of the activation threshold of sensitized Aδ and C fibres. It is thought that the major function of NSAIDs is to prevent peripheral sensitization by inhibiting prostaglandin production, an effect achieved by blocking the action of the enzyme cyclooxygenase (COX).

Peripheral sensitization induces a nociceptive afferent barrage that triggers excitability changes in spinal cord neurons, a response that outlasts the stimulus input. These changes are manifest as changes in RF size, lowered threshold for activation and increased responsiveness, as a direct result of the recruitment of previously subthreshold inputs. Central sensitization is responsible for the secondary hyperalgesia seen after injury. The input from Aβ fibres produces pain by changes in the sensory processing by spinal cord neurons and not by changes in the threshold for activation.

The molecular mechanisms of central sensitization are well understood. Noxious stimuli cause the release of the fast excitatory transmitter glutamate that acts at ionotropic (α-amino-3-hydroxy-5-methyl-4-isoxazolepropionic acid (AMPA), N-methyl-D aspartate (NMDA)) and metabotropic glutamate receptors. Neuropeptides such as substance P are co-released, which produce a slow, progressive, excitatory potential that gives the afferent the opportunity

to produce progressively increased response in neurons when repeatedly activated, due to summation of these slow potentials. They activate second messenger cascades to produce increased intra-cellular calcium levels that depolarize the cell, resulting in phosphorylation of ion channels and receptors, alteration of gene expression, and upregulation of molecules such as prostaglandins and COX enzymes (Fig. 5.10). Not surprisingly, central sensitization can be prevented by drugs that target the NMDA receptor such as ketamine, COX2 selective inhibitors such as rofecoxib, or neuropeptide receptor antagonists such as NK[1] antagonists.

Neuropathic pain mechanisms

Chronic pain is a common symptom of neurological disease, and current pharmacotherapy strategies remain far from satisfactory. This is partly due to the fact that the pathophysiological mechanisms of pain remain incompletely understood. Neuropathic pain can be caused by a variety of insults (Table 5.8) and classified by site of origin (Table 5.9) or response to drug treatments. Recently, clinicians and scientists have begun to address the mechanisms involved in different types of pain. An example of this is the neuropathic pain that occurs in peripheral neuropathy induced by partial nerve damage. This causes a cascade of changes at different sites along the damaged nerve and at the first synapse in the spinal cord that lead to the generation of spontaneous (stimulus-independent) pain or evoked (stimulus-dependent) pain (Fig. 5.11).

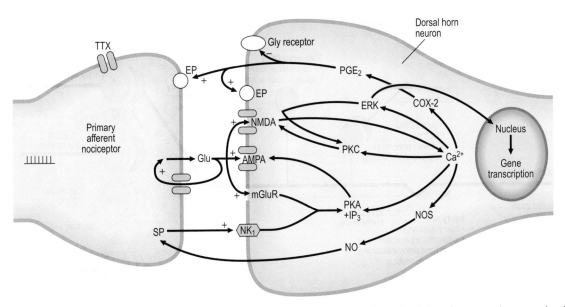

Fig. 5.10 Molecular mechanisms of central sensitization. Prolonged activation of nociceptors results in stimulation of postsynaptic neurons by glutamate and neuropeptide release, leading to activation of multiple signalling pathways that result in the phosphorylation of AMPA and NMDA receptors, leading to central sensitization by lowering the threshold for activation so that subthreshold inputs become suprathreshold and produce action potentials. Cells can regulate their own activity and that of the primary afferent by release of prostaglandin E_2 (PGE_2) and nitric oxide (NO). *AMPA* and *NMDA* (α-amino-3-hydroxy-5-methyl-4-isoxazolepropionic acid and N-methyl-D-aspartate), Ionotropic glutamate receptors; *COX-2*, inducible isoform 2 of cyclo-oxygenase; *EP*, prostaglandin receptor; *ERK*, extracellular signal-regulated kinases; *Gly*, glycine receptor; *IP₃*, inositol triphosphate; *mGluR*, metabotropic glutamate receptors; *NK₁*, neurokinin receptors; *NOS*, nitric oxide synthase; *PKA*, protein kinase A; *PKC*, protein kinase C; *TTX*, tetrodotoxin-sensitive and tetrodotoxin-insensitive sodium channels.

Table 5.8 Causes of neuropathic pain

Cause	Example
Mechanical trauma	Neuropathy, avulsion
Compression	Disk herniation, carpal tunnel syndrome
Inflammation	Arthritis
Infection	Herpes zoster, syphilis
Toxicity	Cisplatin, taxol, vincristine
Disease	Cancer
Ischaemia	Thalamic syndrome, angina
Metabolic	Diabetes
Immune	HIV, multiple sclerosis
Autonomic	Complex regional pain syndrome

Table 5.9 Classification of some common forms of neuropathic pain by site

Peripheral	Spinal	Brain
Neuropathy	Spinal stroke	Stroke
Amputation	Spinal cord injury	Multiple sclerosis
Nerve injury	Multiple sclerosis	Cancer
Avulsion	Cancer	
Radiculopathy	Syringomyelia	
Trigeminal neuralgia	Arachnoiditis	
Cancer	Syphilis	
Herpes zoster		

Several important nervous system mechanisms have been identified.

Peripheral mechanisms include:

1. Ectopic impulse generation (spontaneous activity) occurs at the site of injury (neuroma) or the spinal ganglion or dorsal roots of injured afferents. Abnormal sodium channel expression or redistribution is thought to be responsible for these changes. The pain quality is described as lancinating or shock-like burning pain.

2. Ephaptic connections (involving interactions generated by electrical fields created by neurons) between injured and uninjured nerve fibres, leading to ectopic discharges in injured fibres evoking spontaneous activity in uninjured ones (i.e. amplifying the central signal).

3. Abnormal chemical sensitivity develops in primary afferents (phenotypic switching) so that they become sensitive to substances they were not responding to prior to injury, such as catecholamines.

Central mechanisms include:

1. Central sensitization of spinal cord cells due to the injury barrage, ongoing spontaneous activity in uninjured and injured axons, or release of neuroactive substances from glial cells.

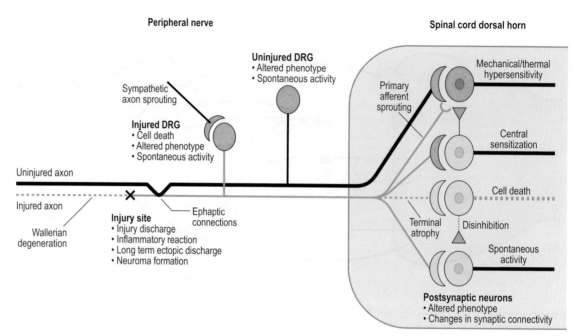

Fig. 5.11 Changes associated with primary afferents after peripheral nerve injury. Axotomy produces a range of effects at distinct sites along the nerve and in the spinal cord that may contribute to pathological pain (see text for further details). *DRG*, Dorsal root ganglion.

2. Disinhibition of spinal cord cells due to afferent cell death, atrophy or decreased supraspinal inhibition, or loss of inhibitory neurotransmitters such as GABA.

3. CNS plasticity in the form of degenerative and regenerative events that result in structural rearrangements of neuronal connections, leading to permanent aberrant connections.

4. Changes at one level of the nervous system leading to subsequent pathophysiological changes at more rostral levels of the neuraxis, for example, thalamus and cortex that can lead to altered sensory perceptions such as phantom limb pain (Box 5.4).

Glial cells and neuropathic pain

Traditionally, the primary role of glial cells is described in terms of neuronal support, especially for their energy demand, as the bioenergetic coupling between neurons and glia (e.g. lactate shuttling and ATP production) is crucial for normal function. However, the past decade has revealed their roles in the development and maintenance of neuropathic pain. Glial cells possess many of the same characteristics as neurons, such as expressing the same receptors and synthesizing and releasing neurotransmitters. Nerve injury and inflammation induce glial cell activation, and recent evidence points to a role for activated glial cells in chronic pain associated with bone cancer and infectious diseases. These conditions change the glia phenotype from having a homeostatic role (described as 'resting') to being a pro-inflammatory phenotype (described

as 'activated'). Once activated, glia produce and release pro-inflammatory cytokines, pro-nociceptive growth factors and prostaglandins that activate pain signalling cascades, disrupt inhibitory circuits and cause neurotoxicity. This also offers another potential avenue for pain control. For example, the drug minocycline, which selectively inhibits activated microglia, is in clinical trials for pain associated with spinal cord injury. Additionally, the expression of specific receptors that can act as biomarkers for these two main glial phenotypes has been identified. Metabolic reprogramming of neurotoxic glial phenotypes by targeting glucose metabolism to modulate their phenotype back toward their normal homeostatic functions may become a future treatment option.

Pharmacology of pain

Pain is a very common symptom that accompanies a variety of pathological states. Therefore analgesia, that is, the relief of pain, is an essential component of many integrated therapeutic strategies. Pain can be acute or chronic, as described in detail above, and its temporal evolution and severity may be unpredictable and pose a real challenge to the clinician. This is exemplified by the case history (see Box 5.1). Unfortunately, at present pain is still managed inadequately in spite of the availability of a wide range of treatments. This inadequacy is due in some instances to the complex nature of pain itself. In other cases, poor pain management is due to misplaced fears as to the adverse effects of analgesics.

The previous review of the pain pathways and of the local circuits involved in nociception and pain shows that multiple neurotransmitter systems, at various levels

Box
5.4
Phantom limb pain

Phantom limb pain occurs in many amputees that suffer a traumatic accident (see Box 5.1). It also occurs in avulsion (i.e. extrusion of nerve roots) injury patients. The sensations occur when an area of the body which is not damaged is touched and elicits pain sensations that feel as though they originate in the amputated region. For example, stroking the face can elicit phantom pain in arm amputees or stimulating the genitalia can elicit phantom pain in lower limb amputees.

For the brain to perceive a phantom it must recognize that a body part is no longer present. This raises the intriguing question of whether the brain has an innate map of the body or if body image is generated from peripheral sensory input. One theory suggests that the brain contains an innate body image—a neural network that is genetically determined but modulated by the environment. If this 'neuromatrix' is deprived of modulating input, it produces an abnormal signature pattern that can result in phantom sensations. This theory can account for phantom sensations in congenital amputees and children, although in these cases the phantoms are rarely painful.

The mechanisms behind phantom limb pain remain incompletely understood but involve plasticity at several levels of the nervous system. This is the remapping hypothesis. Damage to the peripheral nerves causes a deafferentation syndrome (i.e. loss of input). The spontaneous pain is thought to arise from either the nerve neuroma (a disorganised tangle of nerve fibres at the site of nerve damage) or from loss of input to CNS cells causing spontaneous firing in the absence of input. The deafferentation also causes a change in the balance between excitatory and inhibitory inputs to cells. A loss of inhibition leads to an 'unmasking' of preexisting silent synapses of adjacent uninjured nerves that under normal conditions only provide a subthreshold input to cells but are not manifest as part of the normal receptive field. Following injury, these subthreshold inputs become suprathreshold and now evoke action potentials in neurons in response to stimulation of the periphery. The receptive field of such cells in the deafferented spinal cord thus appears to change in response to injury. This remapping procedure occurs at subsequent levels of the brainstem, thalamus and cortex and can be explained in terms of overlap of adjacent afferents from different parts of the body.

The somatosensory and motor cortices contain distorted body maps—the homunculus—for (see Figs. 4.6 and 9.11) sensory input and motor output, respectively. Due to disinhibition of cells caused by the injury, the area of cortex adjacent to the deafferented cortex gradually 'invades' the silent region and

cells become responsive to the new input. In arm amputees, the face somatosensory cortex is adjacent to the arm cortex in the map, and this area now activates the previously arm responsive area of cortex. Thus a stimulus to the face now produces sensations that are perceived as originating from the face and also from the amputated arm (Fig. 5.12). Increased activity from cells in the deafferented motor cortex may be responsible for the cramping-like pain that many patients experience. This is thought to arise because these cells fire impulses to the amputated region but receive no feedback. The strength of the signal increases in order to try to get a response, making the pain worse. Interestingly, clinical studies using electrical motor cortex stimulation or a mirror box to create the illusion of the missing limb, or the use of a prosthetic limb have all been found to reduce the levels of phantom pain in patients.

To conclude, human pain conditions often involve a collection of different mechanisms, often activated concomitantly. Therefore it is unlikely that only one drug can provide relief in complex cases.

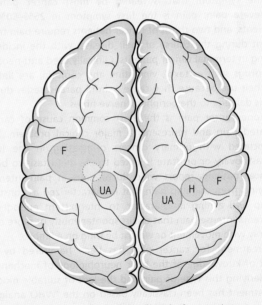

Fig. 5.12 Schematic representation of results from positron emission tomography (PET) studies showing expansion (arrows) of facial somatosensory cortex and upper arm cortical regions into the deafferented hand and forearm cortical regions (dotted circle) following upper limb amputation. On the contralateral side, each limb region has its own distinct cortical representation. *H*, Hand; *F*, face regions of the somatosensory homunculus; *UA*, upper arm.

of the neuraxis, may constitute therapeutic targets in pain management.

Analgesic drugs may affect different aspects of nociception. They may:

- act at the site of injury and decrease the pain associated with inflammatory reactions (e.g. NSAIDs)

- alter nerve conduction (i.e. local anaesthetics)
- modify transmission of nociceptive information in the dorsal horn of the spinal cord (e.g. opioids and antidepressant drugs)
- activate descending inhibitory controls (e.g. opioids)

A general strategy used to control pain is described in the World Health Organization Analgesic Ladder, which was initially introduced in 1986 for patients with cancer pain (Box 5.5). The original ladder has three levels or 'rungs'. On the first rung (i.e. at the first level), aspirin, paracetamol, or other NSAIDs are given to relieve pain. Next, weak opioid drugs can be introduced (such as codeine, tramadol or dextropropoxyphene). Finally, the third rung is represented by strong opioids such as morphine, hydromorphone, fentanyl, buprenorphine and methadone. Other non-opioid drugs can be used in combination with opioids in order to potentiate the pain-relieving effects. This 3-step gradual approach was based on the use of the two main categories of analgesic drugs: non-opioid and opioid drugs. Pain specialists have proposed an update to this, to include a fourth rung (Table 5.10) because of the need for integrating non-pharmacological treatments. The updated ladder focuses on the quality of life and is bidirectional, extending its usefulness to treat acute pain in that the strongest analgesic required can be scaled up or down, according to the intensity described by the patient. However, for chronic pain, the ascending step-wise approach from bottom to top continues.

Box 5.5 Cancer pain

In the UK the likelihood of developing cancer is now more than one in three, and one in four will die from the disease. Cancer mainly affects the elderly, with 65% of cases occurring in those aged over 65 years.

The symptom that is feared by most cancer patients is severe pain; pain is the first symptom in 25%–50% of patients, and two-thirds of cancer patients require pain treatment during the course of their disease, with the incidence rising in terminal cancer patients. Clinically used anti-neoplastic drugs such as taxol, vincristine and cisplatin, are limited in their use because they cause painful paraesthesias due to toxic damage to the peripheral nerve fibres.

Bone cancer pain is the most common cause of cancer-related pain and represents a major clinical problem. Pain associated with primary cancers originating in the lung, breast, ovary or prostate is linked to the metastasis to bone. Cancer patients report wide fluctuations in pain intensity, varying from ongoing pain that is characterized as constant, deep and aching in character, to intermittent episodes of extreme intense pain that occurs spontaneously or more commonly with movement or weight bearing on a limb.

Treatment for cancer pain has been hampered by the lack of knowledge of the basic neurobiology of mechanisms underlying this type of pain and the lack of suitable models. Treatment has been classically based on the 'WHO analgesic ladder', starting with NSAIDs, followed by weak opioids such as codeine and then strong opioid drugs such as morphine (see Table 5.10). However, the efficacy of such drugs is rather limited and they have many unwanted effects. Although cancer pain is treated with opioids to provide round-the-clock analgesia, patients often suffer from 'breakthrough' pain while taking the analgesic medication. Some opioid drug formulations, e.g. ACTIQ® (oral transmucosal fentanyl citrate), have been approved specifically for breakthrough pain. ACTIQ dissolves through the mucous membranes in the mouth and provides rapid pain relief within 5–10 min. Patients find the drug easy to use and effective and they tolerate it well.

Breakthroughs in the understanding of cancer pain mechanisms have arisen with the advent of animal models of bone cancer pain that closely model the human condition. In these models, pain severity is directly related to bone degeneration. Pain is thought to be due to tumour cells releasing cytokines and growth factors that activate T cells and osteoclasts. Osteoclast activity can be controlled by a molecule called osteoprotegerin ligand (OPGL), also known as receptor activator of nuclear factor kappa-B ligand (RANKL), whose receptor is found on osteoclasts. Bone resorption can be blocked by a naturally secreted decoy receptor called osteoprotegerin (OPG), which binds to OPGL and prevents the activation of osteoclasts. Treatment with OPG prevents bone destruction and the secondary associated spinal cord changes and, most importantly, it significantly reduces the breakthrough pain. Bisphosphonates (e.g. zoledronic acid) are another example of drug class that could be used: they induce osteoclast apoptosis. Finally, another approach involves the use of denosumab—a monoclonal antibody that inhibits RANKL and leads to loss of osteoclasts. All these approaches lead to some relief of pain. Bone degeneration is also associated with the release of inflammatory mediators and lowered extracellular pH that lead to the activation and sensitization of bone periosteum primary afferents. This is coupled with neurochemical changes in the spinal cord, particularly increased glial cell activation. Glial cells are known to regulate excitatory amino acid levels and activated cells are also a source of cytokines and growth factors that will alter the surrounding neuronal microenvironment. Ultimately, all these changes lead to the induction of central sensitization, which contributes to pain maintenance.

Table 5.10 Proposed change to the WHO Analgesic Ladder

1. Non-opioid analgesics; if pain persists or increases
2. Weak opioids and non-opioids; if pain persists or increases
3. Strong opioids and non-opioids; if pain persists or increases
4. Invasive and minimally invasive treatments e.g. epidural anaesthesia, PCA pumps, neuromodulation techniques e.g. spinal cord or deep brain stimulation, ablative surgery

PCA, Patient-controlled analgesia.

Opioid receptors and ligands

The terms 'opioid' and 'opiate' are often used interchangeably, although they have a different meaning. 'Opiate' means that a substance is extracted from opium or is similar in structure to natural substances present in opium. Opium is the dried exudate obtained from unripe seedpods of the poppy *Papaver somniferum* and contains morphine, codeine and other alkaloid substances. 'Opioid' is a term that designates substances that are not derived from opium. It refers particularly to opioid peptides, that is, endogenous compounds that bind to opioid receptors and mimic the effect of morphine-like compounds. This term is now used to designate all agents that act on opioid receptors. Morphine, the prototype opioid drug, has been used for many centuries (Box 5.6).

Opioids and opiates bind to opioid receptors, which are G-protein coupled receptors. Three main receptor types have been identified: mu (μ) receptors, divided into the splice variants μ_1, μ_2 and μ_3; delta (δ) receptors, divided into δ_1 and δ_2; and kappa (κ) receptors, divided into κ_1, κ_2 and κ_3 (although for the κ type the receptor subtypes may arise from interaction of a single protein with different membrane associated proteins).

Opioid substances that act as agonists at opioid receptors often have limited selectivity for a given receptor type. Administered systemically, opioid agonists induce a host of effects, which include analgesia. This complex effect profile is a direct consequence of the widespread distribution of opioid receptors in the brain and spinal cord, and also at the periphery. The activation of each main type of opioid receptor can be associated with certain predominant effects, as illustrated in Table 5.11. Although opioid agonists, in particular at mu receptors, can induce significant analgesia, their use is always associated with unwanted effects, some of which may become life threatening, such as respiratory depression. The most prescribed opioid drugs (e.g. morphine, fentanyl, codeine), discussed below, preferentially target the mu opioid receptors. Substances targeting these receptors are responsible for the induction of analgesia and of almost all prototypic opioid unwanted effects such as euphoria, mental clouding, sedation, respiratory depression and cough suppression, pupillary miosis, urinary retention, nausea and vomiting, bradycardia and vasodilation, constipation and histamine release. Opioid agonists reduce neuronal excitability by increasing potassium conductance and can also inhibit neurotransmitter release by decreasing calcium influx that is required for exocytosis.

A range of opioid agonists, partial agonists and also opiate antagonists is available in the clinic. These drugs have unique pharmacokinetic and pharmacodynamic characteristics, as discussed below. The choice of opioid drug used in a patient ideally should take into account all these characteristics but in reality is also influenced by the individual patient response to a particular drug.

Box 5.6 Opium—a trail that goes back to the beginning of medical history

Opium has been known to mankind for millennia. Egyptian papyri mention its medical uses and the Sumerians describe the poppy as 'the plant of joy'. Preparations based on opium extracts have been used to treat cough and diarrhoea. In parallel to this, many cultures have become aware of the addictive properties of opium.

The effects of morphine prompted a search for specific receptors, which culminated with the discovery of opiate receptors in 1973. This discovery was followed in 1975 by the identification of the first endogenous opioid peptides, the enkephalins. All the endogenous opioid substances discovered so far are peptides. Opioid peptides are produced following the general pattern of synthesis of neuropeptides. They are synthesized as part of large protein precursors that undergo extensive posttranslational maturation and, after proteolytic cleavage, release the bioactive peptides.

The three main types of peptides, i.e. the enkephalins, dynorphins and β-endorphin, derive from three different precursors.

- Proopiomelanocortin is the protein precursor of endorphin. Cells expressing this gene are concentrated in the arcuate nucleus of the hypothalamus and β-endorphin projections innervate extensively other hypothalamic nuclei, limbic structures and the raphe nuclei.
- Proenkephalin is the precursor of enkephalins. This precursor is expressed predominantly in interneurons.
- Prodynorphin is the precursor of dynorphins and neoendorphins. Cells expressing the precursor are present in several brain areas, particularly areas involved in nociception, and also in the spinal cord.

Nociceptin/orphanin FQ and nocistatin are opioid-related peptides that are synthesized as part of the orphanin FQ/nociceptin protein precursor. As their name suggests, their effects on nociception appear to be mutually antagonistic. Nociceptin binds to the ORL1 receptor, which shows overall 60% homology with the three main opioid receptor types. Nociceptin can induce strong nociception, whereas nocistatin blocks these effects and has analgesic properties.

Endomorphin-1 and endomorphin-2 are two more additions to the large opioid peptide family. These short peptides have very high affinity and selectivity for mu opioid receptors. Endomorphin-1 appears to be more widely distributed within the brain than endomorphin-2, whereas the latter is more prevalent in the spinal cord.

Table 5.11 Effects associated with the stimulation of opioid receptor subtypes

Effects	Mu receptors	Delta receptors	Kappa receptors
Analgesia			
Supraspinal	+++	+/–	–
Spinal	++	++	+
Respiratory depression	+++	++	+
Pupillary constriction	++	–	–
Reduced gastrointestinal motility	++	++	+
Sedation	++	–	++
Euphoria	++	–	–
Dysphoria	–	–	+++
Dependence	+++	–	+/–

+++, Strong effect; +, weak effect; –, no effect.

Opioid analgesic drugs

Morphine is still the gold standard against which other opioid analgesics are compared. It can be administered via oral, intravenous, intramuscular, or subcutaneous routes. Slow-release preparations are also available. The drug undergoes significant first pass metabolism, so only a small fraction reaches systemic circulation after oral administration. One of the metabolites, morphine-6-glucuronide, is biologically active and induces significant analgesia. The administration of morphine leads to pain alleviation but also to respiratory depression, nausea and vomiting, constipation, sedation, pupillary constriction ('pin-point' pupil) and histamine release. The metabolite morphine 6-glucuronide can accumulate in patients whose renal function is impaired, which increases the risk of respiratory depression.

Heroin (diamorphine) is a prodrug, which is metabolized to morphine (which is ultimately responsible for its effects). Heroin is more lipid soluble than morphine, therefore the effect after intramuscular administration has a more rapid onset. Its properties make it particularly suitable for epidural administration to relieve post-operative pain after major surgery. Its higher solubility also constitutes an advantage for subcutaneous infusion.

Codeine is an analgesic with lower efficacy than morphine (~20% of the potency of morphine). Its analgesic effect is due to demethylation in the liver to morphine. It may be used in combination with aspirin or paracetamol, and it also has a significant anti-tussive (suppression of cough) effect. Like morphine, it induces constipation.

Pethidine is a synthetic substance that is more sedative and has a more rapid onset and a shorter duration of action than morphine. Its metabolite, norpethidine, is active and may accumulate to toxic levels in patients

with renal impairment. Its potency is 1/10th of that of morphine.

Methadone is a synthetic compound with a half-life of 24–30 h. It has significantly higher bioavailability than morphine after oral administration (~80% vs 25%–30% for morphine) and lacks active metabolites. Methadone has activity at the mu opioid receptor; it also inhibits 5-HT reuptake and is an antagonist at NMDA glutamate receptors. It leads to a much milder physical abstinence syndrome than morphine but can induce psychological dependence. Methadone is routinely used in maintenance programs for morphine and heroin addicts.

Fentanyl is a highly potent compound with a half-life of 1–2 h. Fentanyl and related compounds (alfentanil, remifentanil) can be given before or during induction of general anaesthesia. The initial dose can be followed by a prolonged infusion during the surgical procedure. Fentanyl formulations are also used to treat breakthrough cancer pain (see Box 5.5).

Buprenorphine is a very lipid soluble compound, which acts as a partial agonist at mu receptors. It is a potent compound (50 times more potent than morphine) but has less efficacy than morphine. Consequently, it may lead to a re-emergence of pain in patients who have received opioids with higher efficacy such as morphine. It can be used sublingually, and it has a longer duration of action than morphine but is more emetic. It may induce dysphoria and sedation.

Tramadol is an atypical opioid that possesses antinociceptive and anti-hyperalgesic properties. It is an attractive alternative to traditional opioid analgesics because of its improved side effect profile, reduced abuse potential and lack of tolerance and dependence. Tramadol is effective in a broad range of moderate-to-severe types of pain. It acts weakly at mu receptors itself but its metabolite desmetramadol has high affinity for the receptors; tramadol also interacts with monoaminergic systems by blocking 5-HT and noradrenaline reuptake (but less effectively than tricyclic antidepressants).

Opioid antagonists

The opioid antagonist naloxone is used to reverse the effects of opioid agonists. Naloxone is used in the management of opioid overdose or to relieve respiratory depression in apnoeic infants after opioid administration (e.g. pethidine) to the mother during labour. The half-life of naloxone is short (<1 h), therefore repeated injections may be required before reversal of the effect of an agonist (which may have a much longer half-life than naloxone) is achieved.

Important clinical issues in the use of opioid drugs

The use of opioids in the clinic is associated with concerns about tolerance, dependence and addiction, and also other risks posed by the numerous unwanted effects of these compounds.

Tolerance and dependence

Tolerance (i.e. the necessity to increase the dose in order to achieve the same effect) may develop during chronic administration of drugs, and it may be due to both pharmacokinetic and pharmacodynamic changes. Tolerance to opioids can develop rapidly, especially under experimental conditions, when doses are increased steeply. Physical and psychological dependence may also develop. Physical dependence is associated with a withdrawal syndrome when the administration of the drug is stopped abruptly. Psychological dependence leads to craving for the drug. However, it is very important to note that the real risk of tolerance to and dependence on opioids should be assessed during use of opioid drugs in a clinical context. The concept of tolerance can often be misused in pain management, to simply mean the requirement for a higher dose. This only reflects tolerance if the pain has not increased! For example, in pain associated with cancer, the reason for increasing the dose is usually an increase in the pain. Patients can often be maintained on the same oral morphine dosage for months, with no obvious signs of tolerance. Therefore when opioid analgesics are used in appropriate doses to treat pain that is sensitive to such drugs, tolerance is not a prevalent problem associated with chronic opioid drugs. The risk of development of addiction when opioids are used judiciously for the relief of pain is low. However, it is important to note that massively increasing the opioid prescription in the United States led to 30,000 deaths due to opioid overdoses in 2015 alone, therefore there is new concern worldwide about the consequences of misuse of opioids.

Risks associated with the unwanted effects of opioids

The under-use of opioids is sometimes justified by the fear of inducing life-threatening respiratory depression. However, the respiratory depression induced by opioids tends to be short-lived and is often antagonized by the pain. Other unwanted effects of opiates, such as nausea and sedation, may dissipate with prolonged use. If strong opioids are required in a patient, the acceptability of the medication and the patient's response may be much improved by the concomitant management of side effects. For example, if tolerance to nausea and vomiting does not develop after a few days, administration of antiemetic compounds is required (sometimes a combination of such drugs). Pharmacological management may thus become more complex but ultimately provide the patient with a pain-free state.

Mode of administration of opioids

Analgesic drugs are available in a variety of formulations, and the versatility of modes of administration is well illustrated by opioids. As discussed below, each mode of administration has its advantages and drawbacks.

- Oral administration. This is a widely used route and one that most patients prefer. However, it may not always be available (e.g. immediately after surgery), or it can be made difficult by swallowing problems. The occurrence of vomiting will limit the absorption of drugs administered via this route. Furthermore, delays in gastric emptying may also decrease absorption of an orally administered opioid. Even if the drug is absorbed, the metabolism in the gut and liver (first pass metabolism effect) may lead to reduced bioavailability of the drug using this route.

- Sublingual administration. This avoids the first pass metabolism, as absorption of the drug occurs directly into the circulation.

- Rectal administration. First pass metabolism can also be avoided using the rectal route, if acceptable to the patient. Absorption of the drug is slow, but bioavailability is improved overall. It is a mode of administration that can be considered for maintenance of analgesia.

- Intravenous administration. The administration of a bolus of opioids by this route leads to immediate analgesia. However, this route has a higher risk of over-dosage, and the patients must not be left unsupervised for a long time.

- Intramuscular administration. Intermittent intramuscular administration of opioids (e.g. on a 4-hourly basis) is still a standard procedure used worldwide. Pain relief can be achieved satisfactorily but its maintenance at an optimum level requires regular assessment. In addition, repeated injections are painful and the control and adjustment of the doses may not be easy.

- Intrathecal and epidural administration. These techniques allow the use of much lower doses of opioids through spinal catheters. However, side effects do still occur, such as nausea, vomiting and urinary retention, as well as a risk of respiratory depression. Furthermore, local infection or displacement of the catheter may occur.

- Transdermal patch administration. This is a non-invasive mode of administration of the drug and is particularly suitable for lipophilic and potent compounds (e.g. fentanyl).

Clinical experience clearly shows that the patient's response to opioids varies significantly. Ideally, these individual requirements should be taken into account, and this is what the procedure called patient-controlled analgesia (PCA) is achieving today in many centres. PCA relies on a system whereby the patient can administer their own analgesic according to their needs and to the severity of their pain. The patient can administer intermittent boluses of the drug, which is delivered through a catheter, from a lockable programmable pump. The placement of the catheter can be intravenous, intramuscular, subcutaneous, or even epidural. A minimum time period between doses (the 'lock-out' period), as well as a maximum dose of the chosen opioid can be programmed into the PCA device, thus preventing overdose. Experience shows that patients using PCA titrate their analgesia to the point where they are comfortable, without excess demands. The feeling of control over their pain significantly improves the patient's outlook on their condition. Children may use a PCA device with the help of a parent or nurse.

Pain sensitivity to opioids

Different types of pain are differentially sensitive to opioid treatments. Some, such as deafferention pain or muscle spasms, are insensitive to opioid drugs; nerve or CNS compression injury or bone cancer are partially sensitive to opioids, while acute pain, post surgical pain and pain associated with myocardial infarction or other types of cancers can be readily treated with opioids. Lastly, there are some conditions such as irritable bowel syndrome that are opioid sensitive, but opioid consumption is associated with many problems, for example, vomiting, constipation and increased gastrointestinal symptom severity, and a decreased quality of life.

Non-opioid analgesics

NSAIDs represent the most commonly used group of drugs worldwide, most of which are available without prescription. There is significant variability in patient tolerance and response to these drugs. They are mainly used to treat mild or moderate pain, in general associated with inflammatory processes (e.g. rheumatoid arthritis and osteoarthritis). NSAIDs can also be used to treat the severe pain associated with bone metastasis in cancer. The analgesic/antipyretic/anti-inflammatory effects of NSAIDs are largely due to inhibition of COX enzymes and the resulting inhibition of the synthesis of prostaglandins, which are pro-inflammatory. COX has two isoforms: COX-1 and COX-2. COX-1 is a constitutive enzyme, whereas COX-2 is induced at sites of inflammation. Aspirin, paracetamol, ibuprofen and diclofenac are non-selective COX inhibitors. It is the inhibition of COX-1 that underlies the majority of unwanted effects of NSAIDs, such as dizziness, drowsiness and gastrointestinal irritation and bleeding. Nephrotoxicity is due to actions on the constitutively expressed COX-2 enzyme in the kidney. In the stomach, the prostaglandins PGE_2 and PGI_2 inhibit acid secretion and have a gastroprotective action, whereas in the kidney PGE_2 and PGI_2 act as local vasodilators. Therefore, inhibition of their synthesis reduces renal blood flow and may precipitate acute renal failure. In addition,

the prolonged use of non-selective NSAIDs is associated with risk of chronic renal failure due to development of interstitial nephritis. All NSAIDs also have antiplatelet activity, leading to increased bleeding time. More recently, selective COX-2 inhibitors such as rofecoxib and celecoxib have become available. These compounds have similar analgesic efficacy to non-selective COX inhibitors but lack their risk of inducing ulceration and could be used in the treatment of osteo- and rheumatoid arthritis and dental pain. However, following their development it soon became apparent that their use is associated with a very high risk of heart attacks and stroke.

Commonly used NSAIDs include:

- Aspirin (acetylsalicyclic acid) is analgesic, anti-inflammatory and antipyretic. This is due to the irreversible inhibition of the COX enzyme. COX is required for prostaglandin and thromboxane synthesis, peripherally at the site of injury. Aspirin acts as an acetylating agent, that is, an acetyl group is covalently attached to a serine residue in the active site of the COX enzyme. This makes aspirin different from other NSAIDs (such as diclofenac and ibuprofen), which are reversible inhibitors. It is unclear whether the effect of aspirin also has a central component. Aspirin-containing preparations should not be given to children under 12 years because of the risk of development of Reye's syndrome.

- Paracetamol (acetaminophen) is antipyretic and analgesic but with negligible anti-inflammatory effects (so, technically, it is not a NSAID). It is well absorbed after oral administration and does not irritate the gastric mucosa. It was suggested that paracetamol may act as inhibitor of COX-3, a splice-variant of COX-1, but this is now rejected. There is considerable evidence that its analgesic effects are due to activation of descending serotonergic pathways but its primary site of action may still be inhibition of PG synthesis, although this is not associated with an anti-inflammatory action. Its mode of action remains unclear but recent evidence indicates that paracetamol inhibits prostaglandin synthesis in cells with low levels and production of peroxide. At peripheral sites of inflammation with a high peroxide level, its effect may be inhibited. Another suggested mechanism involves the paracetamol metabolite AM404, which is a weak agonist of the cannabinoid receptors CB_1 and CB_2 and a potent activator of the $TRPV_1$ receptor. This suggests that the cannabinoid and $TRPV_1$ signalling pathways play important roles in the analgesic effects of paracetamol. The prolonged use of paracetamol and the ingestion of high doses are associated with significant risk of hepatotoxicity. Paracetamol overdose is treated with N-acetylcysteine.

- Ibuprofen has analgesic and anti-inflammatory properties. Among the non-selective NSAIDs, it is one of the drugs of choice because it is effective and has a relatively low side effect profile. Like other NSAIDs, its mechanism of action is principally through COX-2 inhibition. Alternatives to ibuprofen are: diclofenac, naproxen, piroxicam, ketorolac, indomethacin and mefenamic acid.

Other approaches to pain management

Some types of pain do not respond to either opioid analgesics or NSAIDs, nor can they be managed based only on the principles underlying the World Health Organization Analgesic Ladder. Examples of such types of pain are given below, including their pharmacological management.

Neuropathic pain

Neuropathic pain appears relatively insensitive to opioids. It can be significantly relieved with tricyclic antidepressants (e.g. amitriptyline), anticonvulsant agents (e.g. carbamazepine) or local anaesthetics (Box 5.7). The reason for this diversity of treatment is the pathophysiology of neuropathic pain, which is complex and still incompletely defined (see above). It is well established that neuropathic pain involves changes in the phenotype of the neurons that are part of nociception pathways and also morphological changes within the grey matter of the dorsal horn.

Three commonly prescribed drugs for chronic neuropathic pain associated with diseases such as peripheral (e.g. diabetic) neuropathy, post herpetic neuralgia and fibromyalgia are gabapentin, its analogue pregabalin and duloxetine. Gabapentin was initially developed as a GABA agonist but its mechanism of action is still not fully defined. Research indicates that it binds with high affinity to the $\alpha_2\delta$-1 subunit of voltage-dependent calcium channels and therefore inhibits calcium influx through L and P/Q channels. It also reduces potassium evoked glutamate release and is an agonist at $GABA_B$ receptors. Pregabalin is related in structure to gabapentin and is more potent. It also binds to the $\alpha_2\delta$-2 subunit of the voltage-dependent calcium channel. Pregabalin decreases the release of neurotransmitters such as glutamate, noradrenaline and substance P. Common adverse effects of both include diarrhoea, dizziness, drowsiness and peripheral oedema. Duloxetine is an antidepressant drug that is a selective serotonin and noradrenaline reuptake inhibitor, approved for use in diabetic neuropathy.

Migraine

Pain can affect specifically the craniofacial area. The most common form of this type of pain is generically termed

| Box 5.7 | Local anaesthetics and sodium channels |

Local anaesthetics (e.g. lidocaine, bupivacaine, prilocaine, ropivacaine, tetracaine) are agents which block the initiation and propagation of nerve action potentials by blocking Na^+ channels. Their mode of administration varies with surface anaesthesia, infiltration, spinal or epidural anaesthesia. They are generally used for pain associated with localized surgery, childbirth or in dentistry. A problem associated with local anaesthetics is the risk of systemic toxicity (e.g. hypotension, bradycardia and respiratory depression). The addition of a vasoconstrictor such as adrenaline to the local anaesthetic decreases local blood flow, slowing the rate of absorption and thus prolonging the anaesthetic effect.

The molecular targets of local anaesthetics are voltage-gated Na^+ channels. These channels are present in both nerve and muscle cells. These channels are also the target of the anticonvulsants phenytoin and carbamazepine and some anti-arrhythmic drugs. The main component of Na^+ channels is the α-subunit which forms the ion pore. In mammalian channels the α-subunit is associated with one or two smaller auxiliary subunits designated β_1 and β_2. Na^+ channels have three distinct conformational states. The transition between these states is voltage-dependent. When the membrane depolarizes the channels revert to an open state that conducts ions. This is followed by a non-conducting, inactivated state. When the membrane is in a hyperpolarized state, most Na^+ channels are in closed, resting states, which represent the third conformational state. The selectivity of local anaesthetics for depolarized Na^+ channels is a consequence of the binding of these drugs to the open and inactivated states that predominate at depolarized membrane potentials. These states may be associated with the highest affinity for these drugs. In contrast, the blockade of the channels by tetrodotoxin (TTX)—a powerful toxin extracted from the puffer fish—is independent of the conformational state of the channel.

'headache'. This simple term is deceptive and does not reflect the complexity of this type of pain disorder. The International Headache Society has developed a detailed classification of these conditions, in the form of the International Classification of Headache Disorders, the latest version being ICHD-3. ICHD-3 classifies headache disorders into: (1) primary headaches; (2) secondary headaches; and (3) neuropathies, facial pains and other headaches.

Migraine is a form of primary headache and is the second most prevalent neurological disorder worldwide. In the Global Burden of Disease assessment of 2015, it ranked as the third highest cause of disability worldwide in adults under the age of 50 years. It affects women more than men. Migraine has a significant prevalence in the young (around 9% of children and adolescents) and is associated with missed school days, poorer performance in education and a negative impact on peer interaction and socialization. Migraine can be episodic (affecting the patient on <15 days per month) or chronic (at least 15 days per month and with the characteristics of a migraine on at least 8 days per month, for longer than 3 months). Misdiagnosis and poor management of migraine are significant public health problems worldwide.

Migraine is a disorder that consists of recurrent attacks of severe headache, autonomic nervous system dysfunction, and in some 20% of patients, an aura involving complex neurological symptoms. The aura symptoms develop over 10–30 min and usually last less than an hour. Symptoms can be visual, sensory, or motor but may also involve language disturbances. When a headache follows, it most often occurs within an hour of the end of the aura. Isolated auras without headache (previously called 'acephalgic migraine' or 'silent migraine') may also occur. The most common aura is visual and may consist of visual distortions. Sensory disturbances involve one side of the body and are characterized by descriptions of numbness or tingling on the face and in the hand. The aura often resolves before the onset of the headache. Some patients may experience a combination of migraine attacks: some attacks associated with an aura, and others without aura. Patients may also experience a prodromal phase, hours or days before the headache. Premonitory phenomena may occur in approximately 60% of migraineurs in this phase. These phenomena include psychological, neurological, constitutional and autonomic features. Psychological symptoms include depression, euphoria, irritability, restlessness, mental slowness, hyperactivity, fatigue and drowsiness. Neurological phenomena include photophobia, phonophobia and hyperosmia. The generalized or constitutional symptoms include a stiff neck, a cold feeling, sluggishness, increased thirst, increased urination, anorexia, diarrhoea, constipation, fluid retention and food cravings. Some patients just report a poorly characterized feeling that they know a migraine attack is coming.

The typical migraine headache is unilateral and throbbing. It may be bilateral and constant at first, and later become throbbing. Nausea occurs in up to 90% of patients, and vomiting occurs in about one-third of migraineurs. During the attack many patients experience intense photophobia, phonophobia and osmophobia and seek seclusion in a dark, quiet room. Other symptoms include blurry vision, diarrhoea, abdominal cramps, polyuria (followed by decreased urinary output after the attack), facial sensations of heat or cold, and sweating. Large population studies have shown that 65%–70% of patients have migraine without aura, approximately 18% have migraine with aura, 13% have both types and the remaining minority can have aura without migraine.

Migraine attacks may last 4–72 h. Different combinations of features may occur between patients or even between attacks in the same patient. It is important to note that tension-type headache (the most common form of primary headache) may sometimes present as a throbbing pain but is devoid of the associated features of migraine. It also presents in general bilaterally. and the pain has in most cases a pressing or tightening quality. These differences are important in terms of diagnosis and treatment of the two conditions.

Migraine attacks are triggered by a variety of factors: endocrine changes (e.g. during pregnancy or the menstrual cycle), sleep excess or deprivation, physical exercise, stress or tiredness. Paradoxically, migraine may emerge at a time when the patient feels relaxed. Intriguingly, even in the same patient, it is impossible to predict the sensitivity to common triggers. It is recommended that migraineurs should have regular habits and a balanced lifestyle.

Migraine is a neurovascular disorder, and its pathophysiology is still incompletely characterized; it is viewed as a condition that is associated with an individual's propensity towards brain hyperexcitability. Migraine may involve a primary dysregulation in primary sensory processing in the nervous system. There is a strong polygenic component and susceptibility loci have been found on several chromosomes, for example, chromosomes 1, 2 and 19, and genes associated with migraine include examples such as CACNA1A, SCN1A and KCNK18/TRESK, which are linked to the function of calcium, sodium and potassium channels. Imaging studies have detected activation of the brain stem during migraine attacks. Migraine is associated with a wave of vasoconstriction followed by reactive vasodilatation. The main elements involved in the generation of pain are: the cranial blood vessels, trigeminal innervation of the vessels, and reflex connections of the trigeminal system with the cranial parasympathetic outflow. Convincing mechanistic explanations have recently been proposed for some of the symptoms of migraine (Box 5.8).

As shown in Fig. 5.13, the input from the trigeminal afferents that innervate the meningeal vessels passes through the trigeminal ganglion and synapses with second-order neurons in the trigeminocervical complex. Second-order neurons project to the thalamus. In the pons there is a connection with neurons in the superior salivatory nucleus, which results in a parasympathetic outflow and is mediated through the pterygopalatine, otic, and carotid ganglia. This trigeminal-autonomic reflex exists in normal individuals and is increased in migraine.

Pain is mainly generated at the level of the cranial vessels or in the dura mater. The innervation involved originates from branches of the ophthalmic division of the trigeminal nerve and also branches of the C2 nerve roots (for structures in the posterior fossa). This explains the distribution of pain over the frontal, temporal, parietal, occipital and high cervical (neck) regions. The pain may involve peripheral or central sensitization processes of craniovascular afferents and the activation of vasodilator mechanism. However, migraine is not primarily caused by a vascular event. It is associated with abnormal neu-

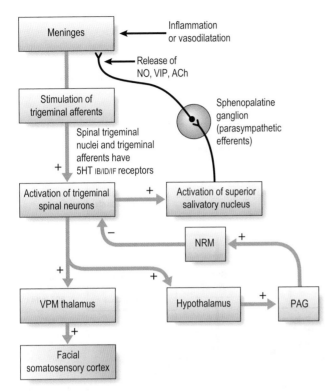

Fig. 5.13 Pathways involved in trigeminovascular activation and pain modulation by serotonin. *Ach*, Acetylcholine; *NO*, nitric oxide; *NRM*, nucleus raphe magnus; *PAG*, periaqueductal grey; *VIP*, vasoactive intestinal polypeptide; *VPM*, ventroposteromedial thalamic nucleus; *5HT*, serotonin; +, excitation.

ronal activity in diencephalic or brain stem nuclei (see Box 5.8).

Evidence accumulated over the last three decades indicates that the neuropeptide calcitonin gene-related peptide (CGRP) has a key role in the pathophysiology of migraine. It is the most abundant neuropeptide in the trigeminal nerve and is expressed in 35%–50% of trigeminal ganglion neurons. Trigeminal activation is associated with CGRP release, which is enhanced during a migraine attack. Very early observations showed that during the attack CGRP serum levels are elevated in the cranial, but not peripheral, circulation indicating an important local effect for this peptide. Successful treatment of a migraine attack concomitantly aborts the pain and the increase in CGRP. The peptide may exert its effects through several different receptors, including the CGRP receptor, calcitonin receptor, amylin receptors, and adrenomedullin receptors. CGRP is expressed in neurons of the cerebral cortex, hippocampus, cerebellum, thalamic and hypothalamic nuclei, and also in brainstem nuclei. At several of these sites there is high expression of the CGRP receptor. The understanding of the crucial role of this peptide has led to the development of new therapeutic agents, as discussed below. Furthermore, recent research suggests that another peptide of interest is the pituitary adenylate cyclase activating polypeptide (PACAP). This peptide exists in two forms—PACAP-27 and PCAP-38—is pres-

ent in the trigeminovascular system and the cranial parasympathetic system, and is co-localized with CGRP. Its release is increased during migraine attacks. The administration of PACAP can trigger the premonitory symptoms of migraine.

Treatment of migraine attacks

The treatment of migraine consists of non-pharmacological and pharmacological approaches. The non-pharmacological strategy consists of the maintenance of a daily routine, which avoids changes in lifestyle and also identifies triggering factors. Pharmacological treatment consists of two strategies: non-specific and migraine-specific treatments.

Non-specific drugs that can be used include aspirin, paracetamol, ibuprofen, diclofenac potassium or other NSAIDs, mild opioids or combination analgesics. These analgesic drugs are also used to treat other types of pain, including tension-type headache—the other major type of primary headache. The administration of drugs that prevent nausea and vomiting (e.g. metoclopramide or prochlorperazine) and are prokinetic, that is, increase gastric motility, increases the efficacy of these drugs. Many migraineurs report a reasonable relief of pain using a combination of mild analgesics. Such combinations may vary, for the same patient, according to the severity of the attack.

Migraine-specific drugs include those that modulate serotonin (5-HT) transmission, that is, the triptan family of drugs and also ergot derivatives. There is ample evidence that 5-HT has a clear link with migraine: very early observations indicated that migraine attacks are associated with increases in the level of the 5-HT metabolite 5-hydroxyindole acetic acid (5-HIAA) and showed that infusion of 5-HT could abort both pharmacologically-induced or spontaneous headaches. The role of 5-HT and some of its receptors is shown in Fig. 5.13.

Ergotamine and dihydroergotamine are ergot derivatives. They bind to at least two receptor classes (adrenergic and 5-HT receptors) and to combinations of different subtypes within these types (e.g. ergotamine binds to 5-HT$_{1A}$, 5-HT$_{1B}$ and 5-HT$_{1D}$ subtypes), and they have complex pharmacodynamics. They induce generalized vasoconstriction, and their use may lead to ergotism—an overuse syndrome—which may include rebound headaches when attempting to stop the drug. These drugs should not be used for the treatment of tension-type headache.

The triptans are a large family of related compounds with a less complex pharmacodynamic profile than the ergot derivatives. Examples of triptans are sumatriptan, almotriptan, eletriptan, frovatriptan, zolmitriptan, naratriptan and rizatriptan. Sumatriptan was the first drug in this category and remains the first choice; it is on the World Health Organisation's List of Essential Medicines. All the triptans have a very similar pharmacodynamic profile. They are 5-HT$_{1B/1D}$ receptor agonists. They can be

Neurobiological mechanisms involved in migraine

Activation of the trigeminovascular system is thought to be responsible for the pain of migraine. The aura symptoms are considered to reflect the onset of cortical spreading depression (CSD). CSD can be triggered by focal activation of the cortex and is more readily seen in the occipital cortex than elsewhere. It is characterized by a slowly propagating wave of strong neuronal depolarization that generates intense neuronal activity, followed by suppressed activity lasting many minutes. This has been confirmed in migraineurs experiencing aura, using blood oxygen level-dependent functional magnetic resonance imaging. CSD produces many changes in the extracellular fluid environment by increasing levels of potassium ions, protons, arachidonic acid (and its prostaglandin metabolites), which can sensitize the meningeal vascular afferents. CSD has also been observed using imaging methods in migraineurs who do not experience aura, but the mechanisms for initiation and propagation of the CSD remain incompletely understood.

An alternative view is that migraine occurs due to dysfunction in brainstem nociceptive circuits such that a defect in pain modulation could result in increased activity in trigeminal neurons making them more susceptible to sensitization (Fig. 5.14).

Identification of mutations in genes that result in defects in ion channels indicates that migraine may be a channelopathy. Most channelopathies are disorders of neuronal excitability, highlighting the importance of activity in the pathogenesis of migraine. In familial hemiplegic migraine there is a defect in the α_1 subunit of P/Q type voltage-gated calcium channels. This channel is expressed in all structures that play an important role in the pathogenesis of migraine. They are known to regulate cortical neuron firing and in mutant mice that are deficient in this gene cortical neurons become hyperactive and may thus contribute to CSD. This channel is also found on cells that regulate the descending inhibitory pain system, and blocking P/Q channels facilitates pain, adding further evi-

dence to dysfunction of brainstem activity being involved in migraine.

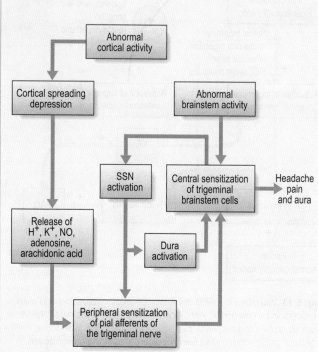

Fig. 5.14 Pathophysiological mechanisms involved in migraine. Abnormal cortical activity leads to cortical spreading depression (CSD) that is the most likely initiating event in stimulating the trigeminal vascular system afferents in migraine. Abnormal activity in trigeminal brainstem neurons involved in the control of facial pain may also contribute to central sensitization of spinal trigeminal neurons (STN) leading to hyperexcitability. When CSD occurs in conjunction with migraine trigger factors, migraine occurs. *SSN*, Superior salivatory nucleus. (Adapted from Pietrobon D, Striessnig J. (2003) Neurobiology of migraine. Nature Reviews Neuroscience 4:386.)

administered non-orally (nasal sprays, suppositories, inhalers, injections). For example, sumatriptan is available in oral, subcutaneous, rectal and intranasal formulations. The oral bioavailability ranges from 14% (sumatriptan) to 69% (almotriptan) or 74% (naratriptan). Triptans have at least three possible sites of action: cranial vasoconstriction (the 5-HT_{1B} component), peripheral neuronal inhibition (the 5-HT_{1D} component) and inhibition of transmission through second-order neurons of the trigeminocervical complex (5-HT_{1B}, 5-HT_{1D} and possibly 5-HT_{1F} component). Triptans remain the 'gold standard' of migraine attack treatment, although their vasoconstrictor profile leads to restricted use in patients with cardiovascular disease. More recently, a 5-HT_{1F} agonist—lasmiditan, a first-in-class drug—has also been introduced for the acute treatment of migraine, but it is associated with a high incidence of adverse events.

The side effects of triptans are tingling, paraesthesias, dizziness, flushing, neck pain, or stiffness. They can constrict coronary arteries, leading to symptoms similar to angina pectoris. Contraindications to use are ischaemic heart disease, hypertension and cerebrovascular disease.

More recently, the extensive characterization of the crucial role of CGRP in migraine pathophysiology has led to the development of the gepants—a new class of drug—which are small molecule antagonists of the CGRP receptor. Ubrogepant and rimegepant were approved in 2019 and 2020, respectively, for the acute treatment of migraine. They prevent vasodilation and can be prescribed especially when the use of triptans is problematic. Gepants are being considered for the prophylaxis of migraine. In parallel, monoclonal antibodies against CGRP (e.g. eptinezumab, fremanezumab) and

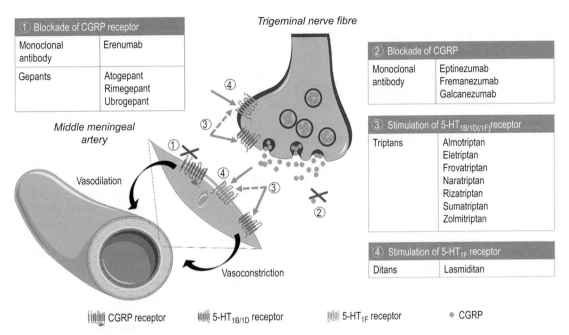

① Blockade of CGRP receptor	
Monoclonal antibody	Erenumab
Gepants	Atogepant Rimegepant Ubrogepant

Middle meningeal artery

Vasodilation

Vasoconstriction

Trigeminal nerve fibre

② Blockade of CGRP	
Monoclonal antibody	Eptinezumab Fremanezumab Galcanezumab

③ Stimulation of 5-HT$_{1B/1D(/1F)}$ receptor	
Triptans	Almotriptan Eletriptan Frovatriptan Naratriptan Rizatriptan Sumatriptan Zolmitriptan

④ Stimulation of 5-HT$_{1F}$ receptor	
Ditans	Lasmiditan

CGRP receptor   5-HT$_{1B/1D}$ receptor   5-HT$_{1F}$ receptor   • CGRP

Fig 5.15 Overview of pharmacological treatment of migraine based on modulation of 5-HT and calcitonin gene-related peptide (CGRP) signalling. (From de Vries T, Villalón CM, MaassenVanDenBrink A. (2020) Pharmacological treatment of migraine: CGRP and 5-HT beyond the triptans. Pharmacology and Therapeutics 211:107528.)

the CGRP receptor (erenumab) have been developed. These are alternatives for the prophylaxis of migraine attacks, but they need to be administered parenterally and their costs are prohibitive for large-scale use, at present.

An overview of treatments focused on 5-HT and CGRP targeting is shown in Fig. 5.15.

Preventive treatment of migraine

If attacks occur at least twice a month, or if there is a clear trend toward an increasing frequency of attacks, preventive treatment may be considered. A variety of drugs belonging to different pharmacological classes can be used as prophylactic treatment. The choice of drug depends on the patient's choice, tolerability and possible interactions with other co-morbidities. All such prophylactic therapies are relatively non-specific and have moderate efficacy and substantial side effects, as illustrated in the examples given below (some of the unwanted effects of the different classes are indicated in parentheses):

- beta-adrenergic receptor agonists—propranolol, metoprolol, atenolol, bisoprolol (tiredness, postural hypotension)
- tricyclic antidepressants—amitriptyline (drowsiness, dry mouth, postural hypotension)
- anticonvulsants—sodium valproate, topiramate (weight gain, hair loss, tremor, hepatotoxicity, teratogenic effects)

- calcium-channel blockers—flunarizine (depression, weight gain, tiredness)
- 5-HT receptor antagonists—pizotifen (drowsiness, weight gain)
- angiotensin II receptor antagonists—candesartan cilexetil (abdominal pain, cough, hypotension)

Overall, novel and better therapeutic targets for the treatment of migraine (acute and chronic) are continuing to emerge from a better understanding of the pathophysiology of migraine, as exemplified by the advent of CGRP-focused interventions and the emergence of PACAP as a new target. PACAP antibodies and antibodies against the PAC$_1$ receptor for PACAP are in development and already being tested in clinical trials.

Finally, it is important to note that there are also non-pharmacological approaches in migraine management, for example, the use of neuromodulation devices. This includes invasive approaches such as deep brain stimulation and occipital nerve stimulation. Other approaches include non-invasive vagus stimulation (e.g. the gamma-Core Saphire is a handheld device which uses set doses of non-invasive stimulation when held onto the skin to either the right or the left branches of the vagus nerve in the neck) or external trigeminal nerve stimulation (e.g. the Cefaly device placed on the forehead) and sphenopalatine neurostimulation. More recently, a remote electrical neuromodulation (REN) device, which involves two surface electrodes set in an armband that stimulate the upper arm peripheral nerves (with the power source being controlled by the patient's smartphone), can trigger a form of central conditioned pain modulation involving the descending pain inhibitory pathways, and has shown promise for the acute treatment of migraine.

Trigeminal neuralgia

Trigeminal neuralgia is characterized by sudden attacks of excruciating pain in the distribution of the trigeminal nerve. It is a condition that has a major impact on the quality of life and ageing increases the risk of developing it. In most cases it affects just one side of the face, mostly the lower part. The pain can be initiated by stimulation of 'trigger zones' (e.g. the cheek, chin or lips), and the attacks can last from seconds to a few minutes. The attacks of pain can be initiated by very ordinary activities, such as washing or brushing the teeth, or eating—mechanical allodynia—such that sufferers do not perform these activities. Attacks may occur many times a day and may last many weeks or months. Some remission may occur but with unpredictable return of the attacks. It is suggested that the cause of this neuralgia is vascular compression (by arteries but also occasionally veins) of the axons of the trigeminal root in the pons. This may be caused by a tumour or an arteriovenous malformation. This may lead to partial focal demyelination, which may alter the electrical activity of trigeminal neurons through ephaptic connections and spontaneous activity.

The first line of treatment of trigeminal neuralgia is pharmacological. The anticonvulsant drug carbamazepine can be used to treat the paroxysmal pain experienced by patients and effectiveness is reported in 60%–80% of cases. Baclofen (a $GABA_B$ receptor agonist) or the anticonvulsants lamotrigine, topiramate, or levetiracetam could also be considered, as well as drugs such as gabapentin or pregabalin. Botulinum toxin injections may be beneficial in some cases. If there is no response or gradual loss of efficacy, surgical procedures could be attempted, such as decompression of the trigeminal nerve root or neuro-ablation via rhizotomy with radiofrequency thermocoagulation. However, there may be recurrence of the pain several years after surgery. Further research is needed to optimize treatment options in trigeminal neuralgia.

Pain in children and in the elderly

A long-held misperception claimed that neonates and young children perceive much less pain than adults because of the immaturity of their central nervous system. This view has been disproven (Box 5.9), and it is clear that the management of pain in children can and should follow the same general principles as those used in adult patients. Young children pose a problem in terms of accurate assessment and rating of their pain, especially when presenting at accident and emergency departments. The use of paediatric rating scales (see Fig. 5.7) can be helpful in categorizing the

---

Box 5.9 Development of pain pathways

The question of whether babies, premature or newborn, feel pain is an important one, as studies show that invasive procedures that would be painful to children or adults are frequently performed on infants admitted to neonatal intensive care units. Premature babies do not 'feel' pain in the truest sense, as pain is a learned experience. However, nociceptive stimuli can have a profound effect on the development of pain pathways.

The newborn nervous system is not a miniature replica of the adult version. Pain-related systems in particular develop during the last trimester and after birth. Much of what we now know about the development of nociceptive systems is based on rodent models, as data from the rat and human post-mortems or abortions are very similar. A newborn rat is similar to a 24-week-old foetus and a week-old rat pup is equivalent to a newborn baby.

Nociceptive afferents are physiologically mature before birth but the nociceptive pathways are not. Thus, the neonatal spinal cord is hyperexcitable due to lack of inhibitory control from spinal cord interneurons and descending pathways. Neurotransmitter receptors are also widely distributed throughout the spinal cord and undergo postnatal refinement, so drugs cannot be given simply scaled down to size. In addition, there are age-related differences in various other systems such as the kidneys and the hepatic enzyme systems, so that dosing intervals are not the same as in adults.

Damage to the newborn nervous system causes profound changes that subsequently alter the development of the pain pathways. For example, neonatal skin damage such as repeated heal lancing for blood can induce skin wounding that produces peripheral sensitization. This can cause release of inflammatory mediators and growth factors that cause skin hyperinnervation on healing and changes in the transmitter phenotype of primary afferents. This change leads to central changes in the spinal cord, such as inappropriate growth or cell death, which may have a permanent effect on neural development. Studies have shown that children who underwent traumatic procedures early in life have lowered pain thresholds compared to those that did not.

---

intensity of pain. Furthermore, children may not be able to articulately ask for pain relief, therefore analgesia maintenance regimes should be considered in order to provide maximum comfort. Once the pain severity has been assessed, treatment can be administered in several ways (Table 5.12). Indirect indices of pain relief can be used: the child could appear less tense and anxious, cry less and sleep better. Oral administration of drugs is a preferred route but the rectal route can be used, as well as use of local anaesthetic-containing creams or intranasal administration of diamorphine. Aspirin should be avoided in children below the age of 12 years, but all other NSAIDs can

Table 5.12 Pain management in the Emergency department

Mild pain (VAS 1–3)	Moderate pain (4–6)	Severe pain (7–10)
Oral/rectal paracetamol 20 mg/kg loading dose, then 15 mg/kg 4–6-hourly or Oral ibuprofen 10 mg/kg 6–8-hourly	As for mild pain plus oral/rectal diclofenac 1 mg/kg 8-hourly (unless already had ibuprofen) and/or oral codeine phosphate* 1 mg/kg 4–6-hourly (over 12 years old) OR Oral morphine 0.2–0.5 mg/kg stat	Consider entonox (50% nitrous oxide and 50% oxygen) as holding measure then Intranasal diamorphine 0.2 mL (0.1 mg/kg) followed by/or IV morphine 0.1–0.2 mg/kg Supplemented by oral analgesics as required

*The Medicines and Healthcare products Regulatory Agency has restricted the use of codeine to those over 12 years of age. Adapted from the National Institute for Clinical Excellence guidelines from the Royal College of Emergency Medicine 2013 document on management of pain in children.

be used, as well as mild or strong opioids, after adequate dose adjustment. Children can also be taught how to use PCA devices. Additionally, it is important to use other non-pharmacological techniques to achieve analgesia. These may include play and distraction, cuddles, or other measures such as attending to the presenting wound/condition.

The provision of analgesia in the elderly also presents specific challenges, especially as we undergo many pharmacokinetic changes as we age. For example, aged adults may have increased body fat and decreased lean body mass, total body water and serum albumin levels that impact the distribution of medications. Additionally, elderly patients may have communication problems and may under- or over-report pain. Careful assessment using observational techniques may be required. The absorption of drugs and their metabolism in the liver may also change in the elderly, in particular as a consequence of decreased hepatic function. A decrease in renal function may also be dangerous, as metabolites (e.g. those of morphine and pethidine) may accumulate. Therefore a reduction in adult doses is often mandatory. Furthermore, the medication taken by the elderly for other diseases may lead to complex drug interactions when analgesics are prescribed. Patients may be particularly vulnerable to side effects such as confusion, sedation and respiratory depression. Smaller, frequently repeated doses of opioids are preferable to larger doses. It is generally accepted that mild pain can be managed by non-pharmacologic methods, for example, heat or ice, or massage; moderate pain with all of these modalities plus over-the-counter (OTC) medications and/or non-opioids; and that severe pain may require intermittent or regular use of opioids, that is, scaling the analgesic ladder.

General comments on pain management

Mild-to-moderate pain can be successfully managed with non-opioid analgesics or opioids with moderate efficacy. Severe pain, acute or chronic, is generally responsive to opioids with higher efficacy. When the latter drugs are used judiciously, they can offer pain relief and significantly improve the quality of life of patients without significant tolerance or dependence. In the case of pain which is opioid-insensitive, additional drugs can be considered, as well as non-pharmacological strategies. Examples of surgical strategies that can be used to control pain are: cordotomy (i.e. lesion of the spinal pathways that mediate nociception and are located in the anterolateral quadrant of the spinal cord), lesioning of the dorsal root entry zone, spinal cord stimulation and motor cortex stimulation. These are important therapeutic alternatives for intractable pain that is resistant to medication.

The complexity of pain management is illustrated by the case presented at the beginning of this chapter (see Box 5.1). Therefore, there is a need for new agents and new therapeutic concepts. For example, research using venomous marine snail toxins has uncovered conotoxins as new drugs for neuropathic pain. Conotoxins comprise a large family of peptides that typically contain 12–30 amino acids. α-Conotoxin Vc1.1 targets nicotinic cholinergic receptors as an antagonist and is effective against peripheral neuropathic pain; it also accelerates functional recovery of injured neurons. Success has already been achieved in the clinic with ziconotide (a synthetic equivalent of ω-conotoxin MVIIA), which suppresses pain through negative modulation of N-type calcium channels. Ziconotide is now a therapeutic option for the treatment of severe chronic pain in patients who have gone through all other forms of treatment, including strong opioids such as morphine. Finally, there has also been much progress in the advanced pharmacological characterization of targets such as the mu opioid receptors, which are G-protein coupled receptors that can support the molecular mechanism of 'biased activation'; this reflects the fact that different agonists at such receptors can stabilize different conformations of the receptor and activate preferentially different pathways. This means that new ligands for this receptor could be synthesized so that they induce exclusive G-protein activation-linked signalling (associated with analgesia) but avoid activation of alternative signalling pathways (such as coupling of the receptor to the intracellular protein β-arrestin), which are responsible for adverse effects such as respiratory depression or tolerance. This could result in drugs with a much-improved profile compared to morphine: high efficacy as analgesics and elimination of risk of major side effects.

Recently, a phase 1 trial was initiated for a non-opioid drug called KCP-506, developed for the treatment of chronic neuropathic pain. KCP-506 is a potent α9α10 nicotinic cholinergic receptor (nAChR) antagonist that has demonstrated robust analgesic, anti-inflammatory and neuroprotective effects across several animal chronic pain models. It offers the potential of a disease modifying therapy that may slow or halt the progression of chronic pain. The $\alpha_9\alpha_{10}$ nAChR drug target is not expressed in the CNS (it is expressed in the dorsal root ganglia and non-excitable tissues) and offers a safer therapy with no centrally mediated toxicities. Unlike other chronic pain therapies, this nAChR antagonist was non-addictive and non-tolerance-inducing in preclinical studies. It may be an effective treatment for many types of chronic pain, including radiculopathy, chemotherapy-induced peripheral neuropathy (CIPN), and diabetic neuropathy.

Self-assessment case study

Mary is a 22-year-old trainee in a City bank in London. She is very fit and rows in one of the top female teams in England. On most weekends, she has training sessions or competitions. One day, as she came home after an intense training session, she developed a severe headache, which seemed to affect only the left side of her head. She had nausea and felt very tired, and went to bed after taking some soluble aspirin. After 3–4 h, the pain had not fully abated, and Mary thought that she was developing a bad cold or influenza. A few weeks after this incident, Mary returned home late in the evening after a long meeting. She felt a tingling sensation in her fingers and sudden nausea, followed after a short while by the same type of severe headache experienced previously. She took paracetamol and tried to relax watching television, but she found the light and the sound unbearable. In the morning she felt tired. Finally, less than a month after this episode, she had a similar throbbing headache and became very sick on a Sunday while she was visiting friends. She decided to consult her general practitioner about these recurring attacks of headache that were disrupting her life.

After studying this chapter, you should be able to answer the following questions:

1. What is the likely diagnosis of Mary's problem?

Considering the described episodes of headache, their characteristics and frequency, Mary is likely to suffer from episodic migraine.

2. What is the optimum treatment for her attacks?

Mary has already tried the first line medication: over-the counter analgesics such as aspirin and paracetamol, but neither helped. So, it is likely that she would have to transition to use of triptans to manage her migraine attacks.

3 What is likely to have caused Mary's condition, and can prophylactic treatment be envisaged?

The migraine attacks may be linked to times of intense effort and fatigue (e.g. sports training or long working hours at the office), which are acknowledged triggers of this type of primary headache. It is likely that the GP or a specialist will continue to monitor Mary, and if the frequency of the episodes increases, a prophylactic treatment will be discussed.

CRANIAL NERVES AND THE BRAINSTEM

6

Chapter summary

1. Twelve pairs of cranial nerves mediate input from special senses, skin, muscles and joints of the head and neck, and parasympathetic innervation to the salivary and tear glands.

2. Each nerve is functionally classified by fibre type as sensory, motor or mixed; each fibre type has specific connections with brainstem nuclei.

3. Individual cranial nerves innervate specific regions of the brainstem, giving it functional significance. The midbrain is associated with cranial nerves II–IV and is involved in eye movements and visual and auditory reflexes. The pons is associated with cranial nerves V–VIII and is involved in mastication, facial expression, facial sensations, eye movements, hearing and balance, salivation, lacrimation and taste. The medulla is associated with cranial nerves VIII–XII and is associated with vital life support functions (cardiovascular and respiration), taste, tongue movements, swallowing, talking, hearing, nausea and vomiting, and coughing responses.

4. The brainstem is topographically organised. Cranial nerve nuclei are located dorsally within the brainstem, descending tracts ventrally, with ascending pathways and the reticular formation sandwiched in between. Sensory cranial nerve nuclei are located laterally, motor nuclei medially and mixed nuclei in between.

5. The reticular formation is a diffuse, multisynaptic meshwork of inter-connected neurons involved in homeostasis, consciousness, alertness, pain, automated cardiovascular and respiratory responses, muscle tone and automated pattern generators (subconscious motor functions).

6. Vascular or physical lesions to cranial nerves or brainstem regions produce distinct clinical signs, which can be diagnosed based on knowledge of brainstem topography and cranial nerve function.

Introduction

To make an accurate diagnosis of the patient's problem, the doctor must carefully evaluate all the neurological findings. To do this, a clear knowledge of the organization and function of the various cranial nerves and tracts within the brainstem is needed. The purpose of this chapter is to build a three-dimensional picture of the organisation of the brainstem. By understanding this arrangement, one can use the signs and symptoms to locate the level of the lesion.

The brainstem resides in the posterior fossa of the skull and comprises the medulla, pons and midbrain. The medulla is continuous with the spinal cord beyond the foramen magnum, and the midbrain connects to the thalamus and forebrain. The brainstem is essential for life; while a human can survive if the cerebral cortex is irreversibly damaged or removed, damage to the brainstem can kill! It is also the origin of conscious perception of different somatic and visceral sensations. The brainstem has three main functions:

1. **Cranial nerve-related functions**. It contains nuclei associated with 11 of the 12 pairs of cranial nerves, and cranial nerves III–XII emerge from its surface.

2. **Conduit functions**. It contains ascending and descending pathways that relay sensorimotor information to and from the cortex, cerebellum and spinal cord, as well as other pathways that originate within the brainstem.

3. **Integrative functions**. Cardiorespiratory activities, complex motor patterns, oculomotor functions, consciousness levels, sleep, alertness and autonomic functions occur via the reticular formation (RF) and the medial longitudinal fasciculus (MLF) that run throughout the length of the brainstem.

Knowledge of the basic organization and various functions of the brainstem is important for understanding brainstem disorders. Signs of primary brainstem injury (coma, irregular breathing, fixed and dilated pupils and loss of oculovestibular reflexes or motor flaccidity) usually imply severe brainstem injury and have a poor prognosis.

Anatomical organization of cranial nerves and their nuclei

Understanding the functional anatomy of the cranial nerves is of great clinical importance. Testing the integrity of the cranial nerves is a part of the neurological examination (see Chapter 3). If a sensory or motor deficit is encountered, it is essential to determine if it is a peripheral or a central problem. If it is a peripheral problem, it is important to establish what nerve(s) are involved, or if it is a central problem, to localize where

---

> **Box 6.1** **Case history**
>
> A student comes into casualty one morning complaining of an inability to see with his left eye. You notice that his left upper eyelid droops. He says that he got very drunk at a party and on the way home, he fell over and hit his head hard on the pavement, losing consciousness for a short while. Initially, he thought the eye closure was due to swelling, but after a week, the eye had still not opened.
>
> On inspection, his left eyelid was shut and, when it was lifted, the eyeball deviated down and out. The left pupil was fixed and dilated, whereas the right pupil responded normally to increased light intensity in either eye. When the student smiled, only minor elevation occurred on the right side of the mouth. Further neurological examination revealed a right-sided Babinski sign, right-sided weakness in the arms and legs and hyperreflexia and hypertonia of the right side limbs. General sensory examination proved normal.
>
> This case gives rise to the following questions:
> 1. Why is the left eye closed and the eye deviated down and out?
> 2. Why does only the right pupil respond to increased light intensity in the left eye?
> 3. Why are there facial paralysis and limb motor deficits?

Table 6.1   Classification of cranial nerves

Pure sensory nerves	Pure motor nerves	Mixed nerves
Olfactory (I)	Oculomotor (III) Trochlear (IV)	Trigeminal (V) Facial (VII)
Optic (II)	Abducens (VI)	Glossopharyngeal (IX)
Vestibulocochlear (VIII)	Accessory (XI) Hypoglossal (XII)	Vagus (X)

the lesion is, and what other systems are affected. To answer these questions, an understanding of the anatomy of the cranial nerves is required.

Cranial nerves have three main functions:

1. to provide the general motor and sensory innervation of the skin, muscles and joints in the head and neck region

2. to mediate special senses (vision, hearing, taste and olfaction)

3. to regulate autonomic (visceral) functions via parasympathetic innervation of autonomic ganglia (e.g. breathing, heart rate, blood pressure, coughing and swallowing)

Cranial nerves are classified as sensory, motor or mixed (containing motor, sensory and autonomic fibres) as summarized in Table 6.1.

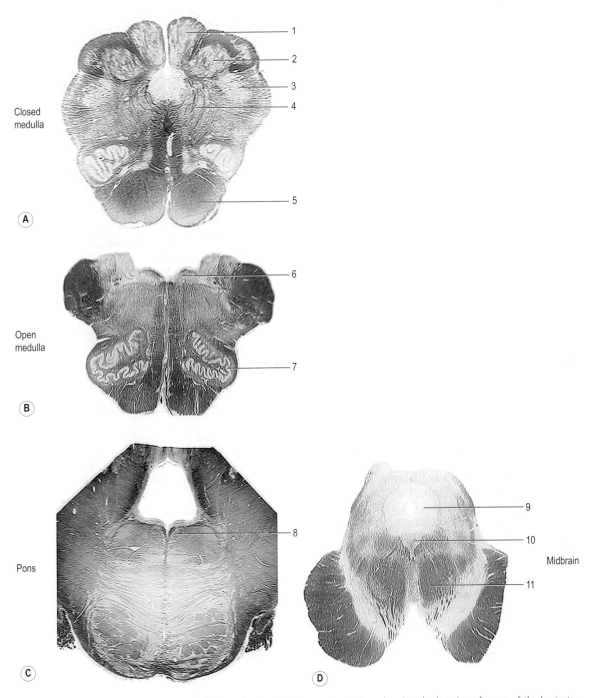

Fig. 6.1 Wiegert-Pal stained transverse sections of different levels of the human brainstem showing the location of some of the brainstem nuclei, and major ascending and descending tracts. *1,* Gracile nucleus; *2,* Cuneate nucleus; *3,* Spinal trigeminal nucleus; *4,* Medial lemniscus; *5,* Corticospinal tract; *6, CN XII,* hypoglossal nucleus; *7,* Inferior olivary nucleus; *8, CN VI,* abducens nucleus; *9,* Periaqueductal grey; *10, CN III,* oculomotor nucleus; *11,* Red nucleus.

Internal organization of the brainstem

The anatomy of the brainstem and organization of different cranial nerve nuclei is extremely complicated. It was traditionally taught by recognizing features in histological specimens from different levels of the brainstem (Fig. 6.1).

However, with modern imaging methods, it is now not necessary to be able to recognize these internal features, which are seen only in post mortem histological specimens; however, one needs to be able to recognize their shape to be able to identify them in medical images such as magnetic resonance images. In order to diagnose brainstem lesions, one has to be familiar with its topographical organization and with the deficits that occur with cranial nerve lesions.

The brainstem is functionally associated with 11 of the 12 pairs of cranial nerves. Cranial nerve I, the olfactory nerve, does not attach to the brainstem but projects directly to the forebrain and is functionally associated with the limbic system. Similarly, cranial nerve II does not directly attach to the brainstem but does have afferent collaterals that terminate in midbrain nuclei. For the other cranial nerves, their inputs are organized sequentially in a rostrocaudal fashion from nerve III to nerve XII (Fig. 6.2A). This gives the different subdivisions of the brainstem functional significance (Table 6.2).

The basic organization of the brainstem is the same for each region. Essentially, it is divided into three sections in the dorsoventral (transverse) axis (Fig. 6.2B). In the dorsal part are located the cranial nerve nuclei; in the ventral part are located fibres of descending pathways; in the middle (called the tegmentum) are located the ascending pathways and various nuclei associated with the reticular formation (see later).

In the mediolateral plane, cranial nerve nuclei are organized with respect to function. Those nuclei associated with purely sensory nerves are located in the lateral brainstem, while purely motor nuclei are located most medially. Cranial nerve nuclei with mixed sensory and motor fibre input are located in between. Each of these nerves has more than one nucleus of origin—at least one sensory and one motor. Sometimes, axons from more than one nerve will terminate in a single nucleus. For example, the sense of taste is shared by three nerves (VII, IX and X) but merges into a single nucleus, the solitary nucleus. Another example is the spinal trigeminal nucleus, which receives general sensations from the face, muscles and ears (cranial nerves V, VII, IX and X).

The ascending tracts are similarly organized in a mediolateral fashion within the tegmentum. Tracts associated with motor function, such as the MLF or the rubrospinal tract, are located more medially to those with sensory functions such as the medial lemniscus (touch and vibration), the spinothalamic tract (pain and temperature) or the lateral lemniscus (hearing). Although their exact location varies at different rostrocaudal levels of the brainstem, the pattern of motor systems being medially located to sensory systems is always preserved.

Fig. 6.3 shows a dorsal view of the brainstem, illustrating the relative mediolateral positions of the cranial nerve nuclei in the brainstem. This is a schematic to demonstrate the overall picture; in reality, some of these nuclei would overlap. There are up to seven different nuclei columns corresponding to the different cranial nerve fibre types based on embryological development (see Box 6.2 and Fig. 6.2B) that can be arranged in a mediolateral row. In reality, the only place this occurs is in the open (rostral) medulla, near its junction with the pons. At the other levels, fewer columns are present.

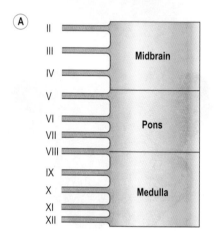

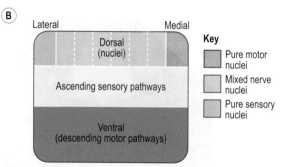

Fig. 6.2 Schematic representations of the brainstem viewed in the rostrocaudal (A) and transverse (B) planes. (A) shows the input of cranial nerves into the different regions of the brainstem. (B) shows the organization of ascending, descending tracts and cranial nerve nuclei within the brainstem.

Table 6.2 Main functions of the brainstem

Brainstem region	Associated cranial nerve input	Main functions
Midbrain	II–IV	Auditory, visual and pupillary reflexes and eye movements Regulates cortical arousal
Pons	V–VIII	Mastication, eye movement, facial expression, blinking, salivation, equilibrium and audition
Medulla	VIII–XII	Equilibrium, audition, deglutition, coughing, vomiting, salivation, tongue movement, respiration and circulation

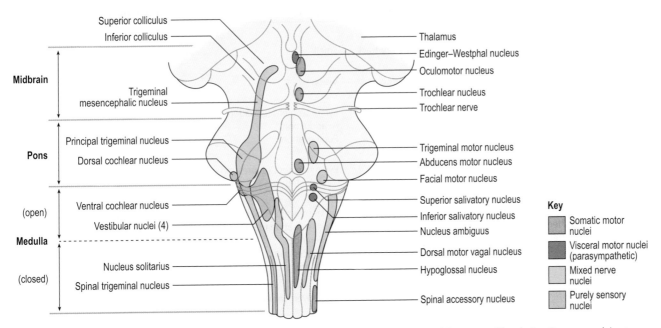

Fig. 6.3 Superior view of the brainstem, showing the schematic organization of cranial nerve nuclei, separated for clarity. Sensory nuclei are shown only on the left side and motor nuclei only on the right side.

What is clear is that sensory nuclei are located laterally to motor ones.

By understanding the basic rules relating to the topographical organisation, the functional significance becomes apparent: (1) that neurons with similar functions are in close proximity and (2) that different functional deficits occur depending on whether the lesion is lateral or near the midline. As the location of ascending and descending tracts and the mediolateral position of cranial nuclei are relatively constant along their rostrocaudal distribution in the brainstem, specific combinations of signs can reliably indicate the site of a lesion. Therefore, analysis of brainstem disorders is simplified by answering two questions:

1. Is it lateral or medial—delineated by the presence/absence of sensory and motor function?

2. What is the level of the lesion—delineated by specific cranial nerves?

In order to determine this, it is important to know what deficits are associated with each cranial nerve and how to test for them. The specific tests for cranial nerves are described in Chapter 3 and deficits associated with specific cranial nerves or their nuclei are shown in Table 6.3.

Reticular formation

Running through the core of the brainstem tegmentum is the RF, which consists of a diffuse network of neurons that exert a widespread influence on central nervous system (CNS) functions. Within this region, cells aggregate to form

Box 6.2 Comparison of spinal and cranial nerves

Functionally, cranial nerves are analogous to spinal nerves in that they contain motor, sensory and visceral afferents but there are differences between cranial and spinal nerves:

- Cranial nerves do not possess dorsal and ventral roots.
- Cranial motor afferent cell bodies are located in brainstem nuclei (not in external ganglia).
- Cranial nerves possess four types of sensory afferents (spinal nerves contain two). In addition to general somatic and visceral afferents, special sensory afferents also innervate specific sensory organs located only in the head.
- Cranial nerves possess three types of motor fibres, whereas spinal nerves contain two (general motor/visceral). General somatic efferents innervate the extra-ocular muscles (nerves III, IV and VI) and intrinsic tongue muscles (nerve XII). General visceral efferents (controlling autonomic effectors) innervate the sweat/tear glands and smooth muscles (nerves III, VII, IX and X). Specialized visceral efferent fibres controlling the striated (skeletal) muscles associated with the facial expression, chewing, neck, larynx and pharynx movements (nerves V, VII, IX, X and XI) are derived from the branchial arches during development.
- Each fibre type projects to, or arises from, a specific brainstem nucleus.

Table 6.3 Cranial nerve summary

Cranial nerve (CN) (fibre type)	Nucleus name	Nucleus location	Function	Symptom/sign of damage
Olfactory (CN I) (special sensory afferent)	Olfactory bulb	Olfactory tract	Smell	Anosmia
Optic (CN II) (special sensory afferent)	Lateral geniculate	Thalamus	Vision	Blindness
Oculomotor (CN III) (general somatic efferent) (general visceral efferent)	Oculomotor Edinger–Westphal*	Midbrain Midbrain	Eye movement (elevation, adduction) Pupil dilation	Eye deviates down and out. Loss of pupillary/ accommodation reflexes
Trochlear (CN IV) (general somatic efferent)	Trochlear	Midbrain	Eye movement (depression of adducted eye)	Diplopia, lateral deviation of eye
Trigeminal (CN V) (general somatic afferent) (general somatic afferent) (general somatic afferent) (special visceral efferent)	Principal Spinal Mesencephalic Motor	Pons Medulla Pons/midbrain Pons	Facial sensation (touch) Facial sensation (pain) and meninges Proprioception Mastication	Facial anaesthesia Loss of facial pain sensation Clinically insignificant Weakness/loss of mastication
Abducens (CN VI) (general somatic efferent)	Abducens	Pons	Eye movement (abduction)	Medial eye deviation
Facial (CN VII) (special visceral efferent) (special visceral afferent) (general visceral afferent) (general sensory afferent)	Motor Solitary Superior salivatory* Principal trigeminal	Pons Pons Pons Pons	Facial expression Taste Salivation, lacrimation Posterior ear skin and outer ear canal	Paralysis of facial muscles; hyperacusis Aguesia (loss of taste to anterior two-thirds of tongue) Dry mouth, loss of lacrimation Loss of sensation
Vestibulocochlear (CN VIII) (special sensory afferent)	Vestibular Cochlear	Medulla Medulla	Balance Hearing	Vertigo, disequilibrium, nystagmus Deafness
Glossopharyngeal (CN IX) (special sensory afferent) (general visceral afferent) (general visceral efferent) (special visceral efferent) (general sensory afferent)	Rostral Solitary Caudal solitary (cardio-respiratory centre) Inferior salivatory* Nucleus ambiguus Spinal trigeminal	Medulla Medulla Medulla Medulla Medulla	Taste Control of blood pressure and general sensations Salivation Stylopharyngeus muscle Innervation of pharynx, posterior one-third of tongue, oropharynx, tonsils, middle ear auditory tube and ear drum	Aguesia (posterior one-third of tongue) loss of blood pressure control and gag reflex Insignificant Loss of gag reflex Loss of sensations to these regions
Vagus (X) (special visceral efferent) (general visceral efferent) (special visceral afferent) (general visceral afferent) (general sensory afferent)	Nucleus ambiguus Dorsal motor vagal* Rostral Solitary Caudal solitary (cardio-respiratory centre) Spinal trigeminal	Medulla Medulla Medulla Medulla Medulla	Swallowing and talking Cardiac, respiratory and GI tract smooth muscle Taste, general sensations of larynx and pharynx, cardio-thoracic and abdominal cavities, blood pressure control Innervation of posterior fossa meninges, pharynx, posterior ear skin and eardrum	Dysphagia and hoarseness of voice; unilateral uvula deviation Tachycardia, loss of cough reflex Aguesia (epiglottis), loss of gag reflex and blood pressure control Loss of sensation
Cranial accessory (XI) (special visceral efferent)	Nucleus ambiguus	Medulla	Pharynx/larynx muscles	Insignificant
Spinal accessory (special visceral efferent)	Spinal accessory	Cervical cord	Neck and shoulder movement	Head turning/shoulder shrugging weakness
Hypoglossal (XII) (general somatic efferent)	Hypoglossal	Medulla	Tongue movements	Atrophy of tongue muscles, deviation on protrusion, fasciculation

*Nuclei associated with the parasympathetic nervous system.

Table 6.4 Function of different parts of the reticular formation

	Location	Function
Ascending reticular activating system (ARAS)	Midbrain	Arousal
Periaqueductal grey region		Rapid eye movement (REM) sleep/pain modulation
Locus coeruleus		Arousal and attention
Raphe nuclei		Wakefulness
Interstitial nucleus of Cajal, nucleus of Darkschewitz, rostral interstitial nucleus of the MLF		Accessory nuclei associated with the vertical gaze centre
Pontine paramedian reticular formation (PPRF)	Pons	Horizontal gaze centre
Micturition centre		Bladder control
Pneumotaxic centre (medial parabrachial nucleus)		Respiration
Salivatory nucleus		Lacrimation/salivation
Supratrigeminal nucleus		Mastication
Pedunculopontine nucleus		Locomotor centre, REM sleep
Dorsal and ventral respiratory nuclei	Medulla	Respiratory centres
Cardiovascular nuclei		Heart rate/blood pressure
Raphe magnus nucleus		Pain modulation
Area postrema		Vomiting pCO_2/pH levels
Chemoreceptor trigger zone		Pattern generators for coughing and swallowing
Lateral reticular nucleus		

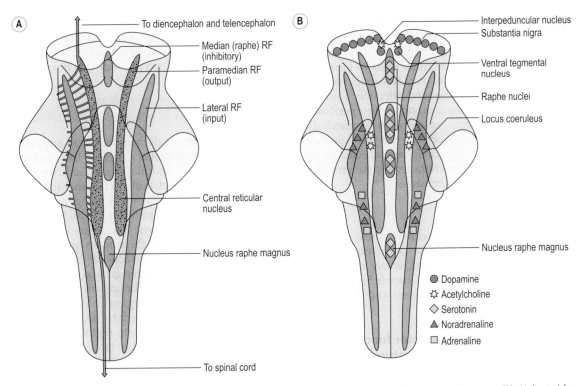

Fig. 6.4 (A) Schematic organization of the reticular formation (RF) showing the location of the various aminergic groups (B). (Adapted from Fitzgerald MJT and Folan-Curran, J Clinical Neuroanatomy & Related Neuroscience, 4th ed. WB Saunders.)

nuclei that are associated with regulating various sensorimotor, cortical arousal and autonomic functions (Table 6.4). They help to regulate, or fine tune, complex behaviours, such as chewing, swallowing, coughing, sneezing, fighting and copulation, using automated pattern generators.

The RF is functionally divided into three regions: a midline region, containing the raphe nuclei, that has a predominantly inhibitory function; a medial (magnocellular) region that provides the output pathways to the spinal cord and forebrain regions; and a lateral (parvocellular) region that receives input from ascending sensory pathways, from the cerebellum, basal ganglia, hypothalamus, cranial nerves and the cerebral cortex (Fig. 6.4). This region provides input to the medial region.

The RF contains sets of neurons that utilize specific amines that function as neuromodulators. The serotonergic (5-hydroxytryptamine [5-HT]) cells have the largest territorial distribution within the CNS and project to the forebrain and spinal cord. Dopaminergic cells in the midbrain project to the basal ganglia and limbic cortical areas. Cells of the locus coeruleus contain noradrenaline and project to the spinal cord and forebrain. Adrenaline-producing cells are rare and confined to the medulla; they project to the hypothalamus and sympathetic preganglionic neurons in the spinal cord. Cholinergic cells of the midbrain project to the thalamus and basal forebrain. An imbalance in aminergic levels is associated with depression, hyperactivity and agitation, or insomnia.

Principal functions of the RF

Mediating behavioural responses: arousal, alertness and affect

The monoamine cell groups of the upper pons and midbrain form the ascending reticular activating system (ARAS) that projects to the cerebral cortex, hippocampus, amygdala, hypothalamus and thalamus. The ARAS regulates sleep and wake cycles, various emotional and behavioural responses, and orientation responses to various stimuli. Clinically, this area is important in regulating levels of consciousness; depletion of serotonin leads to insomnia and tonic firing of locus coeruleus (noradrenaline) neurons regulates general levels of arousal and attention. Damage to the midbrain RF can lead to coma, stupor or a persistent vegetative state. Certain drugs, anaesthetics or metabolic disturbances also affect consciousness levels through their actions on the RF. Levels of RF activity are reflected on an electroencephalogram (EEG) by characteristic patterns that vary with different states of consciousness.

Modulating pain perception

The raphe nuclei and locus coeruleus nuclei contain neurons whose projections synapse onto interneurons in the dorsal horn of the spinal cord, where they mediate stimulus-induced analgesia (see Chapter 5). The RF is also involved in stress-induced analgesia and the diffuse noxious inhibitory control of pain.

Modulating spinal and cranial motor functions (muscle tone, reflexes and body posture)

The RF influences motor activities through reciprocal connections with the red nucleus, basal ganglia nuclei, vestibular nuclei, motor cortex and cerebellum. Activation of the pontine RF and medullary RF has antagonistic roles in the control of body posture, via regulation of flexor and extensor reflexes. The pontine RF gives rise to the medial reticulospinal tract (RST) that facilitates extensor reflexes, inhibits flexor reflexes and increases muscle tone in axial and proximal limb muscles. The lateral RST originates in the medullary RF, facilitates flexor reflexes, inhibits extensor reflexes

and decreases muscle tone in axial and proximal limb muscles. Damage to the brainstem at different levels can result in specific changes in posture, known as decerebrate or decorticate rigidity (see Chapter 9).

Gaze centres in the midbrain and pons control conjugate eye movements in the horizontal and vertical directions via connections with the vestibular and ocular motor nerve nuclei in the brainstem and connections from the frontal and posterior parietal eye fields.

Coordinating motor survival (autonomic) centres

The medulla contains the nuclei that control vital (survival) functions: the respiratory and cardiovascular centres, swallowing, blood pressure and vomiting (Box 6.3). A key nucleus involved in these functions is the solitary nucleus (also called nucleus of the tractus solitarius [NTS]). It is involved in the coordination of swallowing and breathing so that one does not swallow air, or inhale food or vomit. The caudal NTS also receives afferents from stretch receptors in the lungs and from CSF chemoreceptors on the surface of the medulla. These fibres project onto neurons situated in the respiratory centres located in the medullary RF. The NTS also receives information from aortic baroreceptors located in the carotid body in the carotid artery (via cranial nerve IX) and relays this information to the cardiovascular control centres (in the medullary RF) to regulate blood pressure (see Box 6.4).

Blood supply to the brainstem

The entire brainstem derives its blood supply from the posterior (vertebral-basilar) part of the cerebral circulation (Fig. 6.7). The medulla is supplied from the ventral surface by the two vertebral arteries that then join to form the basilar artery, which courses along the ventral surface of the pons. Further rostrally, in the midbrain, the basilar artery diverges to become the posterior cerebral arteries. Branches from these three main arteries supply both the dorsal and ventral surfaces of the brainstem. These branches subdivide into three groups that supply different regions for each part of the brainstem (see Fig. 6.7).

There is a paramedian region on either side of the ventral midline that is supplied by short arteries. Next to this region is an intermediate region, supplied by short circumferential arteries. The lateral zone, which supplies the dorsal aspect of the brainstem, is supplied by branches of long circumferential arteries, such as the posterior cerebral artery. The paramedian and lateral zones are often involved in vascular accidents that give rise to characteristic clinical deficits (see later).

Brainstem reflexes

The brainstem is involved in several reflexes (Table 6.5), and their presence or absence is used to determine brainstem death in a patient (see Box 6.5).

Nausea and vomiting

There are many causes of nausea and vomiting: pregnancy, movement (e.g. travel sickness), vestibular disease, injury and migraine. Treatment is based on the use of anti-emetics. Nausea is easier to prevent than to stop after it has started. Vomiting is coordinated by the vomiting centre located in the lateral medullary reticular formation (Fig. 6.5). This region receives input from the chemoreceptor trigger zone (CTZ), located in the area postrema of the medulla, which is rich in dopaminergic (D_2) and serotonergic (5-HT$_3$) receptors. This region is not protected by the blood–brain barrier (BBB) and is sensitive to circulating toxins or drugs. There is also input from the limbic system (that responds to unpleasant smells or sights), the spinoreticular tract (in response to physical trauma), the NTS (involved in the gag reflex) and the stomach via the vagus nerve and the vestibular system. In motion sickness, nausea is thought to arise due to conflicting signals from the visual and vestibular systems. Output from the vomiting centre is to the spinal motor neurons innervating the abdominal muscles.

Drugs used to fight diseases, such as Parkinson's disease and cancer, frequently cause nausea and vomiting because they activate the CTZ. Dopamine receptor antagonists such as domperidone and metoclopramide can be used to treat nausea. Domperidone does not cross the BBB and has few side effects. Metoclopramide also has an effect on the gut, facilitating the absorption of many drugs, such as analgesics. 5-HT$_3$ antagonists, such as ondansetron, inhibit receptors in the gut and CTZ and reduce nausea but may result in constipation. D_2 and 5-HT$_3$ antagonists are ineffective in preventing motion sickness. Anticholinergic drugs, such as hyoscine (a muscarinic receptor antagonist), or anti-histamine drugs, such as cinnarizine, often prescribed for motion sickness, act directly on the vomiting centre to reduce sickness.

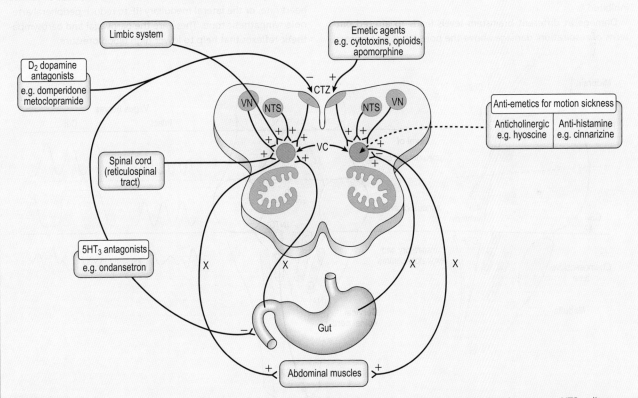

Fig. 6.5 Pathways involved in nausea and their pharmacological modulation. *1*, Excitatory; *CTZ*, chemoreceptor trigger zone; *NTS*, solitary nucleus; *VC*, vomiting centre; *VN*, vestibular nucleus; *X*, vagus nerve; –, inhibitory. (Adapted from Neal MJ. (1997). Medical pharmacology at a glance, 3rd ed. Blackwell Science Ltd.)

Pupillary light reflex

Normally, shining a light into one eye causes both pupils to constrict. In the stimulated eye, this is the direct light reflex, and in the non-stimulated eye, it is the consensual light reflex. Pupil constriction by the pupillary sphincter muscle occurs in response to autonomic parasympathetic stimulation by postganglionic ciliary nerves. This reflex is triggered by stimulation of optic nerve collaterals synapsing in the pretectal nucleus (in the superior colliculus) that, in turn, stimulates neurons in the Edinger–Westphal nucleus. From here, parasympathetic preganglionic fibres

Box
6.4 **Brainstem control of respiration and heart rate**

The medulla houses the respiratory and cardiovascular nuclei of the RF. These control the respiratory and heart rates in response to peripheral stimuli or changes in the partial pressure of oxygen, carbon dioxide and blood pH (Fig. 6.6).

The medulla houses the dorsal (inspiratory) and ventral (expiratory) respiratory groups in the nucleus of the solitary tract (NTS) and nucleus ambiguus, respectively. Their function is to control the basic rhythm of breathing and they can maintain breathing independently of the rest of the brain, as occurs in a persistent vegetative state.

Other centres in the pons are involved in co-ordinating breathing patterns. The pneumotaxic centre, located in the medial parabrachial nucleus, inhibits inspiratory neurons to prevent the lungs becoming over inflated. It limits inspiration and facilitates expiration. When this area is active, breathing rate is more rapid. The apneustic centre stimulates the dorsal respiratory group, prolonging inspiration and reducing expiration. When the pneumotaxic centre is active, the apneustic region is inhibited.

Damage at different brainstem levels leads to altered patterns of respiration: damage above the pons leads to a normal breathing pattern whereas damage between the pneumotaxic and apneustic centres leads to apneusis (breathing with prolonged inspiratory pauses) or Cheyne–Stokes respiration. Damage between the apneustic centre and the respiratory cell groups leads to irregular breathing patterns, and damage below the respiratory groups eliminates the respiratory drive.

Breathing is also regulated by the blood levels of CO_2 and H^+. Chemosensitive cells located in the ventrolateral part of the medulla, close to where the choroid plexus projects through the lateral aperture of the fourth ventricle, detect local acidity or alkalinity changes in the CSF, and strongly increase or decrease respiratory drive via connections with the medullary respiratory centre.

The cardiovascular (baroreceptor) centre is located in the medial NTS and is activated by the carotid sinus stretch (baro-) receptors. Changes in heart rate or blood pressure stimulate these centres resulting in activation of the (autonomic) cardio-inhibitory neurons of the dorsal motor vagal nucleus to reduce heart rate, or the lateral medullary RF to reduce peripheral arteriole sympathetic tone. These are the barovagal and barosympathetic reflexes that help to lower high blood pressure.

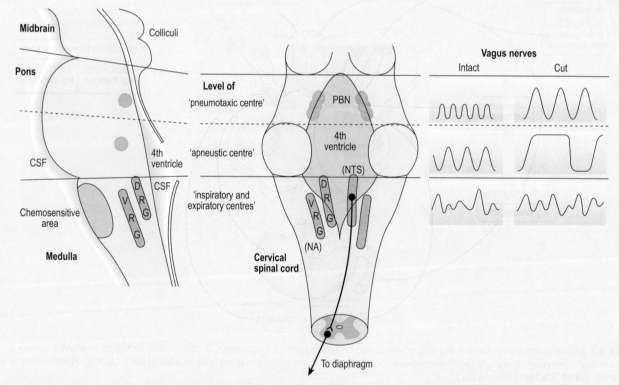

Fig. 6.6 The left and middle diagrams show lateral and dorsal views of the location of brainstem respiratory control neuron groups. The pneumotaxic centre is located in the medial parabrachial nucleus (PBN). The dorsal respiratory group (DRG) located in the solitary nucleus (NTS) and ventral respiratory group (VRG) of neurons located in the nucleus ambiguous (NA) house the inspiratory and expiratory centres, respectively. The right panel shows the breathing patterns seen in decerebrate animals with damage at different brainstem levels. After transection at the upper line, normal breathing can still occur without any influence from above the pons. After transection at the dashed line, the pneumotaxic centre is disconnected from influencing the apneustic centre, so that prolonged inspiration takes place unless inhibition occurs via stimulation of the lung stretch receptors ('vagus intact'). Transection at the lower line removes all influences above the level of the medulla and produces irregular breathing patterns. *CSF*, Cerebrospinal fluid; *V*, ventricle. (Adapted from Jenner S (1989). Human Physiology. Churchill Livingstone.)

travel in the oculomotor nerve to the ciliary ganglion. Dilation of the pupils occurs more indirectly via sympathetic stimulation of the pupillary dilator muscle by postganglionic fibres from the superior cervical ganglion. Damage to the sympathetic nervous system fibres results in Horner's syndrome, characterized by pupil constriction (miosis), decreased facial sweating (anhydrosis) and ptosis (drooping of the eyelid). As the sympathetic pathway has a complex course from the hypothalamus through the brainstem to the T1 thoracic cord, and then on to the superior cervical ganglion before returning to the head,

damage anywhere along this pathway can cause this syndrome. Parasympathetic fibre damage results in dilated pupils (mydriasis), as the fibres are located superficially within the nerve. Ophthalmologists use short-acting parasympathetic-blocking drugs that are derivatives of atropine to dilate the pupil to examine the interior of the eye.

If only the illuminated pupil constricts, then there is damage to the crossing fibres, that is, damage in the

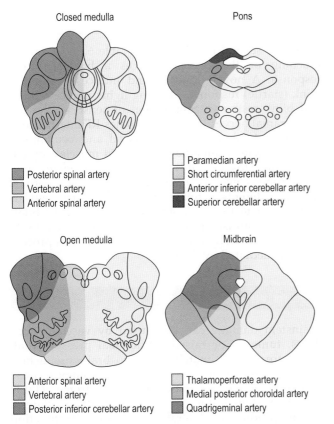

Fig. 6.7 Arterial blood supply to different regions of the brainstem. Only one side is shown for clarity.

Box 6.5 Brainstem death

Brain cells require an adequate oxygen supply to function normally. Prolonged hypoxia or ischemia may be fatal to brain cells. Inadequate or incomplete resuscitation may fail to revive brain functions and thus lead to brain death, whereby all cortical function is lost, but brainstem reflexes and spontaneous breathing are still present. This is termed a persistent vegetative state.

In brainstem death, spontaneous breathing ceases and there is a loss of reflexes. Cardiovascular function can be artificially maintained for a short while but will eventually deteriorate due to loss of function of the brainstem regulatory centres in the medulla. RF cell death leads to the loss of cortical arousal, and thus the lack of brain activity and hence brain death.

Several criteria must be met in order to diagnose brainstem death. There must be no pupillary, corneal, gag, cough, caloric or doll's eye reflex responses or response to painful stimuli applied to cranial nerve territories. Absence of spontaneous breaths can only be confirmed after hypercapnia tests, where the pCO$_2$ is above 45 mmHg.

Brainstem death tests are performed by two doctors either independently or together, and are then repeated, prior to declaration of brain death. Before testing, any analgesic medications, drugs, neuromuscular blockers, metabolic imbalances or lowered body temperature should be allowed to clear or reverse, as these may account for brainstem inactivity. An EEG is not necessary.

Table 6.5 Location and pathways of brainstem reflexes

Reflex	Afferent arc	Efferent arc	Brainstem area
Pupillary light reflex	CN II	CN III (E-W)	Midbrain
Accommodation reflex	CN II	CN III (E-W)	Midbrain
Vestibulo-ocular reflex	CN VIII	CN III, IV, VI	Pons-midbrain
Blinking—sound (startle), light (e.g. flashing lights), corneal touch	CN VIII CN II CN V$_1$	CN VII (eyelid close) CNIII (eyelid open)	Pons Midbrain
Jaw jerk	CN V$_3$	CN V$_3$	Pons
Gag reflex	CN IX	CN X	Medulla

CN, Cranial nerve; E-W, Edinger-Westphal nucleus; V$_1$, ophthalmic and V$_3$, mandibular branches of nerve V.

midbrain. If the optic nerve (afferent input) is damaged on one side, both the direct and consensual reflexes will be lost from the blind eye. The unaffected eye will show both reflexes in response to light. If cranial nerve III (efferent output from the Edinger–Westphal nucleus) is damaged, both reflexes will be lost in the ipsilateral eye and pupillary dilation will be observed in that eye. A unilateral fixed and dilated pupil is suggestive of increased intracranial pressure, pressing on cranial nerve III.

The pupillary light reflex is a very important reflex and occurs even when someone is unconscious. The circuitry involved in these reflexes is detailed in Chapter 7 (see Fig. 7.6B).

Accommodation reflex

The accommodation reflex is associated with cranial nerve III. At rest, the lens is thin to allow the eye to focus on far objects. To focus on near objects, the lens must thicken by a process called accommodation, as described in Chapter 7. Accommodation and convergence of the eyes are mediated by increased tone of the medial rectus muscle and pupil constriction (contraction of the pupillae constrictor muscle), which occur together when a person views a close object. The pathway is as follows: optic nerve afferents travel to the lateral geniculate nucleus and then to the primary visual cortex in the occipital lobe. For the efferent pathway, occipital lobe fibres project to cells of the accommodation centre in the midbrain. From here, they travel to the Edinger–Westphal nucleus. Parasympathetic fibre activation results in ciliary muscle contraction, which shortens the suspensory ligament, allowing relaxation of the lens and causing passive thickening. The accommodation centre also stimulates the somatic motoneurons of the medial rectus muscles, producing convergence of the eyes to a near object, so that focus is maintained (see Chapter 7 and Fig. 7.7C for further details).

Doll's eye (vestibulo-ocular) reflex

This involves conjugate eye movements in response to head movement. The normal response is for the patient's eyes to deviate in the opposite direction to head turning, that is, if the head is briskly extended, the eyes go downwards and if the move is to the right, the eyes move to the left. Normally the cortex inhibits these reflexes, but in a comatose patient, they are disinhibited (see Chapter 8). If present, they show that the pathway (medial longitudinal fasciculus) between the relevant nuclei in the pons and midbrain is intact.

Gag reflex

Stimulation of the uvula (soft palate) or the lateral walls of the oropharynx triggers closing of the trachea. However, under general anaesthesia, this reflex does not work and unconscious patients may vomit. Thus it

is important that no food or drink be consumed for 8–12 hours before an operation, otherwise vomit could enter the trachea, which can be very dangerous.

Jaw jerk reflex

This monosynaptic reflex is the head equivalent of the patella reflex in the spinal cord. It is mediated by the trigeminal nerve, and in normal people, the reflex is weak or absent. It only becomes prominent if there is damage to the descending corticobulbar fibres.

Blink reflexes

There are several blink reflexes (Table 6.5). Unilateral touching of the cornea induces a bilateral blink response. A novel (loud) sound induces a bilateral blink (startle) response. Flashing lights induce a bilateral blink response. Stimulation of sensory afferents from cranial nerves II or VIII activates RF interneurons that project bilaterally to the facial and oculomotor motor nucleus to innervate the eyelid muscles orbicularis oculi (closes eyelid) and evator palpebrae superioris (opens eyelid), respectively. However, corneal sensory afferents activate spinal trigeminal neurons that project to the facial and oculomotor nuclei bilaterally. In contrast, unconscious blinking functions to maintain normal hydration of the eye, and this process is likely mediated by the RF.

Brainstem lesions

Brainstem damage can be caused by vascular accidents, tumours or raised intracranial pressure that, if not treated, ultimately leads to brain tissue herniation. Vascular lesions are the most common cause and produce characteristic clinical syndromes (Table 6.6). Brainstem lesions are unique in that unilateral lesions produce ipsilateral cranial nerve dysfunction and contralateral dysfunction of the ascending tracts (i.e. ipsilateral facial deficits and contralateral body deficits). Certain common symptoms are associated with brainstem lesions depending on their mediolateral location. Unilateral medial lesions in general damage the corticospinal tract, producing contralateral spastic hemiplegia (partial paralysis of muscles, increased muscle tone) and a Babinski sign. Damage to the medial lemniscal pathway results in contralateral loss of light touch, position and vibration senses. The level of a medial brainstem lesion is determined by the involvement of the cranial motor nerves XII, VI and III.

Unilateral lateral lesions, in general, produce five common symptoms that are distinct from medial symptoms:

1. Contralateral loss of pain/thermal sensation (spinothalamic tract damage)

Table 6.6 Unilateral vascular lesions of the medial brainstem

Brainstem area	Possible vascular cause	Specific symptoms (in addition to common symptoms)
Medulla (Déjerine's syndrome)	Anterior spinal/vertebral artery	CN XII: ipsilateral weakness and wasting of the tongue muscles
Pons	Basilar artery branches—paramedian pontine	CN VI: medial deviation of the eye (adduction paralysis) Pontine RF (gaze centre): ipsilateral gaze paralysis Cerebellar systems (pons): ipsilateral limb ataxia (loss of muscle co-ordination) and nystagmus (rapid oscillation of the eyeballs)
Midbrain (Weber's syndrome, Benedict's syndrome)	Posterior cerebral artery	CN III: ophthalmoplegia (eye deviates down and out) Red nucleus: contralateral cerebellar ataxia

Table 6.7 Unilateral vascular lesions of the lateral brainstem

Brainstem area	Possible vascular cause	Specific symptoms (in addition to common symptoms)
Medulla (Wallenberg's syndrome)	Posterior inferior cerebellar artery	CN IX–X Dysarthria, dysphagia (difficulty in talking and swallowing), hoarseness (ipsilateral vocal cord paralysis) Loss of gag reflex Partial loss of taste sensation
Pons	Anterior inferior cerebellar artery	CN V, VII, VIII Deafness or tinnitus Partial loss of taste sensation Ipsilateral facial muscle paralysis, inability to shut eyes Impaired salivation/lacrimation Hyperacusis (abnormally loud sounds) Jaw deviation during opening
Midbrain	Superior cerebellar artery, branches of posterior cerebral artery	Contralateral hemi-anaesthesia (ascending tracts' damage) Intentional tremor (damage to superior cerebellar peduncle)

2. Ipsilateral loss of facial skin sensation (trigeminothalamic tract damage)

3. Horner's syndrome: miosis, ptosis and impaired sweating (descending autonomic fibres injured)

4. Nystagmus, nausea and vomiting (vestibular and dorsal motor vagal nuclei injury)

5. Ipsilateral limb ataxia (cerebellar peduncle damage)

As with medial lesions, the level is determined by the involvement of cranial nerves V–X (see Table 6.7).

Bilateral motor and sensory signs are almost certainly an indication of a brainstem lesion. Vascular occlusion of the basilar artery, which supplies the majority of the ventral part of the brainstem, can be catastrophic, resulting in quadriplegia and often death, due to respiratory failure. It may result in 'locked-in syndrome', where the patient presents with quadriplegia, muteness and facial paralysis. The symptoms resemble coma, but the patient can communicate through eye/eyelid movement (EEG activity is normal). Damage to the basilar artery in the midbrain region produces complex syndromes that

include visual hallucinations, gaze palsies and oculomotor dysfunction.

Damage to the MLF results in a (horizontal) gaze disorder called internuclear ophthalmoplegia. It disconnects the abducens nucleus from the contralateral oculomotor nucleus and is characterized by disconjugate gaze with nystagmus and impaired adduction of the abducting eye (Fig. 6.8). The most common cause in the young, or if damage is bilateral, is multiple sclerosis; in older patients, vascular disease is more likely.

Some brainstem syndromes are more common than others. Wallenberg's syndrome (Fig. 6.9) is the most common brainstem stroke, and many patients show gradual recovery of function after this stroke. Anterior inferior cerebellar artery infarcts are only a tenth of the prevalence of posterior inferior cerebellar artery strokes, and Déjerine's syndrome is rare, accounting for only 0.5% of all brain strokes. Bilateral occlusions are rarer than unilateral occlusions and generally have a poorer prognosis.

Compression injuries of the brainstem by cerebellar or cortical herniation are often fatal (see Chapter 9). In addition, hydrocephalus or a pineal gland tumour (pinealoma) may cause Parinaud's syndrome, which is characterized

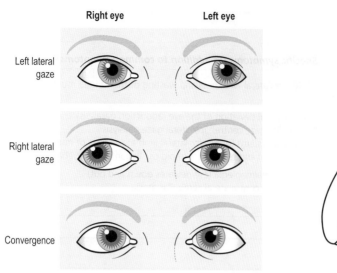

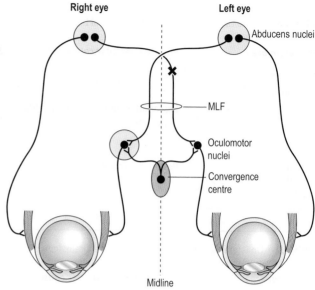

Fig. 6.8 Internuclear ophthalmoplegia results from a lesion in the medial longitudinal fasciculus (MLF) pathway, which connects the abducens nucleus to the contralateral oculomotor nucleus. On the side of the lesion (left MLF, indicated by the 'X'), the person is unable to adduct the eye during contralateral gaze but is able to adduct the eye on convergence, thus distinguishing it from oculomotor nerve palsy. (Adapted from Kingsley RE (2000). Concise Text of Neuroscience, 2nd ed. LWW.)

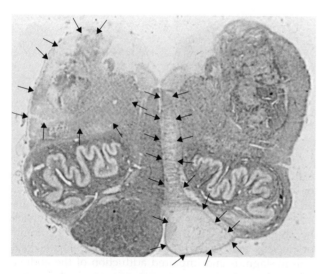

Fig. 6.9 Brainstem lesions resulting from vascular damage. Left side: arrows demarcate damage to the medulla area supplied by the posterior inferior cerebellar artery leading to symptoms associated with Wallenberg's syndrome. Right side: arrows demarcate damage in the territory supplied by the anterior spinal artery.

by compression of the dorsal (tectum) midbrain region, encompassing the superior colliculi and midbrain tegmentum. Symptoms include paralysis of upward gaze and accommodation, fixed pupils and nystagmus.

Comments on the case history

This case (see Box 6.1) is an example of Weber's syndrome caused by damage to the posterior cerebral artery

that supplies the ventral midbrain. This affects the corticospinal and corticobulbar tracts, red nucleus and fibres of the oculomotor nerve.

The oculomotor nerve has somatic fibres that innervate all the extrinsic eye muscles that adduct and elevate the eyeball and upper eyelid, and parasympathetic fibres of the Edinger–Westphal nucleus that innervate the ciliary and pupillary muscles regulating the processes of accommodation and pupil constriction. Damage to this nerve causes the eye to deviate down and out, due to the unopposed action of lateral rectus (abductor) and superior oblique (depressor) muscles innervated by the abducens and trochlear nerves, respectively. Paralysis of the superior levator muscle causes severe ptosis due to the unopposed action of the orbicularis oculi (innervated by the facial nerve). In this case, the left and right optic nerves and right oculomotor nerve are intact, but the left oculomotor nerve (including its parasympathetic component) is not. A fully dilated, non-reactive pupil is due to the unopposed action of the dilator pupillae muscle (supplied by the sympathetic nervous system). Pupils are always monitored during head injury cases because rapidly increasing intracranial pressure (often resulting from an acute cranial bleed) compresses the oculomotor nerve against the temporal bone. Autonomic nervous system fibres reside superficially in this nerve, and these are affected first so that the pupil dilates progressively on the affected side. Pupillary dilation is an urgent indication of surgical decompression of the brain.

The oculomotor nerve forms the efferent arc of two important visual reflexes. The first is the pupillary light reflex that results in constriction of the iris muscle of the pupil to bright light. This reflex involves four sets of neurons. Light activates retinal afferents (CN II) that terminate in the midbrain pretectal nuclei. Axons from this area innervate both Edinger-Westphal nuclei; preganglionic parasympathetic fibres from the Edinger-Westphal nucleus travel in the oculomotor nerve and synapse in the ciliary ganglion, whose postganglionic fibres innervate the constrictor muscle of iris (sphincter pupillae). The second reflex affected in this case is the accommodation reflex. As the pupil is fixed, it fails to respond to changes in depth of the visual field; thus vision is blurred in the affected eye.

The vascular lesion has also damaged the left descending upper motoneuron fibres of the corticobulbar and corticospinal tracts, resulting in muscle paralysis/paresis and abnormal reflexes. This is manifest in the inability to smile voluntarily on the right (contralateral) side. There is no direct damage to the facial nerve because paralysis would affect all the muscles of facial expression, and the other facial nerve motor tests (Chapter 3) would reveal abnormal responses. An upper motoneuron lesion affecting the corticobulbar tract results in contralateral lower facial muscle paralysis/paresis, since the upper facial muscles are innervated by both the contralateral and ipsilateral corticobulbar tracts, and thus remain innervated by the contralateral side. Similarly, impairment of the left corticospinal tract results in right-sided hyperreflexia (due to disinhibition of lower motoneurons), a Babinski sign and increased muscle tone. The prognosis for this patient is poor, and any improvement in functional recovery is unlikely.

Self-assessment case study

A 46-year-old woman, a mother of four who has been taking oral contraceptives for the past 15 years, arrived at Accident and Emergency presenting with nausea and vomiting that had been ongoing for the past few days. Neurologic testing further revealed an absence of a left side gag reflex, dysphagia and Horner's syndrome. Sensory testing showed a loss of pinprick sensation on the left side of her face and the right side of her neck, limbs and trunk. Reflexes were normal, as was muscle strength and tone, but left-sided ataxia was noted in the arm and leg. She was admitted to hospital and discharged a week later. At an outpatient appointment 9 months later, she was asymptomatic.

- Account for the symptoms described in this patient

This patient presents with symptoms that are consistent with lateral brainstem injury, specifically Wallenberg's syndrome. Several cranial nerve nuclei are affected and a dissociated sensory deficit involving the face and body is present. Damage to the spinal trigeminal nucleus/tract results in ipsilateral loss of pain and temperature sensation to the face, and contralateral loss of pain and temperature sensation from the body is due to damage of the spinothalamic tract. Dysphagia and loss of the gag reflex indicate involvement of the glossopharyngeal and vagus nerve nuclei (nucleus ambiguus), while damage to the inferior vestibular nucleus and dorsal motor vagal nucleus produces nausea and vomiting, respectively. Ataxia (loss of coordination) occurs because of injury to the inferior cerebellar peduncle. Horner's symptoms are ptosis (droopy eyelid), miosis (small pupils) and anhidrosis (warm dry facial skin), and are due to damage of the descending sympathetic fibres that run in the lateral part of the medullary tegmentum. Reflexes and motor strength were normal as the pyramidal tract is unaffected.

- What is the most likely cause of the lesion?

The most likely cause is a vascular lesion affecting the posterior inferior cerebellar artery. A tumour is unlikely, as the symptoms are sudden in onset and tumour symptoms present as progressive worsening of affected structures.

- Why is the use of oral contraceptives relevant?

In some patients who suffer brainstem strokes, there are predisposing factors such as hypertension, diabetes and transient ischaemic attacks. In women the use of the pill has been associated with cerebrovascular occlusive disease, especially in women who smoke or have hypertension.

THE VISUAL SYSTEM

7

Chapter summary

1. The eye is a sensory organ divided into two segments. The anterior segment refracts light rays through the cornea and lens into the posterior segment to converge onto the retina, which contains the photoreceptors. The captured image is back-to-front and inverted.

2. The retina comprises of photoreceptors (rods and cones) and bipolar, amacrine and retinal ganglion cells. Rods are sensitive to dim light levels and are monochromatic, while cones use daylight to create colour vision. Cones are concentrated in the centre of the retina (fovea), while rods are more prevalent around the periphery.

3. Visual processing of motion, colour and shape begins in the retina. Processes related to each of these characteristics are relayed as parallel streams to the visual cortex. Information from the nasal side of the retina crosses at the optic chiasm to project onto the contralateral side, while the temporal retina field remains ipsilateral. Retinal ganglion cell axons synapse in the lateral geniculate nuclei (thalamus). From here, information is relayed to the primary visual cortex, so these cells receive information from both eyes. Information is distributed to the visual association cortices to build a picture of the image and to other cortical regions for object identification and location.

4. Damage to the optic nerve produces unilateral, ipsilateral loss of vision; damage at the optic chiasm results in bitemporal hemianopsia (tunnel vision), and after the chiasm causes contralateral homonymous hemianopsia.

Introduction

'Beauty is in the eye of the beholder.' Most of our ideas about our surroundings and our memory of them are based on sight. But how do we see and assign emotional meaning to what we see? Vision is the process by which the brain receives light from the outside world and converts it into a recognizable percept. This is a complex process that starts with the focusing of light rays onto the retina—the specialised sensory component of the eye. This two-dimensional image is then conveyed to regions of the brain that take different properties of the image, such as colour, form, movement and depth, and seamlessly convert them into a three-dimensional percept. Furthermore, objects are recognized in many different orientations, under a wide range of lighting conditions, and, when they are at different distances from the observer, at a variety of sizes. Nearly half of the cerebral cortex is involved in visual processing, suggesting that vision is the most complex task that the brain performs.

As humans are very visually oriented, visual deficits have profound effects on daily life. Depending on the cause, the deficit can be monocular (restricted to one eye) or binocular (affecting both eyes) (Table 7.1). The World Health Organization estimates that 2.2 billion people worldwide have some form of visual impairment. Nearly 60% of these are elderly (>60 years old) and 5% are under the age of 14 years. It is estimated that almost 50% of visual deficits could be remedied with a simple visit to the optician or appropriate drugs.

The three main causes of visual loss in the developed world are uncorrected refractive errors, cataracts and glaucoma; in the less developed world, cataracts and infections such as trachoma and river blindness (onchocerciasis) account for 75% of blindness cases. The latter two diseases cause inflammation of the conjunctiva and scarring of the cornea, which eventually leads to blindness. River blindness affects over 20 million people worldwide, and in parts of Africa produces blindness rates of up to 35%. It can be treated (and prevented for 9 months) with a single dose of ivermectin, a drug which kills the larvae of the *Oncocherca volvulus* filarial worm that causes the disease. Trachoma is easily treated with antibiotics such as tetracycline. Uncorrected refractive errors (e.g. myopia and presbyopia) are common to both adults (see Box 7.1) and children, and the annual global costs of productivity losses associated with uncorrected myopia and presbyopia are estimated to be US$244 billion and US$25.4 billion, respectively.

Structure of the eye

Fig. 7.1 details the structure of the eye. It consists of three layers and two regions: (1) the anterior segment (comprising the cornea, anterior chamber, posterior chamber, and lens) is concerned with light refraction and focusing and (2) the posterior segment, consisting of the choroid and, most importantly, the retina, where light waves are converted into electrical impulses that are transmitted via the optic nerve to the brain.

The eyeball has three layers. The outermost layer is the sclera. This white, opaque, fibrous layer protects the eye and allows attachment of the muscles controlling

---

Table 7.1 Some causes of blindness

Monocular causes	Binocular causes
Vascular	**Trauma to visual pathway (post-chiasm)**
• Transient ischaemic attack	• Stroke
• Amaurosis fugax	• Tumour (e.g. pituitary adenoma)
Inflammation	• Raised intracranial pressure (papilloedema)
• Temporal arteritis	
• Optic neuritis	**Disease**
Trauma	• Diabetes
• Optic nerve damage	• Trachoma
• Retina detachment	• Glaucoma
Disease	• River blindness
• Cataracts	• Macular degeneration (old age)
• Multiple sclerosis	• Cataracts
	Genetics
	• Retinitis pigmentosa (X-linked)

Box 7.1 Case history

Fifty-five-year-old Mr Magoo visits his optician for a sight test, as he is finding it difficult to read with his old pair of glasses and thinks that he may need a new pair. When he was younger, his eyesight was good, except that he was colour-blind and could not distinguish red from green. His optician measures his visual acuity and examines his eye with an ophthalmoscope. He also measures the intraocular pressure. He finds that there are no signs of raised intraocular pressure or visual field defects, but that Mr Magoo's myopia has got significantly worse. He prescribes a new pair of glasses.

This case gives rise to the following questions:

1. What is the structure of the eye, and what are the pathways that convey visual information?
2. Can defects in vision indicate specific defects in the visual pathways?
3. How does the eye respond to light?
4. What is visual acuity, why does it decline with age and how can it be remedied?
5. How is colour perceived and processed by the visual system, and what are the causes of colour-blindness?
6. Which areas of the brain are involved in processing visual information, and how is this information coded?

the movement of the eye—the extraocular muscles. The movement of these muscles is controlled by cranial nerves III, IV and VI. At the anterior pole of the eye, the sclera becomes the conjunctiva (white of the eye), and this merges with the transparent cornea that allows light into the eye. The cornea is the eye's primary refractive surface. It is richly innervated with nociceptive fibres, which, in response to irritation, trigger blinking and the secretion of tears from the lacrimal gland, keeping the cornea free of dust.

The middle layer consists of the choroid, the ciliary body and the iris; together they form the uvea. The choroid lines the whole of the posterior segment, except where the optic nerve leaves the eye. It is a highly vascularized brown membrane. The colour pigment is produced by the melanocytes of the retinal epithelium; these absorb light that has not been detected by the retina and prevents it from being scattered back onto the retina and confusing the image.

At the junction of the anterior and posterior segments of the eye, and continuous with the choroid, is the ciliary body. This consists of radial and circular smooth muscle fibres—the ciliary muscles—which are under autonomic nervous system control and involved in changing the shape of the lens during the process of focusing. The epithelial cells of the ciliary body continually produce and secrete a clear fluid—the aqueous humour—into the small posterior chamber. The fluid then flows through the pupil into the anterior chamber, providing nutrients to the lens and cornea. It eventually drains into the venous blood through the canal of Schlemm, which is a lymphatic-like vessel. Production and reabsorption of this fluid produce the intraocular pressure in the anterior compartment, which is normally 13–29 mm Hg. Blockage of this reabsorption leads to glaucoma by causing ocular hypertension. This reduces blood flow in the retinal capillaries (Fig. 7.2C), and the subsequent ischemia causes damage to the retina and may lead to blindness. The suspensory ligaments extend from the ciliary body to attach to the lens. Contraction of the ciliary muscles pulls on the suspensory ligaments and can change the shape of the lens. In the relaxed eye the suspensory ligaments maintain the lens in a stretched, flattened shape.

The iris is the coloured part of the eye and extends from the ciliary body across the front of the lens, leaving a circular aperture—the pupil—where light passes from the anterior chamber into the lens. The size of the pupil controls the amount of light entering the lens and posterior segment, and this is determined by the contraction of the muscles of the iris.

The lens sits at the junction of the anterior and posterior segments of the eye and is a transparent biconvex structure. It is a secondary refractor of light waves and acts as a fine control for focusing light onto the retina, just like the lens of a camera. As in a camera, the image on the retina is reversed and upside down. The lens is surrounded by a flexible capsule and contains concentric layers of lens fibres, which contain transparent proteins, called crystallins. Cataracts occur when the lens of the eye becomes opaque (Fig. 7.2F). The most usual cause of this is old age, when the crystallin proteins become oxidized and aggregate. Cataracts are treated by surgical replacement of the affected lens with a synthetic lens. High levels of ultraviolet light increase the rate at which the lens becomes opaque; hence the higher prevalence of cataracts in countries at low latitudes.

The posterior segment of the eye is filled with a transparent, thick gelatinous fluid called vitreous humour,

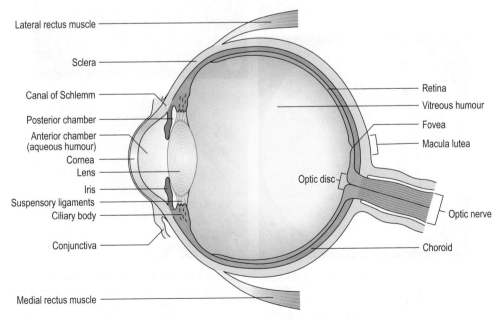

Fig. 7.1 Horizontal section through the right human eye.

composed of fine collagen fibres and large amounts of water. This maintains the shape of the eyeball and also contains phagocytic cells, which remove any debris that might accumulate in the posterior segment and interfere with light transmission.

The innermost layer of the eye—the retina—covers the choroid, ciliary body and posterior face of the iris. The retina can be investigated during examination of the eye (Box 7.2) and consists of two layers. The outer pigmented layer, like the choroid, prevents light scattering and also provides a source of vitamin A, which is needed by the

light-gathering cells. Vitamin A deficiency leads to night blindness (Box 7.3) due to a lack of the protein rhodopsin used by some photoreceptors. The inner neural layer of the retina consists of the light-gathering cells—photoreceptors and associated neurons—as well as glial cells and a dense capillary network. Apart from the photoreceptors, there are four other neuronal types—bipolar and ganglion cells, which are the first- and second-order neurons of the visual pathway, and horizontal and amacrine cells, which are interneurons (see Table 7.5). The centre of the retina is called the macula lutea (yellow spot), which

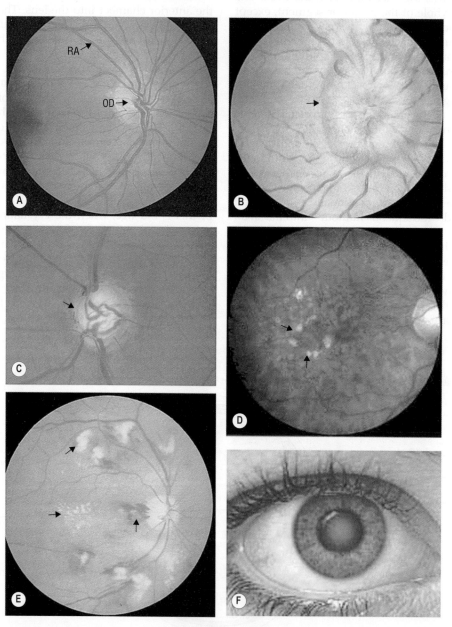

Fig. 7.2 Ophthalmoscope images. (A) A normal eye, showing the optic disc (OD) and the retinal arteries (RA); (B) abnormal fundus, showing papilloedema due to bulging of the optic disc (arrow); (C) glaucoma, where the optic cup is larger and deeper than normal (arrow); (D) macular degeneration, where the macula region is spotty or absent (arrows); (E) cotton wool-like deposits are seen in the eye around blood vessels (arrows) in hypertensive diabetic neuropathy; (F) abnormal lens function—cataract. (A–E, From Munro J, Edwards C (1995). eds. Macleod's Clinical Examination. 9th ed. Churchill Livingstone. D, From www.eyesearch.com.)

Clinical skill: Fundoscopic examination of the eye

Fundoscopy uses an ophthalmoscope to observe the retina. The assessment is best performed in dim light with the subject fixating on a distant object. The ophthalmoscope is adjusted so that the retinal vessels are in focus, and then these are traced back to the optic disc. The clarity of the disc margins is noted, as are the size and shape of blood vessels: arteries are narrower and brighter compared to veins. The presence of retinal vein pulsation is noted, as this can be used as an index of intracranial pressure. It is best observed as the veins cross over the arteries at the disc margins.

Figure 7.2 shows images obtained with this instrument. Because the optic nerve is within the meninges, any changes in pressure in the brain produce a swelling of the optic nerve, called papilloedema, which can be seen in the retina as a swollen optic disc and constricted blood vessels (Fig. 7.2B); it is often asymmetrical. Papilloedema does not normally impair vision, but if left untreated, it will impair the retinal ganglion cell function, leading to blindness because of ischemia of the retinal cells.

Changes in the appearance of the blood vessels, and other changes, such as spots, haemorrhages and dark patches, can indicate the development and progression of conditions such as hypertensive and diabetic retinopathy, subdural haemorrhage or hydrocephalus, and other degenerative changes (Fig. 7.2D and E).

Colour blindness

Most colour blindness, assessed using Ishihara plates, is genetically inherited and due to either a lack of, or the abnormal function of, one or more types of cone cell. However, most colour-blind people can see colour, but they confuse the wavelength and brightness of light over certain parts of the spectrum.

Anomalous trichromats have all three cone populations but an abnormal opsin, so that the wavelengths absorbed are slightly different.

Dichromats lack one of the cone populations:

- protanopes—lack L cones, so are red blind
- deuteranopes—lack M cones, so are green blind
- tritanopes—lack S cones, so are blue blind.

Problems with S cones lead to blue–yellow colour blindness (both appear grey), whereas problems with either M or L cones result in red–green colour blindness, where both red and green are indistinguishable from each other (and appear grey). This red–green colour blindness is X-linked, as the genes for both M and L opsins are on the X chromosome. Therefore this type of colour blindness is more common in men than in women. The S cone defect is located on chromosome 7.

Rare individuals who lack two types of cone have no colour vision, and those who lack cones completely have no photopic vision, and are blind in daylight, when their rods are completely saturated. People who lack rod cells have no peripheral vision and are blind at low light levels—night blindness.

Night blindness (nyctalopia) and vitamin A

According to the World Health Organization, night blindness affects worldwide 5.2 million preschool-age children and 9.8 million pregnant women, due to severe vitamin A deficiency. The incidence is highest in sub-Saharan Africa, which accounts for nearly 50% of the cases. Nyctalopia is an early symptom, which makes doing simple things like going to the bathroom at night or night-time driving difficult. Vitamin A (also known as retinol) is a retinoid compound found in foodstuffs like chicken, beef, liver, eggs, milk, carrots, kale, spinach and orange or yellow fruits that contain β-carotene—an organic pigment—which is the precursor to vitamin A. Vitamin A is needed to produce retinal, which is used by photoreceptors. Lack of retinal causes loss of function, initially in rods but later in cones, as the deficiency develops. This leads to anatomical changes in the photoreceptors followed by neural degeneration. Vitamin A treatment can restore function if given before degeneration occurs. Loss of vitamin A also produces xerophthalmia (abnormal dryness of the sclera and cornea) due to lack of tears.

corresponds to the centre of the visual field and contains the fovea at its centre. This is the region of greatest visual acuity. It lies on a direct line from the centre of the visual field through the centre of the lens. Damage to this region causes macular degeneration (Fig. 7.2D, Box 7.5).

The output of the retina is via the axons of the ganglion cells, which form the optic nerve. They leave the retina at an area called the optic disc. This area has no photoreceptors, so this part of the visual field corresponds to the blind spot. Objects that are projected onto this area of the retina are invisible; however, visual processing fills in the background pattern, so we are unaware of a 'hole' in our vision. Retinal ganglion cell axons become myelinated after the optic disc and form the optic nerve. This is not a true peripheral nerve because it is myelinated by oligodendrocytes, and so is part of the central nervous system. It is an extension of the brain! If damaged, it does not regenerate.

Visual pathways

The visual field corresponds to the visual space seen by each eye, with each eye seeing it from a slightly different angle. This slight disparity provides clues about the distance of the object of interest (depth perception) and has important consequences for the organization of information in the visual regions of the brain: information is compared so that distance can be accurately judged. However, we see only one object, not two. The

brain fuses the image by a process called stereopsis, and this gives us a three-dimensional appreciation of the object. When the eyes cannot fuse an image, the resultant deficit is called amblyopia.

The visual system has to perform three basic functions: (1) see an object clearly, (2) identify it and (3) track it. Different pathways associated with the visual system (Fig. 7.3) carry out these roles.

From each eye, the optic nerves, each containing 0.8–1.5 million axons, travel to the optic chiasm—an X-shaped structure at the base of the brain anterior to the pituitary gland. Here, approximately 60% of the axons from each nerve cross and continue in the opposite nerve as the optic tract. These axons are from the ganglion cells situated on the part of the retina on the nasal side. Beyond the optic chiasm, each optic tract carries the output from the ipsilateral temporal (lateral) retina and the contralateral nasal (medial) retina. This means that all the information from one half of the visual field travels along the contralateral optic tract so that the left hemifield is 'viewed' by the right hemisphere and vice versa.

Most of the optic tract axons travel via its lateral root to synapse with neurons in specific layers of the lateral geniculate nucleus (LGN) of the thalamus (see later). However, approximately 10% of the axons from the medial root terminate in either the superior colliculus or the pretectal nucleus of the midbrain. These fibres are involved in controlling the movement of extraocular muscles and the pupillary light reflexes. A few fibres terminate in the suprachiasmatic nucleus of the hypothalamus and

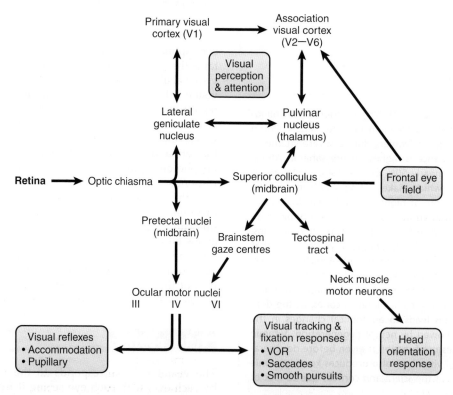

Fig. 7.3 Different functional pathways in the visual system. *VOR*, Vestibulo-ocular reflex.

the reticular formation, where they are involved in the setting of circadian rhythms and in gaze responses.

Axons of LGN neurons project along a tract called the optic radiation to the primary visual cortex, which occupies the areas either side of the calcarine sulcus of the occipital lobe (Fig. 7.4). The axons of the optic radia-tion take two different paths to the inferior part of the visual cortex. One passes directly posterior through the parietal lobe, carrying fibres from the fovea and the lower quadrant of the visual field, while the other courses more laterally through the temporal lobe, before terminating below the calcarine sulcus (see Figs 7.4 and 7.5). This latter pathway is called Meyer's loop, and these fibres represent the upper part of the visual field. The primary visual cortex (Brodmann area 17) is also called the striate cortex because of the prominent horizontal striations caused by myelinated fibres passing through the cortical layers. The remainder of the occipital lobe forms the visual association (or extra-striate) areas. This area also receives input about visual tracking via the superior colliculus and pulvinar nucleus (see Fig. 7.3).

Visual field defects

Because of the organization of the visual pathways, certain types of visual field defects reflect specific lesions. This can be examined by covering one eye and assessing the various quadrants using the visual field confrontation methods described in Chapter 3. Lesions to structures anterior to the optic chiasm produce unilateral defects in the visual field of the corresponding eye, whereas lesions at or posterior to the optic chiasm produce binocular visual deficits (Fig. 7.5 and Table 7.2).

Pupillary light reflexes

Eye pupil size is normally symmetrical. The pupillary reflex causes the pupil diameter to vary between 1.5 mm in bright light and 8 mm in complete darkness in young people. The range is smaller in the elderly. This is achieved by the contraction (and relaxation) of two sets of smooth muscle in the iris, pupillary dilator and sphincter.

Light shone into one eye causes both pupils to constrict. In the stimulated eye, this reflex is called the direct light reflex, and in the non-stimulated eye, the consensual light reflex (Fig. 7.6B). This reflex, and changes due to various pathologies, are described in Chapter 6. Pupil asymmetry can indicate damage to the sympathetic or parasympathetic nervous system (Fig. 7.6A). In a clinical context, whether the symmetry occurs in the dark or the light is important. Asymmetry in the dark implies that the sympathetic nervous system is not functioning properly. Conversely, if it occurs in the light, the parasympathetic nervous system is dysfunctional. Table 7.3 shows the different types of causes of pupil asymmetry.

Administration of morphine interferes with pupil responses, and results in pinpoint pupils. Thus it is not given to head injury patients before primary assessment has been done.

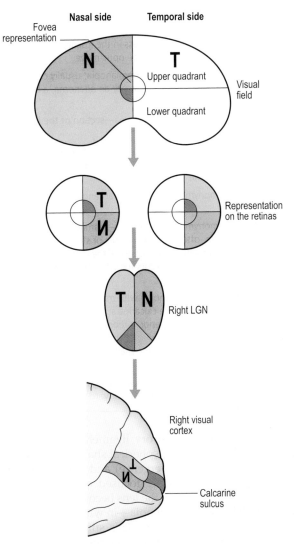

Fig. 7.4 Representation of the visual field projections to the visual cortex. For clarity, only the left visual field is shown. The visual field of each eye is subdivided into four quadrants—left/right and upper/lower—each of which projects to a different area of the visual cortex (above/below the calcarine sulcus) of both hemispheres in a highly organized manner, called retinotopic mapping. Note that the retinal image is inverted both laterally and vertically, so that something on the top left of the visual field falls on the bottom right of the retina. This organization continues to the primary visual cortex. In the optic tract, the foveal input is in the middle of the field, but beyond the lateral geniculate nucleus (LGN), the foveal input moves to the posterior part of the optic radiation and travels through the parietal loop to the posterior part of the visual cortex. The right half of the visual field projects similarly to the left visual cortex. *N,* Nasal side of visual field; *T,* temporal side of visual field.

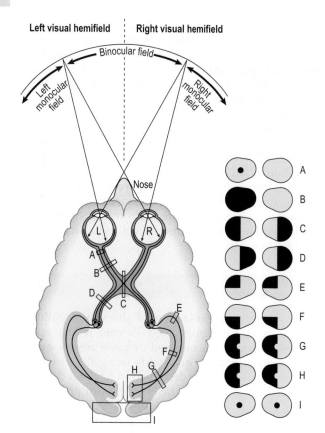

Left visual hemifield | **Right visual hemifield**

Binocular field

Left monocular field

Right monocular field

Nose

L   R

A
B
C
D
E
F
G
H
I

A
B
C
D
E
F
G
H
I

Fig. 7.5 Locations of visual field defects in the visual pathways and the deficits produced by them (see Table 7.2 for a description of each defect). Note the difference in homonymous hemianopsia between lesion D and lesion G, which are on opposite sides of the pathway.

Table 7.2 Visual field defects (see Fig. 7.5) and terminology

- Homonymous—same part of the visual field
- Heteronymous—opposite sides of the visual field
- Anopia—loss of vision
- Hemianopia—loss of vision in half of the visual field
- Quadrantanopia—loss of vision in a quadrant of the visual field
- Scotoma—patch of blindness

A	Scotoma in the ipsilateral (left) visual field—partial lesion of left optic nerve; in young adults, this may be due to multiple sclerosis
B	Complete unilateral blindness in the ipsilateral (left) eye due to complete section of the optic nerve
C	Bitemporal heteronymous hemianopia; usually caused by compression of the chiasm by an adenoma, a benign tumour of the pituitary
D	Right homonymous hemianopia—section of the left optic tract
E	Right homonymous upper quadrantanopia—damage to the right Meyer's loop, possibly caused by a tumour or stroke in the temporal lobe
F	Right homonymous lower quadrantanopia—parietal lobe lesion
G	Right homonymous hemianopia—damage to the optic radiation, often due to tumours or stroke. Classically, following a haemorrhage from the middle cerebral artery, this defect occurs for a number of days, due to oedema
H	Homonymous hemianopia with macular sparing—a lesion above or below the calcarine sulcus, usually due to a stroke in the posterior cerebral artery. The macular sparing is due to sparing of the occipital pole, the most posterior area where the macula is represented
I	Bilateral central scotomas—bilateral lesion in the posterior region of the primary visual cortex, above the calcarine sulcus, often caused by a backward fall or concussion

Focusing of light on the retina

As light passes from the air to the retina, it is first refracted by the cornea, and then by the lens, in order to produce a focused image on the retina. This means that light from a point source must focus onto a single point on the retina, regardless of whether it comes from a distant or near object. Thus the lens must change shape (accommodate) to properly focus the object. Images focused on the retina are inverted and right-to-left reversed due to refraction (Fig. 7.4), and the brain corrects this process.

Accommodation

More than two thirds of the focusing power of the relaxed eye, which is measured in units called dioptres, is produced by the cornea (42 out of 60 dioptres), with the remainder being produced by the lens (Fig. 7.7A). However, while the cornea has a fixed focusing power, the lens, which is elastic, can change its shape, and so can increase the amount by which light is refracted, increasing its focusing power from approximately 18 to 30 dioptres. The contraction of ciliary muscles reduces the tension in the suspensory ligaments and allows the lens to contract to a more spherical shape. This process is called accommodation (vergence) and allows light from near objects to be correctly focused on the retina (Fig. 7.7B). However, with age, the lens becomes less elastic—a condition known as presbyopia—in which there is failure of the accommodation reflex. This stiffening of the lens occurs throughout life but accelerates after 40 years of age; hence the need for 'reading glasses' by most people in later life. By about the age of 60 years, accommodation no longer occurs, as the lens can no longer rebound.

As part of the accommodation reflex, convergence of the eyes occurs so that the point of crossing of the visual axes of the eyes becomes closer and constriction of the pupil occurs to maintain focus. The circuitry for the accommodation reflex is shown in Fig. 7.7C.

Defects in focusing

Normally, the eye is a sphere and parallel light rays, such as those from a distant object, focus on the retina when the

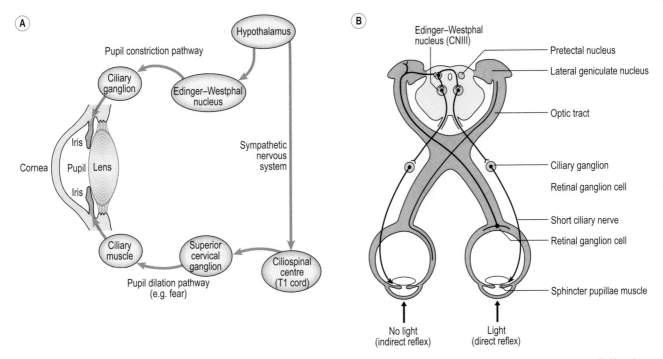

Fig. 7.6 Neural control of pupil size. (A) Autonomic control: hypothalamic stimulation of the sympathetic nervous system causes pupil dilatation. Parasympathetic activation causes the reverse. (B) Pupillary light reflex circuitry. See text for further details.

Table 7.3	Causes of pupil asymmetry	
Name of deficit	**Symptom**	**Cause**
Argyll Robertson	Small pupils that do not react well to light but react equally to accommodation	Pineal tumour Neurosyphilis
Marcus Gunn	Weak direct reflex Strong consensual reflex	Ipsilateral damage to optic nerve
Horner's syndrome	Unilateral asymmetry of pupil (0.5–1 mm difference) Normal direct and consensual reflexes Does not dilate in response to cocaine drops	Oculosympathetic damage
Non-reactive	No response to light or accommodation	Cranial nerve compression Iris disease Brain herniation Acute glaucoma

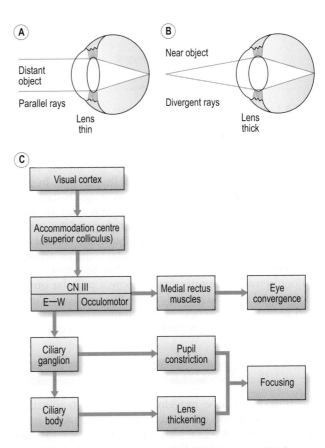

Fig. 7.7 Accommodation for near vision. (A) Unaccommodated eye. (B) Accommodation produces a rounder lens in order to focus on near objects. (C) Neural circuit for accommodation. *E–W*, Edinger–Westphal.

ciliary muscles are relaxed. This is called emmetropia (Fig. 7.8A). In myopia (near-sightedness), the eye is elongated so that the focal point, where the light rays converge into a single point, occurs before the retina. This can be corrected by a concave lens placed in front of the eye (Fig. 7.8C). Hyperopia (far-sightedness) is due to a shortened eye, so the focal point falls behind the retina. Again, this can be corrected by using a convex lens (Fig. 7.8E). Refractive

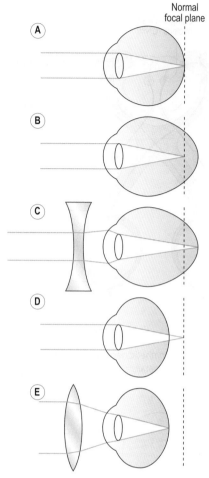

Normal focal plane

(A)

(B)

(C)

(D)

(E)

Fig. 7.8 Eyeballs of different shapes focus light at different points. (A) Emmetropia. (B) Myopia. (C) Myopia corrected. (D) Hyperopia. (E) Hyperopia corrected.

errors can also be caused by the corneal surface being either too curved (myopia) or too flat (hyperopia). In people who have astigmatism, the visual image is distorted due to failure of the light rays to meet at a common focal point. This is because of the irregular shape of the cornea or lens, producing different focal points in the vertical and horizontal planes. It can be corrected by using an artificial lens that is more curved in one plane than the other.

Photorefractive keratectomy is now a popular outpatient corneal surgical procedure used to reduce or correct mild to moderate myopia or hyperopia. This is done by the use of a laser that precisely reshapes the cornea.

Control of eye movements

The purpose of eye movements is gaze stabilization, that is, to keep the eyes stable when the head is moving, or gaze shifting, which allows the fovea to track the visual image when the object of interest is moving. Gaze stabilization involves the vestibulo-ocular and optokinetic systems that deal with fast and slow head

rotational movements, respectively. They both produce conjugate eye movements in the opposite direction to the head movement (see Chapter 8 for details on the vestibulo-ocular reflex), evoking a normal physiological nystagmus response. The gaze shift system has three components: saccades, smooth pursuits and vergence (as part of the accommodation response). Saccadic movements seek out visual targets and smooth pursuit and vergence systems track them as they move.

Saccades are the quick flicks that move the eyes when they jump from one fixation point to another so that new images are captured by the fovea. These can be voluntary, for example, when looking at a portrait painting of a face, the eyes scan across many features of the image to build a picture, and the perception is entirely built up from the repeated scanning of areas of interest in the object. The saccades are not random but are controlled by what a person wants or expects to see. Saccades are also produced reflexively in response to visual, auditory, or somatosensory stimuli, driven by the horizontal (paramedian pontine reticular formation) and vertical (rostral interstitial nucleus of Cajal) gaze centres in the brainstem. Their activity is driven by outputs from the superior colliculus (which turns sensory coordinates into motor coordinates) and frontal eye field (FEF) regions in the frontal lobe, to drive appropriate orientation responses. Stimulation of the right FEF causes eye movement to the contralateral side; damage causes drifting to the ipsilateral side. The FEFs connect to the gaze centres in the pons and midbrain, and to other pursuit centres in the brain (Fig. 7.3). The parieto-occipital centre is part of the visual association cortex and is responsible for involuntary visual pursuit. It is responsible for keeping the eyes fixed on an object after it has been located and bringing it into the fovea by generating a new saccade.

Smooth pursuit movements are voluntary responses (unlike optokinetic reflexes). Signals about object velocity and direction relay from the visual cortex to the medial temporal (MT/V5) cortex (part of the 'where is it pathway'), and from there to the dorsolateral pontine nucleus (DPLN) in the brainstem. This translates velocity into motor commands for the smooth pursuit movement. The DPLN has connections with the vestibulocerebellum to control head following movements to track the speed and direction of the object.

Because of the importance of the eyes in locating and tracking objects, precision control is required. This is performed by the extraocular eye muscles (Fig. 7.9), which control the movement and are innervated by the oculomotor, trochlear and abducens cranial nerves. In order for both eyes to move in parallel, that is, have conjugate eye movements, different muscles contract in each eye. For example, contraction of the lateral rectus in one eye is accompanied by contraction of the medial rectus in the other. The motor neurons fire both statically, to signal about eye position, and dynamically, reflecting eye velocity. The combination of muscles involved in the various movements is different for different eye positions.

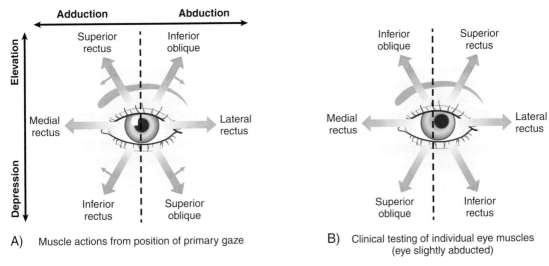

A) Muscle actions from position of primary gaze

B) Clinical testing of individual eye muscles (eye slightly abducted)

Fig. 7.9 Actions of the extraocular muscles when from the position of primary gaze (A) or when isolated during clinical testing (B).

The eye muscles insert into the sclera of the eye. The superior, inferior, medial and lateral recti insert at the front of the sclera in front of the vertical equator of the eye, whereas the oblique muscles insert posterior to the equator. Consequently, by working together, they elevate, depress, adduct or abduct the eye. They also produce rotational movements about the axis of primary gaze; intorsion is rotation of the top of the eye towards the nasal side whereas extorsion is towards the temporal side. When the eyes are looking straight ahead, parallel to the mid-sagittal plane, this is the primary position of gaze. In order to move in different directions, the muscles work as groups. Figure 7.9A shows the muscles that are the prime movers in specific directions (although other muscles contribute to some movements). Extraocular muscles work in synergy with each other. For example, to adduct and elevate the eye, the superior rectus is the prime mover, while the medial rectus helps to adduct the eye, and the inferior rectus helps to elevate the eye. Thus, most often, the muscles work as pairs: adduction/abduction via the medial and lateral rectus, respectively, elevation involves contraction of the superior rectus and inferior oblique, while depression involves the superior oblique and inferior rectus. The normal functioning of individual muscles cannot be assessed from the primary position of gaze. Therefore, to clinically isolate each muscle, the eyeball must be adducted or abducted slightly, so that the angle of gaze coincides with the angle of insertion of the eye into the orbit (23 degrees lateral from the midline for the superior and inferior rectus, and 51 degrees for the superior and inferior obliques). The specific function then becomes apparent (Fig. 7.9B, Table 7.4).

The eyes are normally parallel in all positions of gaze except convergence. When they are not, a squint is present and double vision (diplopia) ensues. This is where the patient is aware of two images of the same object simultaneously. It is usually due to the limited move-

Table 7.4	Functions of extraocular muscles		
Muscle	**Normal action from position of primary gaze**	**Nerve supply**	**Eye position after nerve injury**
Medial rectus	Adduction (inwards)	Oculomotor	Depressed after abduction (down and out)
Superior rectus	Elevation after abduction (up and out) Intorsion increases with adduction	Oculomotor	
Inferior rectus	Depression after abduction (down and out) Extorsion increases with adduction	Oculomotor	
Inferior oblique	Elevation after adduction (up and in) Extorsion increases with abduction	Oculomotor	
Superior oblique	Depression after adduction (down and in) Intorsion increases with abduction	Trochlear	Elevation after abduction (up and out)
Lateral rectus	Abduction (out)	Abducens	Adducted (in)

ment of one eye, a 'lazy eye'. This may be due to either nerve or muscle damage, or a restriction in the mechanical movement of the eye, such as occurs if the orbit is fractured. A weakness in a particular muscle produces diplopia in the direction of movement of that muscle, with an image that is further out from the affected eye.

Testing of eye movements can identify damage to the cranial nerves. Damage to the oculomotor nerve causes the eye to deviate down and out because of unopposed action of the lateral rectus and superior oblique muscles, while damage to the other nerves produces different effects (Table 7.4). The oculomotor nerve also controls the superior levator muscle, which opens the eyelid. Oculomotor nerve damage causes severe drooping of the eyelid (ptosis), due to the unopposed action of the orbicularis oculi, controlled by the facial nerve.

Structure and function of the retina

The retina contains five types of neurons arranged in three nuclear (inner, outer and ganglion) and two synaptic (plexiform) layers (see Fig. 7.10 and Table 7.5). The retina also contains two types of glial cell—Müller cells and astrocytes—which provide structural and metabolic support.

The layers of the retina are arranged with the photoreceptors lying closest to the pigment epithelium, and the capillaries and nerve axons lying on the inner (choroid) surface, so light has to pass through these other

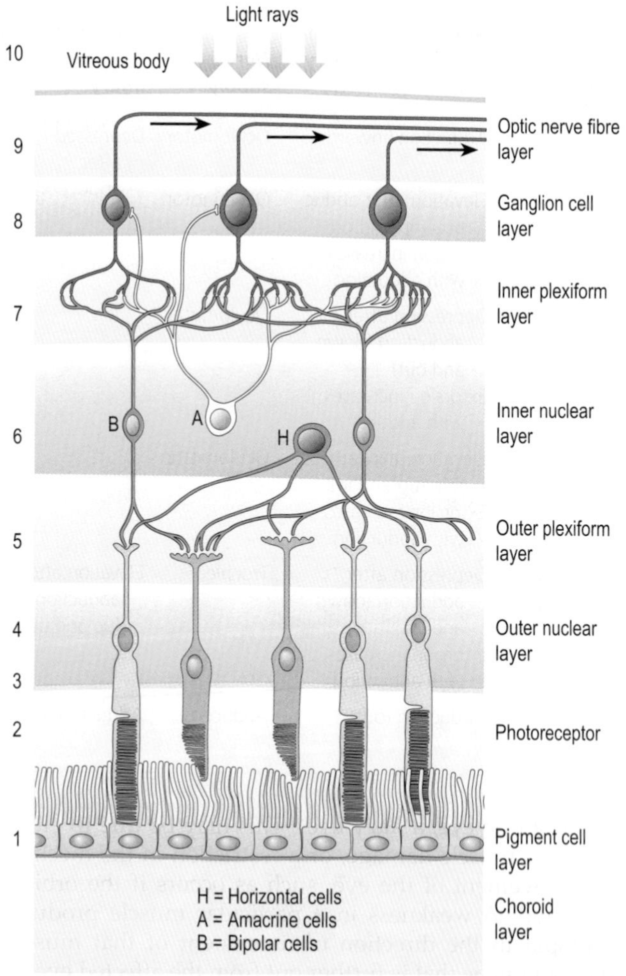

Fig. 7.10 Diagrammatic representation of the retina. For clarity, Müller cells and astrocytes are not shown.

layers before it is detected by the photoreceptors. A detached retina occurs when the pigment epithelial cell layer comes away from the photoreceptor layer, which is mechanically unstable. This causes the photoreceptors to stop working and die, resulting in blurred vision.

Visual processing begins in the retina. Photoreceptors are stimulated by light photons, and the signal is then transmitted and processed by bipolar cells before being conveyed to the brain via the axons of retinal ganglion cells in the optic nerve. Light falling on the retina produces changes in membrane potential in the photoreceptors and bipolar cells, but only ganglion cells fire action potentials; the other cells respond with graded potentials, which release graded amounts of neurotransmitter. Mechanisms exist within the retina to increase contrast and increase colour detection, but the graded potentials allow subtle changes in the light levels falling on the retina to be detected.

Photoreceptors and the detection of light

Rods and cones are the photoreceptors; they have a broadly similar structure but different functions. The human eye has approximately 12 million rods and 6 million cones. Rods are very sensitive to light, and can detect light at very low levels, over a wide range of wavelengths. They are effective in dim light but can only 'see' shades of grey. This is scotopic vision. Nocturnal animals have retinas composed of mostly, or entirely, rods. Their high sensitivity is because they collect light over a longer period and from a larger area than cones, but this also means that they cannot detect very fast-flickering light.

Cones are less sensitive to light than are rods, and so can only work in relatively high light levels; this is photopic vision. There are three different types of cone, each sensitive to a pattern of wavelengths due to the different types of opsin (cone pigments). Humans are trichromats, as they use a three-cone system to absorb light of different wavelengths that correspond approximately to red, green and blue (violet); between them, cones are able to detect colour (Fig. 7.11). The peak wavelengths of the

Table 7.5	Functions of retinal visual cells
Cell type	**Function**
Photoreceptors (rods and cones)	Signal transducers—scotopic and photopic vision
Bipolar cells	Relay cell
Retinal ganglion cells	Output cell
Horizontal cells	Interneuron—contrast detection via lateral inhibition
Amacrine cells	Interneuron—signal modulation Presynaptic to bipolar cells Postsynaptic to retinal ganglion cells

cones do not correspond exactly to red, green and blue, so cones are better described as long- (L), medium- (M), and short-wavelength (S) cones. Colour vision depends on the difference between different signals from different cone populations. Degeneration of photoreceptors because of vascular or genetic conditions causes specific visual deficits (Boxes 7.4, 7.5 and 7.6).

Rods and cones have a differential distribution across the retina; cones are concentrated in the fovea (Fig. 7.12), providing high-acuity colour vision. Furthermore, in this area, the overlying capillaries and nerve axons are displaced, so the cones receive the maximum amount of light. Rods distribute more peripherally and are preferentially sensitive to movement. Overall, there are fewer

S cones (with none in the fovea), and L and M cones are distributed in patches across the retina, so colour vision is grainy.

Rod cells are much more sensitive to light than are cone cells, to the point where they are saturated and unresponsive in normal daylight. Upon transition from light to dark, vision is initially reduced for 10–15 minutes but then recovers as the rod cells become unsaturated and more sensitive over a period of approximately 30 minutes. This is called dark adaptation and is due to chemical changes in the rods. The light stimulates the regeneration of rhodopsin and, as rhodopsin regenerates in the rod, the eye becomes adapted to the lower light level. In reverse, light adaptation is much faster. Rod cells are much less sensitive to red light than L cones, as shown by the distance between the curves in Fig. 7.11. This property is used by people who work in low light conditions, such as astronomers, who wish to retain the maximum dark adaptation of their scotopic vision.

In each retina, rods outnumber cones by ~20:1. There are many more rods and cones (100 million) than bipolar cells, which are more numerous than ganglion cells (1 million). This means that ganglion cells receive convergent input from more than one photoreceptor. The pattern of connection varies between rods and cones. A group of rods projects to a smaller number of bipolar cells, which projects to a smaller number of ganglion cells. This enables the collected light from many rods to be integrated, in order to affect a single ganglion cell, allowing scotopic vision to have low acuity but high sensitivity. In contrast, cones are linked to fewer bipolar cells and input from cones is much less integrated. This non-convergence is highest in the fovea, where single cones connect to single bipolar and single ganglion cells, increasing the acuity of this region. Additionally, in the

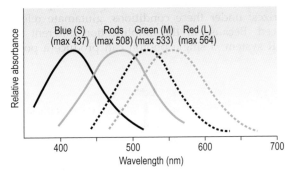

Fig. 7.11 Spectral sensitivities of rods and cones. *L*, Long-wavelength cones; *M*, medium-wavelength cones; *S*, short-wavelength cones. Adapted from Longstaff A. (2005). Instant Notes in Neuroscience. 2nd ed. Taylor and Francis Group.

Box 7.6   Retinitis pigmentosa

This is an inherited visual defect that affects approximately 1 in 4000 people. Symptoms start with night blindness and a loss of peripheral vision and can develop into complete loss of vision. There is narrowing of the retinal blood vessels, and clumps of disrupted retinal pigment are seen, often associated with the vessels. It is a heterogeneous disorder, whose different forms may be inherited as an autosomal-dominant, autosomal-recessive, or X-linked disease. Some of the forms are due to defects in the rhodopsin molecule, while others are due to defects in the Cyclic guanosine monophosphate (cGMP) phosphodiesterase or ion channels in the photoreceptors. The loss of night and peripheral vision is due to the initial loss of rods, after which, patients are completely dependent on cones (photopic vision). However, the cones also progressively degenerate, leading to eventual blindness. In many patients, the mutation responsible is in the rod (e.g. in rhodopsin), but why this should lead to a loss of cones as well as rods is a mystery. Over 100 mutations in opsin genes are associated with this condition. Animal studies also suggest that defective phagocytosis of disc segments by retinal pigment epithelial cells also contributes to this condition.

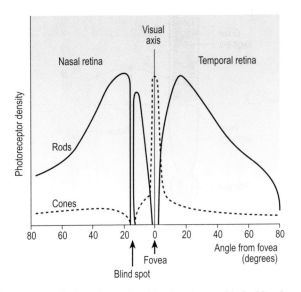

Fig. 7.12 Distribution of rods (solid lines) and cones (dashed lines) across the retina. Adapted from Longstaff A. (2005). Instant Notes in Neuroscience. 2nd ed. Taylor and Francis Group.

fovea, the cone photoreceptors are narrower, allowing even more cones to pack together.

Mechanism of phototransduction by photoreceptors

Both rods and cones consist of outer and inner segments (Fig. 7.13). The outer segments of cones have multiple invaginations of the plasma membrane, while rods contain layers of flattened discs. The discs are continually shed from the outer segments and are phagocytosed by the pigment epithelium (3–4 discs per hour), while new ones are generated from the base, as photoreceptors cannot undergo mitosis. Defects in this process can lead to retinitis pigmentosa (see Box 7.6). The outer segments are specialized for phototransduction, while the inner segment contains the nucleus and biosynthetic machinery.

The outer segment discs contain visual pigments, proteins that absorb specific wavelengths of light called chromophores. The eye chromophore is called retinal (derived from vitamin A). Rods contain more pigment than cones, enabling them to capture more light. Rod cells contain rhodopsin, and there are three different opsins in the cone cells. Rhodopsin consists of an opsin, a G-protein-coupled (GPCR) receptor (see Chapter 2), and a molecule of retinal, which is in the 11-cis form in the dark but is converted to the all-trans isomer by light in the disc membranes. The opsin detects the conformational change and allows transducin—a G-protein—to become activated and to bind GTP in place of GDP. The α-subunit of transducin then dissociates from the βγ-subunits and activates the enzyme cyclic GMP phosphodiesterase. The effect of light is thus to decrease the concentration of cGMP in the photoreceptors, that is, light is an inhibitory stimulus (Fig. 7.14). Deficits in these processes can lead to visual defects (Box 7.6).

In the dark, the resting membrane potential (RMP) of a photoreceptor is approximately −40 mV. This is more depolarised compared to other neurons in the nervous system where the RMP is more hyperpolarised at around −65 mV (see Chapter 2). This is because the membranes are 'leaky' and depolarized by the movement of Na^+ ions that are actively pumped out from the inner segment to enter through open cation channels in the outer segment. This is the dark current. Because of depolarization, glutamate is constantly released in the dark to activate bipolar cells. However, these channels are kept open by cGMP, so, in the presence of light when the cGMP concentration falls, these channels close, and the photoreceptor hyperpolarizes; under these conditions, glutamate release is reduced. Because of the amplification inherent in the GPCR system, a single photon can produce a potential

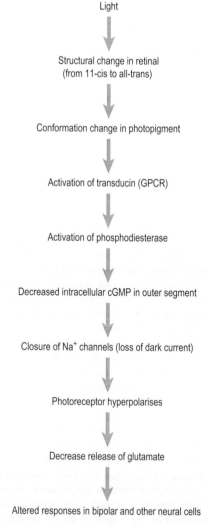

Light

Structural change in retinal
(from 11-cis to all-trans)

Conformation change in photopigment

Activation of transducin (GPCR)

Activation of phosphodiesterase

Decreased intracellular cGMP in outer segment

Closure of Na^+ channels (loss of dark current)

Photoreceptor hyperpolarises

Decrease release of glutamate

Altered responses in bipolar and other neural cells

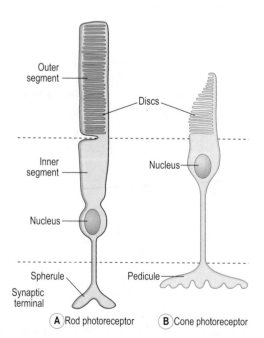

Fig. 7.13 Structure of rod photoreceptor (left) and cone photoreceptor (right).

Fig. 7.14 Sequence of events during phototransduction in rods and cones

change of approximately 1 mV (by blocking the entry of approximately 1 million Na^+ ions). Thus, the overall response of the photoreceptor depends on the light intensity; more light, less neurotransmitter. Rods/cones are paradoxically most active during complete darkness! The cascade is stopped by several mechanisms:

- The intrinsic GTPase activity of transducin converts GTP to GDP. The inactivation of transducin occurs by a protein called RGS9 (regulator of G-protein signalling 9). Inactivated transducin then recombines with the βγ subunits, stopping the action of phosphodiesterase.

- Photon-excited rhodopsin molecules are inactivated by phosphorylation by rhodopsin kinase, and by the binding of arrestin, a protein whose sole function is to block interactions between rhodopsin and transducin.

After prolonged exposure to light (a few seconds), the link between rhodopsin and retinal is hydrolysed and the all-trans-retinal dissociates. This is called bleaching, and the retinal is converted to retinol (vitamin A). Vitamin A is reconverted to 11-cis retinal by retinal isomerase in the dark, and this then binds with the opsin to reconstitute rhodopsin. This restores the sensitivity of the photoreceptor and underlies dark adaptation.

Contrast detection in the retina: 'on' and 'off' channels

One crucial element in object recognition by the visual system involves identifying the edges of objects, usually by changes in light levels. Connections between bipolar cells, horizontal cells, and ganglion cells act to increase contrast between light and dark areas. Therefore, bipolar cells perform the initial data processing in the retina. They receive input from groups of rods or a single cone.

There are two populations of cone bipolar cells, called 'on' and 'off' bipolar cells. These respond to input from cone cells in different ways: 'on' cells depolarize and 'off' cells hyperpolarize in response to light. Along with the horizontal cells, they enhance contrast.

There are two types of bipolar cell based on their structure and response:

- Invaginating bipolar cells form specialized synapses, called triad ribbon synapses, with the base of the photoreceptors. The triad consists of the dendrites of the bipolar cell and two horizontal cells. These 'on' bipolar cells are depolarised by light, due to the reduced glutamate release from the photoreceptor. These cells detect patches of brightness.

- Flat bipolar cells form basal synapses with photoreceptors. In response to light, these 'off' bipolar cells hyperpolarize. These cells detect dark regions of the image.

Cone bipolar cells are termed midget bipolar cells, as they are smaller than rod bipolar cells and depolarize in response to light. All bipolar cells respond to a reduction in glutamate release, but their different responses are due to the different types of glutamate receptor (metabotropic in 'on' cells and ionotropic in 'off' cells) present in their cell membranes.

Cone bipolar cells synapse with ganglion cells that have the same response pattern. That is, 'on' bipolar cells produce an increase in action potential firing rate in their ('on') ganglion cells, and 'off' bipolar cells reduce the firing rate in their ('off') ganglion cells. This leads to two channels. In response to light, the 'on' channel increases the ganglion cell-firing rate, and the 'off' channel reduces ganglion firing. So, in the dark, glutamate release inhibits the 'on' channel and excites the 'off' channel. In the light, the reverse happens; a reduction in glutamate excites the 'on' channel and inhibits the 'off' channel.

Each retinal ganglion cell is affected by light falling on its circular receptive field (RF). The ganglion cells show different responses depending on whether light falls in the centre of the field or in the surrounding ring (Fig. 7.15). An 'on' ganglion cell increases its firing rate in response to illumination of the centre of its field and decreases it in response to illumination of its periphery. In diffuse illumination of both the centre and surround, there is no change in the firing rate. For an 'off' ganglion cell, firing increases with surround illumination, stops with light on the centre, and is unaffected by diffuse lighting. This property of ganglion cells is shared by their bipolar cells, but because bipolar cells do not fire action potentials, it is their graded potentials that vary. This centre–surround antagonism is mediated in part by horizontal cells, which, although they do not synapse directly on bipolar cells, affect the glutamate release from photoreceptors onto bipolar cells.

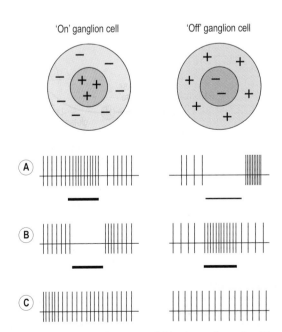

Fig. 7.15 Centre–surround receptive fields of ganglion cells. (A) Centre illumination. (B) Surround illumination. (C) Diffuse illumination.

Horizontal cells increase the contrast in the retina by a mechanism called lateral inhibition. Horizontal cells connect the outputs from neighbouring photoreceptors. In the dark, they are excited by glutamate released from the photoreceptors, which stimulates γ-aminobutyric acid (GABA) release onto neighbouring photoreceptors. GABA inhibits photoreceptors, reducing their glutamate release (Fig. 7.16). This means that in response to centre illumination, a neighbouring photoreceptor, which will continue to release glutamate, will excite the horizontal cell. This inhibits glutamate release from the centre photoreceptor, allowing bipolar cells to depolarize further than they would without the horizontal cell effect. When the surround is illuminated, the reduction in glutamate release from the surround photoreceptors reduces GABA release from the horizontal cell, and so the centre photoreceptor releases more glutamate, causing the centre

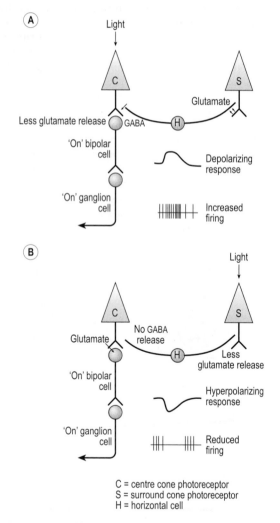

C = centre cone photoreceptor
S = surround cone photoreceptor
H = horizontal cell

Fig. 7.16 Horizontal (H) cells reduce glutamate release from neighbouring photoreceptors. (A) Centre illumination: GABAergic inhibition by horizontal cells enhances the bipolar and ganglion cell responses; (B) surround illumination: no GABA is released from the horizontal cell, so the 'on' channel is suppressed. *C,* Central cone; *S,* surrounding cone.

bipolar cell to be inhibited. The function of centre–surround inhibition is to exaggerate contrast at borders.

Rod cell signalling via amacrine cells

Rods are connected to depolarizing 'on' bipolar cells that are connected to ganglion cells via amacrine cells. Amacrine cells are a very diverse population of interneurons whose neurites have properties of both axons and dendrites and use a wide variety of neurotransmitters to modify synaptic transmission. They are implicated in rod signalling, surround inhibition, and the detection of the direction of motion, particularly in peripheral vision.

Rod signalling depends on light intensity; at high light levels, rods are saturated, and all signalling occurs through the cone cells 'on' and 'off' channels. In lower light levels, such as at dusk, in the dark-adapted eye, changes in rod membrane potential are transferred to neighbouring cone cells through gap junctions to boost cone function, to maintain colour vision and visual acuity at low light levels. However, at very low light levels, this boosting of cone cells is insufficient to maintain colour vision, and all vision occurs via rod–amacrine cell pathways.

Colour responses of retinal ganglion cells

Like bipolar cells, ganglion cells show 'on' and 'off' surround inhibition, but they differ from bipolar cells in producing action potentials, and thus their responses are described in terms of action potential rate, not graded depolarization. They are also spontaneously active. Therefore, inhibition of these cells decreases the resting rate of action potentials and their centre–surround organization makes these cells extremely sensitive to moving stimuli.

Ganglion cells can also be distinguished by their responses to colour. Studies in monkeys (which have a similar visual system to humans) have shown that there are two major populations of ganglion cells, distinguished easily by their size, destination (see below), and response characteristics. The most numerous cells (80%) are small parvocellular (P) cells; these are found near the fovea. Magnocellular (M) cells are larger and less common (10%), and the remaining 10% are small, non-M, non-P (K, or koniocellular) cells, which have low spatial resolution. The RFs of P cells are smaller than M cells, and they often show sustained responses compared with the transient responses of M cells. However, the most striking difference is that they respond differently to coloured light. This is because P cells obtain their input from single cones (or a group of cones with the same wavelength sensitivity—S, M or L), while M cells receive their input from rod cells. M cells are more sensitive than P cells to low-contrast stimuli and are used for motion detection and object fixation, while P cells can distinguish fine detail and are important for spatial discrimination. This separation of functional detection of different features of the image at the first stage in the visual pathway is maintained throughout the visual pathway.

Some non-M, non-P cells receive their input from M and L cones together (but not S) and have larger RFs, so they are good at measuring the brightness. The centre–surround inhibition lets 'on' M cells respond best to green (M cones) and red (L cones) light in the centre, while 'off' M cells fire when the light illuminates the surround.

The output of P ganglion cells shows colour opponency, that is, they are excited by one cone population and inhibited by another (Fig. 7.17). There are two populations of colour opponent P cells. The most common are single red–green opponent.

There are four different possible responses, depending on whether the ganglion cell is an 'on' or 'off' cell (Fig. 7.17A):

- red 'on' centre, green 'off' surround
- green 'on' centre, red 'off' surround
- red 'off' centre, green 'on' surround
- green 'off' centre, red 'on' surround.

Blue-yellow opponency compares input from S cones with that of M and L combined (as the combined input from M and L cones gives the perception of yellow). These cells do not show a centre–surround response but are either excited by blue light and inhibited by yellow or vice versa (Fig. 7.17B) and are associated with K ganglion cells.

Perceived colour is based on the relative activities in different ganglion cells, whose RF centres receive input from the three different cones. This is easily demonstrated, for example, by staring at a red, green or blue square for 30–60 seconds to fatigue the appropriate cone. Then, if one stares at a white box, something strange

happens. Staring at this white box leaves the opponent colour unopposed, and so the white background becomes that colour. For blue, the white background becomes yellow; for red, it becomes green and vice versa.

Recently, a few retinal ganglion cells have been discovered that have melanopsin as their pigment rather than rhodopsin or cone pigments. These cells' axons project to the suprachiasmatic nucleus in the hypothalamus and are associated with endocrine and circadian rhythm functions.

Processing of visual information

Retinal ganglion cells are not mere relay cells for visual information; they extract different aspects of the image. What we 'see' depends on the features extracted in the retina, and how this information is integrated and interpreted by the brain. In the retina, the visual information splits into two streams, one for colour and one for form and motion. This is parallel processing and is important because we view the world with two eyes, providing two parallel streams of information, albeit from slightly different angles. In the central visual pathways, these streams are compared to give information about object depth, contrast and movement, as well as image resolution. Because we use two eyes, there are two separate images in the brain, and somewhere in the visual cortex they are merged (this is known as the binding problem).

Visual processing in the lateral geniculate nucleus

The LGN has six layers (Fig. 7.18) which receive inputs from the M and P ganglion cells. The two ventral layers, called the magnocellular layers (M1–2), are composed of large cells and innervated by M ganglion cells (layer 1 from the contralateral eye, and layer 2 from the ipsilateral eye). The more dorsal parvocellular layers (P3–6) are composed of small cells and receive input from the P ganglion cells, with layers 3 and 5 ipsilateral and 4 and 6 contralateral. In between these layers are even smaller cells, which comprise the K layers that receive input from non-M, non-P cells that signal average illumination.

Just like the retinal ganglion cells, the LGN cells have circular RFs and show the same centre–surround inhibition and colour opponency as the ganglion cells to which they connect. Each layer shows precise topographical mapping of the retina, with the majority of each layer occupied by input from the fovea. The maps are in register, so at any vertical point through the LGN, the same RF is represented. As only input from one half of the visual field goes to each layer of the LGN, there are no binocular responses.

There are two types of neuron in the LGN: geniculostriate neurons, which project to the visual cortex, and a population of small interneurons. As well as receiving input from the retinal ganglion cells, these neurons

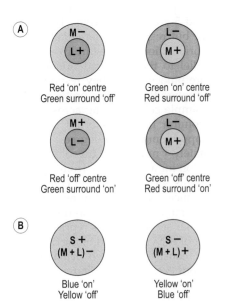

Fig. 7.17 Colour opponency in ganglion cells. (A) Red–green single opponent cells. (B) Blue–yellow opponent cells.

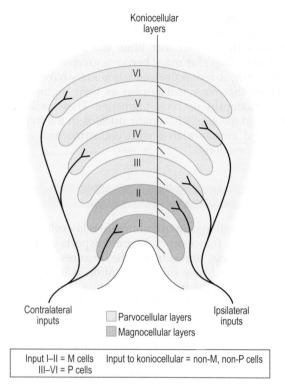

Koniocellular
layers

VI

V

IV

III

II

I

Contralateral
inputs

Parvocellular layers
Magnocellular layers

Ipsilateral
inputs

| Input I–II = M cells | Input to koniocellular = non-M, non-P cells |
| III–VI = P cells | |

Fig. 7.18 Layers in the lateral geniculate nucleus. Magnocellular layers (1 and 2) are shown shaded. Inputs I and II: M cells. Inputs III–VI: P cells. Input to koniocellular layer: non-M, non-P cells.

receive input from the visual cortex and reticular formation, so they may play a role in visual attention (see below).

Visual attention selectively filters out irrelevant information so the relevant detail is consciously perceived. The circuitry involved in attention is similar to that involved in oculomotor control. The FEF; parieto-occipital-temporal, primary visual (V1), and association area (V2, V4) cortices; and SC are also involved (Fig. 7.3). The earliest attentional activity occurs in the FEF neurons, suggesting that this is the source of the attention-control signals. Experimental evidence also suggests that three thalamic nuclei—the LGN and pulvinar and thalamic reticular nuclei (TRN)—are also strongly involved in controlling attention. The pulvinar nucleus seems to be very important, as it has neurons that respond to colour, motion, and orientation. It receives input from the LGN and SC and has reciprocal connections with the visual cortex, and so can directly modulate the efficacy of input from one region to another. Moreover, it modulates cortical neuron firing and so can synchronise firing of different neurons involved in the parallel processing of colour, motion and depth. This may be how the brain solves the binding problem by integrating the parallel streams of information to produce a visual percept of the object. Pulvinar lesions lead to disturbances in visual attention.

Brain imaging studies also show that the LGN is important in visual attention. As outlined in Chapter 1, the thalamus is the 'gatekeeper' to the cortex and the inhibitory TRN is the sentry to the thalamus. The TRN receives input from the prefrontal and visual cortices, as well as the SC. Attentional stimuli decrease TRN inhibition of the LGN. Additionally, corticothalamic activation of LGN from the FEF, V1 and V4 regions excite LGN neurons, so that specific features from the M, P and K cells can be selected for attention. In this way, the LGN fulfils the gatekeeper role for vision.

Organization and response properties of cells in the visual cortex

The V1 has six layers, each with specific inputs from the parallel streams derived from the M, P and K layers of the LGN. The different pathways carry information regarding form, movement, colour and visual attention in a topographic fashion. In this map, the fovea is disproportionately represented, and peripheral vision has little representation. V1 is the first region in which input from both eyes is combined.

Unlike neurons in the retina and LGN, those of the visual cortex do not have circular RFs but respond to lines of a particular orientation. Like many other regions of the brain, the visual cortex is arranged in functional columns. In a given column, which is 30–100 μm across, all the neurons spanning layers 1–6 respond to bars of light of a particular orientation; hence, the name orientation column. In each orientation column (Fig. 7.19), there are two types of cell. Simple cells are found in layers 4 and 6. They have small, centre–surround RFs and respond to stationary bars of a certain orientation from a single visual field; that is, they are monocular and highly sensitive to the position of a stimulus on the retina. In layers 2, 3 and 5 are complex cells. These are not direction sensitive but respond preferentially to bars of light of the same orientation as the simple cells moving across the RF, parallel to the preferred orientation. However, these cells are binocular, as they respond to input from both eyes, although they show a preference for the visual field of the simple cells. Moving across the cortex, each successive column has a preferred orientation, which changes by approximately 15 degrees. Across a distance of approximately 1 mm, there are columns for each possible orientation for a single eye, from a given part of the visual field. This set of orientation columns is called an ocular dominance column. Columns with the same orientation are organized as stripes in the cortex. Parallel to this are a similar set of columns representing input from the same part of the visual field of the other eye. The area of the cortex consisting of two ocular dominance columns, one from each eye, is called a hypercolumn (Fig. 7.19) and represents all of the input from a part of the visual field to the primary visual cortex.

Arranged within the ocular dominance columns are columns of complex cells, which are wavelength-sensitive.

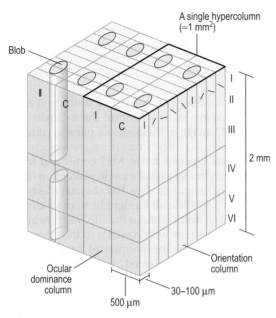

Fig. 7.19 Simple and complex cells are arranged in orientation columns, and these form ocular dominance columns and hypercolumns in the visual cortex. *C*, Contralateral; *I*, ipsilateral.

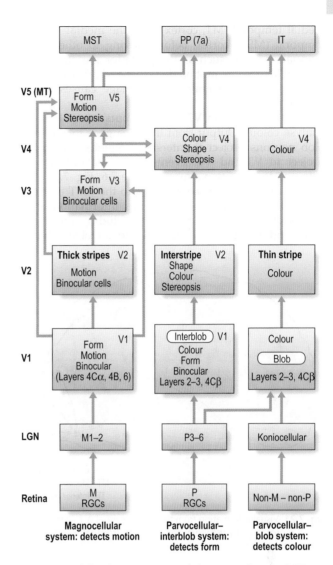

Fig. 7.20 Modelling how we see. *IT*, Inferior temporal cortex; *MST*, medial superior temporal cortex; *MT*, Medial superior temporal cortex; *PP*, posterior parietal cortex; *RGC*, retinal ganglion cell. Integration of parallel processing of the different streams of information. (Adapted from DeYoe, Van Essen. TINS. 1988;11:219–226.)

These colour-sensitive cells are arranged in cylindrical regions called blobs (based on metabolic staining with cytochrome oxidase); they receive convergent input from the parvocellular and koniocellular LGN layers. The areas between the blobs are the interblob regions. The RFs of most of the blob neurons are circular and show varying types of colour opponency. The most complex of these are the double opponent cells, which signal colour contrast. There are four types, depending on the preferred stimulus. For example, one type has a maximal 'on' response to a red spot on a green background and an 'off' response to a green spot on a red background. The other red–green type is the reverse, and a similar combination occurs for blue and yellow.

Parallel processing in the visual cortex

The different streams of input from the LGN—motion, form, and colour—are processed simultaneously in different layers of the visual cortex (Fig. 7.20). Inputs from the M cells of the LGN, which synapse in different sublayers of layer 4 to P cells, concern motion but not colour. Inputs from P cells of the LGN are processed in two streams. One stream in the parvocellular–blob pathway mediates colour vision, while the other—the parvocellular–interblob pathway—performs high-resolution analysis of form. These complex cells are binocular but not wavelength sensitive. They are also important for depth perception.

Outputs from the primary visual cortex

Visual perception involves many different (extra-striate) association regions of the occipital cortex that receive output from the V1 (striate) cortex. In monkeys (and by inference, humans), there are numerous areas known to be involved in further processing of visual input (Fig. 7.21). Many of these areas have some form of retinotopic map, and there are complex interconnections between these regions.

The parallel processing of different information streams continues beyond V1. Many outputs go to the secondary visual cortex (V2, Brodmann area 18), which, on staining for cytochrome oxidase—a metabolic activity marker—shows a pattern of thick and thin stripes. V2 has reciprocal connections with V1. Information leaving V2 splits into two streams (Fig. 7.21). V2 thick stripes receive inputs from the M pathway (via V1 layer 4) and analyse motion. This information is further processed in other regions, V3 and then V5 (also called the medial temporal, MT, cortex), and the medial superior temporal (MST) cortex, before moving to other visual association areas such as the posterior parietal cortex. Cells in V5 are key motion detectors and are also important for depth perception. V5 damage causes loss of motion perception.

The thin stripes of V2 receive inputs from blobs and analyse colour. Output from this area goes to V4. Inter-blob neurons project to interstripe regions, which also project to V3 and V4. Eventually, visual information gets divided into two streams (Table 7.6, Fig. 7.21). The 'where' stream is carried dorsally, to the MST and posterior parietal cortices, and carries information about an object's location and motion, including one's own body and its spatial relationship to an object (visual guidance and reaching movements). The ventral 'what' stream projects to the inferotemporal (IT) cortex, which can identify or recognize an object, pattern, or specific face. V4 projects to V6 and activates cells that respond to complex shapes and have a role in object shape recognition.

The effects of selective lesions to the different areas and functional imaging studies confirm the existence of these two streams. Damage to the posterior parietal cortex causes optic ataxia, where patients can recognize objects but cannot grasp them. Damage to the MST cortex and MT visual cortex results in loss of visual motion perception (akinetopsia) in different directions. This has obvious lifestyle implications: think how difficult it might be to cross a busy road or even to pour a drink without the cup overflowing.

In contrast, patients with damage to the IT cortex have visual agnosia, where the position of an object is recognized, but it cannot be named or a copy drawn (except from memory). In a particular form of this condition, called prosopagnosia, patients cannot recognize individual faces, however familiar. For example, a married person with this condition would not recognize their spouse visually but would recognize the sound of their voice. Alexia is the inability to read written words. Damage to V4 results in loss of colour vision—achromatopsia—while damage to V6 causes an inability to distinguish two-dimensional patterns.

In a particular condition called blindsight (cortical blindness), patients who are totally blind due to the bilateral loss of V1 can still navigate to some extent through space without colliding with objects that they reportedly cannot see. This occurs due to a pathway which goes from the magnocellular neurons of the LGN directly to the thick stripes of V2, providing input to the 'where' pathway.

However, eventually the two streams (Table 7.6) integrate to produce a coherent image of a three-dimensional

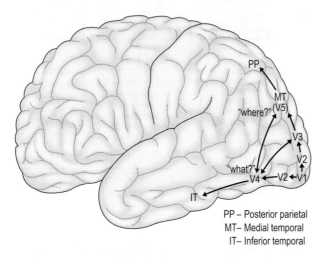

PP – Posterior parietal
MT– Medial temporal
IT– Inferior temporal

Fig. 7.21 Visual information from the primary visual (V1 or striate) cortex is processed by the visual association (extra-striate) cortical areas as two streams.

Table 7.6 Separation of visual information

	Pathway	
	Dorsal stream: 'Where things are or how they move'	Ventral stream: 'What things are or are like'
Function	Motion perception and spatial location Visual guidance of hand and eye movements	Colour and shape perception Object recognition
Retinal ganglion cell type	M cells (non-macular)	P cells (fovea)
LGN cell layers	M1–M2	P3–P6
Cortical input area	V1	V1
Visual association areas	V2, V3, V5, MST cortex, posterior parietal cortex	V2, V4, V6, anterior inferior temporal lobe
Other cortical area involvement	Dorsolateral prefrontal cortex Frontal eye fields	Ventrolateral prefrontal cortex Medial temporal lobe
Effect of lesion	Optic ataxia Ocular apraxia Akinetopsia	Visual agnosia Prosopagnosia Achromatopsia Alexia

LGN, Lateral geniculate nucleus; MST, medial superior temporal.

world. This processing of information in parallel streams can explain how some visual illusions are produced. For example, depth perception is much reduced in computer-generated pictures if the shading is produced by colour contrast as opposed to luminance. This suggests that depth information is processed by the magnocellular pathways.

Summary

The visual system is a complex system designed to extract different features of an image: its colour, motion and shape (Fig. 7.20). Some of this separation occurs early in the pathway and information is processed in parallel throughout the rest of the pathway. For example, colour is detected by cones, which activate P cells that project via parvocellular LGN layers to blob regions of the visual cortex, and onwards to V4. Rods, on the other hand, see only in black and white, work best at low light levels, and are excellent motion detectors. This information travels via the M layers of the LGN to interblob regions of the visual cortex and is forwarded to V5 and the posterior parietal cortex. The parvocellular–interblob pathway is specialized for shape perception, as cells in this pathway are sensitive to the orientation of edges. Within the cortex, there are many complex interactions between the many different visual association regions. We get visual input from two eyes, and the visual image is inverted and back-to-front in the visual cortex. Somehow, somewhere in the cortex, through the interactions between the various visual centres, the image is inverted again to appear the 'right way up', and binocular input is transformed into one seamless three-dimensional percept of the outside world.

Self-assessment case study

A 35-year-old man reported blurred vision and headaches. The ophthalmoscopic examination is normal, with no signs of papilloedema or retinopathy. There are no signs of cataracts or other opacities. Direct and consensual pupillary reflexes are normal as are conjugate eye movements. However, there is mild diplopia. Visual field examination shows a bitemporal heteronymous hemianopia (tunnel vision). A magnetic resonance imaging (MRI) MRI scan is scheduled and a blood sample is taken for endocrine evaluation.

After studying this chapter, you should be able to answer the following questions:

1. Where is the lesion located?

As the visual field deficit occurs in both eyes, the lesion must occur at, or posterior to, the optic chiasm. Any lesion occurring after the optic chiasm produces a homonymous deficit, so this patient has a lesion at the level of the optic chiasm. Compression of the optic chiasm affects only those fibres that decussate. These fibres arise from the nasal side of the each retina, so the part of the visual field affected is the temporal visual field in both eyes. The patient does not notice this extensive lesion, as the temporal visual field of one eye appears in the nasal visual field of the other eye. Examination of each eye separately reveals the deficit.

2. What is the possible cause of the compression and what will the investigations show?

The optic chiasm lies above the pituitary gland, and tumours of the pituitary cause compression of the optic chiasm. Pituitary adenomas are mostly benign and are classified as either non-secretory (more common) or secretory, depending on whether they produce anterior pituitary hormones such as prolactin, growth hormone and ACTH. In this patient the symptoms seem to be entirely due to the presence of a mass, which suggests a non-secretory tumour. The headaches are caused by the stretching of the dura mater, whilst diplopia can be caused by pressure on the ocular motor nerves (3rd, 4th and 6th) due to the lateral extension of the tumour. Imaging of the brain using MRI will show any significant pituitary mass. Analysis of hormone levels in blood will show whether this is a secreting or non-secreting tumour. Non-secreting tumours may also present with inadequate hormone secretion—hypopituitarism.

HEARING AND BALANCE: THE AUDITORY AND VESTIBULAR SYSTEMS

8

Chapter summary

1. The auditory and vestibular systems both use mechanosensory hair cells to transduce stimuli.

2. The outer ear collects and funnels sound waves to induce vibrations of the tympanic membrane. The sound waves are converted into mechanical vibrations by three middle ear bones (malleus, incus and stapes) that amplify the signal. The stapes transfers the sound waves to the inner ear via the oval window where they are converted to fluid pressure waves that stimulate the sensory apparatus.

3. The cochlea contains three fluid filled chambers. The outer two contain perilymph and the inner one contains endolymph. The outer two provide a pathway for pressure waves to flow through the system while the inner chamber contains the auditory sensory apparatus, the organ of Corti.

4. The organ of Corti contains rows of hair cells that sit on the basilar membrane. They have stereocilia that project into the chamber or embed into the tectorial membrane. When the fluid waves cause the basilar membrane to vibrate, the stereocilia bend. Adjacent cilia are connected by tip links and tensing these links opens mechanosensitive K^+ channels, causing the cell to depolarise and release glutamate to stimulate cochlear afferents.

5. The basilar membrane is tapered in shape to provide a spatial map based on resonance frequency. This tonotopic map is preserved along all the neural relay pathways to the auditory cortex (via the brainstem and thalamus).

6. The vestibular system detects head movements. It has three semicircular canals arranged at right angles to each other and two otolith organs that detect changes in rotational and linear

movements, respectively. The system also produces compensatory eye movements during head movement for image stabilization and object tracking.

7. Vestibular sensory hair cells are also connected by tip links that open or close K^+ channels when they are displaced by endolymph fluid.

8. Damage to the auditory system results in conduction or sensorineural deafness. Specific tests are used to assess the functional integrity of the auditory system.

9. Damage to the vestibular system results in vertigo, nausea and nystagmus. The integrity of the system can be assessed in several ways (e.g. vestibulo-ocular reflex, caloric test and Hallpike's manoeuvre).

Introduction

Hearing is one of our most important senses, because of its roles in the perception of speech and the ability to communicate. Hearing deficits are common, particularly in the young and the elderly, and the prevalence increases with age. In the UK, approximately one in six of the population have some form of hearing impairment; 8 million are aged over 60 years and 900,000 have profound deafness, including 50,000 children. Worldwide, the World Health Organization reports that 432 million adults and 34 million children have 'disabling' (>35 dB loss in their good ear) hearing loss, and these numbers will drastically increase by 2050. Nearly 80% of people with disabling hearing loss live in low- and middle-income countries. The symptoms of hearing loss—earache, tinnitus (ringing in the ears), vertigo and otorrhea—are associated with ear problems.

Hearing loss is hardest for young children. They are deprived of the normal acquisition of speech and consequently require other forms of communication (e.g. sign language or lip reading). Acute deafness in adolescents can have a significant psychological impact, as it deprives them of social contact with their peers. In the elderly, deafness causes increased isolation and estrangement from family and friends. People with hearing loss ranging from mild to severe are termed 'hard of hearing'. They usually communicate through spoken language and can benefit from hearing aids, cochlear implants and other assistive devices. 'Deaf' people mostly have profound hearing loss, which implies very little or no hearing. They often use sign language for communication.

The vestibular system is intimately involved in maintaining balance, and the most frequently reported symptoms of vestibular disorders are dizziness, unsteadiness when walking, vertigo and nausea. These symptoms can range from mild, lasting minutes, to severe, resulting in total disability. As the vestibular system interacts with many other parts of the nervous system, symptoms may manifest as problems with vision, movement, thinking and memory. Vestibular disorders occur frequently and affect people of all ages. Balance disorders are increased in frequency in the elderly and, by the age of 75 years, become one of the most common reasons for visiting the doctor. In many cases the cause lies in the inner ear.

The impact of deafness and balance disorders in society is significant in terms of financial and emotional costs: the cost of diagnosis and treatment, hearing aids, speech therapy or vestibular rehabilitation, and lost work potential. This chapter reviews the anatomy and physiology of the auditory and vestibular systems and describes clinical signs and symptoms associated with their dysfunction (Box 8.1).

Auditory system

The auditory system is a specialized sensory system with two main functions: to detect and localize sound and to decode sounds into meaningful language. It comprises the cochlea, the afferent auditory pathways and the auditory cortex in the temporal lobe and can detect frequencies from 20 Hz to 20 kHz. The auditory pathway uses both ears to detect and signal the location of the sound. Complex inhibitory circuitry magnifies the differences in the timing and intensity of sounds that occur between the two sides during normal hearing.

Case history

A 63-year-old retired road construction labourer has had progressively worsening tinnitus for the past several years, as well as episodes of feeling unwell. On several occasions he reported that the room span around like a merry-go-round. In the last 6 months he has begun to stagger to the right when walking and has had difficulty in coordinating his right hand. A month ago he noticed muscle weakness on the right side of his face. On examination the doctor detected a right-sided hearing deficit. The patient also had no ability to wrinkle his forehead or retract the right side of his face when asked to smile. There was no corneal reflex on the right side. He had trouble coordinating his right hand and had intentional tremor on finger-to-nose testing and heel-to-shin testing of the right upper and lower limbs. The doctor immediately referred the patient to an ear, nose and throat (ENT) specialist at the local hospital for further tests. Audiometry tests revealed a high-tone hearing loss of 20 dB on the right. The examination also showed that the patient had a wide-based gait and inability to tandem walk. There was no nystagmus on caloric stimulation of the right ear. The ENT specialist sent the patient for a magnetic resonance imaging (MRI) scan, which revealed a tumour in the right posterior fossa at the cerebellopontine angle.

This case gives rise to the following questions:

1. What are the possible causes of deafness?
2. What are the causes of this patient's symptoms?
3. What is the rationale underlying the different tests for deafness?
4. What are the links between hearing and balance disorders?

Anatomy of the ear

The ear apparatus comprises three main regions: the outer, middle and inner ear (Fig. 8.1), each of which has specific functions (Table 8.1).

The outer ear (auricle or pinna) collects sound waves with the help of the external folded cartilaginous structures, such as the lobule, helix and concha regions. Sound waves are collected and funnelled along the sigmoid-shaped external auditory canal to the middle ear. The tympanic membrane (myringa, also known as the eardrum) separates the middle ear from the outer ear. It is a thin (0.1 mm), translucent membrane with an area of approximately 18 mm^2, shaped like the diaphragm of a loudspeaker. It is exquisitely sensitive to sounds and can vibrate at 0.01 nm at the minimum hearing threshold. Importantly, once sound waves stop, so do the tympanic

Table 8.1 Characteristics of the auditory system

Division	Mode of operation	Functions
Outer ear	Air vibration	Protection, sound localization
Middle ear	Mechanical vibration	Impedance matching, pressure equalization, amplification, inner ear stimulation
Inner ear	Mechanical, hydrodynamic and electrochemical	Sound filtering, signal transduction
Central auditory nervous system	Electrochemical	Signal transmission and information processing

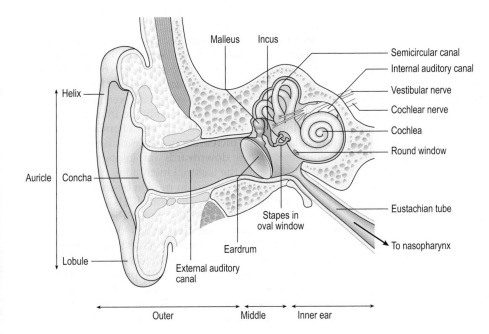

Fig. 8.1 Cross-section showing the outer, middle and inner ear divisions.

Malleus Incus

Semicircular canal
Internal auditory canal
Vestibular nerve
Cochlear nerve
Cochlea
Round window

Helix

Eustachian tube

Auricle Concha

Stapes in
oval window

To nasopharynx

Lobule

Eardrum

External auditory
canal

Outer   Middle   Inner ear

vibrations. Resonance of the eardrum by sound waves drives the movement of the middle ear ossicles: the malleus, incus and stapes. In order for pressure differences not to impede the vibrations produced by the sound, the middle ear atmospheric pressure is the same as that in the outer ear. This is achieved by the eustachian tubes, which open automatically during swallowing, linking the middle ear to the atmosphere via the nasopharynx (see Fig. 8.1).

The middle ear converts the air pressure waves into fluid vibration in the inner ear by movement of the oval window, an elastic membrane separating these compartments. The specific configuration of the bones amplifies tympanic membrane vibrations by 30% and focuses the movement of the stapes in the oval window to overcome the inner ear fluid inertia. Additionally, as the oval window is only one-sixth of the area of the tympanic membrane, the size differential between these membranes also compensates for impedance mismatch between air and the cochlear fluid. In this way, the sound signal is amplified 22-fold in the middle ear. Two muscles, the tensor tympani and tensor stapedius, innervated by the trigeminal and facial nerves, respectively, move the ossicular chain.

The inner ear houses the cochlea and vestibular apparatus, which are contained within the bony labyrinth of the temporal bone (Fig. 8.1). Inside the bony labyrinth, surrounded by perilymph, is the membranous labyrinth, a series of ducts and cavities filled with potassium ion-rich endolymph that contains the sensory apparatus. Hearing receptors are located within the cochlea, while the balance receptors are located in the semicircular canals and vestibule. Movement of the endolymph in the inner ear activates the sensory hair cell receptors.

The cochlea is shaped like a snail's shell, consisting of three fluid-filled spaces (Fig. 8.2A) enclosed in a bony core called the modiolus:

1. scala vestibuli, which runs from the oval window

2. scala tympani, which ends at the round window

3. scala media (cochlear duct)

The scala vestibuli and scala tympani contain perilymph (similar to cerebrospinal fluid) and are continuous with each other at the apex (also called the helicotrema) of the cochlea. The cochlear duct contains endolymph (similar to the intracellular cytoplasm of cells), which is necessary for auditory and vestibular hair cells to function normally; it is unique to the vestibulocochlear system. Within the cochlea, a delicate continuous (Reissner's) membrane is suspended within the bony labyrinth, creating a second chamber within the first. This is the membranous labyrinth (cochlear duct/scala media) that houses the organ of Corti (Fig. 8.2B).

Auditory receptors and their role in sound transduction

The organ of Corti contains inner hair cells (IHCs) and outer hair cells (OHCs), distinguished by their location, function, innervation and their supporting cells. These cells sit on the basilar membrane. There are ~3,500 IHCs, arranged in a single row, and they are the primary sound transducers. Each IHC is innervated by ~20 myelinated (type I) afferent fibres. There are ~12,000–20,000 OHCs organized in three rows at the base, to five rows at the apex of the basilar membrane. OHCs are innervated by unmyelinated (type II) afferents, each of which synapses with ~10 OHCs. OHCs represent only ~5% of the nerve output. The cochlear nerve contains ~30,000 type I and 3000 type II afferents.

Hair cells have bundles of stereocilia that act like antennae (Fig 8.2C); their base is tapered so they can move like hinge joints. The cilia protrude through the reticular lamina, which provides structural support and a physical barrier to ion movement between the endolymph and perilymph. IHC cilia sit freely in the surrounding endolymph, whereas OHC cilia are embedded in the tectorial membrane. Adjacent cilia are stepped in height to form ranks that are connected by tip links connected to mechanosensory transduction (MET) channels. Some of these channels are open at rest, meaning type I cochlear afferents have a low tonic firing frequency. Endolymph displacement causes the cilia to sway back and forth. When the shorter hairs push towards the taller cilia, the tip links stretch and become tense; with movement in the opposite direction, they become slack. When the links tighten, K^+ channels open, allowing these ions to flow down their concentration gradient (endolymph has a concentration of ~150 nmol/L, whereas perilymph is ~4 nmol/L). This generates a strong voltage difference, the endocochlear potential. Entry of K^+ into the hair cell causes depolarisation and opening of Ca^{2+} channels (Fig. 8.2C). This produces release of glutamate to increase the discharge rate in the cochlear afferents. K^+ ions exit the cell via basal ion channels and are recycled back to the stria vascularis via the spiral ligament.

As described earlier, sound waves collected by the outer ear and relayed through the middle ear cause the stapes to induce vibrations of the oval window that set the perilymph fluid of the scala vestibuli in motion. The round window serves as a pressure valve, bulging outwards as pressure rises in the inner ear. The increased peri-lymphatic pressure in the scala vestibuli is transferred across the vestibular membrane into the cochlear duct. However, endolymph in this chamber is incompressible, so the increased pressure causes the basilar membrane to flex downwards impinging on the scala tympani. Because the tectorial membrane sits on the basilar membrane, it too is set in motion by displacement of endolymph fluid. Both OHCs and ICHs are stimulated, but the way IHCs and OHCs respond is very different. When the basilar membrane bends downwards, IHC stereocilia bend away from the tallest cilia, decreasing tip link tension and closing MET channels so that type I afferents become silent. When the pressure in the scala vestibuli decreases and increases in the scala media, the basilar membrane rebounds and the IHC stereocilia move towards the tallest rank. This tenses the tip links,

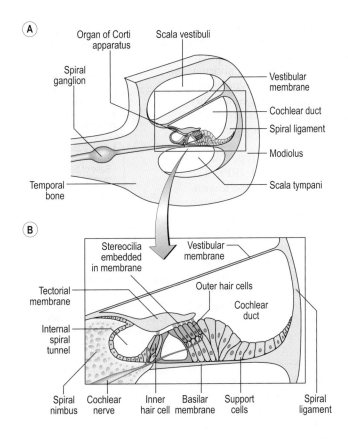

(A) Transverse section labels: Organ of Corti apparatus, Scala vestibuli, Spiral ganglion, Vestibular membrane, Cochlear duct, Spiral ligament, Modiolus, Temporal bone, Scala tympani

(B) Stereocilia embedded in membrane, Vestibular membrane, Tectorial membrane, Outer hair cells, Cochlear duct, Internal spiral tunnel, Spiral nimbus, Cochlear nerve, Inner hair cell, Basilar membrane, Support cells, Spiral ligament

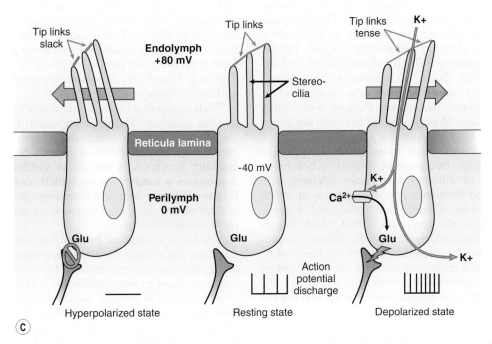

Tip links slack — Endolymph +80 mV — Tip links — Tip links tense — K+ — Stereocilia — Reticula lamina — Perilymph 0 mV — -40 mV — Glu — Ca²⁺ — Glu — K+ — Glu — K+ — Action potential discharge — Hyperpolarized state — Resting state — Depolarized state

Fig. 8.2 Anatomy of the cochlea. (A) Transverse section through one turn of the cochlea helix. (B) Magnified view of box region in (A), showing the organ of Corti. (C) The role of hair cell stereocilia in mechanosensory transduction. Arrows point to the direction of flow of endolymph that results in the opening or closing of mechanosensory K⁺ channels by changing the tension in tip links. This causes either the release or inhibition of glutamate release by hair cells to activate vestibular afferents.

opening the MET channels, causing afferents to robustly fire (Fig. 8.2C). OHCs respond to changes in movements of the tectorial membrane. In contrast to IHCs, depolarization of OHCs causes the cell to contract and shorten, pulling the tectorial membrane down. OHC hyperpolarization lengthens the cell. OHC shape changes amplify sound-induced basilar membrane movements, creating a cochlear amplifier that sharpens the frequency tuning of the cochlea.

The range over which a sound excites a type I auditory afferent determines its receptive field (RF). The frequency at which the neuron is excited with the lowest-intensity sound is its 'characteristic frequency'. Sound frequency is measured in Hertz (Hz). However, with supra-threshold stimulation, the type I afferents respond to a wider range of frequencies. Many auditory afferents respond to sounds at frequencies below their best frequency when the sounds are loud, and so the RFs overlap. The greatest sensitivity to sounds occurs over 1–4 KHz, which closely matches the frequency range of speech (250–4000 Hz).

Auditory encoding

Sounds are due to variations in air pressure over time creating longitudinal waves of compression and rarefaction that vary in intensity and frequency. The amplitude of the waves determines the intensity of the sound: the louder the sound, the greater its amplitude. Sound intensity is measured on a log scale in decibels (dB). A 10-dB increase in sound represents a 10-fold increase in intensity. Sounds cause discomfort at approximately 120 dB. They are painful above 140 dB and may cause acute auditory damage. The intensity of jet engines is approximately 140 dB, while that of whispering is 20 dB, talking is 50 dB and factory noise is 100 dB. Prolonged exposure to loud sounds kills hair cells and causes deafness or a hearing deficit. The louder the sound, the quicker the loss, with higher frequencies lost first. Most people fail to notice the deficit until they cannot hear someone else's speech.

Sounds are recognized as tones when the pressure waves have a single frequency or as noise when many irregular waves of different frequencies interfere with each other. Sound frequency specifies the rate at which the alternate phases of rarefaction occur, and it determines the pitch of the perceived sound. Most sounds are mixtures of frequencies (and so are called complex tones); the particular mixture determines the timbre. Timbre gives characteristic information about the nature of the sound. For example, it allows us to distinguish the sounds of two different musical instruments playing the same note.

Hair cells sit on the basilar membrane, and the shape of this membrane changes along its course in the cochlea. The width of the basilar membrane increases from the base to the apex, allowing different parts to resonate at different frequencies along its course. In addition, the

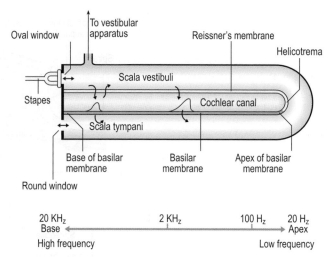

Fig. 8.3 Tonotopic organization of the 'unwound' basilar membrane. Vibration of the stapes causes displacement of the scala vestibule perilymph that is transmitted through Reissner's membrane to cause endolymph movement within the cochlear canal. This causes the basilar membrane to resonate at different positions along its length according to frequency. High-frequency sounds travel along the basilar membrane and dissipate energy at the narrow, taut end, whereas low-frequency sounds propagate towards the apex of the membrane before dissipating their energy. This sets up a frequency map along the length of the membrane.

base is taut, while the apex end is more flexible, making it differentially sensitive to vibration. Consequently, the highest frequencies (and pitch) set the narrow (base) end resonating, while lower (characteristic) frequencies set the apex in motion. This means that the properties of the basilar membrane result in a frequency gradient, a tonotopic map of sound frequency, along its length (Fig. 8.3). This map is faithfully repeated at relay stations along the auditory pathway.

Pitch is encoded in the firing of specific populations of cochlea afferents. The most important factor is its position along the basilar membrane. This mechanism, which contributes to perception of sounds over much of the auditory spectrum, is known as auditory place coding. It provides a mechanism by which complex sounds are fragmented into individual frequencies, relaying information about their relative intensity and timing to the central nervous system.

Loudness is signalled by two mechanisms. The louder the tone, the greater the firing frequency of the hair cell along the basilar membrane. However, the dynamic range of most primary afferents is only 20–30 dB, not nearly enough to account for the 120-dB range for loudness discrimination. The existence of a subpopulation (about 20%) of high-threshold primary afferents, which innervate the IHC with a widely distributed range of thresholds, accounts for the latter. In this subpopulation, the number of active neurons and their firing frequency signal loudness.

Auditory pathways

The central circuitry of the auditory pathways is very complex and organized to discriminate the three important parameters of hearing: location, intensity and timing. Accurate sound localization requires bilaterally intact auditory pathways. The ascending pathways are organized as two main systems: one is tonotopically 'hard-wired' according to frequency, providing a fast, secure pathway to the cortex; the other surrounds this system and is less precisely organized with respect to frequency but is additionally sensitive to the timing and intensity of the sound. This pattern is maintained all the way to the cortex. Parts of this surrounding system are organized to preserve binaural (i.e. involving both ears) hearing.

The cell bodies of the cochlear nerve afferents are located in the spiral ganglion. Their peripheral processes synapse with the hair cells, and their central processes converge with the central processes of the vestibular nerve, to form the vestibulo-cochlear nerve in the internal auditory canal (Fig. 8.1). Cochlear nerve afferents terminate in the cochlear nucleus located at the border of the medulla and pons. The cochlear nucleus divides into dorsal and ventral nuclei that extract different features of the incoming sound. The sound is split into two streams with different functions: one for location and one for quality (akin to the visual system, where motion and form processing are separated). The ventral cochlear nucleus (VCN) has two main cell types that are specialized for encoding intensity (stellate cells) and timing (bushy cells), thus providing information about sound location, while the dorsal cochlear nucleus (DCN) encodes pitch information and analyses the quality of sound. The DCN dissects the tiny frequency differences that make words like 'hat' sound different from 'hot', 'hut' and 'hit'. Each cochlear nucleus gives rise to a separate, 'parallel' ascending pathway that conveys specific attributes of the sound to higher centres.

The majority of DCN axon collaterals cross the midline to form the contralateral lateral lemniscus (LL), which ascends to the contralateral inferior colliculus (IC) in the midbrain. Other axon collaterals ascend ipsilaterally in the LL to the IC. Similarly, VCN fibres enter both the LL via the superior olivary nucleus (SON) and the trapezoid body (TB). Axons from the SON go to the LL nuclei and to the IC. From the IC, auditory fibres travel to synapse in the main auditory nucleus of the thalamus, the medial geniculate nucleus (MGN). From there, thalamocortical axons travel to the primary auditory cortex (AI or Heschl's gyrus) in the temporal lobe via the auditory radiation of the internal capsule (Fig. 8.4). Auditory cortical cells receive input from both ears but preferentially respond to input from the contralateral ear. Surrounding the AI are the association areas of hearing, which are involved in decoding sound into language.

Like the basilar membrane, the IC, MGN and AI are all tonotopically organized. For example, in the AI, high tones are represented posteromedially and low tones

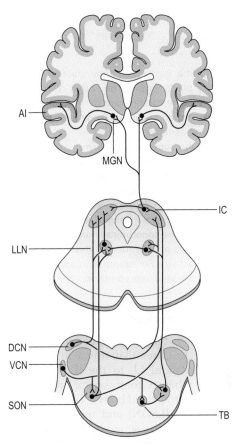

Fig. 8.4 The auditory pathways. *AI*, Primary auditory cortex; *DCN*, dorsal cochlear nucleus; *IC*, inferior colliculus; *LLN*, lateral lemniscus nucleus; *MGN*, medial geniculate nucleus; *SON*, superior olivary nucleus; *TB*, trapezoid body; *VCN*, ventral cochlear nucleus. Connections of one side only are shown for clarity.

anterolaterally. Additionally, cells in the AI are organized into separate columns based on whether sound from the ipsilateral ear excites or inhibits them (similar to ocular dominance columns in the visual system). These columns are perpendicular to the tonotopic frequency columns in the AI. Tonotopic maps are not immutable; they can be modified by experience or damage (Box 8.2).

Sound localisation is determined by its coordinates in the vertical (elevation) and horizontal (azimuth) planes. Different mechanisms are used to determine these coordinates. When sounds arrive in the vertical plane, the pinna and external auditory canal act as direction selective filters due to the shape of the pinna and the plane of the tympana. Sound waves stimulate the eardrum either directly or indirectly, resulting in different timing patterns that depend on the elevation of the sound source and its course through the external auditory canal. The ability to perceive speech is critically dependent on discriminating the timing and pattern (Box 8.3).

The central auditory pathways are unlike other ascending pathways because of the presence of three pairs of accessory nuclei (between the cochlear nuclei and the IC) that modulate the input and the bilateral representation of auditory impulses.

The brain is not a 'hard-wired', immutable structure but is, in fact, a highly plastic organ. The cortex contains many maps of the body's image for different perceptual functions: vision, touch, movement and hearing. These maps can be altered by experience and damage.

Located in the supratemporal gyrus of the temporal lobe are the structures involved in hearing and language comprehension. They consist of the primary auditory cortex (AI) and its association areas. Studies have shown that the AI is the region responsible for sound localization, whereas the association areas are more important in language functions (See Box 8.3).

AI cortical cells are tonotopically organized based on sound frequency, but the organization of this map can be altered by experience or activity. For example, in auditory learning tasks there is an increased representation for those frequencies that are used during training. In patients with chronic tinnitus, magnetic resonance imaging analysis has shown that there is a change in the map in the auditory cortex as compared with healthy subjects, in that the tinnitus frequency expands into adjacent frequency regions. This has been likened to an auditory phantom and may involve mechanisms akin to those proposed for phantom limb pain (see Box 5.4).

Deaf patients also show considerable plasticity in the auditory cortex. Recent functional imaging studies have shown that a significant amount of cross-modality plasticity occurs in the temporal lobe. For example, in congenitally deaf people the auditory cortical regions do not respond to sound but instead to visual cues in response to sign language. Tactile sensitivity can also activate this region, reflecting increased attention to a stimulus.

Superior olivary nucleus

The SON receives bilateral sound input (via the VCN) and gives rise to fibres that travel in both the ipsilateral and contralateral LL to the IC. Ipsilateral inputs are excitatory, whereas contralateral ones are inhibitory (mediated by the trapezoid body). The SON has two subnuclei, the lateral (LSON) and medial (MSON) nuclei, that are used to localise sounds. The SON complex uses two methods to localise sounds in azimuth: interaural level differences and interaural time differences to detect differences in intensity and timing between sounds entering the ears simultaneously (Fig. 8.5).

Trapezoid body

Axons from the VCN that decussate run through the TB. This structure helps locate the spatial direction of the sound by exaggerating differences in sound intensity through crossed inhibition of LSON cells (Fig. 8.5B). Some collaterals from the TB enter the facial and trigeminal nerves to form part of the efferent pathways of the acoustic reflexes.

Lateral lemniscus nuclei

The lateral lemniscus nuclei (LLN) are located in and adjacent to the LL, and send axons to both the ipsilateral and contralateral LL. They receive input from collaterals of the SON. There are reciprocal connections between the nuclei on the two sides. They are thought to participate in acoustic reflexes.

Inferior colliculus

The IC is an important auditory centre receiving input from three main sources: the LL, the contralateral IC and descending axons from AI. Its efferents project to the MGN and to the contralateral IC (inhibitory function), the superior colliculus and the reticular formation.

Functionally, the IC integrates spatial information from the SON, intensity information from the VCN, and pitch information from the DCN. It participates in acoustic reflexes whereby its connections with the superior colliculus form an auditory space map that is synchronised with the retinotopic map so that unexpected auditory responses coordinate head and eye movements towards the sound source.

Brainstem acoustic reflexes

Reciprocal connections exist between all of the relay nuclei in the auditory pathways that allow for auditory modulation. Brainstem reflexes function mainly to prevent damage to the auditory system and to distinguish selective sounds from background noise. Collaterals from the LL connect to interneurons of the reticular formation and to cranial nerve motor nuclei, to produce reflex arcs. The efferent fibres from these regions innervate the middle ear muscles.

1. Fibres enter the Vth and VIIth motor nuclei to link with motor neurons supplying tensor tympani and stapedius muscles, respectively, in the middle ear. These muscles exert a damping action on the middle ear ossicles. The tensor tympani is activated by one's own voice and the stapedius by external sounds. Damage to these nerve branches may lead to hyperacusis (hypersensitivity to sounds).

2. Unexpected or high-intensity sounds evoke acoustic reflexes manifest as a startle response and a stapedial reflex. The auditory component of the startle response evokes bilateral blinking and activates the limbic (arousal) system to prepare for fight or flight responses, mediated by reticulospinal fibres that connect to the motor nucleus of cranial nerve VII and the spinal cord. The stapedius reflex is a bilateral response involving stiffening of the

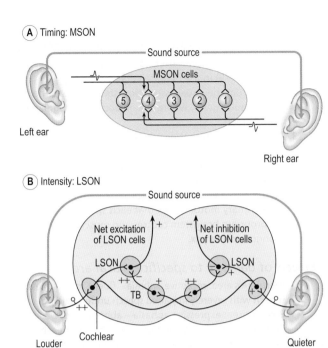

(A) Timing: MSON

Sound source

MSON cells

5 4 3 2 1

Left ear

Right ear

(B) Intensity: LSON

Sound source

Net excitation of LSON cells +

− Net inhibition of LSON cells

LSON

LSON

TB

Louder

Cochlear

Quieter

Fig. 8.5 Sound localization: the role of the superior olivary nuclei. (A) The medial SON (MSON) participates in coincidence detection via timing differences. Sound travels different distances to reach the right and left ears. The MSON neurons are maximally excited when action potentials from both ears activate the cells simultaneously. Different neurons are sensitive to different interaural time delays, created by receiving input from cochlear axons of different lengths, and so create a spatial map based on sound location. MSON cells can detect delays as short as 10 microseconds. (B) The lateral SON (LSON) participates in localization via interaural intensity differences. A sound reaching the nearer of the two ears is perceived to be loudest because of stronger excitation of the ipsilateral LSON cells as compared to the contralateral LSON (++ vs. +) from the cochlear nuclei. Input to the contralateral LSON is relayed via inhibitory cells of the trapezoid body (TB) and so inhibits cells of the contralateral SON. The LSON cells only encode sounds arising from the ipsilateral side, and both nuclei are needed to represent the full range of positions in the horizontal plane. Sounds emanating near the midline produce lower firing rates on the ipsilateral side because of enhanced inhibition from the contralateral side so that, at or beyond the midline, the contralateral TB input can completely silence the LSON neurons.

stapedius muscle as a protective (inhibitory) response to protect the cochlea from damaging stimuli by reducing the vibration of the eardrum. Clinically, it is used as a measure of middle ear function, as muscle contraction is directly related to stimulus intensity, and so can measure the reflex threshold for each ear.

3. Cholinergic efferent fibres originating from cells located near the SON form the olivocochlear bundle, which preferentially innervates OHCs. When activated, the OHCs contract, pulling the tectorial membrane down towards the organ of Corti. This may produce an increase in the amplitude and frequency sensitivity of the IHCs. This provides a feedback mechanism for regulating selective attention to certain sounds, for example, being able to extract sound from the surrounding noise.

Auditory perception

The sounds that a person hears are a construct of the brain, as sound waves make no noise! As well as being very sensitive to air pressure changes, the auditory system is adept at perceiving many different sounds at once. For example, when listening to music, one is able to pick out all the different instruments contributing to the song, and the singers. However, certain sounds convey meaning, and the analysis of sounds that convey meaning is more complex than the detection of sound. Detecting sounds is the function performed by the AI, while assigning meaning is the function of the association auditory cortex (AII). Decoding sounds into language is the main function of Wernicke's area, which is located in the dominant (usually the left) hemisphere of the brain in humans. The non-dominant hemisphere deals with non-verbal tasks, such as musical appreciation and comprehension.

As in the visual system, auditory information streams into a dorsal 'where' pathway, for where things are, and a ventral 'what' pathway, for what things are, so that we can identify objects by sound. For example, sirens are associated with fire engines, police cars and ambulances, and ring tones with mobile phones. These patterns of activity are relayed from the AI and AII areas, and further processed via the 'what' pathway in the inferior temporal lobe, sending information to the prefrontal cortex. Information about spatial tuning and sound-guided movement is relayed from the AI and AII via the 'where' pathway to the posterior parietal cortex and then onto the motor cortex in order that responses can be made to the sound. For example, when the telephone rings during the middle of the night, we automatically know where the phone is and reach to pick it up without thinking. In fact, the hand automatically makes the appropriate shape to pick up the receiver based on the sound heard.

Functional imaging studies have shown that auditory information is processed in other parts of the brain, such as the nucleus accumbens, amygdala and medial prefrontal cortex, which are associated with putting emotional labels on sounds or tunes.

Clinical signs associated with damage to the cochlear nerve

The clinical signs of damage to the auditory nerve are deafness and tinnitus. Lesions to the auditory pathway within the brainstem, thalamus or cortex do not produce significant hearing loss; rather, they produce difficulty in locating or discriminating the sound, especially during difficult auditory tasks. Hearing problems associated with lesions central to the cochlear nucleus are poor speech discrimination, poor sound localization, poor selective attention and poor auditory short-term memory. Unilateral hearing loss indicates damage to the ipsilateral ear or nerve. Deafness can be of two types:

Relationship between hearing and speaking

The language areas in the brain are located in the dominant hemisphere. When these areas are damaged, the resultant clinical syndrome is called aphasia. Thus there is a clear neuroanatomical basis for language.

The basic unit of speech is the phoneme, that is, the smallest speech sound. For example, pin has three phonemes: p, i and n. Morphemes are combinations of phonemes that provide meaning (words). Syntax represents the rules governing word sequences (grammatical structure), and semantics is the way in which language governs meaning.

Basic circuit for understanding spoken language (Fig. 8.6)

1. When a person hears a sentence, this is transmitted via the auditory apparatus to the primary auditory cortex in the temporal lobe.
2. This then connects to Wernicke's area (in the temporal lobe), which decodes the language into meaning.
3. If the sentence is to be repeated, or replied to, the information has to be transmitted forwards to Broca's area (expressive speech) in the frontal lobe (via the arcuate fasciculus).
4. Broca's area then produces speech via the motor programmes of the motor cortex, which activate the tongue and laryngeal muscles.

Basic circuit for understanding written speech

1. Visual input is transmitted to the visual cortex (areas 17–19) in the occipital lobe.
2. Input from the visual association area is sent to the left angular gyrus, where the objects are recognized and named.
3. Input then goes to Wernicke's area, where words are assembled into sentences, and the appropriate messages are sent via the arcuate and superior longitudinal fasciculi to Broca's area.
4. Broca's area activates motor programmes in the primary motor cortex that elicit speech via appropriate brainstem centres and muscles of the tongue and larynx.

Effects of damage to specific cortical areas

- Wernicke's area: receptive aphasia – fluent meaningless speech with severely impaired speech understanding.
- Broca's area: expressive aphasia – abbreviated, ungrammatical but meaningful speech, but speech understanding is impaired where syntax conveys meaning.
- Arcuate fasciculus: conduction aphasia – speech deficiencies are similar to those in receptive aphasia but, because comprehension remains intact, the patient attempts to say the right words.
- Angular gyrus: alexia (inability to read) with agraphia (inability to write), but the patient can comprehend speech and speak normally.

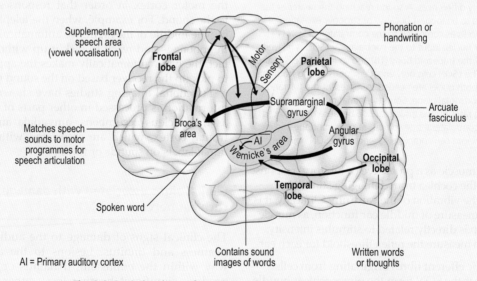

Fig. 8.6 Cortical pathways for understanding language (see text for details).

- Conduction deafness results from any interference with the passage of sound waves through the external or middle ear that prevents them from reaching the cochlea (e.g. wax build-up in the outer ear or middle ear infections). Sound wave propagation still occurs via bone conduction. Conduction deafness is never complete or total.

- Nerve (perception or sensorineural) deafness results from damage to the receptor cells of the organ of Corti or the cochlear nerve or nucleus.

The defect is in the segment of the auditory mechanism common to both air and bone conduction, thus hearing failure in both routes occurs. The amount of loss depends on the degree of damage to the organ or nerve.

Clinical tests

There are two simple tuning fork tests, the Rinne and Weber tests, which together can distinguish conduction from perception deafness. Both depend on the differences between air conduction and bone conduction of sound. Sound transmitted by air conduction depends on the integrity of the middle ear, while bone conduction can bypass the middle ear and activate the basilar membrane of the inner ear directly. These tests are described in Table 8.2.

Other hearing tests

Audiometry

Auditory acuity is measured with an audiometer. The device produces pure tones at specific frequencies using headphones and each ear is tested separately. The auditory threshold for a range of tones is determined by decreasing the volume of each tone until a person no longer hears it. Audiometric tests can identify the frequencies lost: in middle ear disease, low-frequency loss is common, whereas cochlear nerve damage is associated with high-frequency impairment.

Tympanometry

This procedure measures the impedance of the middle ear and it helps to determine the cause of conductive hearing loss. It does not require the active participation of the person being tested and is commonly used in children. A small plug inserts into the ear canal, measuring eardrum vibration, how much sound passes through the middle ear and how much is reflected as pressure changes in the ear canal. The results indicate whether the problem is a blocked eustachian tube, fluid in the middle ear or disruption in the ossicular chain. Tympanometry also detects changes in contraction of the stapedius muscle. This muscle contracts in response to loud noises as part of the acoustic reflex, protecting the inner ear. The acoustic reflex changes if the hearing loss is neural. When the acoustic reflex is decreased, the stapedius muscle cannot remain contracted during continuous exposure to loud noise.

Electrocochleography

Electrocochleography measures the activity of the cochlea and the auditory nerve. This and the auditory brainstem response test are used to measure hearing in people who cannot, or will not, respond voluntarily to sound. For example, these tests can identify whether infants and children have profound hearing loss and whether a person is faking or exaggerating hearing loss (psychogenic hypoacusis). Sometimes the tests can help determine the cause of sensorineural hearing loss. Under anaesthesia, a recording electrode is inserted through the tympanic membrane to lie close to the round window to record the nerve compound action potentials to different frequencies.

Auditory brainstem response

This is a test for neural hearing loss. It measures nerve impulses in the brain resulting from stimulation of the auditory nerves by calibrated clicks presented to the ear. Computer averaging of scalp-evoked potentials produces an image of the wave pattern of the nerve impulses. This technique evaluates deficits due to trauma or disease involving the brainstem, especially in children. Children labelled as 'slow learners' have been shown to actually have hearing deficits rather than being mentally retarded. The auditory brainstem response can also be used to monitor certain brain functions in people who are comatose, or in those undergoing brain surgery.

Main causes of hearing loss

Infection

Prenatal causes

Viruses, such as German measles (rubella) or cytomegalovirus (CMV) during pregnancy, can cause com-

Table 8.2 Comparison of the Rinne and Weber hearing tests

Test	Method	Normal response	Conduction deafness	Sensorineural deafness
Rinne	Place a vibrating tuning fork in contact with the mastoid process, and then close to the pinna. Compares air conduction with bone conduction and determines their relative sensitivities in each ear separately	Sound is heard louder and longer by air conduction because sound energy travelling through bone dissipates more quickly	Bone conduction is better than air conduction on the affected side	Air conduction is better than bone conduction in the affected ear. Sound is loudest in the unaffected ear
Weber	Place a vibrating tuning fork in the middle of the forehead and ask the patient in which ear the tone is heard. It detects relative hearing loss differences between the two ears	Sound is heard equally well on both sides	Sound is louder in the affected ear	Sound is louder in the unaffected ear

plete destruction of the cochlear nerve in the foetus. Meningitis also leads to deafness by destroying IHCs.

Perinatal causes

Middle ear infections, such as otitis media, which is a bacterial infection, cause swelling and bulging of the tympanic membrane and pain and pus collection in middle ear. These are most common in children, as the eustachian tubes are not fully formed and do not drain well into the nasopharynx. 'Glue ear'—otitis media with effusion—is the primary cause of hearing loss in children, affecting more than 20% of 2-year-olds and 15% of 5-year-olds in winter, often as a complication of acute ear infections and respiratory illnesses. Ear infections are easily treated with antibiotics such as amoxicillin and analgesic drugs such as paracetamol and ibuprofen.

Ototoxic agents

Prolonged use of particular drugs (see Table 8.3) such as aminoglycoside antibiotics can be ototoxic and can affect both divisions of the vestibulocochlear nerve. Antibiotics predominantly affect the organ of Corti by accumulating at high concentrations in the endolymph. Hair cell damage causes subsequent retrograde degeneration of auditory neurons. The risk of ototoxicity is enhanced by persistently elevated plasma concentrations of the drugs. Repeated courses of therapy continue to damage more cells, leading to more vestibulo-cochlear dysfunction.

Hereditary diseases

More than 100 genes essential for normal hearing and deafness have been detected on 19 out of 23 human chromosomes. Genetic causes are responsible for more than half of all cases of congenital deafness and the most common mutation is in the connexin 26 protein that regulates K^+ flow in and out of hair cells. Genes for approximately 20 hereditary forms of deafness have been cloned; they are involved in making hair cell bundles and the tip link connections between hair cells, and transforming sound energy into electrical activity. Otosclerosis is the most common adult cause of hearing loss and is an autosomal-dominant genetic disorder. It is characterized by fusion of the stapes to the oval window, causing difficulty in movement, followed by eventual cessation of ear ossicle movement. It is amenable to microsurgery (stapedectomy).

Gradual hearing deterioration

This is commonly associated with the work environment. Persistent loud sounds, such as aircraft or pneumatic drills, cause deterioration of hearing by destroying both IHC and OHCs (frequency- and intensity-dependent). Any noise >85 dB is potentially damaging. The perception of higher frequencies is affected first, and then that of lower ones. The amount of damage depends on exposure time, so reducing the intensity and length of exposure to loud sounds limits the damage. Presbyacusis is the progressive hearing loss that occurs with normal ageing. High frequencies (18–20 kHz) are lost first, and lower frequencies (4–8 kHz) later.

Trauma and tumours

Head injuries that fracture the temporal bone may cause hearing damage. Bleeding from the ear and Battle's sign (postauricular haematoma) are common symptoms associated with these fractures. Slow-growing acoustic tumours usually arise in the vestibular division of cranial nerve VIII (Fig. 8.7). They affect both divisions of the vestibulocochlear nerve. Tinnitus, vertigo, deafness and symptoms of damage to cranial nerves VII and V are associated with these tumours (see Box 8.3), as they emerge from the internal auditory meatus at the cerebellopontine angle to impinge on the brainstem. Surgery is required to remove them.

Treatment for hearing deficits

Treatment depends on the cause. For example, if fluid or wax blocks the outer or middle ear, the fluid is drained or the wax removed. For sensorineural deafness, often no cure is available, and in these situations

Table 8.3 Common ototoxic drugs	
Neomycin	Most potent of all antibiotics in destroying the organ of Corti
Streptomycin or gentamycin	Affects the vestibular part of nerve more than cochlear part
Salicylates (e.g. aspirin metabolites)	Reversible hearing loss and tinnitus
Quinine and its synthetic substitutes	Produce permanent deafness
Anti-cancer drugs	E.g. cisplatin (common) or vincristine (rare) – typically bilateral and sensorineural

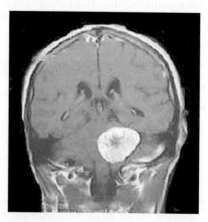

Fig. 8.7 Magnetic resonance image showing an acoustic neuroma compressing the cerebellopontine angle. From the British Acoustic Neuroma Association.

treatment involves compensating for the hearing loss. Most affected people use a hearing aid. Rarely, a cochlear implant is used.

Hearing aids

Hearing aids help people with conductive or sensorineural hearing loss. These people do not hear softer speech sounds—usually, consonants as opposed to harder vowel sounds—or the higher frequency components of speech. Hearing aids use a microphone to collect sounds, an amplifier to magnify the softer sounds while limiting the louder sounds and a speaker to transmit the sounds so that they are heard. The original hearing aids were of the analogue variety and these essentially amplify all sounds (e.g. speech and noise) in the same way. Nowadays, digital hearing aids are commonly available and these convert sounds into a series of numbers, which are mathematically processed, before converting them back into analogue signals. This non-linear processing means that they amplify soft sounds more, medium sounds similarly to any other hearing aid but loud sounds less. This makes for better sound quality and listening is easier, especially in noisy environments.

Cochlear implants

This is a type of hearing aid for profoundly deaf people and consists of several parts. An internal coil is surgically implanted in the skull behind and above the ear, and electrodes are implanted in the cochlea. An external coil is held in place by magnets on the skin over the internal coil. The speech processor is connected to the external coil by a wire and is worn in a pocket or special holster. The microphone is placed in a hearing aid worn behind the ear. Children who receive these implants and intensive speech therapy can acquire speech and language skills.

Tympanostomy tubes (grommets)

Grommets are indicated for recurrent (5–6 episodes/year) infections such as chronic otitis media with effusion (glue ear), recurrent acute otitis media and complications of acute otitis media in children. These infections are caused by blockages of ventilation in the inner ear canal, leading to bacterial infection or fluid build-up. The tubes are surgically implanted and left in place for 8–12 months but often fall out on their own. They profoundly improve hearing and language-learning abilities in young children and reduce the frequency of infection.

Stem cells

Scientists in the USA are exploring the potential of using stem cells to restore hearing. For example, researchers at Stanford University are surgically implanting stem cells into the cochlea to become hair cells, while researchers at Rutgers University-New Brunswick are using inner ear stem cells and converting them to auditory neurons as a potential way to reverse hearing loss. The aim is to ultimately use a patient's own adult stem cells and genetically reprogram them to treat hearing loss. As yet, no clinical trials have begun using this approach.

Vestibular system

The functions of the vestibular system relate to posture and balance (equilibrium), specifically the following:

1. detection and conscious perception of head position and movement

2. coordination of compensatory eye movements during head movement, providing stabilization of the visual image and target fixation

3. compensatory postural adjustments of the trunk and limb muscles following head movement

In order to accomplish this, the vestibular system is connected with the spinal cord (via the medial and lateral vestibulospinal tracts [VSTs]), the cerebellum (via the flocculonodular lobe and fastigial nucleus) and cranial nerve nuclei (III, IV and VI) associated with ocular movements.

Anatomy

The vestibular apparatus, like the cochlea, is contained within the membranous labyrinth of the inner ear and comprises the semicircular canals and the vestibule, which contains the utricle and the saccule (Fig. 8.8). There are five sense organs: the utricle, the saccule and, at the base of each semicircular canal, the ampulla. These house the sensory hair receptors, the otolith organs (in the utricle and saccule) and the cristae (in the ampullae). They are innervated by the peripheral axons of vestibular ganglion cells, whose axons run in the vestibulocochlear nerve that synapses with the vestibular nuclei in the brainstem. Some vestibular afferents terminate directly in the flocculo-nodular lobe of the cerebellum.

These vestibular receptor organs monitor two components of motion: (1) angular acceleration, that is, the detection of rotational movements such as shaking or nodding the head and (2) linear acceleration, that is, detection of motion with respect to gravity such as the sensation when a lift suddenly goes into free-fall or what happens when the body begins to lean to one side.

Semicircular canals

The semicircular canals detect angular acceleration/deceleration of the head. The motion of the endolymph fluid informs the brain whether one is moving. The semicircular canals, in conjunction with the visual and skeletal systems, have specific functions that determine an individual's orientation in space.

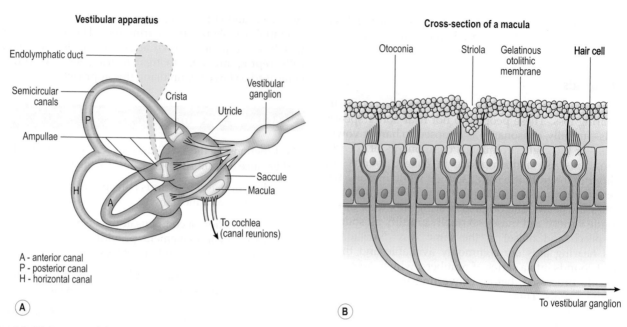

Fig. 8.8 (A) Anatomy of the vestibular apparatus. (B) Cross-section of a sensory macula.

There are three canals, oriented perpendicular to each other in the horizontal, anterior and posterior planes, so that each canal detects motion in a single plane. Horizontal canals are in the same plane and function synergistically. Similarly, the anterior canal on one side and the posterior canal on the other side (and vice versa) are in the same plane and form a synergistic pair. The orientation of the synergistic pairs of canals is important. With the line of sight in the horizontal plane, the horizontal canals are tilted upwards by 25–30 degrees. Each pair of vertical canals is orthogonal to the other and oriented approximately 45 degrees to the right and to the left, respectively. The semicircular canals signal the brain regarding the direction and speed of rotation of the head such as when nodding the head up and down or looking from right to left. Each canal is a continuous endolymph-filled hoop (Fig. 8.9). The sensory hair cells are located in a small swelling at the base of the canals called the ampulla. The lateral ampulla is activated by turning the head to the left or right; head flexion activates the superior ampulla and the inferior ampulla is active during head extension.

The sensory epithelium containing the hair cells embeds into a gelatinous mass, the cupula, which is pushed up into a crest, the crista. When the head rotates in the plane of the canal, the inertia of the endolymph causes it to wash over the cupula, deflecting the hair cells. The same arrangement is mirrored on both sides of the head. Each tuft of hair cells is polarized. If deflected one way, it will be excited; if deflected the other way, it will be inhibited (Fig. 8.9). The transduction mechanism is the same as in the cochlear hair cells, that is, adjacent cilia are connected by tip links and movement of stereocilia tense or relax the tips, opening or closing K^+ ion channels to produce depolarization or hyperpolarization of the cell. Thus the canals on either side of the head operate in a push–pull rhythm; when one is excited, the other is inhibited. Specifically, excitation occurs in the direction of rotation. However, if, for example, both sides push at once, debilitating vertigo and nausea ensue. This is why infections of the endolymph or damage to the inner ear can cause vertigo. In cases of severe intractable vertigo, this can be relieved by cutting one vestibular nerve so that the brain gradually gets used to receiving input from one side only.

Utricle and saccule

The utricle and saccule detect linear acceleration and the pull of gravity. Each organ has a sheet of hair cells and supporting cells—the macula—whose cilia are connected by tip links and are embedded in a gelatinous mass, just like the semicircular canals. Unlike the canals, however, this gel has small crystals of calcium carbonate embedded in it, called otoliths (or otoconia). The otoliths provide the inertia so that when movement to one side occurs, the otolith–gel mass causes the hair cells to deviate (Fig. 8.10). The hair cells are excited (or inhibited) by the bending of the stereocilia towards (or away from) the kinocilium, just as for hair cells of the semicircular canals. Once movement reaches a constant speed, the otoliths come to equilibrium and the motion is no longer perceived.

Hair cells of the utricle and saccule are polarized towards a central shallow groove—the striola (see Fig. 8.8B)—which divides each into medial and lateral halves. The kinocilia are arranged in different directions on either side of the striola so that a single sheet of hair cells can detect motion forwards and back, and side to side. In the

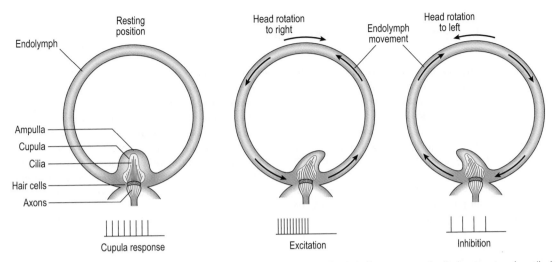

Fig. 8.9 Anatomy of a semicircular canal. Head rotation causes endolymph movement, which causes cupula displacement and vestibular afferent discharge on head rotation. Hair cells are normally spontaneously active, and rotation in one direction causes an increased discharge, while rotation in the opposite direction causes decreased firing.

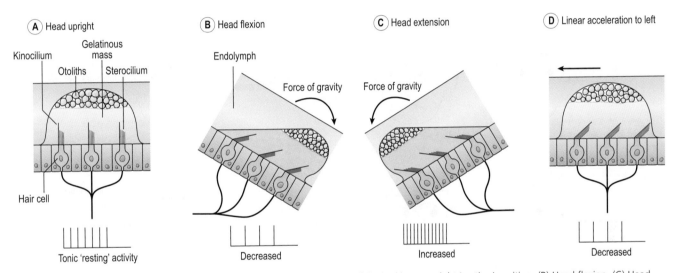

Fig. 8.10 Effects of different head movements on the activity of the macula. (A) Head in an upright 'resting' position. (B) Head flexion. (C) Head extension. (D) Linear acceleration.

utricle the deflection of kinocilia towards the striola excites the hair cells, while in the saccule, deflection away from the striola excites the hair cells. Each macula can therefore cover two dimensions of movement. The utricle lies horizontally in the ear and detects motion in the horizontal plane. The saccule is oriented vertically, so it detects motion in the sagittal plane (up and down, forwards and back). The saccule and utricle maculae are functionally antagonistic on the two sides of the head, so that, for example, tilting the head laterally to one side has opposite effects on the corresponding hair cells of the two utricular maculae.

A major role of the saccule and utricle is to keep the head vertically oriented with respect to gravity. If the head and body start to tilt, such as when a student falls asleep in a lecture, the vestibular nuclei will automatically compensate with the correct postural adjustments via activation of the VSTs. This is the head-righting reflex.

Vestibulo-ocular reflex

An important role of the semicircular canal system is to keep the eyes still while the head moves. When the head is nodded, shaken or swivelled, there is no difficulty in staying focused on an image, but if the image is moving rapidly and the head is still, the eyes are unable to keep pace with the quick movements. This is because the semicircular canals exert direct control over the eyes so that they can directly compensate for head movements but not vice versa. This compensatory reflex is the vestibulo-ocular ('doll's eye') reflex (VOR). This reflex keeps the eyes fixed on a particular object when the rest of the body is moving. It works automatically by sensing head rotations and elicits a compensatory adjustment in the opposite direction. As it is a reflex, it also works in the dark or if the eyes are shut and can be used to assess brainstem integrity in comatose patients (Box 8.4).

Clinical applications of the vestibulo-ocular reflex

The vestibulo-ocular reflex (VOR) can be used to assess the level of brainstem damage in a comatose patient. While the unconscious patient is lying in the supine position, the head is rotated from side to side or tilted up and down. Normally, the eyes will rotate in the opposite direction, giving the impression that the gaze is fixed straight ahead, much like the eyes in a toy doll. This is known as the doll's eye reflex.

This reflex can also be elicited using the caloric test (Fig. 8.11). In a normal patient, cool water decreases the temperature of the endolymph and inhibits the hair cell activity on that side. This produces nystagmus of the eyes with the slow phase (S) towards the side of irrigation and the fast phase (F) away from the irrigation. With warm water irrigation, the opposite happens. This can

be remembered by the pneumonic 'COWS'—cold opposite, warm same. In unconscious patients whose cortex is non-functional but whose brainstem is intact, there is no F phase (due to lack of signal from the gaze centres), so now cold irrigation leads only to a slow deviation to the side of irrigation—'cold same'—whereas warm irrigation produces the opposite response. Bilateral irrigation of the ears with cold water produces downward eye movements, while the opposite occurs with bilateral warm water irrigation.

If the medial longitudinal fasciculus (MLF) is damaged, irrigation results in lateral deviation of the eye only on the less active side. Pons or low midbrain brainstem damage or vestibular nerve damage produces no eye movement.

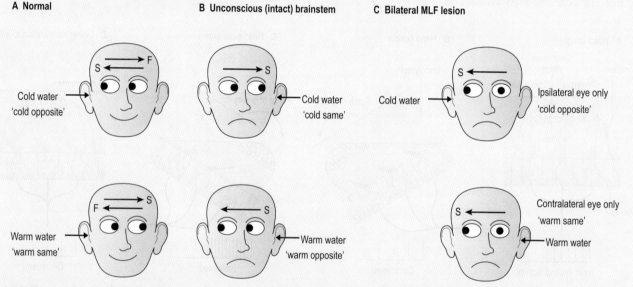

A Normal　　　　　　　**B Unconscious (intact) brainstem**　　　　　　　**C Bilateral MLF lesion**

Fig. 8.11 Ocular responses to caloric stimulation of the semicircular canals. Caloric testing involves the patient lying supine with the head tilted backwards at an angle of 30 degrees so that the horizontal canal is vertically orientated. Water is flushed into the ear and this sets up convection currents in the semicircular canal endolymph that cause movements of the eyes. (A) Normal patient (conscious). (B) Unconscious patient (brainstem intact). (C) Unconscious patient with a bilateral medial longitudinal fasciculus lesion.

The VOR moves the eyes in response to head movements and involves the three pairs of extraocular eye muscles: the medial–lateral rectus pair (adduction/abduction), the inferior rectus–superior oblique (depression and extorsion, elevation and intorsion) and the superior rectus–inferior oblique (elevation and intorsion, depression and extorsion). These pairs of muscles align closely to the planes of orientation of the semicircular canals. It is easiest to explain how the VOR works by using the medial–lateral rectus pair coupled to the horizontal canal as an example (Fig. 8.12).

When the head rotates to the left, the left horizontal canal is excited and the right is inhibited. To keep the

eyes fixed on an object of interest, the right lateral rectus and the left medial rectus muscles must contract in order to move the eyes to the right. On the other side, the right horizontal canal is wired to the complementary set of muscles. Since it is inhibited, it will not excite its target muscles (the right medial rectus and the left lateral rectus), nor will it inhibit the muscles that must be used (the right lateral rectus and the left medial rectus). Eventually, as the eyes track to the right, they end up at the limit of right lateral gaze. Under the influence of a signal arising from the lateral gaze centre in the cortex, they then rapidly flick back to the centre of the visual field as they lose contact with the object of interest, ready to track another object.

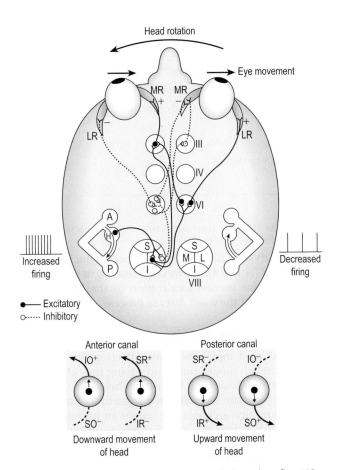

Fig. 8.12 Neuronal circuitry involved in the vestibulo-ocular reflex. When the head turns to the left, the eyes move to the right, causing increased firing in the left horizontal canal and decreased response in the right. Cells that receive information from the left horizontal canal are excited relative to the right canal and stimulate cells in the vestibular nuclei of the brainstem. Neurons from the left medial vestibular nucleus project to the abducens nucleus (VI) on the right side to stimulate the right lateral rectus muscle. They also project to the oculomotor nucleus (III) on the left side to stimulate the left medial rectus muscle. The same vestibular cells also inhibit the opposing muscles (the right medial rectus and the left lateral rectus via connections with the left abducens and right oculomotor nuclei; if eye movement was in the vertical direction, the trochlear nucleus [IV] would also be involved, in place of the abducens nucleus). Actions of the various extraocular eye muscles resulting from stimulation of the semicircular canals are shown. *A*, Anterior canal; *H*, horizontal canal; *P*, posterior canal. Muscles: *IO*, inferior oblique; *IR*, inferior rectus; *LR*, lateral rectus; *MR*, medial rectus; *SO*, superior oblique; *SR*, superior rectus.

This slow drift to one side and rapid re-centring of the eye is called nystagmus and is a normal physiological event.

The axonal connections between the vestibular and oculomotor nuclei that mediate the VOR travel in a tract called the medial longitudinal fasciculus (MLF) in the brainstem. The integrity of this tract is crucial for the normal functioning of the VOR (see Box 8.4). It is occasionally damaged by medial brainstem strokes.

Nystagmus can occur by rapidly spinning someone around in a barber's (Bárány) chair for a brief period, thereby evoking the VOR. For example, consider spinning to the right. At onset, the head and labyrinths

accelerate to the right, causing the endolymph to flow to the left, and the cupulae of both horizontal semicircular canals deflect to the left. The hair cells of the right horizontal canal are excited and so increase their rate of firing, while those of the left canal are inhibited. A VOR occurs, leading to a rhythmic back and forth movement of the eyes, slow to the left and fast to the right. This (rotatory) nystagmus is the attempt by the vestibular system to provide for continued visual fixation on a target during rotatory movement of the head and body. The direction of nystagmus is specified by the direction of the fast phase. Thus rotation to the right produces a right lateral nystagmus.

When the spinning abruptly stops, because of its inertia, the endolymph does not stop as quickly in the horizontal canals. This equates to a flow of endolymph and cupula displacement in the direction of the previous rotation, that is, to the right. For the left horizontal canal, endolymph flow is towards the utricle, and for the right horizontal canal, it is away from the utricle. Thus the firing frequency of vestibular nerve afferents increases on the left and decreases on the right. This is the pattern of excitation and inhibition that would occur if the subject were being rotated to the left and the brain interprets this signal as such. Consequently, for a brief period after stopping rotation, a postrotatory nystagmus occurs in the opposite direction; the eyes move slowly to the right and, when they reach the limit of lateral gaze, quickly to the left. This effect lasts for 20–30 seconds after cessation of rotation. Many will be familiar with the disorientating effects when getting off a merry-go-round at the funfair.

If the subject tries to reach out and touch an object during the period of post-rotatory nystagmus, the movement will miss the target in the direction of the slow phase of nystagmus, that is, to the right in this case. This inaccuracy is called past pointing and occurs because the brain perceives that a leftward rotation is occurring, due to the inputs from the semicircular canals. Therefore, it considers this and automatically compensates for the movement by adding a few degrees of motion to the right. This causes the object to be missed to the right. In terms of the muscles of posture and balance, the direct effect is also to compensate for the perceived rotation.

During post-rotatory nystagmus there is a perception of spinning or falling in the direction of the nystagmus, that is, to the left. This sensation is called vertigo. Any attempt to walk during the perception of vertigo can lead to a fall. Since the perception is one of falling to the left, there will be an attempt to compensate with a fast, voluntary contraction of the extensor muscles on the left. This can lead to an abrupt fall to the right. Therefore the consequences of suddenly stopping rotation to the right are nystagmus and vertigo to the left, and past pointing and falling to the right.

Central pathways of the vestibular system

Vestibular primary afferents terminate mainly in the vestibular nuclei. A small number of fibres project directly into the vestibulocerebellum (flocculo-nodular lobe and

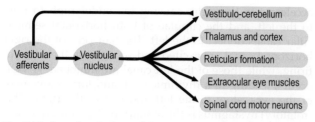

Fig. 8.13 Central projections of the vestibular apparatus.

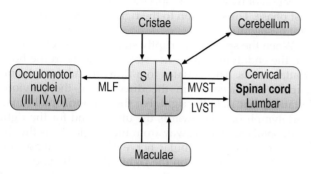

Fig. 8.14 Connections of the vestibular nuclei. *I*, inferior vestibular nucleus; *L*, lateral vestibular nucleus; *LVST*, lateral vestibulospinal tract; *M*, medial vestibular nucleus; *MLF*, medial longitudinal fasciculus; *MVST*, medial vestibulospinal tract; *S*, superior vestibular nucleus.

Table 8.4	Symptoms of balance disorders
A sensation of dizziness or vertigo	
Falling or a feeling of falling (towards the dysfunctional side)	
Light-headedness or feeling woozy (syncope)	
Visual blurring	
Disorientation	
Spontaneous nystagmus	
Ataxia	

uvula). Vestibular afferents terminate in four subnuclei—the superior, inferior, lateral and medial nuclei—and axons from these subnuclei project to five areas (Figs 8.13 and 8.14) to participate in reflexes.

The superior and medial nuclei receive input from the cristae and are involved in the VOR via connections with the ocular nuclei, reticular formation, gaze centres and tectal nuclei. Input from the maculae goes to the lateral, inferior and medial nuclei. These nuclei project to spinal motor nuclei via the lateral and medial VSTs, which are involved in postural balance. The lateral VST facilitates the action of the anti-gravity (extensor) muscles, while the medial VST mainly influences the activity of the axial muscles of the head and neck (head-righting reflex). The superior and lateral vestibular nuclei also interact with the flocculo-nodular lobe of the cerebellum. Damage to the vestibular nerve or its nuclei often results in balance disorders.

Other second-order axons project to the contralateral ventral posterior nucleus of the thalamus, and from there to the somatosensory cortex (area 3a) and the posterior parietal cortex (area 5). These connections account for the conscious appreciation of our equilibrium and head position. The precise location of the cortical area (primary vestibular cortex) for the conscious perception of vestibular function is unknown but is thought to be just caudal to the facial somatosensory area, as electrical stimulation of this area elicits sensations of vertigo. Functional imaging in caloric testing in volunteers also shows that the insula and temporoparietal areas are involved.

Vestibular system damage: balance disorders

Vestibular dysfunction produces rather distinct signs and symptoms (Table 8.4). However, these signs may not be very useful for precise localization of the lesion or for identification of the exact disease process.

Causes of balance disorders

Infections, head injury, ischemia affecting the inner ear or brain, certain medications and ageing may change our balance system and result in disequilibrium. A conflict of signals to the brain regarding the sensation of movement can cause motion sickness (e.g. when an individual tries to read while riding in a car). Symptoms of motion sickness include dizziness, sweating, nausea, vomiting and generalized discomfort.

Examples of balance disorders

Common syndromes cause 70% of cases of vertigo:

1. Benign paroxysmal positional vertigo (BPPV) is a brief (60-second), intense sensation of vertigo that occurs because of a specific positional change of the head, for example, when getting out of bed in the morning. It is the most common cause of vertigo. The exact cause is unknown, although it is thought to be due to a dislodged otolith from the utricle, which gets stuck in the ampulla, making it sensitive to gravity. In certain positions it stimulates the cupula, causing abnormal sensations. These persist until the crystals relocate elsewhere or disperse. Inner ear infections, head injury, ageing or drugs may trigger BPPV.

2. Ménière's disease is an inner ear fluid balance disorder that causes episodes of vertigo, fluctuating hearing loss, tinnitus and the sensation of fullness in the ear. It is probably caused by an imbalance between the production and reabsorption of endolymph, which eventually ruptures the membranes, causing changes in ion concentrations of the solute; these lead to depolarization of the endolymph fluid, ultimately killing the hair cells. There is no cure for this condition.

3. Labyrinthitis is an infection or inflammation of the semicircular canals causing dizziness and loss of balance.

4. Vestibular neuritis is a (viral) infection of the vestibular nerve.

5. Perilymph fistula is leakage of inner ear fluid into the middle ear. It can occur after head injury or physical exertion or is idiopathic.

Diagnosis of balance disorders

The diagnosis of a balance disorder is complicated because there are many types of balance disorder and because other medical conditions, including ear infections, blood pressure changes and vision problems, or some medications, may contribute to the problem. Examples of diagnostic tests are:

1. Hallpike's manoeuvre. With the patient lying in the supine position, the head is lowered quickly below the horizontal plane of the table and turned to one side. The patient then sits up and the test is repeated, turning the head to the other side. If there is vestibular dysfunction, the patient will develop nystagmus and complain of vertigo within 10 seconds of head movement.

2. Audiometry.

3. The caloric test—weak nystagmus or the absence of nystagmus may indicate an inner ear disorder.

4. Imaging of the head and brain.

5. Posturography—this requires the individual to stand on a 'tilt table' capable of movement within a controlled visual environment; body sway is recorded in response to movement of the platform and/or the visual environment.

Treatment of balance disorders

There are various treatments for balance disorders. If the balance disorder is secondary to another disorder, the primary cause is addressed. Vestibular rehabilitation can be attempted, whereby exercises include movements of the head and body specifically developed for the patient. For people with Ménière's disease, dietary changes, such as reducing the intake of sodium, alcohol and caffeine, and/or avoiding nicotine may be helpful; drugs such as anti-histamines that are prescribed for vertigo are also helpful. Some aminoglycoside antibiotics, such as gentamicin and streptomycin, are specifically used to treat Ménière's disease to kill hair cells, thereby disabling the vestibular apparatus. However, these also affect the cochlear hair cells and cause hearing loss. In cases that do not respond to medical management, surgery may be indicated, for example, insertion of a shunt in Ménière's disease to drain the excess fluid or section of the vestibular nerve to relieve chronic vertigo.

Comments on the case history

This case history (Box 8.1) describes a large acoustic neuroma that has emerged from the internal auditory canal into the skull cavity and is compressing cranial nerves V and VII, the nerves of facial sensation and expression. This accounts for the loss of facial sensation and corneal reflex, and the inability to smile or wrinkle the forehead. Acoustic tumours are benign and develop slowly over a period of years. They expand in size at their site of origin and, when large, displace normal brain tissue. The tumour does not invade the brain but compresses the hindbrain as it enlarges. The tumour becomes pear-shaped with the small end in the internal auditory canal. Large tumours (>2.5 cm) can be life-threatening when they cause severe pressure on the hindbrain, which may manifest as severe headaches, clumsy gait and mental confusion. This is a life-threatening complication requiring urgent treatment. In the worst case, it may cause severe raised intracranial pressure leading to tonsillar herniation. Unless the tumour is removed, the prognosis for this patient is poor.

Early symptoms are easily overlooked, making diagnosis more difficult. However, there are symptoms pointing to the possibility of an acoustic neuroma. The first symptom in 90% of acoustic neuroma patients is a unilateral hearing deficit, often accompanied by tinnitus. The loss of hearing is often subtle and worsens slowly, and there may be a feeling of fullness in the affected ear. These early symptoms are sometimes mistaken for normal hearing changes due to ageing. The patient may compensate by talking more loudly.

Since the vestibular portion of cranial nerve VIII is most commonly where the tumour arises, unsteadiness and balance problems may occur during growth of the neuroma. The heel-to-shin and finger-to-nose tests assess motor coordination and are associated with the cerebellum. A wide-based gait indicates some cerebellar dysfunction, and absence of nystagmus on caloric stimulation indicates damage of the vestibular connection to the oculomotor nuclei.

Treatment options for this patient include radiotherapy and surgery. Radiotherapy arrests tumour growth; some tumours shrink, but they rarely disappear. Follow-up of these patients is important because ~20% of tumours continue to grow after radiosurgery or at some time in the future.

Only surgical removal of the tumour can cure the patient. Removal can be either partial or total, depending on its size and the risk of complications in the patient. Preservation of the facial nerve is the primary task if there is to be a successful outcome to the surgical procedure when hearing is already lost. In this patient, if the tumour is removed, the facial nerve symptoms may resolve but the deafness is likely to be permanent.

Self-assessment case study

A tired-looking young, single, working mother arrives at the doctor's surgery with her 10-month-old baby boy. The child is crying and has a runny nose. According to your records, it is the third time during the winter that you have seen the baby. The boy is pyrexic at 44.25°C (102.8°F), and the mother tells you that the temperature has been raging for 36 hours, with vomiting and some diarrhoea. The baby cries almost continuously and has been constantly pulling at the left ear. She has been giving him a half-teaspoon of baby Calpol (infant paracetamol) every 4 hours, which seems to help. Otoscopy reveals a swollen and inflamed eardrum, with signs of pus accumulation. The doctor prescribes a course of amoxicillin and makes a follow-up appointment for 2 weeks' time. The doctor also asks the mother whether she would consider seeing an ear, nose and throat specialist to check the baby's hearing, and about the possibility of having grommets fitted. She asks why?

After studying this chapter, you should be able to answer the following questions:

1. What are the common causes of ear infections?

This case is an example of acute otitis media. Although otitis media can occur in people of all ages, it is most common in young children, particularly those between the ages of 3 months and 3 years. Usually, this disorder develops as a complication of the common cold and may arise 4–7 days after the onset of a cold. The eustachian tube swells during a cold and can become blocked, providing a breeding ground for trapped viruses or bacteria from the throat.

2. What are the symptoms and how are they treated?

Usually, the first symptom is a persistent, severe earache due to pressure build up in the middle ear, pressing on the eardrum. Temporary hearing loss may occur, as the eardrum cannot vibrate. This may cause long-term damage unless quickly treated. Young children may have nausea, vomiting, diarrhoea and a temperature of up to 105°F. The eardrum is inflamed and may bulge. If the eardrum ruptures, discharge from the ear may be bloody at first, then change to clear fluid and finally to pus. Serious complications include infections of the surrounding bone (mastoiditis), sinuses, or infection of the semicircular canals (labyrinthitis), paralysis of the face, hearing loss, inflammation of the covering of the brain (meningitis) and brain abscess. Signs of an impending complication include a headache, sudden profound hearing loss, vertigo and chills and fever. A doctor examines the ear to make a diagnosis. If pus or some other discharge is draining from the ear, a sample is sent to a laboratory and examined to identify the organism causing the infection. The infection is treated with oral antibiotics. Amoxicillin is often the first choice of antibiotics for people of all ages.

3. Why is the doctor worried about hearing loss and suggesting the insertion of grommets?

As the eustachian tubes are not fully developed and so do not drain well into nasopharynx, the infection may develop into 'glue ear'—otitis media with effusion—which is the biggest single cause of hearing loss in children. As the eardrum is swollen, temporary hearing loss may occur, as the eardrum cannot vibrate; this may cause long-term damage in terms of speech development and learning ability, unless quickly treated. Grommets inserted into the eardrum allow pressure equalization between the outer and middle ears, effectively reducing the incidence of infection and improving hearing quality. Grommets are suggested after recurrent infections that are resistant to antibiotic treatment.

MOTOR SYSTEMS I:
DESCENDING PATHWAYS AND CEREBELLUM

9

Chapter summary

1. Behaviour involves conscious and unconscious motor activity that arises from multiple brain regions.

2. Unconscious motor activity involves the autonomic nervous system, which regulates smooth muscle functions. The actions are mostly reflex responses regulated by the hypothalamus. Postural control is also regulated non-consciously from the brainstem.

3. Conscious movements are controlled by two separate systems: the upper motor neurons (UMNs) of the cortex and brainstem that plan and generate commands to make voluntary movements and the lower motor neurons (LMNs) of the spinal cord and brainstem whose function is to produce skeletal muscle contractions. The action of these systems is coordinated by the cerebellum and basal ganglia nuclei. The four component parts are hierarchically ordered, connected by tracts and somatotopically organised.

4. UMNs and LMNs are distinguished by their location and axonal projection territories: UMN axons never leave the CNS and synapse with interneurons or LMNs, whereas LMN axons travel in the peripheral nervous system and terminate at the neuromuscular junction.

5. A reflex response is the simplest form of movement. They are automated, involuntary responses triggered by sensory input that are not directly controlled by the brain. Reflexes can be classified in many ways, for example, using clinical criteria (superficial, deep, visceral, somatic, pathological), anatomical location (segmental, suprasegmental, intersegmental, spinal, cranial), functional role (flexor withdrawal, crossed extensor, postural, righting), developmental aspects (innate, i.e. genetically determined, or acquired, i.e. learned) or by the number of synapses involved (monosynaptic, disynaptic, polysynaptic).

6. Descending motor pathways are divided into two main classes: pyramidal or extrapyramidal. Pyramidal pathways arise from the cortex and control voluntary movements of the contralateral limbs, while extrapyramidal pathways arise from the brainstem and control postural adjustments in response to voluntary movements and balance.

7. Damage to UMNs results in positive neurological signs such as spasticity, hypertonia, hyperreflexia and muscle paresis in groups of muscles, whereas LMN damage results in muscle atrophy, hypotonia, paralysis and hyporeflexia in individual muscles.

8. The cerebellum has three lobes, three different functions, three pairs of cerebellar peduncles, three pairs of deep nuclei and three cerebellar cortex layers. The cerebellum is involved in motor learning and the coordination of multi-joint movements. It acts in two main ways: feedback mode as a comparator of the actual movement with the intended movement, and feedforward mode for the execution of well-rehearsed, rapid movements where it runs a programme that predicts the consequences of the intended movement.

9. Damage to the cerebellum produces ataxia, hypotonia, nystagmus, dysarthria, asynergia and intentional tremor on volitional limb movements.

Introduction

Movements, whether involuntary or voluntary, are elicited by coordinated and graded patterns of muscular contractions, orchestrated by the motor neurons of the spinal cord and brainstem. A major function of the brain is to control motor behaviour, which is manifested as coordinated movements of the eyes, mouth, limbs and body. For example, consider a person playing tennis. In order to serve an ace to an opponent, the player must first assess where the opponent is standing, and then throw the ball up into the air and coordinate the arm to use the racket to hit the ball in a particular predetermined direction so that the opponent cannot return the serve. Coupled to this are the postural adjustments required to maintain appropriate balance so as not to foot fault while serving, and to coordinate the movements of the various muscles of the body to produce sufficient power and racket speed to hit the ball at the top of the throw.

To perform all these different functions concomitantly would not be possible without the coordinated efforts of four distinct but interactive systems, which are hierarchically ordered (Fig. 9.1). The first of these are the lower motor neurons (LMNs) of the spinal cord ventral horn and the brainstem, whose axons innervate the striated muscles (via neuromuscular junctions) of the body and head, respectively. LMNs receive sensory input from proprioceptors, which, together with other spinal cord and brainstem interneurons, act to modulate LMN activity and coordinate the movement of different muscle groups.

The activity of LMNs is modulated by the second system—the upper motor neurons (UMNs)—whose cell bodies lie in the cortex and brainstem. The axons of UMNs form the descending motor pathways that synapse with interneurons or LMNs in the brainstem or spinal cord; they never innervate muscles directly. Traditionally, UMN axons are divided into two descending systems: the pyramidal and extrapyramidal tracts. The pyramidal tract arises from the motor cortex and is essential for planning, initiating and directing voluntary movements and complex spatiotemporal sequences of movements. The extrapyramidal tracts, which are evolutionarily older, arise from the brainstem. They play an important role in postural control, usually involving many muscle groups, particularly anti-gravity muscles, and navigation movements. This also means that the brainstem contains cell bodies of both LMNs (associated with cranial nerves) and UMNs (origins of the extrapyramidal tracts).

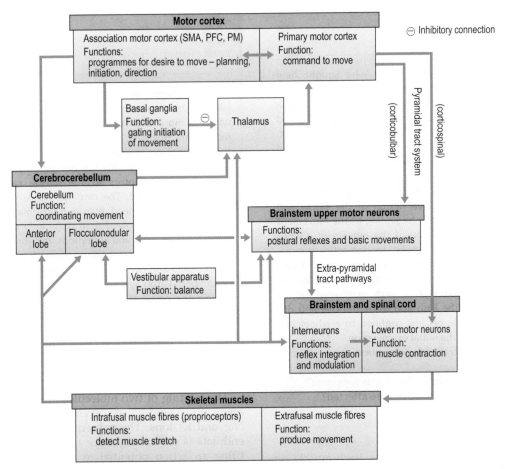

Fig. 9.1 Schematic representation of circuits involved in motor function. *PFC,* Prefrontal cortex; *PM,* premotor cortex; *SMA,* supplementary motor area.

The third and fourth systems are arranged in parallel with the hierarchical organization of LMNs and UMNs. These are the cerebellum and basal ganglia, which are large collections of nuclei that modify movement on a minute-to-minute basis. They do not project directly to LMNs but are important for successful motor performance. Their output regulates the activity of UMNs. The basal ganglia and cerebellum receive information from the motor cortex and both structures send information back to it via the thalamus. The output of the cerebellum to the motor cortex is excitatory, while the basal ganglia are inhibitory (in that they reduce thalamic activation of the motor cortex, see Chapter 10). The balance between these two systems allows for smooth, coordinated movement. The cerebellum acts as a motor performance error detector, whereas the basal ganglia function to suppress unwanted movements as well as to prepare the motor cortex for the initiation of movements (see Chapter 10). All levels of the motor hierarchy, except the basal ganglia, receive information from somatic proprioceptors that continually inform the motor system about the position and movement of the body and limbs. Disturbances to any of these structures lead to paresis (weakness), paralysis or spasticity of movement, as demonstrated in the case history described in Box 9.1.

Involuntary motor control of smooth muscle is performed by the autonomic nervous system (ANS). The LMNs of this system reside outside the spinal cord, in the paravertebral and prevertebral sympathetic chain ganglia, in the parasympathetic postganglionic ganglia near the target organ, or in the gut wall itself in the case of the enteric system. Their function is controlled by the hypothalamus, brainstem reticular formation and spinal cord autonomic centres. The importance of autonomic control of organs, such as the heart, bladder and sexual organs, and the pharmacological means of modulating its function makes visceral motor control systems an important topic in clinical medicine (see Chapter 1).

In order to understand how voluntary motor behaviour is produced, it is necessary to begin by considering the interaction between LMNs and skeletal muscles.

Skeletal muscle contraction

Voluntary movements occur by the active contraction of skeletal muscles. Striated muscles make up approximately 40% of the mass of an adult human and attach to the skeleton by tendons. They act in pairs, with the contraction of one muscle being associated with the relaxation

Box 9.1 Case history

David is a 63-year-old retired actor who sought help because of progressive weakness of his arms and legs, along with slurred speech. He complained of frequent muscle cramps in his legs. Neurological examination showed bilateral loss of strength in his arms, shoulders and feet. There was some wasting of the muscles of the hands and of the feet and fasciculations were observed in the tongue. Stretch reflexes were hyperactive in his arms and legs, and the Babinski sign was present bilaterally. There was increased resistance to passive flexion of the elbow and knee, which was strong at the beginning of the movement but collapsed towards the end of the movement. Clonus was present in response to Achilles' tendon reflex stimulation. All sensations and mental status were normal. David was prescribed the drug riluzole. He became progressively weaker during the next 3 years, with increasing atrophy and fasciculations in the limb and trunk muscles and difficulty in breathing. He became confined to a wheelchair and died 4 years after the initial examination.

This case gives rise to the following questions:

1. What are the causes of the various symptoms?
2. What nervous system regions are affected?
3. Why was David given riluzole?

Box 9.2 Diseases of the neuromuscular junction

Normally, large amounts of acetylcholine (ACh) are released from motor neurons with each action potential, which is more than enough to ensure excitation of the motor unit. However, there are certain conditions in which this does not occur and muscle weakness ensues. In myasthenia gravis auto-antibodies are produced that destroy nicotinic ACh receptors so the muscle cannot respond to the ACh released. The cardinal sign is variable muscle weakness with the head, eyes and proximal muscles being more commonly involved than distal limb muscles. Muscle tone, reflexes, bulk and sensations are normal. Treatment consists of using acetylcholinesterase inhibitors, such as neostigmine and pyridostigmine, and immune suppression. In Lambert–Eaton syndrome, auto-antibodies are directed against the presynaptic voltage-dependent Ca^{2+} channels, which allow the influx of Ca^{2+}, triggering exocytosis of vesicles containing ACh. This reduces the amount of ACh released. Patients present with proximal weakness, and sensory and autonomic disturbances.

of the opposing (antagonistic) muscle. Each muscle consists of muscle fibres and each muscle fibre receives input from a single LMN.

When the LMN axon reaches the muscle, it branches, and each branch forms a specialised synapse called the neuromuscular junction (NMJ). Upon stimulation, the LMN axon releases acetylcholine (ACh) into the synaptic cleft. The region of the muscle that lies under the synapse is the motor endplate and contains a high density of nicotinic acetylcholine receptors (nAChRs).

The NMJ is an unusual synapse compared with other synapses in the vertebrate central nervous system (CNS). It releases only a single type of neurotransmitter onto a single type of postsynaptic receptor (in invertebrates and in the ANS more than one neurotransmitter is released), and each action potential releases a large number (200–300) of vesicles into the synaptic cleft.

The release of so many vesicles leads to a rapid rise (within 200 µs) in the concentration of ACh to approximately 1 mM. The postsynaptic membrane of the endplate is highly folded and contains abundant nAChRs and an enzyme—acetylcholinesterase (AChE)—which is responsible for the breakdown of ACh released into the cleft. It is present as both soluble and membrane-associated forms and, by hydrolysing ACh into choline and acetate, reduces the concentration of ACh back to baseline levels within 1 ms. The choline is then transported back into the motor axon, where it is recycled to produce ACh.

The binding of two molecules of ACh to each nAChR opens this ligand-gated ion channel to allow the flow of Na^+ and K^+ ions. The subsequent depolarization of the endplate is sufficiently large to exceed the threshold for firing an action potential in the muscle plasma membrane and this triggers Ca^{2+} release from intracellular stores, in sufficient amounts to cause muscle contraction. In some diseases auto-antibodies bind to the nAChR to prevent activation (Box 9.2).

Blocking activity at the neuromuscular junction

Activation of the NMJ can be affected by ACh antagonists, which act either presynaptically or postsynaptically. Certain toxins, such as the botulinum toxin, from the bacterium *Clostridium botulinum*, can prevent presynaptic ACh release. It prevents the exocytosis of ACh vesicles, by destroying the proteins that allow fusion of the vesicle to the presynaptic membrane, thus paralysing the muscle. Severe botulism can be fatal and recovery takes several weeks. Today, local Botox injections are used by cosmetic surgeons to paralyse facial muscles, thus reducing wrinkles, and by clinicians to treat enduring muscle spasms and spasticity.

The poison curare, used by indigenous South American hunters, is a mixture of plant alkaloids that act by inhibiting the postsynaptic nAChRs of the NMJ. A similar mechanism of action occurs in cobra snakebites. Here, one of the peptides in the venom—α-bungarotoxin—binds tightly to the nAChRs, taking days to be removed from the receptor. Both produce muscle weakness and respiratory arrest. Prey caught in this way can be safely eaten as neither poison is absorbed in the gut. One of the alkaloids in curare—tubocurarine—was first used to produce blockade of skeletal muscle during surgery but has now been replaced by other similar drugs (e.g. gallamine, pancuronium, vercuronium, atracurium, rocuronium, cisatracurium and mivacurium), which vary in their duration of action (15–60 min). All are competitive antagonists of ACh that bind to nAChRs to prevent the depolarization of the motor end plate and are therefore called non-depolarizing blocking agents. They also act on presynaptic receptors, interfering with Ca^{2+} influx, which causes inhibition of the release of ACh. These agents do not cross the blood–brain barrier. Their action can be rapidly reversed by the administration of AChE inhibitors, such as neostigmine. This prevents breakdown of ACh released into the cleft, effectively increasing the local concentration of ACh, which can then compete with the blocking agent. Neostigmine is considered the drug of choice for routine practice in the reversal of neuromuscular blocking agents in the paediatric population.

Another class of drugs used to induce neuromuscular blockade are agonists of nAChR. These drugs, which have some structural similarity to ACh, act by producing a sustained depolarization of the endplate and are therefore called depolarizing blocking agents. This makes the muscle unresponsive to stimulation, as the voltage-sensitive Na+ channels that produce the muscle action potential are all inactivated. The only clinically relevant member of this group is suxamethonium (Box 9.3). Its blocking action occurs in two phases. In phase 1 there is an initial brief depolarization of the skeletal muscle fibres, causing small contractions (fasciculations), and repolarization is inhibited. In phase 2, desensitization blockade occurs. After the drug has been present for a period of time, the motor endplate loses its sensitivity and depolarization cannot occur. Desensitization continues for several minutes, even after drug is no longer present. Therefore this dual block effect delays recovery.

The motor unit

The smallest functional component of the motor system is the motor unit. This consists of the LMN and the muscle fibres that it innervates. Although each muscle fibre is supplied by only one motor neuron, each motor neuron innervates between three and a few thousand muscle fibres (precision vs power functions). This is the innervation ratio, which determines the precision with which a muscle is controlled. Muscles with a low innervation ratio, such as the extraocular muscles (ratio of three fibres per motor neuron), which control eye movements, are very finely regulated, whereas muscles with a high ratio, such as the gastrocnemius (ratio of 1000–2000 fibres per motor neuron), are less precisely regulated. Additionally, this organization reduces the chance that damage to one or a few motor neurons will significantly affect the muscle action. If a single LMN dies, some of the muscle fibres that were innervated by the motor axon

Suxamethonium and genetic variability

Suxamethonium chloride is the gold standard neuromuscular blocking agent (NMBA) used in clinical anaesthesia. It is used as a muscle relaxant to facilitate endotracheal intubation, mechanical ventilation and a wide range of surgical and obstetric procedures, due to its rapid onset of effect (3060 s) when injected intravenously, and short duration of action (2–6 min), despite adverse effects such as anaphylaxis, hyperkalaemia and malignant hyperthermia. It is rapidly hydrolysed by non-specific cholinesterase enzymes, called pseudocholinesterases, present in plasma and normally its effect wears off within 5–10 min as the drug is metabolized. However, in approximately 1 in 3000 individuals the effects are longer lasting and may continue for many hours. This is due to an autosomal-recessive genetic variation that causes the production of a form of plasma cholinesterase that cannot metabolize suxamethonium. In this case the patient requires ventilatory support. Suxamethonium should be used with caution in patients with atypical plasma cholinesterase or with muscle diseases.

In 2008 sugammadex was approved in the UK for use in clinical practice as an alternative drug to neostigmine because it could rapidly reverse neuromuscular blockade of the longer-lasting, non-depolarising paralysing agents roncuronium and vercuronium. This means that roncuronium can be given at sufficiently high doses to work quickly and reliably (for situations such as laryngeal surgery where the laryngeal muscles are relatively resistant to neuromuscular blockade) without the adverse effects of suxamethonium. However, sugammadex is costly compared with other NMBAs and this limits its routine use. If sugammadex becomes cheaper and more widely available, it is possible that rocuronium will become the only non-depolarising NMBA used and sugammadex will become the reversal agent of choice.

become innervated by an adjacent motor neuron, which sprouts new connections and takes over control of the denervated muscle fibres. Thus the average size of the motor units in the muscle increases but with functional consequences: instead of smaller motor units with finer control there are now fewer, but larger, units and muscle precision decreases.

The types of motor unit can be distinguished by the properties of the muscle fibre and the firing characteristics of its LMN. The most numerous are slow muscle units, which innervate muscle fibres rich in haemoglobin. They are found in muscles that are important for activities requiring sustained contractions, such as postural control (anti-gravity muscles). Prolonged activation of these units produces little reduction in muscle force even after an hour or more. Fast muscles have less haemoglobin, appear paler and fatigue more quickly. These contain fast fatigue units, whose activity is important for muscle contractions that require large forces, such as during activities like jumping and sprinting. Repetitive activation of these units causes a rapid decline in the force of contraction after approximately 30 s. In addition, some motor units are fast-fatigue-resistant and can sustain activity for approximately 5 min before declining. These different motor units allow the nervous system to produce movements appropriate to the circumstances and also help to explain the different types of structural composition of muscles. For example, the muscle of a 100-m sprinter contains more fast-fatigue muscle fibres—essential for producing power—than those of a marathon runner, whose muscles are conditioned for endurance and therefore have more slow muscle fibres.

Slow muscle fibres are innervated by small α-motor neurons, while fast fibres are innervated by large α-motor neurons. This relationship is important, as soma size determines the order in which motor units are recruited during a voluntary movement: the smallest ones first, then fast-fatigue-resistant and finally fast-fatigue. This is known as the size principle. Motor neurons are deactivated in reverse order as the voluntary movement is terminated. Recruiting an increased number of motor units generates the increased force of contraction. During a submaximal contraction of each muscle, each motor unit fires a small burst of action potentials and then rests. Greater force is generated by having more motor units active and reducing the pause time. For finely controlled movements, such as hand movements, small motor units are used; for more powerful ones, such as quadriceps activation, larger motor units are recruited.

A single impulse in the motor neuron causes a single contraction in the muscle, a twitch (Fig. 9.2). This lasts much longer than the refractory period of the action potential so if a second impulse arrives before the muscle relaxes; the second twitch is superimposed on the first. This generates more force in the muscle. Trains of action potentials will cause twitches to summate. At low frequencies (12 Hz), this will produce a force that oscillates about a plateau value (unfused tetanus) but as the frequency increases (30 Hz) the force becomes smooth and reaches a plateau that is the maximum force attainable by that motor unit. This is called a fused tetanus and there are no longer peaks and troughs corresponding to individual twitches evoked by the motor neuron action potential. Asynchronous firing of different motor neurons produces a steady-state input to muscles, causing the contraction of a relatively constant number of motor units, and averages out the changes in muscle tension due to contractions and relaxations of different motor units. This allows movements to be executed smoothly. The firing frequency of motor neurons also regulates the muscle tension produced by motor units.

Motor pools

The motor neurons that innervate the same muscle are called a motor pool and the various motor neuron pools are topographically organised: LMNs innervating flexors are separate from extensors and LMNs innervating distal muscles are spatially separate from those innervating proximal muscles (see Fig. 4.4B). The force of contraction of a whole muscle depends on the frequency of firing of the individual motor neurons and also the proportion of the motor pool that is active. Initially, increases in force are brought about by increases in firing rate but larger increases in force are provided by increasing the number of active motor units. This is called recruitment. All the neurons within a motor pool are excited by common inputs in the spinal cord. Which neurons fire first will depend on both their size and the specific arrangement of synaptic inputs. Smaller neurons are more easily excited than larger ones and neurons with more inputs are excited more easily than more sparsely innervated ones.

There are two types of LMN found in the same pool: α- and γ-motor neurons. α-Motor neurons are larger and innervate the striated (extrafusal) muscles that generate the forces needed for movement and postural balance. γ-Motor neurons are smaller and only innervate the muscle spindle sensory receptors embedded within capsules in the muscle, called intrafusal fibres. Their function is to regulate the tension of the muscle spindle by setting the muscle fibres to a set length (see later).

Reflexes

A reflex is the simplest motor response to sensory input. The reflex directly couples the sensory signal to a motor output to produce simple, stereotyped responses to particular sensory inputs. Reflexes occur in both the autonomic and somatic nervous systems. The neural pathways involved are called reflex arcs and, in their simplest form, consist of a sensory neuron and a motor neuron; this is called a monosynaptic reflex. Sensory receptors have their cell bodies in the dorsal root ganglion of the peripheral nervous system (PNS) and synapse on the cell bodies of LMNs in the spinal cord or brainstem. The axons of the LMNs travel in the spinal nerve of the same spinal segment, and axon collaterals may travel up and down the spinal cord to affect motor neurons in adjacent segments.

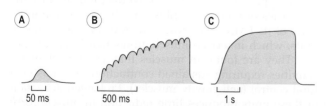

Fig. 9.2 Summation of muscle contraction. (A) Single twitch. (B) Unfused tetanus (12 Hz). (C) Fused tetanus (30 Hz).

Monosynaptic reflexes

In humans there is only one type of monosynaptic reflex, called the stretch (or the myotatic or deep tendon) reflex (Fig. 9.3). It occurs when the tendon of a muscle is hit using a reflex hammer (see Chapter 3) with adequate force to cause stretching of the muscle. This elicits a brief contraction of that muscle via activation of the intrafusal and extrafusal muscle fibres. The reflex acts to prevent rapid muscle stretch when the force on it increases rapidly and returns the muscle back to its original length. This reflex is most prominent in extensor (anti-gravity and postural) muscles and is most easily seen in the knee-jerk reflex. When the patellar ligament is tapped just below the knee there is a rapid contraction of the quadriceps muscles, which swings the lower leg forward. The contraction is stimulated by input from the muscle spindles, which are embedded in the muscle and act directly on the large α-motor neurons supplying the muscle. As there are no other synapses between the sensory neuron and the motor neuron the reflex is very rapid and is all or none, that is, once initiated it cannot be stopped. Tendon reflexes are used to assess the functional integrity of the spinal cord at specific levels (Table 9.1). All stretch reflexes are ipsilateral, so any reflex testing must be performed on both sides to determine if there is a difference.

Muscle spindles

The extrafusal muscle fibres form most of the muscle bulk and produce the contraction. In parallel with these are specialised sensory receptors called muscle spindles (Fig. 9.4). These detect the force acting on the muscle and provide sensory input to the spinal cord about the length and rate of change of length (velocity) of the muscle.

Muscle spindles consist of a small capsule containing a small number (~8–10) of modified muscle fibres called intrafusal fibres, which have a central region that is non-contractile and around which the ends of sensory nerves are wrapped. Intrafusal fibres are arranged in parallel with the extrafusal muscle fibres. There are two types of intrafusal fibre: nuclear bag fibres and nuclear chain fibres.

Nuclear bag fibres are modified multinucleated muscle fibres, swollen in the middle to form a non-contractile bag-like structure. They are innervated by myelinated afferent nerves. There are two types of nuclear bag fibre: dynamic

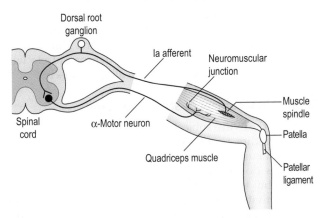

Fig. 9.3 The stretch reflex arc. Stimulation of the patellar ligament stretches the quadriceps muscle, exciting the muscle spindle, which fires action potentials to stimulate the α-motor neuron in the lumbar spinal cord. The motor axon releases acetylcholine at the neuromuscular junction causing the homonymous muscle to contract.

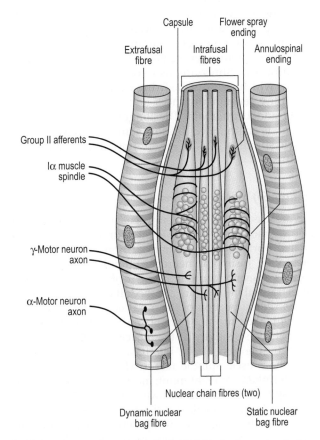

Fig. 9.4 Anatomy of a muscle spindle (simplified). A muscle spindle contains two types of intrafusal fibre: nuclear bag fibres and nuclear chain fibres. Bag fibres are innervated by Ia spindle afferents while chain fibres are innervated by group II muscle afferents. Intrafusal fibres have their own motor innervation from γ-motor neurons. α-Motor neurons synapse on extrafusal fibres.

Table 9.1	Main deep tendon reflexes
Muscle (joint) assessed	**Spinal level assessed**
Supinator (wrist)	C5–C6
Biceps (elbow)	C5–C6
Triceps (elbow)	C7
Quadriceps (knee)	L3–L4
Gastrocnemius (ankle)	S1

primary Ia afferents, which are large in diameter (~16 μm), and static secondary (II) afferents, which are smaller in diameter (8 μm). These differ in their responses to muscle stretch: static fibres are stiffer than dynamic ones and so signal muscle length rather than velocity. Ia fibres are rapidly adapting, whereas group II fibres are non-adapting and so fire even though the muscle has stopped moving. The peripheral endings of Ia afferents are called annulo-spiral endings, while those of the group II muscle spindle afferents are called flower spray endings.

Nuclear chain fibres are slender and have nuclei arranged along their length in a chain-like fashion. They are innervated by both Ia and II afferents. They are stiff, like static fibres, and respond to length.

Each muscle spindle contains at least one dynamic and one static fibre and a variable number (3–5) of chain fibres. The distal portion consists of striate muscle with contractile properties. It is the group II static afferents that allow the brain to know the position of the muscle when it is still, such as when you are holding your arms outstretched with your eyes shut (unconscious proprioception).

When the tendon is tapped, the rapid, phasic component of the monosynaptic reflex is triggered by the stretching of the dynamic Ia afferents in the central non-contractile part of the muscle spindle so that they fire action potentials that are relayed to the spinal cord. Subsequently, as the non-contractile pole ends of the intrafusal fibres are also stretched, they elongate slowly, which reduces the firing of the Ia neurons. The remaining tension produces static responses in both the Ia and II afferents. The longer-lasting tonic component is maintained by the static responses of the muscle spindles. This is very important in maintaining posture.

Gamma (γ) motor neurons

The muscle spindle is the only sensory receptor to have its own motor supply. γ-Motor neurons innervate the striated portions of the intrafusal fibres, and are therefore called fusimotor neurons. Stimulation of γ-motor neurons does not cause movement of the joint to which the extrafusal muscles are attached. It only places tension on the central portion of the intrafusal fibres. Therefore, although they are not part of the stretch reflex *per se*, they set the sensitivity of the muscle to stretch by regulating the tension of the intrafusal fibres; that is, they keep the muscle spindle taut. γ-Motor neurons receive little peripheral afferent input; most of their input is from supraspinal descending pathways, such as the reticulospinal and vestibulospinal pathways.

Appreciating the relationship between extrafusal and intrafusal fibres is important in understanding motor function. As the extrafusal fibres of the muscle contract, stretch on the muscle spindles is reduced and sensory information from the muscle spindles stops unless the muscle spindles themselves also shortened. During intentional activity, at the same time as the α-motor

neurons fire to produce shortening of the extrafusal fibres, the γ-motor neurons are stimulated to shorten the intrafusal fibres. This α-γ co-activation ensures that the muscle spindle is shortened at the same rate as the muscle and the sensitivity of the muscle spindles is maintained despite shortening of the muscle. γ-Motor neurons conduct action potentials more slowly than α-motor neurons. This means that the intrafusal fibres will contract fractionally later than the extrafusal fibres, allowing time for the sensory systems to respond.

Reciprocal and synergistic innervation

Skeletal muscles act in antagonist pairs. Contraction of one muscle is prevented by the tone of the opposing muscle, unless that muscle is simultaneously relaxed. During the knee-jerk reflex, as well as stimulation of α-motor neurons supplying the quadriceps muscles, there is reciprocal inhibition of the hamstring muscles at the back of the thigh. This occurs via an inhibitory interneuron in the spinal cord, which is stimulated by the sensory input from the muscle spindles of the quadriceps. This is a disynaptic reflex.

The quadriceps muscle group comprises four leg extensor muscles that function synergistically to extend the lower leg about the knee joint. The majority of the muscle spindle input is to the motor neurons in the same motor pool (the homonymous muscle). However, approximately 40% of the synapses occur with motor neurons going to all the other leg extensors. Thus activation of the muscle spindles in one extensor muscle will produce synergistic contractions in all four muscles.

Supraspinal control of stretch reflexes

Stretch reflexes are subject to descending modulation via direct or indirect connections between UMNs and α- and γ-motor neurons. Most of the axons from descending pathways do not form synapses directly with α-motor neurons but terminate on these interneurons. Alterations in the activity of these pathways may affect the size or threshold for activation of the reflex. For example, the amplitude of the reflex can be reinforced by various measures, including clenching of the teeth, pulling interlocked fingers (Jendrassic manoeuvre; see Box 9.4) and general distraction of attention. These measures only work when the reinforcement is at a higher level than the reflex being tested, and the reinforcement is thought to be due to the removal of tonic inhibition from the LMNs.

Golgi tendon organs

As well as muscle spindles, muscles have a second type of sensory organ called the Golgi tendon organ (GTO) that is found in the tendons. These are placed in series with the muscle fibres and measure muscle tension. An increase in muscle tension activates a negative (autogenic) feedback reflex of the homonymous muscle called the inverse myotactic reflex (Fig. 9.5), which prevents further increases in tension. This reflex protects the

Jendrassic manoeuvre

In patients with reflexes that are difficult to elicit or appear absent, the use of reinforcement techniques may be helpful in observing a response. This is the Jendrassic manoeuvre. It is most often used when testing lower limb reflexes; the patient is asked to interlock their fingers and try to pull their hands apart while keeping the fingers interlocked. Clenching the teeth can be added to this task if necessary. The tendon is struck during this process. A positive response (if none was present before) or an enhanced response (f the response was weak previously) is to be expected in the absence of any pathology. This indicates that the reflex is under some level of supraspinal inhibition. The main idea behind the reflex is that when the brain is asked to focus on a specific, focal voluntary movement such as pulling the hands apart, it 'forgets' about other body regions and so the descending drive is reduced. The reinforcement task must be at a neurological level above the reflex to be tested. Remember that most descending motor axons do not directly activate α-motor neurons but synapse with inhibitory interneurons that regulate the size of the reflex. When this inhibition is temporarily reduced, the reflex gets bigger, and this is reminiscent of what is seen in patients with stroke or other upper motor neuron lesions.

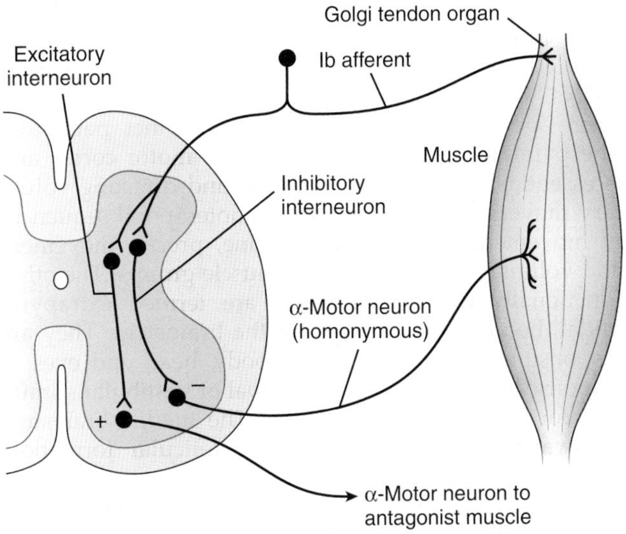

tendon from being injured by too much tension. It also plays a role in mechanisms related to muscle fatigue and joint hyperextension/flexion.

GTOs consist of collagen fibres that contain the endings of Ib afferent neurons at the tendon-muscle interface. GTOs are relatively insensitive to passive stretch but are sensitive to active contraction when most of the force acts directly on the tendon. When muscle tension increases the collagen fibres are stretched, causing Ib afferents to fire. The frequency of firing is proportional to the level of tension. These afferents synapse onto interneurons, which, in turn, synapse onto the α-motor neurons of both the homonymous (inhibitory action) and antagonistic (facilitatory action) muscles. Thus the function of this reflex is to 'switch off movement' and allow the muscle to relax.

The sensory inputs involved in the myotactic and inverse myotactic reflexes affect the same motor neurons but with opposite effects (Fig. 9.6). Sometimes, in pathological situations, these two systems get trapped in a loop where they alternatively trigger each other. This causes the muscle to alternately contract and relax several times a second. This is termed clonus. It can be seen in ankle stretch reflexes where the foot oscillates about the ankle.

Control of muscle tone (stiffness)

All muscles are under some degree of stretch and this is responsible for resting tension in the muscle called muscle tone. The stretch reflex, which maintains muscle length in response to increased load, and the inverse myotactic reflex, which maintains a constant tension, work in opposition. When the load on a muscle is increased, either the mus-

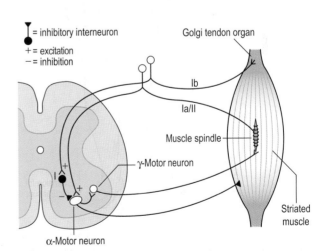

Fig. 9.5 Inverse myotactic reflex arc. The Golgi tendon organ fires in response to an increase in tension and activates spinal cord interneurons that inhibit the α-motor neurons innervating the homonymous and synergistic muscles, thereby relieving excess muscle tension and relaxing the muscle. At the same time connections with other sets of interneurons allow excitation of α-motor neurons innervating the antagonistic muscles, causing their contraction (not shown). +, Excitation; -, inhibition.

Fig. 9.6 Cooperation of myotactic reflexes. Activity of Ia and group II fibres produces α- and γ-motor neuron co-activation, which produces muscle contraction while maintaining its sensitivity during contraction. Stimulation of the Golgi tendon organ (Ib) fibre inhibits α-motor neurons (and γ-motor neurons), producing relaxation. Differences in the conduction velocity (Ib fibres are slower than Ia/II fibres) and the presence of inhibitory interneurons allow contraction and relaxation to occur.

cle must lengthen or the tension must increase. Working together, these reflexes control the tone of the muscle. If the load on a muscle increases but the length is maintained, the contraction is isometric. This is normally the case for postural muscles. Alternatively, if the load is moved by shortening the muscle, this isotonic contraction maintains a constant tension. Damage to LMNs or descending pathways will change the level of tone within muscles.

Polysynaptic reflexes—Flexor and crossed extensor reflexes

These two linked reflexes are stimulated by noxious stimuli, both actual (such as a sharp object) and perceived (such as threatening behaviour). These polysynaptic reflexes trigger a complex set of actions (Fig. 9.7).

The flexion reflex is an important protective reflex. Stimulation produces a withdrawal of the entire threatened limb from the harmful stimulus on the ipsilateral side, with a compensatory extension of the opposite side. These reflexes

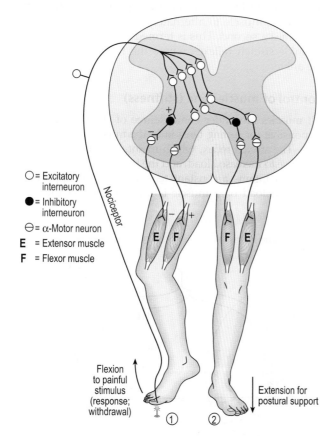

O = Excitatory interneuron
● = Inhibitory interneuron
⊖ = α-Motor neuron
E = Extensor muscle
F = Flexor muscle

Flexion to painful stimulus (response; withdrawal)

Extension for postural support

① ②

Fig. 9.7 The flexor (1) and crossed extensor (2) reflex arcs. These are polysynaptic reflexes. The flexor withdrawal reflex has a protective function. A noxious stimulus activates nociceptors that stimulate spinal cord interneurons in several spinal segments to excite the ipsilateral flexor α-motor neurons, which withdraw the limb from the stimulus. At the same time, the antagonistic extensor muscles are inhibited. The crossed extensor reflex is a contralateral response to an ipsilateral stimulus to maintain balance. Here, nociceptors activate interneurons that excite the α-motor neurons of the extensor muscles of the contralateral leg, while inhibiting the flexors of that leg.

may be important in maintaining balance as the centre of gravity changes. For example, treading on a sharp object produces a withdrawal of the foot with extension of the other leg in order to support the extra weight (see Fig. 9.7).

Flexion reflexes differ from myotactic reflexes in that they involve several interneurons between afferent axons and motor neurons. This gives the brain opportunities to override, modulate or control these reflexes via activity in descending pathways. This is impossible for the monosynaptic and synaptic reflexes from proprioceptors. Damage to descending pathways can alter flexion reflexes.

Spinal motor function

A considerable amount of local processing of sensory information occurs in the spinal cord and this influences motor output. Motor reflexes are simple patterns generated in the spinal cord but the spinal cord is also involved in producing the complex patterns involved in locomotion. During locomotion, networks of neurons produce cycles of activity in order to contract groups of muscles in a carefully timed sequence. These networks, which are called central pattern generators, are initiated by descending input and are modified by reflexes. They are more prominent in quadrupeds than in bipeds, as is evidenced by the observation that when the spinal cord is transected in animals such as cats and rats, there is greater recovery of locomotion than in humans.

Descending pathways

As outlined in Chapter 4, several descending motor pathways that originate in the brain and brainstem modulate LMN function (Table 9.2). The name of the individual tract indicates where it originates and terminates. Unlike LMNs, they use glutamate as their neurotransmitter. There are three main functionally distinct pathways. The pyramidal pathway arises in the motor cortex and is essential for planning, initiating and directing voluntary movements and complex spatiotemporal sequences of movements. It provides for fine, precise movement and voluntary control of distal muscle groups. The other functionally distinct pathways are termed extrapyramidal, because they arise from the brainstem. They are responsible for orientating the body, head and eyes in response to somatic, auditory, visual or vestibular stimuli and for regulating muscle tone. The medial brainstem pathways arise from cells in the reticular formation, vestibular nuclei and tectum. These motor pathways provide for reflex movements related to posture and balance, usually involving many muscle groups—particularly anti-gravity muscles—to prevent the body or head from being destabilised. A lateral brainstem pathway originates in the red nucleus and provides for voluntary movements of the arms but not the individual digits.

Each of these main motor pathways terminates in the spinal cord in a different pattern, which reflects the modality of movement controlled by that motor pathway (Fig. 9.8).

Table 9.2 Summary of the main functions of the descending tracts

Motor system	Tract	Origin	Decussation (where appropriate)	Distribution and cord levels	Main action on lower motor neurons (LMNs)		Function
					Excitatory to	Inhibitory to	
Pyramidal	Lateral corticospinal, Anterior corticospinal	Motor cortex	Spinomedullary junction, Spinal cord	Crossed, Bilateral, All levels	Hand and finger flexors, Trunk flexors	Hand and finger extensors, Trunk extensors	Control of fine voluntary movement
	Corticobulbar	Motor cortex	Pons and medulla, Midbrain and pons	Bilateral, Crossed	Mixed cranial nerve motor nuclei (V, VII, IX, X, XII), Oculomotor nuclei (III, IV, VI)	Mixed cranial nerve motor nuclei (V, VII, IX, X, XII)	Control of brainstem motor nuclei
Extra-pyramidal: lateral	Rubrospinal	Red nucleus of midbrain	Midbrain, Ventral tegmentum	Crossed, Cervical cord	Limb flexors	Limb extensors	Control of gross limb movements
Extra-pyramidal: medial	Medial reticulospinal	Pons	—	Ipsilateral, All levels	Axial and proximal limb extensors	Proximal limb flexors	Facilitates extensor reflexes, inhibits flexor reflexes, and increases muscle tone in axial and proximal limb muscles
	Lateral reticulospinal	Medulla	—	Bilateral, All levels	Proximal limb flexors	Axial and proximal limb extensors	Facilitates flexor reflexes, inhibits extensor reflexes and decreases muscle tone in axial and proximal limb muscles. Autonomic activation of ANS preganglionic LMNs
	Lateral vestibulospinal	Lateral vestibular nucleus	—	Ipsilateral, All levels	Axial and proximal limb extensors	Axial and proximal limb flexors	Stimulates extensor and inhibits flexor muscles to aid postural control of the body (balance)
	Medial vestibulospinal	Medial and inferior vestibular nuclei	—	Bilateral, Cervical cord	Axial ipsilateral	Axial contralateral	Stabilises head position while body is moving (balance)
	Tectospinal	Superior colliculus	Midbrain, Dorsal tegmentum	Crossed, Cervical cord	Neck extensors	Neck flexors	Coordinating head and eye reflex responses to auditory, visual and somatic cues

ANS, Autonomic nervous system; LMNs, lower motor neurons.

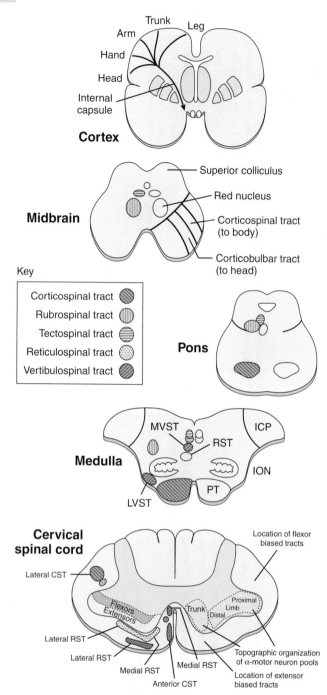

Fig. 9.8 Location of the descending pathways along the neuraxis. The locations of the main descending pathways in the spinal cord in relation to the topographic organization of muscles are shown schematically. Pathways that act mainly on extensor motor neurons are located in the ventral funiculus, while those acting on flexor motor neurons run in the lateral funiculus. The schematic positions of these pathways at higher levels of the neuraxis are shown. *ICP*, Inferior cerebellar peduncle; *ION*, inferior olivary nucleus; *LVST*, lateral vestibulospinal tract; *MVST*, medial vestibulospinal tract; *RST*, reticulospinal tract.

The pyramidal system comprises the corticospinal and corticobulbar tracts. Approximately 60% of the neurons are in the primary, supplementary and premotor areas of the frontal lobe. The rest are in the somatosensory cortex (30%) and the posterior parietal cortex (10%). Their axons pass through the internal capsule (genu and posterior limb) and descend in the basal part of the brainstem but they differ in their termination sites. Corticobulbar fibres terminate on LMNs in the brainstem and control facial movements. Corticospinal axons bypass the brainstem LMNs and terminate in the spinal cord to control limb movements. Corticospinal tract (CST) axons are often called pyramidal tract axons (after the area in the medulla where the axons cross the midline—the spinomedullary junction—Fig. 9.9). The CST is concerned with generating voluntary movements of the hands (see Table 9.2) that require precision, speed and agility. It has very little effect on the lower limbs.

At the spinomedullary junction 85% of the corticospinal axons decussate to form the lateral CST. The remaining 15% are uncrossed fibres that form the anterior CST, and these fibres decussate in the spinal cord at the same segmental level where they synapse. Both tracts are excitatory and most of these axons synapse with spinal cord interneurons; some lateral CST axons synapse directly with α-motor neurons, especially those involved in movement of the fingers whereas the anterior CST axons synapse bilaterally on interneurons to control voluntary movements of the axial muscles. The terminal distribution of the corticospinal motor pathway partly overlaps with those of the other lateral and medial extrapyramidal pathways.

The rubrospinal tract is a small contralateral pathway that ends on interneurons in the spinal cord; these convey motor commands to cervical motor neurons for the control of limb muscles (see Table 9.2). As an evolutionary old pathway, its function differs across species. In quadrupeds, like rodents, it is involved in intra- and inter-limb coordination during locomotion. In primates its function is associated with skilled forelimb movements. In humans rubrospinal axons are intermingled with those of the lateral CST and the function of the rubrospinal tract has largely been taken over by the latter. The majority of red nucleus axons do not project to the spinal cord but relay information to the motor cortex from the cerebellum via the thalamus and inferior olivary nucleus (ION) and are involved in complex cognitive-motor functions, such as motor learning, error encoding, timing and control of ongoing movement (see later).

The medial brainstem motor pathways are represented by the anterior CST, reticulospinal, vestibulospinal and tectospinal tracts. They are associated with balance and postural control via the temporal and spatial coordination of movements. Their axons travel in the brainstem tegmentum (and are therefore spatially separate to the pyramidal system) and the spinal cord ventrolateral funiculus (see Fig. 9.8) and end mainly on interneurons in the medial third of the spinal cord grey matter. These interneurons carry the motor commands

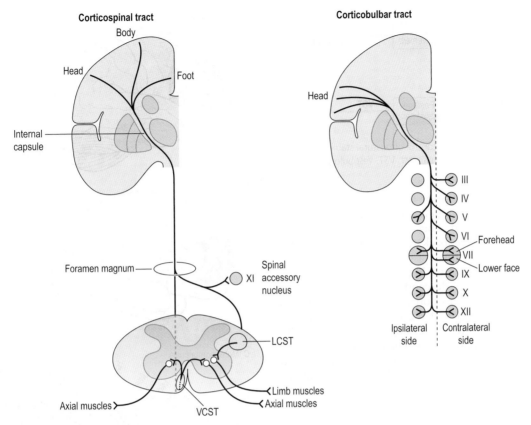

Fig. 9.9 Course and termination sites of the corticospinal and corticobulbar tracts. Both tracts pass through the posterior limb of the internal capsule. Non-ocular brainstem lower motor neurons (LMNs) are supplied bilaterally by the head area of the primary motor cortex, except for the lower facial muscles of the facial motor nucleus, which are supplied only by the contralateral motor cortex. Contralateral input is greater than ipsilateral input. Ocular motor neurons receive only contralateral input. The corticospinal tract bypasses the brainstem cranial LMNs. It decussates at the spinomedullary junction to form the lateral and ventral corticospinal tracts that innervate the LMNs of the spinal cord. *LCST*, Lateral corticospinal tract; *VCST*, ventral corticospinal tract.

to α- and γ-motor neurons that innervate proximal limb, trunk and axial muscles (see Table 9.2).

The reticulospinal tract (RST) has lateral and medial components (see Fig. 9.8). They function in postural control via the regulation of flexor and extensor reflexes through antagonist mechanisms (see Table 9.2). The lateral RST has a predominantly inhibitory effect on segmental reflexes while the medial RST has a facilitatory effect on extensor motor neurons.

The vestibulospinal tract (VST) is also divided into medial and lateral tracts (see Fig. 9.8). The medial VST descends to the cervical and upper thoracic spinal cord and acts on interneurons that facilitate activity in neck muscles, keeping the head steady to provide a platform for eye movements. It is involved in postural reflexes in response to gravity, or to changes in acceleration of the head. For example, the head-righting reflex occurs when the head droops towards one side. The change in head position is sensed by the vestibular system semicircular canals, which then stimulate the medial pathway to activate motor neurons to lift the head back to the correct position by increasing muscle tone in the appropriate anti-gravity muscles. The ascending components of the medial pathway coordinate activity of the vestibular and oculomotor nuclei.

The lateral VST arises from the lateral vestibular (Dieter's) nucleus in the medulla and descends in the ventral funiculus to all levels of the spinal cord. Its function is to maintain balance by acting on the extensor motor neurons (see Table 9.2), to keep the centre of gravity between the feet. It also has important connections with the cerebellum, to regulate posture.

Both the RST and the VST provide information to the spinal cord for the maintenance of posture in response to changes in stability or body position. This involves both feedforward and feedback mechanisms (Fig. 9.10). Postural control involves an element of anticipation in some muscle groups when a movement is to be made. Prior to an intended movement, its effect on postural stability is evaluated and used to generate a change in the activity of muscles that may not necessarily be involved in the movement. For example, consider reaching forwards to open a door. This shifts the centre of gravity and destabilises the body. Increased compensatory activity occurs in the calf muscles to counter-balance the intended arm movement and re-establish body

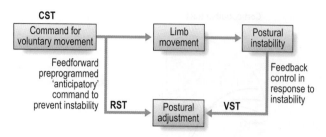

Fig. 9.10 Circuitry involved in the control of postural stability. *CST*, Corticospinal tract; *RST*, reticulospinal tract; *VST*, vestibulospinal tract.

stabilization. This occurs prior to reaching for the door-knob and is a preprogrammed action carried out by the RST. On the other hand, once postural instability has occurred, a corrective feedback system acting via the VST returns the system to normal.

The tectospinal tract (see Fig. 9.8) originates in the superior colliculus and descends to the contralateral cervical spinal cord to act upon the axial motor neurons of the neck on both sides of the cord. This pathway is important in generating orientating movements of the head and eyes in response to visual, auditory or somatic stimuli (see Table 9.2). The superior colliculus also receives input from the corticotectal tract whose axons arise from the ipsilateral frontal and visual association cortices.

The motor cortex

The cortex is involved in the planning and execution of movements, which is a 'ready, steady, go' process. Depending on which cortical area is involved, movements can be conscious (involving premotor cortex) or unconscious (involving posterior parietal cortex) but both produce movements that look similar. The level of conscious awareness depends on the amount of skill required. The more skilled we become, the less planning required. For example, when we first learn to drive we are consciously aware of looking in the mirror (mirror, signal and manoeuvre) before pulling out onto the road, looking at the gearstick when changing gear or looking for turns, cars or pedestrians on the road. As we become more confident, seasoned drivers, these movements become second nature and become unconscious responses when we drive.

The motor cortex consists of three reciprocally interconnected regions: the primary motor cortex (MI), premotor (PM) area and supplementary motor area (medial premotor or SMA) (Fig. 9.11A, B). The latter two form the secondary (association) motor cortex and all contribute axons to the pyramidal tract. The areas are functionally distinct. The MI cortex, located in the precentral gyrus, has a topographical representation of the body surface, with the head, lips and hands represented laterally and the legs and feet represented medially (Fig. 9.11C), similar to the homunculus that exists in the primary somatosensory cortex (see Fig. 4.6). In this region the more complex the

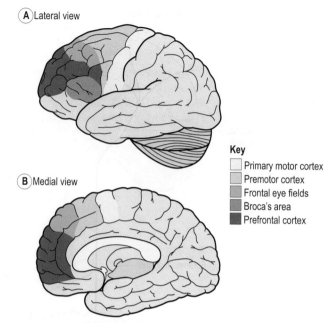

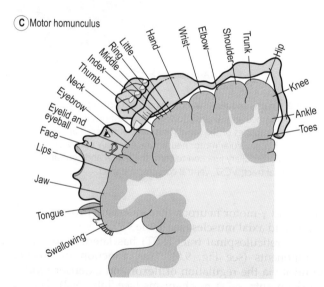

Fig. 9.11 Functional areas of the motor cortex viewed from the lateral (A) and medial (B) surfaces. (C) Homuncular map of the body surface in the primary motor cortex. Note the distorted representation of the cortex for the lips and hands, which require fine control.

movement of a particular body part, the more motor cortex is devoted to it. Thus the lips, tongue and hands, which we use to explore and communicate, have distorted representations due to the variety and complexity of the movements. This topographical representation is also found in the association motor areas.

The MI cortex is involved in the voluntary control of movements by carrying the motor command to the LMNs. This is the 'go' part of 'ready, steady, go'. The PM area is involved in planning movements (i.e. the 'steady' part, where the plans are held until needed) that involve external sensory cues. Activity in PM cells is temporally

Box 9.5   Apraxia

Apraxia is the loss of ability to carry out familiar learned purposeful movements in the absence of sensory or motor impairment. Patients with apraxia have normal reflexes and tone, and no muscle weakness, but they have difficulty in performing complex motor tasks such as brushing their hair, cleaning their teeth or dressing themselves.

There are several different sites for initiation of movement in behavioural contexts. The premotor cortex has links with the homologous area on the contralateral side and the ipsilateral posterior parietal cortex via commissural pathways. Damage to these pathways results in different types of apraxia. Ideomotor apraxia occurs when a person cannot perform a previously learned movement, or mimic movements of a limb when shown by another person. It is a transient phenomenon, as the contralateral side takes over the role of the damaged side. Constructional apraxia is a failure to comprehend the spatial relationships of objects in space and may be identified by asking a patient to reconstruct a three-dimensional object using building blocks. It is often due to a lesion in the superior longitudinal fasciculus, which connects the parietal and frontal lobes.

linked to movements. Here, cells are active when there is an intention to make a movement rather than during the movement. The PM area is about six times larger than the MI and receives a rich sensory input (tactile and visuospatial) from the parietal lobe. It deals with learned motor activities of a complex and sequential nature by coordinating contractions of specific groups of muscles; for example, it is active during writing. The SMA is also involved in planning movements but is concerned with internally generated commands or cues. Its cells are active while an intended movement is being thought about. The SMA is crucial for the performance of complicated tasks involving both sides of the body, for example, two-handed tasks such as typing. Damage to the PM or SMA results in apraxia (Box 9.5).

The frontal eye field region of the motor cortex controls voluntary scanning movements of the eyes, such as during reading. This region has connections with the superior colliculus and the gaze centres located in the paramedian pontine reticular formation. Stimulation of this region causes conjugate deviation of the eyes towards the opposite side to the stimulation, whereas damage to this region induces a transient conjugate deviation of the eyes towards the side of the lesion.

The prefrontal cortex relays input from the limbic system to the motor cortex about the desired goal of the movement. The MI cortex is involved in a motor loop with the cerebellum, while the SMA forms a loop with the basal ganglia. These loops allow the cortex to recruit and coordinate specific motor programmes.

Limb movements are controlled by the contralateral MI cortex but LMNs controlling muscles in the trunk or head that normally act in unison, such as those involved in chewing, swallowing and talking, have bilateral innervation. All non-ocular brainstem LMNs, except those of the lower facial muscles, have bilateral corticobulbar innervation (see Fig 9.9B). Lesions of the internal capsule, which damage the corticobulbar and corticospinal tracts, produce pronounced contralateral lower facial weakness but only transient impairment of the function of other brainstem LMNs.

Actions of upper motor neurons

UMNs have several regulatory functions. They can modulate the activity of α- and γ-LMNs either directly (monosynaptically) or indirectly (via interneurons). This activity can be either excitatory (monosynaptically) or inhibitory (via inhibitory interneurons). In this way the magnitude of the reflex is gated. Thus damage to descending pathways can alter the strength of a reflex. Another important function is efference copy. UMN signals are conveyed to other motor areas of the brain to inform them that an active movement is happening. Cells in the pontine nuclei, for example, receive a copy from the pyramidal tract neurons and relay it to the cerebellum to keep it informed of the intended movement. UMNs can activate the intrinsic pattern generators that produce stereotyped movements. Finally, UMNs terminate not only on LMNs and interneurons but also on other UMNs. For example, corticobulbar axons terminate on neurons of the RST, VST and rubrospinal tracts. The cells of the medial brainstem descending pathways are also richly interconnected. This is important because the brain must be able to switch off selective postural systems to accomplish some types of movement. Disconnection of the cerebral cortex from the brainstem motor centres controlling postural pathways affects the postural responses of the limbs to stimuli and can be used as an indicator of the level of brainstem damage in comatose patients (Box 9.6).

Clinical importance of reflexes

Reflexes are extremely important and inform the doctor about the segmental functioning of the nervous system. The stretch reflex is most important and is routinely tested in the neurological examination. The scoring of tendon reflex responses is shown in Table 9.3. Flexion reflexes are rarely tested, except in unconscious patients or where an UMN lesion may be suspected.

If the axons of LMNs are severed, the muscle contraction becomes weakened to the point of paralysis, depending on how many axons are damaged. The strength of the reflex therefore decreases (hyporeflexia). Complete absence of a reflex (areflexia) results in flaccid (floppy) paralysis of a muscle. Within 3 weeks of denervation the muscle undergoes atrophy (wasting) due to lack of use. In response to denervation the muscle

Box
9.6
Decorticate and decerebrate rigidity

When physical or vascular damage to the brainstem produces functional disconnection between the red nucleus (midbrain) and the vestibular nuclei (pons), patients show an increase in extensor muscle tone called decerebrate rigidity. It is caused by tonic activity in the lateral vestibulospinal and reticulospinal tracts that act on the extensor motor neurons and the loss of rubrospinal inhibition of extensor motor neurons. This leads to the appearance of the positive neurological signs of increased muscle tone and hyperactive stretch reflexes. In response to a startling or painful stimulus both the arms and legs extend and pronate (Fig. 9.12A). The cerebellum also plays a role in decerebrate rigidity because ablation of the anterior cerebellar lobe enhances decerebrate posturing due to the loss of inhibitory input to the lateral vestibulospinal tract. Lesioning the lateral vestibular nucleus or stimulating the anterior cerebellum inhibits this rigidity.

If damage to the brainstem occurs above the level of the red nucleus, decorticate rigidity may ensue due to the loss of corticobulbospinal control. Here, the arms flex and the legs extend in response to the stimulus (Fig. 9.12B). This posturing occurs because of activity in the brainstem flexor facilitation pathways. The red nucleus now controls posture and this pathway counteracts the activity of the lateral vestibulospinal and reticulospinal tracts that activate extensor muscles. Since the rubrospinal tract only extends to the cervical spinal cord it most strongly influences the arms (excites flexors, inhibits extensors) and therefore counteracts the extension of the arms (by the lateral vestibulospinal and reticulospinal tracts) but not the legs.

Damage to the medulla below the level of the vestibular nuclei disconnects the motor neurons from tonic vestibulospinal and reticulospinal tract activity, resulting in flaccid paralysis, hypotonia, loss of respiratory drive and quadriplegia. Essentially, there are no reflexes and this state resembles the early stages of spinal shock, as there is a complete loss of

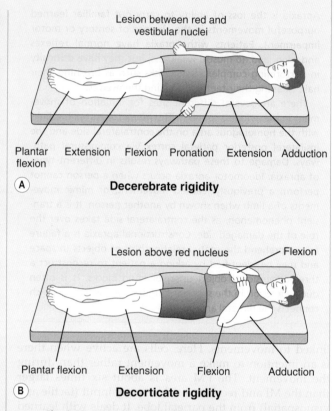

Decerebrate rigidity

Lesion between red and vestibular nuclei

Plantar flexion | Extension | Flexion | Pronation | Extension | Adduction

(A)

Decorticate rigidity

Lesion above red nucleus — Flexion

Plantar flexion | Extension | Flexion | Adduction

(B)

Fig. 9.12 Decerebrate (A) and decorticate (B) posturing.

activity in the motor neurons. Subsequently, over time, some segmental reflexes may recover but these will be hyperactive due to loss of descending motor control. An easy way to remember the difference between the two postures is to remember that decerebrate has an extra 'e' for 'extension'.

Table 9.3 Scoring of deep tendon reflex responses

Normal	+
Brisk	++
Very brisk (+ clonus)	+++
Absent	0
Present with reinforcement	+/−

synthesises large numbers of ACh receptors, which are distributed over the whole surface of the muscle rather than being restricted to the NMJ. This means that the muscle becomes hypersensitive and in response to circulating levels of ACh will show fasciculation (spontaneous, small contractions of muscle fibres). If the damaged

nerve can be repaired surgically, LMN axons can regrow, at the rate of a few millimetres a day, to eventually reinnervate the muscle. Physiotherapy of muscles artificially moves the muscle, thereby preventing atrophy.

The absence of a limb reflex indicates either a failure of afferent input to reach the LMN or failure of the efferent output from the LMN to reach the muscle. Most often, decreased reflexes reflect damage to the PNS (nerves or roots) or muscles. In other cases it may reflect NMJ disease (see Box 9.2). Loss or reduction of the stretch reflex is the only clinical sign needed to localise a lesion involving LMNs. Damage to LMNs also results in other signs and symptoms (Table 9.4).

While damage to LMNs leads to flaccid paralysis, damage to UMNs results in spasticity and can be caused by damage to the spinal cord, brainstem, motor cortex, or the tracts connecting them. The spasticity is more

Table 9.4 Comparison of symptoms associated with upper motor neuron (UMN) and lower motor neuron (LMN) lesions

	UMN lesion	LMN lesion
Location	CNS	PNS or CNS
Common cause	Stroke, trauma, infectious disease, multiple sclerosis, amyotrophic lateral sclerosis	Trauma, stroke, tumour, diabetes, polio, alcoholism, amyotrophic lateral sclerosis
Classical description	Spastic paralysis/paresis	Flaccid paralysis
Structures involved	Motor cortex, internal capsule, pyramidal tract	Brainstem or spinal cord LMNs or their axons
Distribution	Groups of muscles, never individual muscles	Segmental, limited to muscles innervated by damaged motor neurons or their axons
Effect on voluntary movement	Paralysis or paresis, especially of skilled movements	Paralysis
Effect on muscle tone	**Increased (hypertonia)**	Decreased (hypotonia)
Effect on stretch reflex	**Hyperactive**	Hypoactive to point of absence
	Clonus	
Effect on cutaneous reflexes	Decreased	Decreased
Effect on muscle	No (or slight) atrophy	Pronounced atrophy
		Fasciculation and fibrillation
Muscle strength	Decreased	Decreased

Positive neurological signs are in bold type.
CNS, Central nervous system; PNS, peripheral nervous system.

marked when the lesion is in the brain, as opposed to the spinal cord.

UMN damage leads to either positive or negative neurological signs (see Table 9.4). Negative UMN signs are the loss or absence of function caused by the loss of monosynaptic connections to LMNs. A major negative sign of UMN damage is weakness in the limbs. Weakness in both limbs on one side is called hemiparesis (hemiplegia) and can indicate a brain lesion, most often in the internal capsule where the descending fibres are grouped closely together. Here, a relatively small lesion can have a widespread effect. Cerebral strokes affecting the middle or anterior cerebral arteries rarely cause hemiplegia because of the somatotopic organization of the motor homunculus (Fig. 9.11C). If the weakness occurs in both lower limbs, it is termed paraparesis and usually indicates a spinal cord lesion (often anterior spinal artery occlusion). This weakness has a characteristic pattern because in the upper limb the flexors are stronger than the extensors and in the lower limb the reverse is true. This means that the greatest weakness will be shown in the arm extensors and the leg flexors. Some muscle groups, such as the axial trunk muscles and brainstem motor nuclei, receive bilateral descending innervation and are therefore protected from complete loss of function by stroke.

In contrast, some lesions cause the appearance of signs not normally present or cause an increase in function; these are referred to as positive neurological signs and are most often due to disinhibition. Hyperreflexia and spasticity (hypertonia) are typical examples of positive neurological signs that usually accompany UMN lesions (see Table 9.4). Patients complain of stiffness, inability to relax and jerky movements. Loss of descending inhibition

results in the development, after initial flaccid paralysis, of spastic paralysis. The spinal reflexes remain intact but are no longer subject to control from the motor cortex. Owing to the muscle activity triggered by reflexes, the muscles do not atrophy, there is no fasciculation, and there is a general increase in tone, which is most easily seen in the stronger muscles. This leads to a clasp-knife effect; in response to passive movement of a joint against a background of increased extensor muscle tone, there is a sudden collapse in the resistance to movement due to the inhibition of extensor motor neurons by GTOs and free nerve endings in the muscles and tendons.

The Babinski (extensor plantar) response is a pathological polysynaptic reflex. It is evoked by noxious cutaneous stimulation of the sole of the foot and normally consists of a flexion withdrawal response. The stimulus causes the toes to curl down, adduct together and withdraw from the stimulus. This reflex tests the integrity of spinal cord segments L4–S2. In cases when the descending input from the cortex is disrupted, either through damage to motor areas of the cortex or through damage to CSTs, the plantar reflex changes to an extensor reflex with dorsiflexion of the big toe and fanning of the other toes, known as the Babinski sign. This abnormal response is normal in children under the age of 2 years, before they learn to walk, and reflects the immaturity of the CST connections with LMNs. This cardinal sign indicates reliably the loss of descending control from the CST and reflects UMN damage.

A common misconception is that all the signs and symptoms of a UMN lesion equate with damage to the pyramidal system and result in spasticity. Pure pyramidal tract lesions in humans are rare. Studies in primates have shown that selective CST lesions produce weakness, hypotonia, loss of fine distal hand movements, the Babinski sign and loss of the cremasteric and abdominal reflexes. The other signs of UMN damage—hypertonia, hyperreflexia and clonus—must reflect damage to the medial brainstem descending pathways. Spasticity probably occurs through the loss of inhibitory control in the VST and RST. Experimental evidence shows that lesioning the lateral vestibular nucleus reduces spasticity, as does sectioning the dorsal roots, implying that spasticity represents an increase in the gain of the stretch reflexes due to loss of descending inhibition. A similar explanation is proposed to explain clonus.

There are several degenerative diseases that affect motor neurons such as motor neuron disease, amyotrophic lateral sclerosis (ALS; Box 9.7), poliomyelitis (Box 9.8), spinal muscular atrophy, progressive muscular atrophy and progressive bulbar palsy.

ALS (also known as Lou Gehrig's disease in the USA) is the most common disease affecting motor systems. It is characterised by the progressive degeneration of LMNs and UMNs, particularly in the pyramidal tract, resulting in spastic paraparesis or tetraparesis with stiffness and weakness of the hands, muscle cramps and discomfort. As the disease progresses, the hand muscles atrophy, reflexes increase and the weakness spreads to the trunk and head muscles (except for the extraocular muscles). Onset is around the age of 50 years and the disease affects 1/100,000 of the population. It is fatal and most patients die within 6 years of onset (see Box 9.7).

ALS is the disease described in the case history in Box 9.1. David shows the classic positive signs of UMN damage: spasticity, hyperactive stretch reflexes and the Babinski sign. He shows the clasp-knife effect and clonus, which are further indications of damage to UMN pathways. Negative signs of muscle weakness—muscle atrophy and fasciculation—indicate damage to LMNs. As the UMN and LMNs continue to die, David's symptoms get worse. He is prescribed riluzole, which is currently the only drug approved for treating ALS. Riluzole has a complex pharmacology but one of its effects is to block glutamate activity. However, it prolongs the life of the patient only marginally. Another drug—gabapentin—is sometimes also given to slow the progression of muscle weakness.

Spinal muscular atrophies are hereditary diseases that are also associated with motor neuron death. There is a mutation in the survival motor neuron (SMN1) gene that results in spasticity and muscle weakness. The incidence is 8 cases per 100,000 live births, the mortality rate is high during infancy and no known treatment exists. Death is caused by severe and progressive restrictive lung function.

The cerebellum

The ultimate executors of movements are the LMNs and they are under the command of the UMNs. However, it

---

Genetics of amyotrophic lateral sclerosis

Most patients with amyotrophic lateral sclerosis (ALS) have the sporadic form of the disease and have no apparent family history of the disorder. Between 5% and 10% have familial ALS. This is associated with genetic mutations. The most well known gene encodes the superoxide dismutase type 1 enzyme (SOD1) and is located on chromosome 21. This enzyme acts as a free radical ion scavenger and there are more than 90 mutations in SOD1 associated with familial ALS. Recent evidence indicates that mutant SOD1 promotes apoptosis by binding to the anti-apoptotic protein bcl-2, and by sequestering the heat shock proteins HSP27 and HSP70, which have neuroprotective roles in motor neurons. Mutant SOD1 is recruited into mitochondria and this leads to their death. However, mutations in SOD1 account for only 15%–20% of familial cases. SOD mutations are not seen in ALS sufferers with the sporadic form. More recently, two loci on chromosomes 16q and 18q have also been identified in familial ALS patients. Other genes now known to be involved in ALS include C9orf72, found on chromosome 9, which causes defects in presynaptic terminals by the production of hexa-nucleotide repeats that results in abnormal protein aggregation. This gene is also associated with frontotemporal dementia (FTD). At least 65 different mutations in TARDBP (Tar DNA binding protein) which affects the production and (mis)folding of a key nuclear protein TDP-43 protein are known to cause ALS. This can also result in FTD. Likewise, there are 85 known mutations in the FUS gene (FUS RNA-binding protein) which affect mRNA processing resulting in abnormal protein aggregation in motor neurons but this is not associated with FTD.

Several pathogenic pathways may be involved in the death of neurons seen in ALS: (1) autoimmunity to some forms of Ca^{2+} channel (e.g. L-type); (2) increased oxidative stress; (3) excitotoxicity due to the loss of glutamate transporters, and overstimulation of glutamate receptors due to reduced reuptake; and (4) excessive neurofilament accumulation within the motor neuron. Abnormal editing of the glutamate AMPA receptor GluR2 has been found in ALS patients, whereby a change in the second transmembrane domain drastically alters the Ca^{2+} permeability of the receptor, from impermeable to permeable.

---

is not sufficient to simply command the muscles to contract in order to produce smooth, coordinated movements. This requires additional control mechanisms to order the correct sequence of muscle contractions. This important task is performed by the cerebellum. In order to accomplish this task, the cerebellum receives sensory information about balance, posture and limb position from the ascending tracts (Table 9.5) and compares it with information from the PM and SMA. In effect, it acts as a comparator of movement and if there is a mismatch between what the muscles should be doing and what the signals from the muscles show them actually doing, it sends signals (via the motor thalamus) to the primary motor cortex to correct the movement so that it is performed in a smooth, coordinated fashion. Different parts of the cerebellum coordinate movement in different parts of the body. Movements are not initiated in the cerebel-lum. It can be thought of as a subordinate to the motor systems of the motor cortex and basal ganglia.

Circuitry of the cerebellar cortex

The general gross anatomy of the cerebellum is described in Chapter 1. The cerebellar cortex consists of numerous small gyri and a core of white matter, within which are embedded the deep cerebellar nuclei. As the cerebellar cortex has a regular structure, neural processing is thought to be the same in all parts. The cortex has three layers and contains five cell types that form a simple circuit that is repeated many times. The outer layer is the molecular layer and is almost cell-free. It consists mainly of the axons and dendrites of various cerebellar neurons. The middle layer is a single layer of large neurons called Purkinje cells, which are the main output cells of the cerebellar cortex. Below this layer is the granular layer, which is densely populated with small neurons called granule cells. Its organization is shown in Fig. 9.13 and consists of two motor loop circuits, one excitatory and inhibitory, that sculpt movements.

Two sets of afferent fibres provide excitatory input to the cerebellar cortex: mossy fibres and climbing fibres (see Table 9.5). Mossy fibres form the main input to the cerebellum, targeting the deep cerebellar nuclei to stimulate the deep excitatory loop. They are the axons of second-order neurons from the spinal cord, brainstem and cerebral cortex that convey proprioceptive information. These inputs are topographically organised, producing somatotopic maps in the cerebellar cortex that are retained in the deep cerebellar nuclei. A whole-body representation is found in the anterior lobe and two half-body representations, one from each side, are found in the posterior lobe. The head regions of these maps overlap and receive visual and auditory information as well. The presence of these maps has been confirmed by PET scans.

Collateral branches from mossy fibres form an inhibitory cortical loop that inhibits the afferent input by making excitatory connections with the dendrites of granule cells in synaptic complexes called glomeruli. Each mossy fibre innervates approximately 600 granule cells and each granule cell receives input from up to four mossy

---

Box 9.8 Polio and post-polio syndrome

Infection with the poliomyelitis (polio) virus results in several different bodily responses. The most common form (90%) is asymptomatic or evokes only minor malaise. There are two other forms, non-paralytic and paralytic polio, which produce transient (2–10 days with complete recovery) or permanent muscle weakness and paralysis, respectively. In the latter, patients suffer flaccid paralysis of muscles and painful spasms in non-paralysed muscles. The amount of paralysis is inversely proportional to the motor neuron loss. The virus enters through the mouth and travels in the bloodstream to various central nervous system targets such as the cerebellum, vestibular system, motor cortex and reticular formation. It can travel along peripheral nerves to infect lower motor neurons. Polio occurs most often in children. The affected muscles become atrophied and the limb is flaccid and small.

In approximately one-third of patients who have previously had polio a late-onset post-polio syndrome occurs 30–40 years after the initial illness. This post-polio syndrome is characterised by muscle weakness, muscle pain and increasing muscle fatigue. The disease is not caused by reactivation of the polio virus (as occurs in shingles) or by re-infection but appears to be due to deterioration of the remaining motor units due to their overuse.

Nowadays, in the western hemisphere, polio has been eradicated by a WHO vaccination programme. Children receive three oral polio vaccinations of a live attenuated version of the virus to enable them to develop antibodies to the virus. The first is administered at 2 months (with the DPT vaccination), and there are further vaccinations at 4, 6 and 18 months of age. Paralytic polio is still endemic throughout the Indian subcontinent and in Africa and Asia.

Table 9.5 Input pathways to the cerebellum

Pathway	Origin	Peduncle	Fibre type	Function
Spinocerebellar	Clarke's nucleus	ICP	Mossy	Proprioceptive and cutaneous sensation from trunk and legs
Cuneocerebellar	Accessory cuneate nucleus	ICP	Mossy	Proprioceptive and cutaneous sensation from arms and neck
Trigeminocerebellar	Trigeminal nuclei	ICP	Mossy	Proprioceptive and cutaneous sensation from face and jaw
Olivocerebellar	Inferior olivary nucleus	ICP	Climbing	Motor skills learning
Vestibulocerebellar	Vestibular nuclei	ICP	Mossy	Balance
Pontocerebellar	Pontine nuclei	MCP	Mossy	Cognitive, visual and motor input from cortex

ICP, Inferior cerebellar peduncle; MCP, middle cerebellar peduncle.

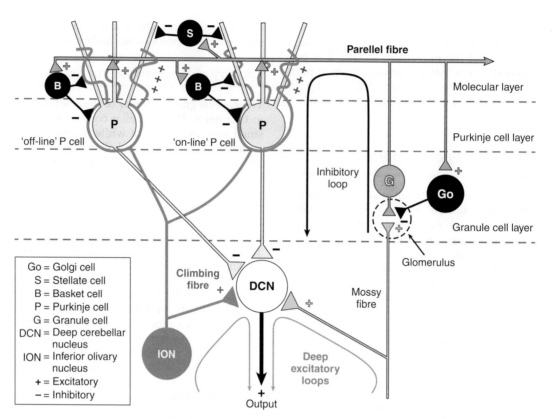

Fig. 9.13 Microcircuitry of the cerebellar cortex.

fibres. The axons of the granule cells, the only excitatory cells in the cerebellar cortex, ascend into the molecular layer, bifurcate to form a T-shape and run parallel to the surface. For this reason they are called parallel fibres; each fibre synapses only once with 2000–3000 Purkinje cell dendrites and each Purkinje cell receives input from approximately 20,000 parallel fibres. Thus the input from granule cells to Purkinje cells is very weak. Mossy fibres have high background firing rates that are altered by sensory inputs. Stimulation of mossy fibres evokes repetitive firing of single action potentials in Purkinje cells, termed simple spikes. The net effect is to cause the Purkinje cells to increase their firing rate, enabling them to signal across a wide range of mossy fibre inputs.

Climbing fibres are less branched than mossy fibres and synapse directly on each Purkinje cell body, winding around it and the proximal dendrites, like ivy climbing a trellis, to make many (~300) synapses. They also make direct synapses with deep cerebellar nuclei to stimulate the deep excitatory loop. All climbing fibres arise from the contralateral ION. Climbing fibres also activate the cortical inhibitory loop by the stimulation of Purkinje cells. Because of their robust synaptic connection, climbing fibres evoke a burst of depolarisation, called a complex spike, which causes the Purkinje cell to become inactivated after stimulation (postsynaptic depression). This process is involved in motor learning behaviour (see later).

The Purkinje cells are the output cells of the cerebellar cortex. They are inhibitory GABAergic neurons whose axons project to the deep nuclei, which give rise to the cerebellar output to other brain regions. Each Purkinje cell has an intricate, extensive dendritic tree. Purkinje cells are tonically active at rest but change their firing frequency as movements occur and this modulates the output of the deep cerebellar nuclei.

There are three types of inhibitory interneuron: stellate, basket and Golgi cells. Axons of stellate cells target the Purkinje cell body and so exert a powerful inhibitory effect, whereas basket cells target the Purkinje cell dendrites (see Fig. 9.13). When stimulated by granule cells, the stellate and basket cells function by focusing the excitatory input from mossy fibres onto strongly excited 'on-line' Purkinje cells through lateral inhibition of the weak responses (from other parallel fibres) to adjacent 'off-line' Purkinje cells. This lateral (surround) inhibition produces spatial focusing of cerebellar cortical output. The activation of the on-line Purkinje cells results in the selective inhibition of neurons within the corresponding deep cerebellar nucleus. Golgi cells participate in glomeruli synapses to inhibit granule cells, thereby regulating the gain of granule cell input to the Purkinje cells. The net effect of this modulation is to regulate the temporal firing of mossy fibres to produce only a brief firing of Purkinje cells. Together, these inhibitory neurons restrict Purkinje cell output in time and space, allowing them to fire only transiently.

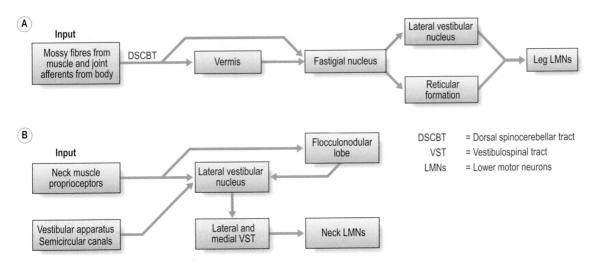

Fig. 9.14 Circuitry of the vestibulocerebellum involved in (A) posture control and (B) head balance.

Deep cerebellar nuclei

The deep nuclei of the cerebellum receive inhibitory input from Purkinje cell axons. They also receive excitatory collateral input from mossy and climbing fibres. The net output is excitatory and goes to different regions of the brainstem: the reticular formation, red nucleus, spinal cord and motor thalamus.

The most prominent of the deep nuclei is the dentate nucleus. It lies most laterally in the white matter core and is functionally associated with the posterior lobe. Most medial are the fastigial nuclei; they are functionally associated with the flocculonodular lobe. Between the fastigial and dentate nuclei are the interposed nuclei, comprising the more medial globose and more lateral emboliform nuclei; they are functionally associated with the anterior lobe.

Functional organization of the cerebellum

In the sagittal plane the cerebellum forms three functional areas—the vestibulocerebellum, spinocerebellum and cerebrocerebellum—based on their afferent input. Each division is associated with a pair of deep cerebellar nuclei. The paired flocculus and midline nodulus form the flocculonodular lobe or vestibulocerebellum. They receive input from vestibular nuclei and muscle spindles, GTOs and joint afferents in neck muscles (via the cuneocerebellar tract). The vestibulocerebellum functions to maintain the stability of the head on the body. It acts on the neck muscles via the lateral VST to maintain a steady head position despite movements of the body, thereby maintaining visual fixation on distant objects, such as when a person is running or in a moving vehicle.

The midline cerebellar cortex is called the vermis. This region coordinates the balance and posture of the body as a whole. Its posterior part is also associated with eye movements, in response to vestibular input, via the vestibulo-ocular reflex. Damage to the flocculonodular lobe results in nystagmus.

The vestibulocerebellum receives ipsilateral input from the postural muscles of the legs via the dorsal spinocerebellar tract (SCBT) of the spinal cord. These axons synapse in the fastigial nucleus and the vermis. The fastigial nucleus receives the output of vermis Purkinje cell fibres and sends axons to the reticular formation and Dieter's nucleus. Thus the output to the postural muscles is via the spinal projection of the VST (bilaterally) and RST (Fig. 9.14, Table 9.2) to control muscle tone. Head balance and body balance are interrelated and there are many cross-connections between the flocculonodular lobe and the vermis.

The spinocerebellum coordinates locomotor and other voluntary movements of the arms and legs. Anatomically, it corresponds to the anterior lobe, and the vermis and the area immediately lateral to it, to the paramedian region of the posterior lobe. The latter region is not anatomically differentiated from the vermis but is functionally different because it is interconnected with the interposed deep cerebellar nuclei.

The paramedian region coordinates locomotor and other voluntary movements of the distal limbs. It is the only part of the cerebellum that receives direct input from the spinal cord via the dorsal and ventral SCBTs. It monitors the muscle spindles, tendon and joint afferents, and the state of spinal reflexes. Output from the interposed nuclei is to the contralateral red nucleus, which gives rise to the contralateral rubrospinal tract, thereby functionally activating mainly ipsilateral flexor motor neurons (Fig. 9.15).

The largest part of the cerebellum is the cerebrocerebellum, which corresponds to the lateral parts of the posterior lobe. These regions control motor skills associated with speech, hand–eye coordination, independent limb movements and cognitive eye movements. Cognitive eye movements are those in which the eyes move actively to scan an object of interest. For example, while you are

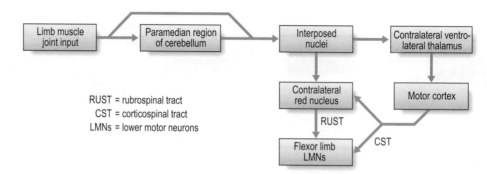

Fig. 9.15 Circuitry of the spinocerebellum involved in the voluntary control of limb movement.

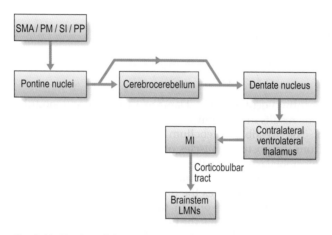

Fig. 9.16 Circuitry of the cerebrocerebellum involved in speech and cognitive movements. *LMNs*, Lower motor neurons; *MI*, primary motor cortex; *PM*, premotor cortex; *PP*, posterior parietal cortex; *SI*, primary somatosensory cortex; *SMA*, supplementary motor cortex.

reading this, your eyes are jumping from one fixation point on the line to another, under the control of the cerebral cortex. The cerebellar hemispheres are connected to the dentate nucleus, whose efferent axons project to the contralateral ventro-lateral thalamus and from there to the motor cortex (Fig. 9.16). There are also reciprocal connections with the red nucleus. The hemispheres receive input from the premotor, supplementary, primary motor somatosensory, posterior parietal and visual cortices via the pontocerebellar tracts from the pontine nuclei.

Cerebellar function in the control of movement

The cerebellum coordinates complicated multi-joint movements and is involved in learning new motor tasks (Fig. 9.17). In terms of circuitry, the cerebellum operates in both feedback and feedforward modes. The feedback mode is a corrective error mode, in that the cerebellum compares the motor intention with the actual motor performance. Any mismatch between the two signals generates a signal to make the error smaller. A motor error occurs when the position of a limb is not the intended one, causing an unpredicted muscle stretch that activates the muscle afferents. This unexpected proprioceptive activity is relayed to the cerebellum by the spinocerebellar mossy fibres activated by the movement error, to excite Purkinje cells, which then inhibit the deep cerebellar nuclei that drive the red nucleus and ventrolateral thalamus. This feeds back to the motor cortex to prevent the erroneous movement.

For the execution of well-rehearsed, ballistic (rapid) movements, such as a tennis serve, there is not enough time for feedback correction of errors. In this situation the cerebellum operates in a feedforward mode, running a programme that predicts the consequences of the motor action. Any unexpected disruptions that occur when the cerebellum is in feedforward mode cannot be corrected for and so impair the motor performance (resulting in a foul serve in this case).

The predictions inherent in feedforward operation must be learnt during attempts to perform the task. This is motor learning and involves the climbing fibres of the ION. For example, consider learning to juggle with three balls. The idea is to throw the balls in the air and catch one while the other two are in the air. This requires good hand–eye coordination. During the early attempts, many balls will be dropped. As you get better, fewer balls are dropped and eventually you learn to juggle. During the learning phase the climbing fibres are very active and send motor error signals via the olivocerebellar tract to the cerebellum. Climbing fibres, unlike mossy fibres, strongly excite Purkinje cells, overriding the mossy fibre input by modifying the AMPA glutamate receptors, which mediate fast synaptic transmission at the level of the parallel fibre–Purkinje cell synapse. The net effect is to weaken the inhibitory loop. Gradually, as the new task is learnt, the error rate is reduced, the activity of climbing fibres is reduced and performance is enhanced. This mechanism is probably used for all acquired voluntary movements, such as learning to walk, skip or ride a bicycle. Damage to the ION in humans results in deficits in both short-term adaptation (error correction) and long-term motor learning tasks.

Cerebellar diseases

Cerebellar syndromes have a variety of causes (Table 9.6) and some are genetic. Seven genes have been linked to spinocerebellar ataxias. In mutant mice these gene deletions

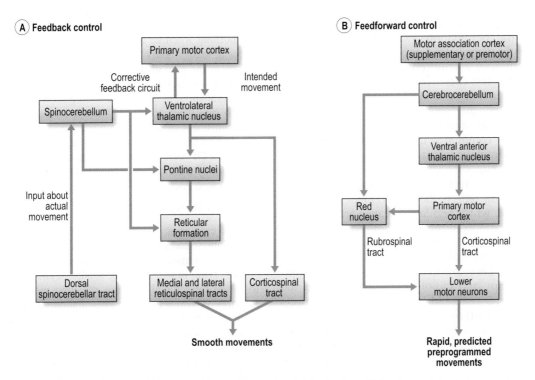

Fig. 9.17 Cerebellar control of movement. The cerebellum can operate using (A) feedback or (B) feedforward circuits to correct errors or predict movement respectively.

Table 9.6	Causes of cerebellar diseases

Genetic (e.g. Friedreich's ataxia [autosomal recessive], spinocerebellar ataxia [autosomal dominant])

Stroke

Primary (e.g. medulloblastoma) or secondary tumours

Trauma

Degeneration

Toxicity and metabolic disturbances (e.g. alcoholism, anticonvulsant drugs, hypothyroidism, vitamin E deficiency)

Miscellaneous (e.g. hydrocephalus, multiple sclerosis)

Developmental (e.g. cerebral palsy, Dandy-Walker malformation)

lead to loss or disturbed migration of granule and Purkinje cells in the cerebellum. Lesions of the cerebellum must be quite large before obvious symptoms appear, as there is much functional redundancy within the cerebellum due to the multiple somatotopic maps present.

Damage to the cerebellum does not produce paralysis or muscle weakness, or affect the ability to start or stop movements, but does affect the precision and coordination of movements. This is termed ataxia. Focal lesions of the cerebellum produce deficits on the same side of the body as the lesion. The signs of cerebellar damage are as follows:

• asynergia: loss or decomposition of coordinated movement

• dysarthria and dysphonia: speech deficits such as slurring due to errors in the timing of impulses to the muscles controlling speech; articulation problems: words become broken down into individual syllables and flow becomes 'explosive' or 'scanning'

• intention tremor: swaying to and fro of the limb perpendicular to the direction of movement; this is present only during reaching movements and not at rest

• nystagmus: involuntary oscillating eye movements in horizontal, vertical or circular directions

• dysmetria: alteration in the rate and force of movement, for example, over- or under-reaching for an object

• dysdiadochokinesis: the inability to perform rapid alternating movements such as pronation and supination of the hand

• hypotonia: loss of muscle tone due to decreased activity in γ-motor neurons

Other signs may include titubation, a rhythmic tremor of the head in an up-and-down ('yes-yes') or side-to-side ('no-no') motion. Pendular (slow) reflexes may also occur, but they are of little use as localizing signs.

The cerebellum is particularly susceptible to the effects of alcohol. Drunkenness is associated with many of the symptoms of mild cerebellar damage! For example, slurred or incoherent speech, incoordination, ataxic gait, clumsiness and double vision are all signs of cerebellar damage. These disorders reflect the role of the cerebellum in the coordination of skilled movements.

Lesions of the vermis lead to truncal ataxia. This is most commonly seen in children and is due to a tumour called a medulloblastoma, which grows from the granule cell layer to invade (and block) the fourth ventricle. Morning headache, dizziness, vomiting (due to raised intracranial pressure affecting cranial nerve function) and lethargy are common symptoms, and on physical examination, a dramatic feature is the inability to stand upright without support. Attempts to walk result in a wide-based gait with reeling and swaying from side to side. Truncal ataxia reflects the involvement of the flocculonodular lobe, which regulates balance and the coordination of the para-axial muscles. Symptoms are often absent when the child is lying down. These tumours are highly malignant and can spread to other parts of the nervous system. They are treated surgically, and adjuvant chemotherapy and radiotherapy (except when the child is less than 5 years old because of adverse effects on brain development) are used to prevent reoccurrence. Survival rates are 60%–85% at 5 years after diagnosis, depending on how aggressive the post-radiation chemotherapy is. Prognosis is poorer for surgery only, as the tumour re-emerges.

Lesions of the anterior lobe result in gait ataxia. This is commonly seen in chronic alcoholics, where alcohol abuse causes neuronal degeneration of granule and Purkinje cells, resulting in cortical atrophy of the anterior lobe. This affects the coordination of the lower limbs, resulting in a staggering, drunken gait, even when the person is sober. As the degeneration progresses, loss of control in trunk and arms and eventually speech may ensue. The person also suffers from dysdiadochokinesis and the heel-to-shin test is almost impossible to perform, as the patient will have sensory ataxia (positive Romberg sign) due to peripheral neuropathy.

Damage to the posterior lobe commonly results from stroke, tumours, degenerative disease or traumas that affect a cerebellar hemisphere, peduncle, midbrain or pons. Symptoms manifest as incoordination of voluntary movement and loss of muscle tone. The patient presents with tremor of the limbs, dysmetria and dysdiadochokinesia, resulting in clumsiness of movements. There are often speech impediments with regard to phonation and articulation.

Self-assessment case study

Bryan, a 7-year-old boy, is brought to the GP by his mother who is worried by his recent behaviour. For the last month he has been suffering on and off from headaches, particularly in the morning when he awakens. He has been resting a lot and sleeps at least 9 hours a day. He also appears lethargic. In the past week the pain of the headaches has been so severe he has been sick several times and has been complaining of dizziness. On examination, motor system testing shows him to sway from side to side when standing. There is nystagmus and diplopia and clumsiness of movement when asked to grab things. The doctor suspects a brain tumour and sends him to the local hospital for a CT scan. The results confirm the suspicion. Bryan is immediately admitted to hospital and scheduled for brain surgery the next day.

1. Explain the signs and symptoms

This case is an example of childhood medulloblastoma. Medulloblastoma presents with the usual symptoms of a posterior fossa tumour. The symptoms are often absent when the child is lying down. Morning headache and vomiting are due to raised intracranial pressure affecting meningeal afferents. Lethargy is also a common presentation. On physical examination, cerebellar signs dominate, e.g. truncal ataxia (reeling/swaying, wide-based gait) and other signs of cerebellar dysfunction, e.g. loss of balance and clumsiness are common as the tumour enlarges. Raised intracranial pressure may cause hydrocephalus resulting in papilloedema and visual difficulties. Dizziness occurs as the flocculonodular lobe that is connected to the vestibular apparatus and is involved in balance is affected, and nystagmus also indicates that the flocculonodular lobe is affected.

2. Explain the pathophysiology of the brain tumour

Medulloblastomas are highly malignant and tend to seed along the neuraxis following the CSF pathways. They arise from the granular layer of cerebellar cortex and invade the 4th ventricle. They can block CSF flow, yielding hydrocephalus.

3. What treatment options are available and what is the prognosis?

These tumours are treated surgically and, in most cases, complete macroscopic removal is possible. Occasionally the tumour is attached to the floor of the 4th ventricle, in which case a sheet of tumour cells have to be left behind. In these cases the tumour often returns. Adjuvant therapy is then essential. Chemotherapy and radiotherapy are used, as medulloblastomas are radiosensitive. Radiation of the entire neuraxis is performed, as these are extremely malignant tumours that can spread to secondary sites such as the spinal axis.

Current treatments result in a 60%–85% survival rate 5 years after diagnosis depending on how aggressive the post-radiation chemotherapy is. Prognosis is poorer for surgery only treatments as tumours often reappear elsewhere.

MOTOR SYSTEMS II:
THE BASAL GANGLIA

Chapter summary

1. The basal ganglia are a group of subcortical structures that include the striatum (caudate and putamen), globus pallidus (internal and external), substantia nigra (SN) and subthalamic nucleus. These structures have a role in the initiation and maintenance of movement. The striatum receives major cortical glutamatergic input, and its activity is modulated by dopaminergic input from the SN. The output from the basal ganglia is directed towards the thalamus, which sends projections to the cortex, thus closing the corticobasal ganglia-thalamocortical loop.

2. Several pathways connect the cortex and the basal ganglia nuclei: the direct, indirect and hyperdirect pathways. Neurodegenerative processes in the basal ganglia lead to imbalance in the activity of these pathways and emergence of hypokinetic disorders, such as Parkinson's disease, or hyperkinetic disorders, such as Huntington's disease.

3. Parkinson's disease is characterized by rigidity, tremor and bradykinesia, and a range of non-motor symptoms including depression, cognitive dysfunction and autonomic nervous system dysfunction. There is a marked loss of dopaminergic cells in the SN and presence of widespread aggregates of the protein α-synuclein in Lewy bodies and Lewy neurites. As the disease evolves, the neurodegeneration progresses from the subcortical to the cortical level and affects multiple cell types and neurotransmitter systems. Pharmacological management is based on the principle of dopamine replacement therapy using the precursor L-DOPA and dopaminergic agonists. Treatment is symptomatic and associated with long-term complications.

4. Huntington's disease is an inherited autosomal dominant disease associated with a mutation in the gene encoding the protein huntingtin. The neurotoxic consequences of this mutation lead to loss of cells in the cortex and striatum and loss of striatal efferents. The disease is characterised by involuntary choreic movements and cognitive and psychiatric symptoms. Treatment is symptomatic and based on the principle of reducing dopaminergic signalling.

5. Neuromodulatory techniques, such as deep brain stimulation, can be used to address the complications of treatment in Parkinson's disease. Stimulation of the subthalamic nucleus leads to alleviation of dyskinesias induced by dopaminergic stimulation and allows a marked reduction in drug dosage.

6. Non-pharmacological treatments currently being explored for neurodegenerative diseases of the basal ganglia include the use of graft cells that could replace the degenerating circuits, and blockade of the effect of mutated genes, for example, using antisense-based therapies.

Introduction

The smooth execution of movements involving the trunk and the limbs, and the maintenance of posture, balance and normal gait, would not be possible without the coordinated activity of supraspinal centres, in particular, the upper motor neurons (UMNs) of the corticospinal pathway, the lower motor neurons (LMNs) of the spinal cord ventral horn and an intact neuromuscular junction and muscle. Disturbances in the function of the major descending motor pathways are associated with paresis, paralysis or spasticity. In parallel, several other structures provide the irreplaceable central input required for normal motor activity and are involved in its continuous control and coordination. The basal ganglia and cerebellum are the main structures fulfilling these roles. They are at the interface between the intention and execution of movement. Neuronal activity in these structures is correlated temporally with motor activity in a complex manner. This chapter is dedicated to the basal ganglia and illustrates how their dysfunction leads to specific alterations in motor performance, which can be severely debilitating (Box 10.1). Disorders of the basal ganglia can lead to either hyperkinetic or hypokinetic manifestations.

Basal ganglia: structure and organization

General organization

The basal ganglia consist of several subcortical interconnected nuclei that are involved in the initiation and execution of movement. They comprise the caudate nucleus, putamen and globus pallidus (in the telencephalon), subthalamic nucleus (in the diencephalon) and substantia nigra (SN; in the mesencephalon). The relative locations of these structures are described in Chapter 1.

The caudate nucleus and the putamen are two nuclei that are interconnected and form the striatum. The globus pallidus has an internal (or medial) and an external (or lateral) division (termed GPi and GPe, respectively). The striatum receives afferents from the neocortex, thalamus and SN. The globus pallidus receives projections from the striatum and subthalamic nucleus. The major output of the basal ganglia, which represents mainly projections from the GPi and SN, is directed to thalamic nuclei (in particular, the ventral anterior, ventral lateral and centromedian nuclei), which project to motor and prefrontal cortical areas. A smaller contingent of efferent fibres project to the pedunculopontine nucleus in the brainstem tegmentum and to the superior colliculus. The SN can be subdivided into substantia nigra pars compacta (SNpc) and substantia nigra pars reticulata (SNpr). The pars compacta contains neurons that project to the striatum, whereas the pars reticulata receives striatal input and provides the nigral output.

Circuits and neurotransmitters

The basal ganglia form a network of parallel loops and circuits that integrate the neuronal activity in various cerebral regions (motor, oculomotor, limbic and associative), the basal ganglia nuclei and the thalamic nuclei. Lesion or degeneration in the basal ganglia leads to diseases that present with a range of characteristic motor

Case history

Gavin Porter, a 57-year-old recently retired businessman, came to the doctor with his wife because of 'trembling' that affected his hands, in particular the right hand. Over the last year, the trembling had become worse, and he sometimes felt that his legs trembled very slightly too. He had also become rather slow in his movements, and sometimes sat for hours in an armchair with a rather expressionless face. His wife found this irritating; she thought that his general mood had changed and he had become more withdrawn. He was finding it increasingly difficult to button and unbutton his shirt and tie his shoelaces. He had recently suffered two falls, one of which had resulted in a serious skin laceration on his head. When asked, he could not pinpoint a specific cause for these falls. He was otherwise in good health. He had taken early retirement in order to enjoy other activities, such as gardening and voluntary work. Gavin seemed to be deeply worried about his progressive physical incapacity. In his moments of anxiety about the future, the trembling was much worse.

This case gives rise to the following questions:

1. What is the cause of the symptoms (i.e. tremor, rigidity, slow movements, altered gait and balance)?
2. Would confirmation of the diagnosis require additional tests?
3. Are there any risk factors for developing this disease?

symptoms. Fig. 10.1 summarizes the functional organization of the basal ganglia and shows the major neurotransmitters present in afferent and efferent pathways.

The striatum is a heterogeneous structure consisting of two main compartments: the matrix and the striosomes. These compartments can be identified by the differential distribution of various neurochemical markers such as the various subtypes of opioid receptors (mu [μ], delta [δ] and kappa [κ]) or the enzyme acetylcholinesterase. The majority of neurons in the matrix and striosomes are medium-sized projection neurons, which have highly collateralized axons and dendrites endowed with dense spines. These cells are the medium spiny neurons.

The cortex provides glutamatergic excitatory input to all striatal projection neurons. The cortical projections are organized somatotopically, innervating both the matrix and the striosomes. The cortex is connected with the globus pallidus and the SN through several distinct pathways: direct, indirect and hyperdirect (see Fig. 10.1A).

1. The projection of the striatal medium spiny neurons to the GPi and SNpr is known as the *direct pathway*. The main neurotransmitter in this projection is γ-aminobutyric acid (GABA), which is colocalized with peptides such as substance P and dynorphins. GPi and SNpr neurons project to the thalamus and are also GABAergic. Thalamic neurons, which contain glutamate, project to the cortex, thus closing the loop.

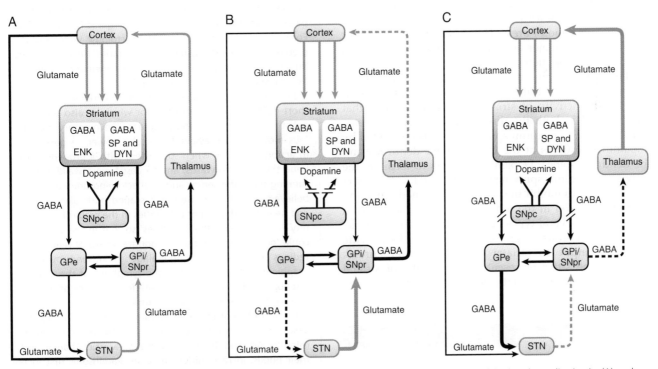

Fig. 10.1 Functional organization of the basal ganglia. The diagrams illustrate the functional organization of the basal ganglia circuits (A) under normal conditions, (B) in Parkinson's disease and (C) in Huntington's disease. Thin and broken lines indicate pathways that are hypoactive, and thick lines indicate pathways that are hyperactive. *DYN,* Dynorphin; *ENK,* enkephalin; *GABA,* γ-aminobutyric acid; *GPe,* external globus pallidus; *GPi,* internal globus pallidus; *SNr,* substantia nigra reticulata; *SNpc,* substantia nigra pars compacta; *SNpr,* substantia nigra pars reticulata; *SP,* substance P; *STN,* subthalamic nucleus.

2. In the *indirect pathway*, striatal GABAergic medium spiny neurons (which also contain enkephalins) project to the GPe. These pallidal neurons are GABAergic and project to the subthalamic nucleus (STN). The STN has glutamatergic neurons that project to the GPi and SNpr. The circuit is ultimately completed through the GABAergic nigrothalamic projection and the glutamatergic thalamocortical projections, as in the case of the direct pathway. Another link between the direct and indirect pathways is provided by neurons of the GPe, which establish contact with the GPi and SNpr through axon collaterals.

3. The third projection, the *hyperdirect pathway*, is monosynaptic and glutamatergic. It links the frontal cortex to the STN bypassing the striatum, thereby facilitating faster stopping behaviours. In a similar way to the indirect pathway, it has a net inhibitory action on the thalamus and cortex.

Through these three pathways the cortex modulates, for example, increases (direct pathway) or decreases (indirect and hyperdirect pathway) the excitatory thalamocortical projections. The presence of GABA as a main transmitter in the striatal efferents indicates that the striatal projection neurons will have an inhibitory effect on target cells in the SN and globus pallidus. In contrast, the STN is a source of excitation through glutamatergic transmission. Thus through parallel loops and the balance between excitation and inhibition, the basal ganglia are involved in the transfer of information from the neocortex to the motor areas, in particular the premotor and supplementary motor areas. This results in facilitation or inhibition of the major descending motor pathways (e.g. corticospinal projection).

The SNpc contains neurons that produce dopamine and project to the striatum, exerting a modulatory influence on the activity of striatal projection neurons that are involved in both the direct and indirect pathways. Cortical input to medium spiny neurons is controlled by dopaminergic fibres at the level of their dendrites and the dendritic spines. Dopamine appears to facilitate the activity of medium spiny neurons involved in the direct pathway and to inhibit the activity of the medium spiny neurons involved in the indirect pathway. The striatum also contains several types of interneurons, for example, cholinergic neurons. Nigral dopaminergic cells provide inhibitory input to striatal cholinergic interneurons. Although the latter represent less than 10% of striatal cells, they exert important integrative functions in the striatum.

Parkinson's disease

Symptoms

Parkinson's disease (PD) was first described in 1817 by James Parkinson, a doctor with encyclopaedic interests, who was practising in the East End of London (Box 10.2). He based his monograph, 'An Essay on the Shaking Palsy', on the analysis of six cases. The cardinal features of this disease are motor: tremor (unilateral or bilateral), bradykinesia and rigidity. They may occur in isolation or in any combination (Box 10.3).

Tremor

The most prominent symptom is resting tremor of the extremities and usually accompanies the disease. The tremor has a characteristic frequency of 4–6 Hz and may begin in only one extremity and spread to others. The distal joints of the limbs are preferentially affected. In the hand, the tremor is characteristic and involves the thumb and fingers rolling together. This is called a 'pill-rolling' tremor. The tremor occurs at rest and disappears during intentional movement and sleep. However, in the late stages of the disease, an 'active' tremor may emerge with a frequency of 6–8 Hz. Tremor is exacerbated by anxiety; it primarily affects the hands but can also affect the lower limbs, jaw and lips.

Box 10.2 James Parkinson (1755–1824): a physician and a radical thinker

James Parkinson was a general practitioner, whose medical writings attest to his busy medical career. However, his intellectual interests were much wider. He was a respected palaeontologist, and his two books 'Organic Remains of a Former World' and 'Outlines of Oryctology' were considered reference works by his contemporaries. He also had an interest in politics and social issues, as a member of several 'reform societies' and 'revolutionary clubs'.

In 'An Essay on the Shaking Palsy', Parkinson gives a short definition of the disease, for which he also provides a Latin synonym, 'paralysis agitans': 'Involuntary tremulous motion, with lessened muscular power, in parts not in action and even when supported; with a propensity to bend the trunk forwards, and to pass from a walking to a running pace: the senses and intellect being uninjured.' He believed that the disease had 'escaped particular notice', and he hoped that other colleagues in the medical community would 'extend their searches' so that in the end they could 'point out the most appropriate means of relieving a tedious and most distressing malady'. Parkinson provided a graphic depiction of most of the symptoms of the disease but apparently failed to appreciate features such as the significant muscular rigidity and bradykinesia.

In the 19th century, other important contributions to the description of this disease were made by the French neurologists Armand Trousseau and Jean-Martin Charcot and their pupils. In recognition of James Parkinson's first incisive insight into this pathology, it is the eminent neurologist Jean-Martin Charcot who gave the disease the name of 'Parkinson's disease'.

Case history (continued)

Gavin had a full neurological examination. He was alert and oriented for time and place. Memory and general knowledge were appropriate for his age, but his speech was slow and quiet, rather monotonous and almost devoid of natural voice inflexions. His face was impassive, and he rarely blinked. A mild resting tremor was present in the orofacial musculature, which diminished on speaking or swallowing.

His strength was intact and deep tendon reflexes were normal. There was cogwheel rigidity upon passive movement of the limbs. The 'pill-rolling' 4–6 Hz tremor of the right thumb and index fingers was abolished by volitional movement. Gavin's gait was rather slow. If given an abrupt push, he could not quickly restore his posture, and was at risk of falling. Cutaneous sensation and proprioception were intact.

Gavin was diagnosed with Parkinson's disease and was prescribed L-dihydroxyphenylalanine (L-DOPA) with carbidopa. The doctor discussed the prognosis with Gavin and his wife.

This case gives rise to the following questions:

1. Why was Gavin given L-DOPA with carbidopa and are there any therapeutic alternatives?
2. What is the long-term prognosis for this patient?

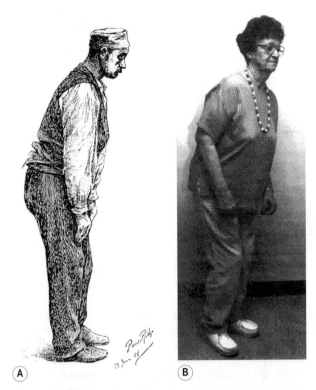

Fig. 10.2 (A) Rigid posture of a patient with Parkinson's disease. (B) Characteristic flexed posture of a patient with Parkinson's disease. (A, Drawn by Paul Richer, a former intern of Jean-Martin Charcot's. From Richer (1888). In Koller, WC, ed. Handbook of Parkinson's Disease. New York: Marcel Dekker Inc., 1987. B, From Hauser RA, Zesiewicz TA. (1996) Parkinson's Disease—Questions and Answers. Merit Publishing International, Basingstoke.)

Bradykinesia/akinesia

Bradykinesia is a slowing of normal movement. In the advanced stages of the disease, the patient becomes akinetic and shows almost no motor initiative. There is reduced arm-swing when walking and reduced blinking, and various simple or complex daily tasks (e.g. washing, brushing the teeth, dressing and writing) can be affected. There is a gradual loss of normal facial movement and expression (Fig. 10.2). Speech is poorly articulated, and the voice is quiet and monotonous. Eating and swallowing become increasingly difficult. This may result in a tendency to drool (sialorrhoea). It is estimated that up to 70% of patients ultimately experience drooling, which may lead to dermatitis and aspiration.

Rigidity

Parkinsonian patients have increased muscle tone in flexor and extensor muscles and typically present resistance to passive movement of the limbs. This rigidity is due to inappropriate sensitivity of the muscles to stretching and an inability to obtain complete relaxation. The increased resistance to movement, combined with tremor, leads to the 'cogwheel' phenomenon. Manipulating the patient's limbs feels like manipulating a lead pipe; hence the term 'lead pipe' rigidity.

Other motor and non-motor manifestations of Parkinson's disease

Abnormalities of posture and gait are associated with this disease and tend to appear at a later stage. The gait of a parkinsonian patient becomes slow and shuffling, and the posture is flexed (see Fig. 10.2). Patients have a marked tendency to fall, which is partly due to the rigidity of limb and trunk muscles but also a consequence of the failure of postural adjustment movements, such as holding out the arms. As the disease progresses, 'freezing' also begins to appear. Patients become 'frozen' when trying to initiate walking, when passing through narrow spaces or when turning. This immobility can be overcome using sensory cues, such as drawing lines on the floor, and asking the patient to step over them.

The patient's handwriting is altered (Fig. 10.3), and as the disease evolves, it becomes small and indecipherable (micrographia). The skin may have a greasy appearance (seborrhoea), and constipation is common. Other autonomic abnormalities, such as urinary dysfunction (in particular, urinary incontinence due to bladder detrusor hyperreflexia), increased sweating and sexual dysfunction, are also encountered in parkinsonian patients.

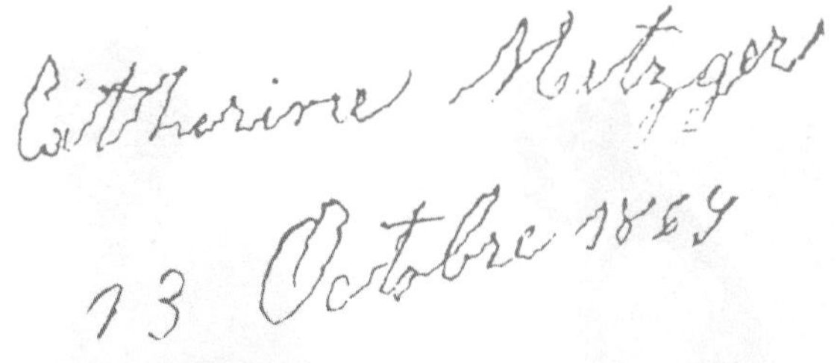

Fig. 10.3 A specimen of the handwriting of a patient with paralysis agitans under the care of Professor Charcot at the Hôpital St Louis in 1869. (From Charcot (1872). In Koller, WC, ed. Handbook of Parkinson's Disease. New York: Marcel Dekker Inc., 1987.)

Box 10.4	Case history (continued)

Gavin continued to take L-DOPA with carbidopa for 6 years. Initially, he complained of nausea and tiredness. The drug improved his motor symptoms, especially during the first year. However, the dose administered had to be increased gradually, and during the last year, he had started suffering from totally unpredictable complete immobility, although he was taking his medication regularly. Sometimes, episodes of immobility alternate with abnormal violent movement of his limbs, which he cannot control and finds extremely embarrassing. His sleep is disturbed, and he complains of nightmares. He has frequent falls, and his wife finds it very difficult to lift him. He has become very apathetic and withdrawn, and has lost interest in any activities that he used to enjoy before he became ill.

Gavin's condition after 6 years of treatment raises the following questions:

1. Was the prescription of L-DOPA with carbidopa the best choice when treatment was initiated?
2. What could have been done to alleviate the additional problems that emerged in this case?

Table 10.1 Classification of parkinsonian syndromes

Idiopathic Parkinson's disease

Secondary parkinsonian syndromes

Infectious/post-infectious (e.g. linked to meningitis or HIV/AIDS)

Toxic (e.g. manganese or carbon monoxide poisoning)

Drug-induced (e.g. MPTP)

Metabolic (e.g. Wilson's disease)

Posttraumatic (e.g. linked to brain injury)

Vascular (e.g. multiinfarct in cerebrovascular disease)

Tumour (e.g. meningioma)

Parkinsonian syndromes as part of other neurodegenerative disorders

Multiple system atrophy

Progressive supranuclear palsy

Corticobasal ganglionic degeneration

Diffuse Lewy body disease

PD patients also present with sleep-wake cycle dysregulation, and, especially in the late stages of the disease, many patients present with memory impairment, confusion and disorientation, and other features of dementia. Cognitive deficits represent a significant clinical problem and may be compounded by the unwanted effects of medication. It is estimated that dementia occurs in approximately 30% of parkinsonian patients, especially when the disease is diagnosed after the age of 70 years. Depression is also very common at any stage of the disease and may be reactive or part of the disease process (Box 10.4). Interestingly, some of the non-motor symptoms can predate the onset of the disease by years or even decades. As the disease evolves, they become increasingly prevalent and significantly affect the patient's quality of life.

The diagnosis of PD is made entirely on symptom presentation and does not involve additional laboratory investigations or imaging procedures. PD is diagnosed by: (1) finding at examination at least two out of several signs of a movement disorder (e.g. rigidity, resting tremor, bradykinesia or problems with posture and gait) and (2) a positive response to dopamine substitution treatment. In the early phase of the disease, misdiagnosis can be quite common. Imaging of the dopamine transporter using a single photon emissoin computed tomography (SPECT) ligand (DaTscan; see Chapter 2) can be used to confirm the diagnosis: a decreased signal reflects decreased dopaminergic innervation.

The presentation in the patient described in Boxes 10.1 and 10.4 is typical of PD. His muscle strength is not affected, but his symptoms reflect difficulties in initiating and coordinating simple motor acts, and impaired posture and gait. The patient has no gross sensory impairment. Furthermore, no muscle weakness, paralysis or spasticity are detected, which rules out a lesion of the UMNs or LMNs. The motor abnormalities have global effects on his performance of motor acts that form part of normal daily activities and also on also his posture. This suggests an abnormality of motor systems that is not strictly localized. The onset of this dysfunction in motor performance is gradual, which rules out a vascular event and is suggestive of a neurodegenerative process. There is no pattern of relapse and remission, and the state of the patient is constantly deteriorating. Thus, as the pathological process is likely to be progressive, it is important to understand the rationale of any treatment attempted and to establish whether therapeutic strategies can at least slow down the neurodegenerative process and improve the patient's quality of life.

All parkinsonian syndromes (Table 10.1) are characterized by akinesia, rigidity and tremor at rest. It is important to differentiate between idiopathic PD (i.e.

Table 10.2 Hoehn and Yahr staging of Parkinson's disease

Stage 1

Signs and symptoms on one side only

Mild symptoms

Inconvenient but not disabling symptoms

Usually presents with tremor of one limb

Friends have noticed changes in posture, locomotion and facial expression

Stage 2

Symptoms are bilateral

Minimal disability

Posture and gait affected

Stage 3

Significant slowing of body movements

Early impairment of equilibrium on walking or standing

Generalized dysfunction that is moderately severe

Stage 4

Severe symptoms

Can still walk to a limited extent

Rigidity and bradykinesia

No longer able to live alone

Tremor may be less than in earlier stages

Stage 5

Cachectic stage

Invalidism complete

Cannot stand or walk

Requires constant nursing care

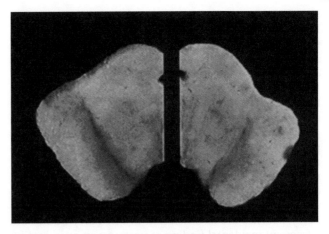

Fig. 10.4 Neurodegeneration in Parkinson's disease. Brain sections from the midbrain of a normal patient (left) and a Parkinson's disease patient (right). The Parkinson's disease hemisphere on the right shows loss of melanized dopaminergic neurons in the substantia nigra. (From Alexi T. et al. (2000). 'Neuroprotective strategies for basal ganglia degeneration: Parkinson's and Huntington's diseases' Progress in Neurobiology 60:409.)

no detectable cause for the disease) and secondary parkinsonism, which may be due to other causes such as vascular lesions in the basal ganglia, carbon monoxide or manganese poisoning, repeated head trauma ('boxer's parkinsonism') or chronic blockade of dopaminergic receptors in the basal ganglia (use of antipsychotic drugs in schizophrenic patients). PD is an irreversible neurodegenerative disease. In the final stages of the disease, patients become bedridden and death occurs due to medical complications (Table 10.2).

Pathology of Parkinson's disease

The pathological hallmark of PD is degeneration of the nigrostriatal dopaminergic pathway. Postmortem analysis of specimens from patients with PD shows a striking reduction in dopaminergic cells in the SN (Fig. 10.4). *In vivo* imaging of dopaminergic neurons, using, for example, a labelled precursor of dopamine or markers of the dopamine neuronal reuptake system, also confirms the loss of striatal dopaminergic terminals (see below). Unfortunately, when the diagnosis is made, it is likely

that more than 50%–60% of dopaminergic neurons in the SN will have been already lost.

Nigrostriatal dopaminergic neurons are tonically active and exert a modulatory influence on the striatum and striatonigral and striatopallidal efferent pathways through D_1 and D_2 receptors, respectively. According to the prevailing model of basal ganglia circuitry, dopamine facilitates the activity of striatal projection neurons in the direct pathway through D_1 receptors and inhibits the activity of striatal projection neurons in the indirect pathway via D_2 receptors. Under normal conditions, as a result of the activity in the two pathways and the neuromodulatory effect of dopamine, there is adequate thalamocortical excitatory input (see Fig. 10.1A) and facilitation of movement.

As illustrated in Fig. 10.1B, the degeneration of dopaminergic nigrostriatal cells leads to an imbalance in striatal output pathways, and there is also evidence of early dysfunction in the STN and an altered cortical drive of the STN in the hyperdirect pathway. The loss of dopamine appears to lead to an increase in the activity of GABAergic striatal neurons in the indirect circuit and a decrease in the activity of GABAergic striatal neurons in the direct circuit. Decreased inhibition in the direct pathway leads to increased activity of inhibitory GABAergic nigrothalamic projections and diminished thalamocortical input, and therefore, less activation of the motor cortex. The slowness of normal movement (bradykinesia) or lack of movement (akinesia) seen in parkinsonism is considered to be a consequence of this increased inhibition of thalamic neurons that project to the cortex. The increased activity in the indirect pathway leads ultimately to a similar consequence through disinhibition of the STN, which provides an excitatory glutamatergic projection to the SN. Therefore, in PD, the excitatory input to cortical areas involved in motor control is reduced. In other diseases of the basal ganglia, such as Huntington's disease, the opposite occurs, leading to a hyperkinetic syndrome (see later in this chapter). However, this is a simplified view of the functioning of the basal ganglia, and the limitations of this functional model become apparent as the disease evolves and as complications of treatment emerge.

PD is characterized by the massive loss of nigrostriatal dopaminergic melanized cells, but the pathological examination also reveals other abnormalities. For example, another characteristic finding in PD, although not pathognomonic, is the presence of Lewy bodies in neuronal cells. These are concentric eosinophilic cytoplasmic inclusions with peripheral halos and dense cores, containing aggregates of the proteins α-synuclein and ubiquitin and also lipids and membranous organelles. Lewy neurites are also detected in PD. Lewy bodies are a frequent incidental finding at postmortem examination in elderly patients. In PD, Lewy bodies and other signs of neurodegeneration can be found in the SN and also in other structures, such as the locus coeruleus, nucleus basalis of Meynert, pedunculopontine nucleus, dorsal motor nucleus of the vagus, cerebral cortex and spinal cord, as the disease evolves. It is important to note that Lewy body pathology initially occurs in cholinergic and monoaminergic brainstem neurons and in neurons in the olfactory system, and ultimately is also found in neocortical areas. Thus there is evidence that the neurodegenerative process in PD does not exclusively affect dopaminergic systems; as the disease evolves, significant changes in noradrenergic, serotonergic and cholinergic neurons can be detected. Thus multiple cell types in the central and peripheral autonomic nervous system are involved in the neurodegenerative processes. In 2003, Braak and colleagues formulated a hypothesis for the spread of the pathology in PD. They proposed that an unknown pathogen (virus or bacterium) could trigger synuclein pathology in the gut, and that this would then be transferred, via the vagus nerve, to the central nervous system, where the spread would gradually affect higher structures in the neuraxis (Fig. 10.5). Synuclein pathology in the gut may be exacerbated by changes in the gut microbiome, which have been reported in PD patients. Later on, Braak suggested an additional point of entry of the pathology, through the olfactory mucosa, and propagation through the olfactory tract. Accumulating in vitro, in vivo and clinical evidence are lending significant support to this hypothesis of a rapidly progressing pathology.

Genetics and pathophysiological processes in Parkinson's disease

PD is one of the most common neurological disorders leading to major disability and ultimately death. It affects 1/1000 of the population and is increasing in both incidence and prevalence due to increased longevity and improvements in treatment. It is at present the fastest growing neurological disorder worldwide. It is more common in men than in women in most populations, and occurs in all races. It is the second most common neurodegenerative disease, affecting 2%–3% of the population above the age of 65 years.

The cause of PD is unknown. There is evidence for a role of both environmental and genetic factors. The increased risk associated with exposure to certain toxic agents, such as manganese or pesticides, and the association of parkinsonism with viral encephalitis lethargica clearly show that external precipitating causes cannot be ruled out. The risk of developing PD is heightened by previous traumatic brain injury. The proportion of risk associated with genetic factors is significant. The progress in identifying genes associated with the disease is due to research on familial PD, which has an

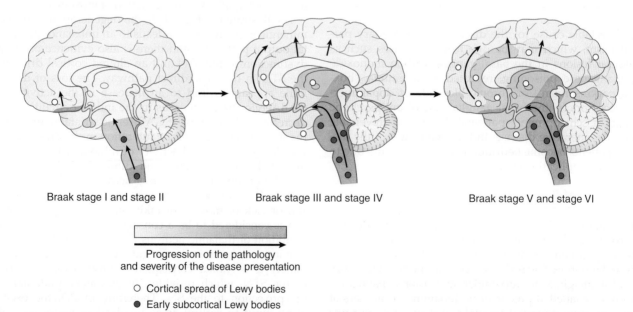

Braak stage I and stage II   Braak stage III and stage IV   Braak stage V and stage VI

Progression of the pathology
and severity of the disease presentation

○ Cortical spread of Lewy bodies
● Early subcortical Lewy bodies

Fig. 10.5 Progression of Lewy body pathology according to the Braak hypothesis. (adapted from Braak H. et al. (2003), Idiopathic Parkinson's disease: possible routes by which vulnerable neuronal types may be subject to neuroinvasion by an unknown pathogen. *Journal of Neural Transmission*, 110:517.)

earlier onset than the sporadic form of the disease and represents a minority of PD cases (~15%). This research has led to the identification of several genes associated with inherited forms of PD—both autosomal dominant and recessive forms. Missense mutations in the SNCA gene encoding α-synuclein, and also copy number variations (duplication or triplication) in this gene, are associated with autosomal dominant forms of PD. Another gene associated with autosomal dominant inheritance is LRRK2, which encodes the protein leucine-rich repeat protein kinase 2 (also named dardarin). Mutations in the PRKN (encoding a ubiquitin ligase) and PINK1 (encoding a mitochondrial serine/threonine-protein kinase) genes are examples of mutations associated with autosomal recessive forms of juvenile-onset PD. It is important to note that there are still many cases of familial and early-onset disease with no known genetic cause. The majority of cases of PD, which are the sporadic and late-onset form of the disease, are not associated with a clearly defined unique genetic determinant. Genome-wide association studies (GWAS) have identified more than 90 independent risk-associated variants, mostly in patients of European ancestry, and much remains to be understood about genetic risk for PD in other populations. GWAS and meta-analyses have shown that sporadic disease-linked common variability exists at loci, such as SNCA, LRRK2 and GBA1 (encoding glucocerebrosidase), all of which harbour disease-causing mutations associated with Mendelian forms of PD. This suggests a clear link between familial and sporadic forms of the disease, especially in terms of commonality of pathophysiological mechanisms. Although the loci identified through GWAS may confer a small risk in isolation, summation of the impact of several loci makes it possible to calculate a polygenic risk score for an individual, thus creating future opportunities for genetics-informed personalized therapy in PD.

Progress in the genetics of PD has contributed to advances in the characterisation of key processes involved in the pathophysiology of the disease. Dopaminergic cell loss in the SN occurs naturally with increasing age, but is accelerated in PD. This may be due to increased oxidative stress or selective neurotoxins, which may preferentially target dopaminergic cells that are rich in neuromelanin. The oxidation of endogenous dopamine leads to the formation of H_2O_2 and highly reactive free radicals (Fig. 10.6). Neuromelanin, which gives nigral dopaminergic cells their characteristic colour, is an oxidation product of dopamine. Postmortem studies show evidence of oxidative damage and decreased activity of complex I of the mitochondrial electron transport chain in the SN in PD. Patients also have increased iron levels in the SNpc and a reduced concentration of the iron-binding protein transferrin, which makes iron more available for oxidation reactions. There is also evidence of increased lipid peroxidation in PD.

The reported development of severe parkinsonian symptoms in young drug addicts following accidental exposure to the toxin 1-methyl-4-phenyl-1,2,3,6-tetrahydro-pyridine (MPTP) not only lends strength to a neurotoxic link in PD, through exposure to environmental neurotoxins, but has also highlighted the role of mitochondria in PD pathophysiology. MPTP can be produced during the synthesis of the opiate pethidine. MPTP is very lipophilic and crosses the blood–brain barrier (BBB) without difficulty. It is converted into a toxic metabolite, the 1-methyl-4-phenylpyridinium ion (MPP^+), through the action of the enzyme monoamine oxidase type B (MAO_B). MPP^+ is taken up by the plasma membrane dopamine transporter into nigral dopaminergic neurons, and selectively destroys them by inhibiting complex I of the respiratory chain in mitochondria (Fig. 10.7). The administration of MPTP in primates replicates all the clinical signs of PD including tremor, rigidity, akinesia and postural instability.

The aggregation of α-synuclein in PD tissue indicates a defect in proteostasis, that is, the cellular pathways that control the formation, maintenance, trafficking and degradation of proteins. The function of this protein is not well understood, but there are indications that it has a role in synaptic vesicle dynamics, mitochondrial function and protein folding processes. α-Synuclein acquires neurotoxic properties during the process of transition from soluble monomeric forms, to oligomers and protofibrils, and ultimately insoluble mature fibrillary deposits. The triggers for aggregation may be the overproduction of protein or mutations that leads to protein misfolding. The cellular mechanisms that ensure degradation of proteins, such as lysosomal-mediated autophagy or the ubiquitin-proteasome system, may be deficient, especially in ageing, and this leads to impaired clearance of the aggregates. Furthermore, there is evidence that aggregated α-synuclein can be released by neurons and ultimately propagated along axonal pathways, thus leading to a widespread dissemination of pathology across the neuraxis. There is also evidence that α-synuclein aggregation and mitochondrial dysfunction may exacerbate each other.

Neuroinflammation, and, in particular, microglial activation, is another element of the pathophysiology seen in PD. There is evidence that neuroinflammation can exacerbate protein misfolding. Interestingly, several genes associated

Oxidative stress in Parkinson's disease

(a) $\quad DA + O_2 + H_2O \xrightarrow{MAO} 3\text{,}4\text{-DHPA} + NH_3 + H_2O_2$

(b) $\quad DA + O_2 \longrightarrow SQ^\bullet + {}^\bullet O_2^- + H^+$

$\qquad DA + {}^\bullet O_2^- + 2H^+ \longrightarrow SQ^\bullet + H_2O_2$

(c) $\quad H_2O_2 + 2GSH \longrightarrow GSSG + 2H_2O$

(d) $\quad H_2O_2 + Fe^{+2} \longrightarrow OH^\bullet + OH^- + Fe^{+3}$

Fig. 10.6 Oxidation processes in the basal ganglia. Examples of reactions involving dopamine, leading to the formation of free radicals, and oxidation of protective substances such as glutathione. *DA*, Dopamine; *H_2O_2*, hydrogen peroxide; *3,4-DHPA*, 3,4-dihydroxy phenylacetaldehyde; *OH^-*, hydroxyl ion; *$OH^\bullet$*, hydroxyl radical; *GSH*, reduced glutathione; *GSSG*, oxidized glutathione; *Fe^{2+}*, ferrous iron; *Fe^{3+}*, ferric ion; *${}^\bullet O_2^-$*, superoxide radical; *MAO*, monoamine oxidase; *$SQ^\bullet$*, quinones.

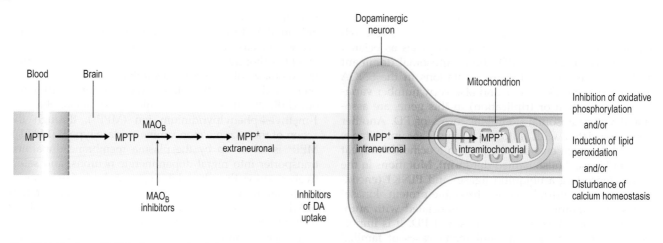

Fig. 10.7 The fate of MPTP after systemic administration and mechanisms underlying its toxicity for dopaminergic neurons. *DA*, dopamine; *MAO$_B$*, monoamine oxidase B; *MPP$^+$*, 1-methyl-4-phenylpyridinium ion; *MPTP*, 1-methyl-4-phenyl-1,2,3,6-tetrahydropyridine.

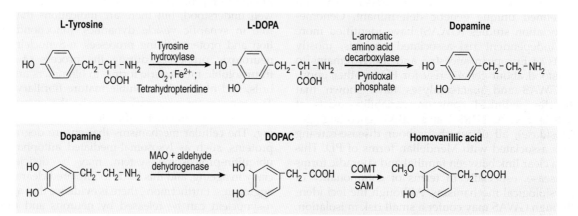

Fig. 10.8 Biosynthesis and metabolism of dopamine. *L-DOPA*, L-dihydroxyphenylalanine; *DOPAC*, dihydroxyphenylacetic acid; *COMT*, catechol-*O*-methyl-transferase; *SAM*, S-adenosylmethionine; *MAO*, monoamine oxidase.

with PD risk encode proteins involved in immune regulation, such as LRRK2. However, neuroinflammation can play a complex role; microglia could phagocytose extracellular aggregates and clear complexes of antibody-bound α-synuclein aggregates, which is the intended result of immunotherapeutic interventions currently being explored for this disease, as discussed below.

Treatment of Parkinson's disease

Pharmacological treatment of PD attempts to compensate for the loss of nigral dopaminergic cells and the imbalance in input thus created in the striatum. Dopamine replacement therapy has been the major principle of treatment for PD for more than five decades (Box 10.3). This therapy and other therapeutic approaches are reviewed below.

Dopaminergic medication

L-DOPA

Dopamine does not cross the BBB; therefore direct systemic supplementation with dopamine is not thera-

peutically useful. L-DOPA (levodopa), a precursor in the biosynthetic pathway of dopamine (Fig. 10.8), can be used to increase dopamine concentrations in the deficient areas. After oral administration, L-DOPA is absorbed into the systemic circulation through the energy-dependent saturable activity of a neutral amino acid transporter in the duodenum. The same transporter also facilitates the passage of L-DOPA across the BBB. In the brain, L-DOPA is taken up into dopaminergic neurons and can be converted into dopamine in the remaining cells in the SN. It is important to note that uptake of L-DOPA will also occur in other dopaminergic cells, such as the cells of origin of the mesolimbic and mesocortical dopaminergic pathways (see Fig. 10.9). Conversion of L-DOPA into dopamine is catalysed by an aromatic amino acid decarboxylase (also called DOPA decarboxylase). This conversion occurs not only in the brain but also at the periphery. The conversion at the periphery can be blocked by co-administration of a DOPA decarboxylase inhibitor such as benserazide or carbidopa. L-DOPA can also be metabolized at the periphery by catechol-*O*-methyltransferase (COMT). The administration of L-DOPA with COMT inhibitors,

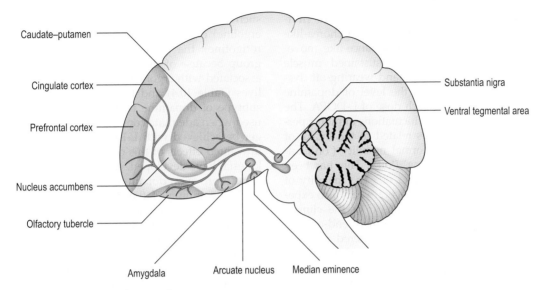

Fig. 10.9 Dopaminergic projections in the central nervous system.

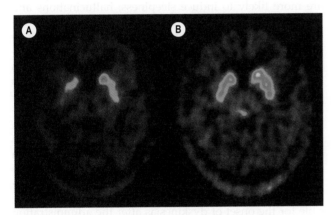

Fig. 10.10 PET studies on [^{18}F]6-L-fluorodopa accumulation in a subject with Parkinson's disease (Hoehn and Yahr stage 3). (A) A scan after administration of L-DOPA without entacapone, (B) a scan at the same level after administration of L-DOPA with entacapone. Note that striatal uptake of fluorodopa is enhanced in the presence of entacapone. (From Olanow C.W. et al. (2000). 'Continuous dopamine-receptor stimulation in early Parkinson's disease.-' *Trends in Neurosciences*, 23(10 Suppl):S117-26.)

Table 10.3 Complications of L-DOPA therapy
Motor fluctuations (end-of-dose deterioration, 'on-off' phenomenon, delayed or no 'on' responses)
Dyskinesias ('on'-period dyskinesia, biphasic dyskinesias, 'off'-period dystonia)
Non-motor complications (tingling, pain, akathisia, autonomic dysfunction)
Neuropsychiatric complications (hallucinations, delirium, mood changes, hypersexuality, sleep fragmentation, nightmares)

such as entacapone, opicapone or tolcapone, significantly improves the central bioavailability of the precursor (Fig. 10.10) and leads to fewer variations in plasma concentration. As other amino acids compete with L-DOPA for intestinal absorption through the same transporter, dietary protein intake can change the bioavailability of L-DOPA.

Prior to the introduction of L-DOPA into clinical use, life expectancy following diagnosis was approximately 10 years. L-DOPA has increased the quality of life, particularly in the early years of treatment, and improved survival. L-DOPA remains the most efficacious antiparkinsonian drug. However, the use of L-DOPA is associated with a wide range of unwanted effects and long-term additional drug-induced problems: nausea, vomiting, postural hypotension, hallucinations and paranoid delusions, and complex acute and delayed motor complications, such as dyskinesias (abnormal involuntary movements) and the 'on-off' effect (Table 10.3).

Nausea and vomiting are due to conversion of L-DOPA into dopamine at the periphery and activation of dopamine receptors in the chemoreceptor trigger zone (in the area postrema in the medulla), which is outside the BBB. This can be largely prevented by co-administration of L-DOPA with DOPA decarboxylase inhibitors such as carbidopa or benserazide (in the case scenario, L-DOPA is given to the patient with carbidopa). Nausea can also be treated with domperidone, which is a dopamine receptor antagonist that does not cross the BBB. Hallucinations are due to the increased production of dopamine in mesolimbic dopaminergic neurons. The motor complications of long-term L-DOPA therapy are particularly disabling (Box 10.4). The pathogenesis of late complications is only partly understood. They occur in 75%–80% of patients taking L-DOPA for more than 4–5 years but can also occur in patients taking it for less time than this. They do not appear immediately after the initiation of L-DOPA therapy but require chronic exposure to L-DOPA with intermittent dosing. Dyskinesias are subdivided into chorea-like movements (hyperkinetic, purposeless dance-like movements) and dystonias (intense and sustained muscle contractions). Peak-dose dyskinesia and wearing-off dystonias are due to fluctuations in the level of dopamine produced intracerebrally after each dose of L-DOPA. The 'on-off' effect refers to dramatic fluctuations in motor performance, which are not always related to the intake of L-DOPA. Patients experience normal mobility ('on') followed suddenly by total 'freezing' ('off'). This has been likened to switching a light on and off. The majority of patients treated with L-DOPA for several years also experience an increasingly rapid wearing-off of the clinical benefit after each dose of precursor, termed 'end-of-dose deterioration'. This may be due to the altered pharmacokinetics of L-DOPA, with exacerbations of peaks and troughs in the concentration of dopamine produced and changes in the sensitivity of dopaminergic receptors. In patients with marked motor fluctuations, benefit may be derived from controlled-release forms of L-DOPA/carbidopa or L-DOPA/benserazide, which compensate for the short half-life of the standard formulation (Table 10.4). Their bioavailability is 70%–80% that of normal L-DOPA/carbidopa or L-DOPA/benserazide combinations. To avoid fluctuations in its level, L-DOPA can be administered continuously by intravenous or intraduodenal routes (using surgical percutaneous tube placement). Surgical intervention may also be attempted to relieve L-DOPA-induced dyskinesia and dystonia (see below). Furthermore, drugs acting at a variety of targets have been explored to specifically treat L-DOPA-induced dyskinesias. These include α_2 receptor antagonists, glutamate receptor antagonists (acting at 4-amino-3-hydroxy-5-methyl-4-isoxazole propionic acid [AMPA], N-methyl-D-aspartate [NMDA] and metabotropic glutamate receptors), 5-HT$_{1A}$ receptor antagonists, D$_4$ receptor antagonists and adenosine A$_2$ receptor antagonists. An example of such a drug is amantadine (a low-affinity NMDA receptor antagonist).

Dopaminergic agonists

Dopamine receptor agonists represent another therapeutic option and compensate for the failure in dopaminergic transmission by directly stimulating dopamine receptors. Agonists are ergot (a fungus that grows on grasses such as rye and wheat)-derived (e.g. bromocriptine, cabergoline) or non-ergot-derived (pramipexole, ropinirole, rotigotine); the prescription preference is for the latter group because of the risk of fibrotic heart valve disease associated with ergot compounds. They have varied half-lives (Table 10.4) and have a higher affinity for the D$_2$ subtype of dopamine receptors (Box 10.5). They can be used when adequate control of the symptoms can no longer be achieved with L-DOPA/carbidopa, or significant unwanted effects of this combination (dystonia and dyskinesia) have developed. A significant number of patients may improve on dopaminergic agonists alone, especially at the beginning of the disease. The early introduction of dopaminergic agonists might be beneficial, especially in younger patients, in delaying the introduction of L-DOPA and the subsequent onset of the dyskinesia and 'on-off' effects seen with L-DOPA. The decision whether to initiate treatment in a patient with L-DOPA or with dopaminergic agonists is based on clinical judgement. The agonists do not have the same efficacy as L-DOPA; thus, ultimately, L-DOPA must be prescribed. Agonists are more likely to induce sleepiness, hallucinations and impulse-control disorders (e.g. binge eating, hypersexuality, gambling) compared to L-DOPA. The latter are likely due to the increased dopaminergic tone in the mesolimbic reward-associated pathway. Dopamine agonists can induce nausea and vomiting, which can be treated with domperidone. They can also induce hallucinations, cardiac arrhythmias and postural hypotension. Their potential for causing dyskinesia and dystonia is much less than that of L-DOPA/carbidopa (Fig. 10.11). Agonists with longer half-lives avoid the peaks and troughs in plasma concentration seen with short-acting compounds such as L-DOPA and other agonists. A pulsatile profile of receptor stimulation is considered to be at least partly responsible for the onset of dyskinesias after the administration of short-acting compounds. Apomorphine is an agonist that can be used subcutaneously (intermittent injection or continuous infusion) in patients who experience major loss of L-DOPA efficacy. Pramipexol and ropinirole are available as extended-release formulations, and rotigotine can be used transdermally as a patch, thus providing continuous drug delivery and added pharmacokinetic benefit compared to agents that need to be taken orally several times a day.

Monoamine oxidase B inhibitors

MAO$_B$ is the isoform of monoamine oxidase (MAO) that is involved in dopamine metabolism (see Fig. 10.8). The inhibition of MAO$_B$ by selegiline (also called deprenyl), rasagiline or safinamide, can increase the levels of dopamine and may also protect against xenobiotics that may be converted into neurotoxic species in a manner similar to MPTP (see above). MAO$_B$ inhibitors are used as adjunctive therapy. Used in conjunction with L-DOPA, selegiline allows a dose reduction and prolongs the duration of L-DOPA action. It can be used as monotherapy only at a very early stage of the disease.

Table 10.4	Half-life of dopaminergic drugs
L-DOPA/carbidopa	1–1.5 h
Bromocriptine	12–15 h
Cabergoline	>24 h
Pramipexole	8–12 h
Ropinirole	6–8 h
Rotigotine	5–7 h

Dopaminergic systems and receptors

Dopamine is a catecholamine neurotransmitter associated with numerous physiological and pathological processes, including motor activity, emotion, cognition, addiction, endocrine regulation, and cardiovascular and renal function. Because of the variety of effects induced by dopamine, one of the major challenges is to develop dopaminergic drugs that selectively affect these processes.

In the central nervous system, dopamine-containing neurons form three main pathways (Fig. 10.9).

1. The nigrostriatal pathway: cell bodies lie in the substantia nigra, and the axons innervate the caudate nucleus and the putamen. This system is mainly involved in the integration of sensory information and the control of movement.
2. The mesolimbic/mesocortical pathway: cell bodies are situated mainly in the ventral tegmental area (which is medial to the substantia nigra), and the axons innervate the nucleus accumbens (considered by some authors to be the most ventral part of the striatum), olfactory tubercle, amygdala and cortex (in particular, the prefrontal and cingulate cortices). This system is associated with reward and reinforcement mechanisms (involved in addiction), emotional behaviour and cognition.
3. The tuberoinfundibular pathway: cell bodies are located in the arcuate nucleus in the hypothalamus,

and the axons project to the median eminence. In this system, dopamine acts as a modulator of the hypothalamic–pituitary axis (e.g. it inhibits prolactin secretion).

Dopamine exerts its effects through five receptor subtypes: D_1, D_2, D_3, D_4 and D_5. These can be grouped into two classes: D_1-like receptors (this includes the D_1 and D_5 receptors) and D_2-like receptors (this includes the D_2, D_3 and D_4 receptors). Additional complexity is conferred by the existence of multiple receptor isoforms within a receptor subtype. All dopamine receptors are G-protein-coupled receptors. They are associated with several signal transduction systems. The two main classes of receptor may exert opposite effects on the same signalling mechanism. For example, D_1-like receptors activate adenylate cyclase, whereas D_2-like receptors inhibit this enzyme. D_1 and D_2 receptors are the predominant dopamine receptor subtypes in the central nervous system. They are present at moderate-to-high densities in the projection areas of the dopaminergic pathways. Dopamine receptors can be located postsynaptically or presynaptically. In the latter case, they may act as autoreceptors, which regulate dopaminergic signalling, but also as heteroreceptors, through their location on non-dopaminergic terminals.

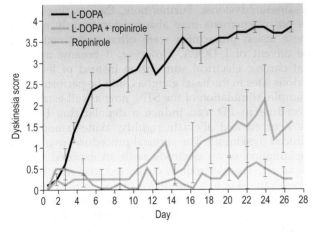

Fig. 10.11 Dyskinesia in 1-methyl-4-phenyl-1,2,3,6-tetrahydropyridine (MPTP)-treated monkeys. Frequency of dyskinesia in MPTP-treated marmosets treated with L-DOPA, ropinirole or L-DOPA with ropinirole. Note the significantly higher dyskinesia score in L-DOPA-treated animals. (Redrawn from Olanow C.W. et al. (2000) Continuous dopamine-receptor stimulation in early Parkinson's disease. *Trends in Neurosciences*, 23(10 Suppl):S117-26.)

Non-dopaminergic medication

Anticholinergic agents

Anticholinergic medication is used in order to redress the potential dopamine–acetylcholine imbalance that may

develop in the parkinsonian striatum. Dopamine exerts an inhibitory effect on striatal cholinergic cells. Therefore, cholinergic hyperactivity may be due, at least in part, to this loss of inhibitory control. Antimuscarinic agents, such as benzhexol, benztropine and procyclidine, are particularly effective in reducing tremor. They produce only a minor improvement in bradykinesia. Their side effects include dry mouth, difficult micturition, constipation and confusion. Their use is very problematic in the elderly, as they increase the risk of confusion and cognitive impairment.

Amantadine

Amantadine was initially developed as an antiviral compound, and its antiparkinsonian effects were discovered serendipitously. It appears to increase dopamine release, and it can inhibit dopamine uptake and block NMDA glutamate receptors. It is well absorbed and has a half-life of approximately 24 hours. Its efficacy is moderate. Its side effects include confusion, hallucinations, nightmares, ankle oedema and livedo reticularis (an erythematous rash of the lower extremities).

Other strategies

Surgical intervention

Surgical procedures were first attempted in PD in the early 20th century (Box 10.6). The introduction of

Box 10.6 Surgery and neurostimulation in Parkinson's disease (or finding the right answers through trial and error)

Surgical intervention was relatively common in the management of Parkinson's disease before the introduction of L-DOPA. In 1930, L.J. Polack and L. Davis performed posterior rhizotomies (cutting of sensory nerve roots), which led to some improvement in rigidity but no improvement in tremor. Later on, Paul Bucy excised Brodmann's cortical area 4, which led to decreased tremor but was accompanied by contralateral hemiparesis. In the 1950s, lesions to the caudate, ansa lenticularis and pallidum led to a reduction in tremor and rigidity in 40%–70% of patients but with high mortality rates. In 1952, while attempting a pedunculotomy in a parkinsonian patient, Irving Cooper damaged and then ligated the anterior choroidal artery. This led to a reduction in tremor and rigidity, which was attributed to an ischaemic lesion in the medial pallidum, ansa and fasciculus lenticularis, and the ventrolateral nucleus of the thalamus. This focused attention on two important targets for lesioning or stimulation: the thalamus and the medial pallidum. Alim-Louis Benabid in the mid-1990s showed that stimulation of the subthalamic nucleus was an equally interesting approach. In recent years, continuing advances in stereotaxic procedures, brain imaging and electrophysiological recording have gradually made surgery much more precise and accurate. Deep brain stimulation (DBS) is now an established technique and, since the 1990s, more than 160,000 patients have undergone the procedure. DBS is based on the implantation of electrodes linked to an implantable pulse generator (similar to a pacemaker) to provide long-term, continuous stimulation. The immediate effects of DBS involve an alteration of firing patterns in neural circuits, but it is likely that there are also other longer-term effects involving alterations in neurotransmitter dynamics and gene expression, and possibly neurotrophic aspects. DBS is used in Parkinson's disease, essential tremor and dystonia. Other indications include treatment-resistant epilepsy, depression and obsessive-compulsive disorder.

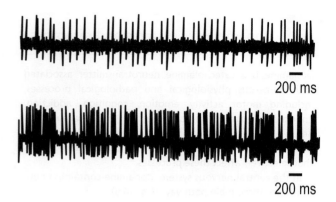

Fig. 10.12 Changes in neuronal activity after experimental nigrostriatal lesion: firing of neurons in control rats (top) and rats whose nigrostriatal projections are lesioned unilaterally using 6-hydroxydopamine (bottom). Note that the lesion changes the spiking activity from a regular pattern of discharge to bursting activity. From Hirsch E.C., et al. (2000) 'Metabolic effects of nigrostriatal denervation in basal ganglia'. *Trends in Neurosciences*, 23(10 Suppl):S78-85.

L-DOPA therapy led to a relative loss of interest in surgical intervention. However, more recently, this approach has been playing an increasingly important role in the management of advanced PD, especially in patients with motor complications due to pharmacological treatment.

The rationale for surgical treatment is based on the alterations in neuronal firing in the basal ganglia that accompany the degeneration of nigrostriatal neurons. The loss of nigral cells, combined with intermittent stimulation of dopamine receptors, may lead to abnormal firing patterns in striatal output pathways. There may be reduced activity of neurons in the GPe, in parallel with a significant increase in the activity of neurons in the SNpc, GPi and STN. For example, after nigral lesion, neurons in the STN change their activity from a

spiking pattern to a bursting pattern (Fig. 10.12). PD is associated with increased rhythmicity and synchrony of neural activity and oscillations. These abnormalities may underlie parkinsonian symptoms, and the dyskinesia/dystonia induced by long-term L-DOPA replacement therapy. Stereotactic lesions can be performed in the thalamus or GPi. Targeting the thalamus may prove particularly useful in patients with intractable tremor, whereas pallidotomy may alleviate rigidity and L-DOPA-induced dyskinesia/dystonia. Furthermore, the wearing-off and 'on-off' phenomena may also be significantly reduced. These lesion procedures were often performed before the advent of L-DOPA. However, it became apparent that chronic electrical stimulation instead of lesions at various sites in the basal ganglia could be performed. For example, stimulation of the STN, now a well-established procedure in PD, can induce a depolarizing block of the neurons and alleviate rigidity, akinesia and drug-induced dyskinesia. The surgical procedure involves the implantation of an electrode with an exposed tip into the target. The electrode is connected to a wire running beneath the skin to a stimulator placed in the chest. The stimulator can be adjusted externally using a programmer. If a side effect occurs due to electrical stimulation, the stimulation can be reduced. Fig. 10.13 illustrates these techniques and the clinical improvement associated with their successful use. The improvement can last for years and may allow a very significant reduction in the doses of drugs taken by the patient. Bilateral deep brain stimulation (DBS) of the STN can lead to an approximately 50% improvement in activities of daily living and the motor score, compared with the preoperative state; drug dosage and dyskinesia are reduced by more than 60%. Therefore, although this neurostimulation treatment is not used routinely in a large number of patients, it offers a valuable option in the management of advanced disease.

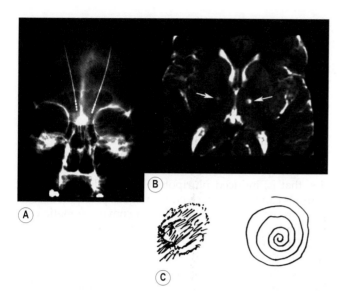

(A)
(B)
(C)

Fig. 10.13 Surgical intervention in Parkinson's disease. (A) Bilateral implantation of electrodes for stimulation of the subthalamic nucleus. (B) Bilateral pallidotomy (arrows indicate the lesions). (A and B, Courtesy of Dr S. Karanth.) (C) Improvement in handwriting in a patient who received a unilateral thalamic lesion. (After Narabayashi C. (1990). Surgical treatment in the levodopa era. In Stern G, ed. Parkinson's Disease. The Johns Hopkins University Press, 609.)

Cell replacement therapies

It has been hypothesised that the neurodegenerative processes in PD could be counteracted by the provision of neurotrophic factors that could support the failing neurons (Box 10.7). However, in spite of promising experimental results with factors such as GDNF and neurturin (a factor related to GDNF), translation to the clinic has not been successful. Considering the significant localized neurodegeneration in the midbrain in PD, use of neural grafts would appear to be a particularly well-suited strategy for the replacement of lost dopaminergic cells. Cell replacement therapies for PD began more than 50 years ago and have evolved significantly over the last three decades of the 20th century, as summarized in Table 10.5, providing a solid base for present cell replacement research. In experimental animals, autologous foetal dopaminergic cells transplanted into the striatum survive and adopt a morphology and neurochemical phenotype consistent with dopaminergic reinnervation. Initial attempts in patients involved the use of homografts of adrenal medulla, which contains catecholamine-secreting cells. However, follow-up studies showed poor survival of the grafts, modest clinical improvement accompanied by numerous side effects and a high level of morbidity and mortality. Human embryonic nigral grafts were subsequently attempted, and the accumulated observations so far show that they can lead to significant and long-lasting clinical improvement. Furthermore, positron emission tomography (PET) studies have provided evidence of regulated dopamine release from such grafts. As illus-

---

Box 10.7 Neurotrophic factors

Neurotrophic factors are endogenous substances that control cell proliferation and differentiation in the nervous system. Trophic effects are essential during development, but also at the adult stage, in the immediate aftermath of injury and during regeneration. Many neurotrophic and growth factors are present in the substantia nigra and/or the striatum. Experimental evidence shows that several of these neurotrophic factors support the survival and differentiation of mesencephalic dopaminergic neurons. These factors include epidermal growth factor (EGF), basic fibroblast growth factor (bFGF), brain-derived neurotrophic factor (BDNF), glial cell line-derived neurotrophic factor (GDNF) and neurturin, which is related to GDNF. Neurotrophic factors reverse dopaminergic deficits in animal models. However, neurotrophic factors are large molecules that do not cross the BBB after systemic administration. Direct injection of these factors into the cerebral ventricles or parenchyma is unlikely to become a routine clinical procedure. An alternative is the cerebral implantation of encapsulated cells engineered to produce and secrete neurotrophic factors, or the use of viral vectors (e.g. adeno-associated virus or lentivirus). Encapsulation would protect against a host immune response and counter the danger of abnormal growth. Studies carried out so far with neurotrophic factors have not led to any significant clinical benefits in PD.

Table 10.5 Cell-based therapies in Parkinson's disease

1970–72	Experimental adrenal medulla and foetal nigral cell grafts in the anterior eye chamber
1979	Experimental grafts of foetal nigral cells in animals with nigrostriatal lesions
1985	Adrenal medulla grafts in patients with Parkinson's disease
1988	Foetal nigral grafts in patients with Parkinson's disease
1997	Foetal pig nigral grafts in patients with Parkinson's disease
1998	Experimental grafts of embryonic stem cells in animals with nigrostriatal lesions

trated in Fig. 10.14, in the case of a patient who unilaterally received ventral mesencephalic tissue from four human embryos in the anterior, posterior and middle putamen, clinical improvement was paralleled by improvement in dopamine storage capacity, as reflected in the accumulation of DOPA. Furthermore, PET analysis with the use of [^{11}C]raclopride, an in vivo marker of D_2 receptors, showed that the endogenous dopamine produced by the graft can be released by agents such as methamphetamine and thus displace the marker from the receptors, which further confirms the functionality

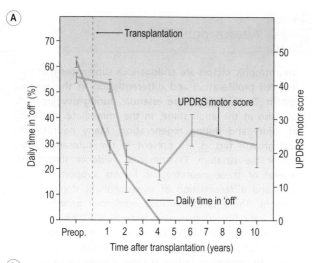

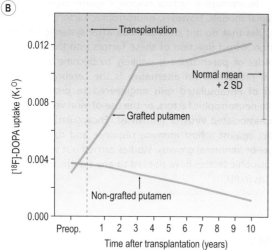

Fig. 10.14 Effect of nigral transplants in PD. (A) Percentage of the day spent in the 'off' phase and motor examination score on the Unified Parkinson's Disease Rating Scale (UPDRS), preoperatively and after intrastriatal grafting. (B) [^{18}F]DOPA uptake before and after transplantation. Note the concomitant increase in [^{18}F]DOPA uptake and clinical improvement after grafting. (From Piccini P. et al. (1999). 'Dopamine release from nigral transplants visualized in vivo in a Parkinson's patient.' *Nature Neuroscience*, 2(12):1138.)

of the graft. Retrospective studies on postmortem tissue from patients who survived for more than 10 years after receiving their grafts in the 1990s clearly showed that most of the transplanted neurons remained healthy and functional, but there was, in some cases, evidence of Lewy body pathology in the graft, suggesting that host-to-graft transmission of PD pathology is possible.

Other grafting attempts have involved the use of dopaminergic xenografts from porcine donors and non-neuronal cells engineered to secrete dopamine-synthesizing enzymes (thus acting as a pump that provides the deficient amine). However, more recently, efforts have been focused on the use of stem cells derived from the blastocyst stage of the embryo, before implantation in the uterus. They are capable of multiple divisions

and can differentiate into a variety of cell types, including dopaminergic neurons. After transplantation, stem cells can integrate into the host tissue and differentiate into neurons and glia. Their high plasticity offers enormous potential, but their unrestrained and uncontrolled growth could lead to tumour formation. This can be obviated by transforming the cells into more differentiated cells before transplantation. It is now possible to collect non-neuronal, somatic cells from a patient (e.g. skin fibroblasts) and re-programme them using a combination of transcription factors, to achieve stem-cell characteristics, that is, induced pluripotent stem cells (iPSCs), and neurons can then be derived from these pluripotent cells. It has recently become possible to convert somatic cells directly into neurons, without the intermediate stem cell step. This approach has all the advantages of cell therapy without the risk of allogeneic approaches based on the use of cells from other donors, which require immunosuppression. Furthermore, the cells can also be edited for specific deleterious genetic mutations; exploratory studies are focused at present on editing mutations in the GBA gene. Therefore autologous neuron replacement therapy is providing new hopes in the field of grafting.

The experimental and clinical observations of intracerebral cell grafts suggest that the cells used for transplantation should have the capacity to: (1) grow neurites, (2) establish connections with the appropriate neurons in the host tissue (e.g. in PD, the grafts are placed ectopically in the striatum), (3) differentiate successfully into dopamine-releasing cells and (4) resist destruction by any neurotoxic latent process.

General management strategy and long-term prognosis in Parkinson's disease

There is currently no cure for PD, as progression of the neurodegenerative process is irreversible. The evolution of the disease is highly variable between individuals. Some patients maintain reasonable function 12–15 years into the disease, while others experience rapid worsening of symptoms very early on. Current approaches to classification into subtypes are not optimum, and consensus on patient stratification is lacking. Current treatments are only symptomatic but have improved the patients' overall quality of life, especially in the early years of treatment, and have increased average life expectancy. Patients usually experience improvement in symptoms when L-DOPA therapy is first introduced. The response is relatively stable throughout the day, and this is probably due to the ability of remaining nigrostriatal neurons to produce dopamine from L-DOPA, and store it and release it in a relatively physiological manner. It is particularly important to stress the need to take the medication 'on time and every time' in this disease, thus minimising fluctuations in drug levels. However, in spite of the medication, degeneration continues and disability becomes more severe. This leads to a tendency to increase the dose of dopaminergic drugs. However, the number of nigral residual cells is very small, and the levels of dopamine produced from L-DOPA supplementation will start to fluctuate widely. Patients first notice a much shorter duration of improvement after taking a dose of medication and also develop peak-dose dyskinesias. At this point, further increasing the doses of drugs leads to more severe dyskinetic episodes, which are not necessarily accompanied by significant improvement in the dyskinesia-free intervals. The importance and complexity of successfully managing a patient who presents with a combination of akinesia and dyskinesia cannot be overstated, and the strategies chosen depend on the preference and experience of the specialist in charge of the case (see example in Table 10.6). In parallel with pharmacological adjustments, the surgical options are important additional options in such cases.

A significant number of patients develop dementia and also experience major postural problems. Postural imbalance is not improved significantly by drugs, is a cause of morbidity and mortality and increases the strain on the carers. Dopamine agonists often offer only transient improvement of motor symptoms. In the early phases of the disease, the stigma of tremor may be restrictive and a serious threat to employment. Thus each aspect of the disease requires careful consideration and specific rehabilitative management. A view that has emerged recently is that the optimum management of

---

Table 10.6 Treatment recommendations for motor fluctuations and dyskinesias in Parkinson's disease including akinetic crisis

1. End-of-dose deterioration (wearing-off)
   Take L-DOPA well before meals (30–60 min)
   Add dopamine agonist
   Add selegiline
   Change to, or add, L-DOPA administration and reduce size of individual doses to avoid overdosage
   Take the first L-DOPA dose immediately on rising
   Eat a low-protein diet during the day
   Take L-DOPA as a dispersible or liquid formulation for early-morning or afternoon akinesia

2. Paroxysmal 'on-off'
   See the preceding recommendations on wearing-off
   Fewer, higher doses of L-DOPA, however, may be preferable in some patients
   Administer apomorphine by subcutaneous intermittent injections or continuous infusion (mini-pump)

3. Peak-dose mobile dyskinesias
   Discuss with the patient whether the dyskinesias are an acceptable price to pay for mobility (mild to intermediate dyskinesias often bother the carer more than the patient)
   Discuss whether the patient prefers more time 'on' with dyskinesia or less time 'on' with less dyskinesia
   Suggest intake of drug with meals (may help peak-dose dyskinesias)
   Adding a long-acting dopamine agonist should help reduce 'troughs' of dopaminergic stimulation; it may also permit lower doses of L-DOPA to be used and hence often reduce the severity of dyskinesias
   Try controlled-release L-DOPA preparations (peak-dose dyskinesias can increase)
   Administer subcutaneous apomorphine by injection or infusion pump
   Add amantadine

4. Biphasic dyskinesia
   Overlapping doses of L-DOPA and use of controlled-release preparations often result in permanent dyskinetic chaos
   May be worsened by protein meals
   Take higher doses less often, going through complete cycle to 'off' again before taking next dose

5. Off-period dystonia
   Dispersible L-DOPA preparation or apomorphine injection, especially as a first dose, eliminate early-morning dystonia
   Controlled-release L-DOPA during day or at bedtime
   Add agonist during day or at bedtime
   Add anticholinergic
   Local administration of botulinum toxin in selected cases

6. Akinetic crisis
   Intensive care facilities should be available
   Ancillary measures: parenteral fluids with electrolyte and caloric substitution, anti-thrombotic prophylaxis, physiotherapy, skin care
   Restart L-DOPA at a slightly lower dose than before and increase gradually to the previous dose over 1–2 days if akinetic crisis is the result of L-DOPA withdrawal
   Increase L-DOPA dose by 100–200 mg/daily until response is observed if akinetic crisis is due to underdosing
   Administer single injection of apomorphine by subcutaneous continuous infusion (initially 1–2 mg/h; increase by 0.5–1 mg every 12 h with an 8–12 h break at night; maximal daily dose 170–240 mg). If domperidone cover is required, give 20 mg three times daily before staring apomorphine; in emergencies, give 50–60 mg domperidone 30–60 min before apomorphine, if necessary via nasogastric tube

From Möller J.C., Bandmann O. and Oertel W.H. (1999). 'The therapy of the parkinsonian syndrome.' *Deutsch Med Wochenschr*, 124(8), 219-222.

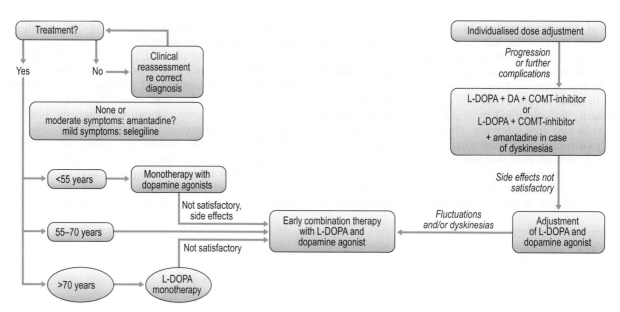

Fig. 10.15 Algorithm for treating akinetic rigid Parkinson's disease patient. COMT, catechol-O-methyltransferase; DA, dopamine agonist. (Adapted from Braune HJ, Moeler JC, Oertel WH. (1999) In LeWitt PA, Oertel WH, eds., Parkinson's Disease: The Treatment Options. London: Martin Dunitz, 251.)

young (i.e. 50–60-year-old) patients and elderly patients may differ. Fig. 10.15 offers a possible algorithm of differential treatment to illustrate this point. In particular, the introduction of L-DOPA is delayed as much as possible in younger patients, because L-DOPA-induced dyskinesias and dystonias seem to be more marked in young patients. Therefore, for younger patients, symptomatic therapy may be better initiated using a dopamine agonist. In the case presented here, it may have been wiser to delay the introduction of L-DOPA therapy. The complications could be initially treated with a controlled-release L-DOPA preparation, with or without a dopaminergic agonist.

Dopamine agonists may adequately control symptoms for several years, after which L-DOPA introduction becomes inevitable. Finally, it is important to stress that the successful management of parkinsonian patients, particularly in the middle and late stages of the disease, involves a multidisciplinary approach combining medical treatment with physiotherapy, speech therapy and occupational therapy (Table 10.7), and also the provision of specialist nursing care. For example, it has been shown that boxing exercises (e.g. jabbing and hook punches) can lead to improvement in balance, gait, walking speed, stride length, step width, 'get-up-and-go' time and ability to reach forward, after only 3 months of practice. It has been suggested that sustained multidisciplinary therapy may support neuroplasticity.

One of the most promising areas of research is focused on the development and validation of biomarkers that would allow diagnosis of the disease at an early, prodromal stage. It is likely that PD pathology is present at least 10–15 years before motor symptoms become apparent. At this early stage, many patients may present with non-motor symptoms, such as hyposmia, constipation and rapid eye-movement sleep behaviour disorder (a form of sleep disturbance during which individuals may act-out dreams). Research diagnostic criteria that can be used for prodromal stage interventions will have significant value for the exploration of compounds with neuroprotective and preventive potential. Other biomarkers could be used to assess disease risk; for example, it has been found that increased levels of serum or plasma uric acid are associated with a decreased risk of developing PD. Furthermore, aggregates of α-synuclein can be detected in the skin of patients with PD, raising the possibility of the future diagnostic use of skin biopsies.

As the aggregation of α-synuclein is a key pathological event in PD, there is intense research focus on new immunological therapeutic approaches based on passive or active immunization against α-synuclein; antibodies against α-synuclein aggregates could become the first disease-modifying therapies in PD.

Huntington's disease

Huntington's disease (HD) is a hereditary neurodegenerative disease that affects the striatum and the cortex and is characterized by motor, cognitive and psychiatric symptoms. HD is associated with prominent atrophy of the cortex, which mostly affects the motor and premotor areas, and a loss of (enkephalinergic) striatal spiny GABAergic neurons, which are the origin of the striatal efferent pathways. MRI and CT scanning show that in advanced HD there is atrophy of the caudate, putamen and cerebral cortex. In some cases, brain weight may be reduced by one-third (Fig. 10.16). There is early massive loss of striatopallidal neurons, followed by loss of striatonigral neurons. Striatal interneurons are

Table 10.7 Motor control deficits and corresponding physical therapy in Parkinson's disease

Motor control deficits	Corresponding physical therapy
Truncal stiffness	Exercises involving trunk movements
Mis-scaling of movement amplitude	Use large-amplitude movements
Respiratory complications and impairment	Breathing exercises with relaxation techniques
Slowed gain, stepping cadence	Gait exercises, especially varying walking cadence exercises
Stride length	Rhythmic auditory stimulation
Balance instability, falling	Self-initiated and external perturbations
	Side-to-side rocking motion and facilitation of anterior/posterior motion
	Pregait-type activities
Problems with simultaneous and sequential movements	Repetitive practice of functional activities, simultaneous sequencing of different motor programmes, rising from seated position
Impaired prediction of movements, inability to start movements ('freezing')	Rhythmic activities with cueing signals, polysensory cueing
	Selection of proper cueing frequencies
Hastening	Biofeedback and relaxation techniques
Dyskinesia and dystonia	Slow stretching exercises
Tremor	Upper-body karate training
	External damping device for the upper extremity
Speech impairment	Delayed auditory feedback device, prosodic exercises, rhythmic stimulation
Dysphagia	Reclining neck at 60 degrees with head support
Psychological symptoms and problems	Relaxation and cognitive restructuring, training in social skills specifically adapted to Parkinson's disease, teaching programmes for relatives

From Pohl M, Mrass GJ, Oertel WH, Rehabilitation in Parkinson's disease (1999), In LeWitt PA, Oertel WH, eds. Parkinson's Disease: The Treatment Options, London, Martin Dunitz.

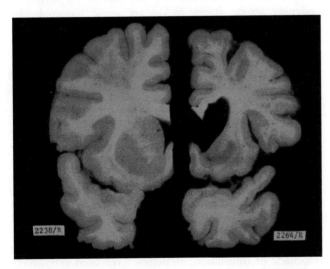

Fig. 10.16 Neurodegeneration in Huntington's disease: brain sections taken through the caudate putamen of a normal patient (left) and a Huntington's disease patient. The Huntington disease hemisphere on the right shows degeneration of the caudate nucleus adjacent to the lateral ventricle, which has enlarged in response to striatal atrophy. (From Alexi T. et al. (2000). 'Neuroprotective strategies for basal ganglia degeneration: Parkinson's and Huntington's diseases.' Progress in Neurobiology, 60:435.)

relatively spared. HD is an autosomal dominant disease due to a mutation in a gene present on the short arm of chromosome 4, which encodes the huntingtin protein. A DNA test can identify the mutation. Individuals at risk can be offered genetic testing after suitable counselling. Prenatal genetic testing can also be carried out. The onset of the disease is in mid-life, and progression to death takes place over 15–20 years. The disease occurs in 5–10/100,000 of the population. Transmission can occur through parents of either sex and is fully penetrant.

The function of huntingtin is unknown. It is a large protein that may act intracellularly as a scaffolding protein, thereby providing a platform to facilitate interactions between various proteins involved in multiple cellular pathways. The protein is present in all tissues and is essential for life, as homozygous knockout mice are not viable. The mutation in exon 1 of the huntingtin gene leads to an abnormal number of repeats of glutamine (encoded by the CAG codon) in the N-terminal region of the protein. The mutated protein is expressed early in life, but the disease becomes apparent in mid-life. Interestingly, several other neurological diseases are associated with the expansion of a CAG repeat in the genome. Examples are spinobulbar muscular atrophy, dentatorubropallidoluysian atrophy (DRPLA) and different types of spinocerebellar ataxias. Huntingtin (as well as the other proteins containing polyglutamine repeats) can directly interact with transcription factors and thus modify the expression of multiple genes. Interestingly, only specific subsets of neurons are vulnerable in each of these diseases, although the affected proteins are present throughout the brain and other organs.

The length of the polyglutamine tract varies between individuals. The number of repeats is inversely correlated with age at onset of the disease. Individuals with more than 40 repeats will invariably develop adult-onset disease, whereas the presence of 55 repeats or more leads to onset at an age of less than 20 years. The disease has several stages: the first stage is characterized by mood changes, cognitive deficits and subtle motor changes. Subsequently, abrupt, involuntary movements (chorea) become dominant, and swallowing, speech and gait deteriorate. In the last stage of the disease there is significant weight loss, emerging bradykinesia and rigidity, and death becomes imminent.

The cortex of HD mutation carriers shows progressive thinning up to 15 years before the onset of motor symptoms. Ultimately, the disconnection of corticostriatal afferents is likely to play a major role in the dysfunction that occurs downstream in striatal projections. Initially, it is likely that there is increased glutamate release and over-excitation of striatal spiny neurons, followed by silencing of the striatal neurons in the late stages of the disease. The triplet expansion mutation in exon 1 of the huntingtin gene leads to a toxic 'gain of function', which is ultimately associated with a host of pathophysiological changes, such as abnormal energy metabolism, disrupted neurogenesis, reduced axonal transport and protein trafficking and disrupted production of brain-derived neurotrophic factor (BDNF). Proteins with polyglutamine repeats can aggregate and form fibrils similar to the amyloid β-fibrils in Alzheimer's disease. The mutant protein can be found in the cytoplasm and is also present in large intranuclear inclusions. Striatal projection neurons receive significant glutamate input from the cortex; therefore, they may be at an increased risk of excessive stimulation of glutamate receptors and subsequent uncontrolled rises in cytoplasmic Ca^{2+}, leading to cell death. Therefore, it has been suggested that excitotoxicity is involved in striatal cell loss. The intrastriatal administration of excitatory amino acids, such as kainic acid, ibotenic acid or quinolinic acid, leads to massive striatal neurodegeneration. Agonists at the NMDA glutamate receptor such as quinolinic acid, injected intrastriatally in experimental models, lead to a pattern of neuropathology that is very similar to the pattern found in HD. Mitochondrial poisons such as 3-nitropropionic acid, which compromise energy metabolism, also lead to striatal degeneration. It cannot be ruled out that metabolic compromise leads to secondary excitotoxicity through uncontrolled release of glutamate. It is also known that in HD astrocytic glutamate transporters are deficient, and also that the ability of astrocytes to buffer potassium is impaired, which leads to prolonged depolarisations and underlies the increased neuronal

excitability. However, there are still missing links in the pathophysiology cascade, between the production of the protein with expanded CAG repeats and the triggering of multiple deleterious effects including transcriptional dysregulation, mitochondrial dysfunction, altered proteostasis, oxidative stress, disrupted axonal transport and synaptic dysfunction.

As illustrated in Fig. 10.1C, the loss of striatal efferent pathways leads to disinhibition of the glutamatergic thalamocortical input and the emergence of abnormal movements that define a very characteristic hyperkinetic syndrome. The patients affected present with chorea, that is, an involuntary, jerking movement that affects the limbs and axial muscle groups. Patients try to suppress these movements and incorporate them into more purposeful ones. It is important to note that chorea can be due to a variety of causes. It can be associated with a hereditary disease (e.g. HD) but can also be induced by drugs (e.g. antiparkinsonian drugs and oral contraceptives) or alcohol or have an immunological or metabolic cause. Sydenham's chorea is post-infectious and associated with rheumatic fever.

Chorea must be differentiated from hemiballismus, in which movements are more violent and jerky and affect only one side of the body as a result of damage to the subthalamic nucleus on the contralateral side. Writhing movements are also associated with athetosis, which is another dyskinesia. In this case, movements are slower and reflect gradual transitions from one dystonic posture to another. Athetosis is typically encountered in cerebral palsy.

The cortical changes and loss of striatal efferent pathways are accompanied by dopaminergic hyperactivity, especially in the earlier stages. Anti-dopaminergic medication, for example, dopaminergic antagonists such as haloperidol, can alleviate the symptoms. Depletion of vesicular amine stores in dopaminergic terminals, by drugs such as tetrabenazine, may also help. Many patients develop depression, which responds to antidepressant medication (e.g. selective serotonin reuptake inhibitors or serotonin-noradrenaline reuptake inhibitors). It has been suggested that antidepressant drugs not only improve mood but also may have some neuroprotective effects.

HD is an irreversible neurodegenerative disease, and in the last stages of the disease, cardiovascular and respiratory complications due to increased debility are a common cause of death. One of the possible strategies for treating this disease is based on the principle of inhibition of expression of the mutant allele at the DNA or RNA level. However, inhibition of the mutant allele must not disrupt the parallel expression of the normal allele, which is required for development. Antigene (i.e. blockade of transcription) or antisense oligonucleotide (blockade of translation) strategies have been extensively explored. Encouraging observations suggest that an antisense oligonucleotide-based approach can be effective in humans. The nature of the degenerative process in HD has also led to much research on cell replacement strategies, as in PD. For recovery of normal movement, complete restoration of striatal efferent circuits is required. Foetal striatal cells have been commonly used for transplantation in animal models of HD. Encouraging results have led to trials in patients using autografts or xenografts (porcine donors). There is evidence that grafts of foetal striatal cells implanted in the striatum of patients with HD may survive and lead to long-lasting cognitive and motor improvement. The use of stem cells, including induced pluripotent stem cells, is also under investigation and offers additional hope for the treatment of this devastating disease.

Self-assessment case study

A 37-year-old shipyard welder was brought to the general practitioner by his wife. He had always been very good-natured and of an even disposition. According to her, his behaviour had altered a lot lately: he had become irritable and aggressive, especially with his close family, and had memory lapses. He had also started moving his arms and hands in a strange, jerky, unpredictable manner. His 82-year-old mother said that he reminded her of his paternal grandfather, who had 'turned funny' at about the same age, and showed similar symptoms before he died in a car accident.

On examination, the patient seemed slightly disoriented, but speech, comprehension and memory appeared normal. There were no abnormal eye movements, and pupils were equal and reactive to light. Vision and hearing were normal. His facial expression was symmetrical. Deep tendon reflexes were normal. His hands, legs and feet were affected by jerky movement, which gave him a 'dance-like' appear-ance. Superimposed on these jerky movements was a slow, writhing movement of the arm. He was obviously trying to hide the existence of these movements, pretending that they were part of normal, purposeful ones.

After studying this chapter, you should be able to answer the following questions:

1. What is the most likely cause of this patient's symptoms, and what is the diagnosis?

It is likely that this patient has Huntington's disease, judging by the specific type of abnormal movements displayed. There is a clear indication of an inherited aspect of his condition.

2. What are the treatment options for this patient?

At present, treatment options are mostly symptomatic. The loss of striatal efferent pathways is accompanied by a hyperdopaminergic state, particularly in the earlier stages of the disease. Tetrabenazine, a synaptic vesicle monoamine transporter inhibitor, could be used to decrease dopaminergic tone. Dopaminergic antagonists could also be used to this effect. Antidepressant drugs can be used throughout the disease.

3. What is the expected course and prognosis of this disease?

This is a terminal neurodegenerative disease. The patient will deteriorate gradually, and death will occur approximately 15–20 years after diagnosis.

STROKE AND HEAD INJURY

11

Chapter summary

1. Stroke is a generic term for a brain injury that has a vascular origin. The majority of strokes are ischaemic and the consequence of a loss of blood supply in various areas of the central nervous system (CNS). A minority of stroke presentations are due to haemorrhage. Both types of strokes are associated with significant and long-lasting consequences for individuals. The neurological deficits are a reflection of the functions associated with the brain areas where the vascular supply is disrupted by ischaemia or haemorrhage. Temporary disruptions in blood flow, such as in transient ischaemic attacks (TIAs), lead to temporary deficits.

2. Blood is supplied to the brain via anterior and posterior arterial circulations; the former supplies the supratentorial structures, whereas the latter supplies the posterior fossa structures. Venous drainage occurs through superficial and deep veins that drain into the various venous sinuses and the internal jugular vein.

3. The pathophysiology cascade of stroke includes a wide range of different mechanisms, for example, excitotoxicity, increased oxidation, disruption of cerebral metabolism and neuroinflammation, which compound the initial cell loss and expand the area which is initially compromised by the vascular accident.

4. Several factors can modify the risk of stroke. They include atrial fibrillation, hypertension, smoking, a diet rich in saturated fat, age, sex, ethnicity and previous strokes or TIAs.

5. Head injury can present with various levels of severity. One of the immediate consequences of traumatic injury to brain tissue incurred during a head injury is the swelling of brain tissue. Cerebral oedema can be vasogenic or cytotoxic. The increased cranial pressure associated with oedema can lead to herniation and ultimately death, because of compression of the brainstem and the compromise of

vital functions. The pathophysiology of traumatic brain injury shares many similarities with the pathophysiology of stroke.

6. Traumatic brain injury, even as a single occurrence, can enhance the risk of neurodegenerative disease later in life. Repetitive mild concussion, such as that incurred during sports or in a military context, for example, upon repeated exposure to blast waves linked to explosions, can lead to chronic traumatic encephalopathy, a distinct form of neurodegeneration which is accompanied by major changes in mood, behaviour and cognition.

7. The acute period following a stroke or traumatic brain injury offers a window of opportunity for intervention with neuroprotective agents. However, various compounds that have shown efficacy in experimental studies have failed to show efficacy in clinical trials. Specialist rehabilitation regimes, which harness brain plasticity and compensatory mechanisms, can support the recovery of some neurological function after stroke or traumatic brain injury.

Introduction

The blood supply to the brain provides it with oxygen, nutrients and a means to excrete metabolic waste. If the blood supply is interrupted in any way, devastating consequences can ensue. The brain has high metabolic demands and the capacity for anaerobic metabolism is minimal; interruption of the oxygen supply for a few minutes can cause irreversible damage. The vascular system is a supporting system, and diseases of vascular origin will cause secondary alterations in other systems such as the central nervous system (CNS). Vascular disease is often identified by its characteristic temporal profile of sudden onset, with the rapid appearance of specific combinations of neurological symptoms.

A stroke, or cerebrovascular accident, is characterized by a temporary, or permanent, loss of function of brain tissue caused by disruption of the vascular supply. Brain infarctions (ischaemic stroke) account for approximately 85% of strokes, and cerebrovascular haemorrhagic accidents, such as subarachnoid or intracerebral haemorrhages, account for the remaining 15%.

Stroke is the second largest cause of death worldwide and the fourth in the UK. Approximately one third of stroke patients die within a year after stroke. In the UK, someone has a stroke every 5 min, and approximately 100,000 people have a stroke each year, 38,000 of whom will die. In the USA there are approximately 750,000 strokes per year, with 160,000 deaths. The incidence and mortality rate are higher in older patients and the mortality rate increases with subsequent strokes. There

Box 11.1 Case history

Mr Arthur Attack is a 71-year-old who arrives at Accident and Emergency accompanied by his wife. Mrs Attack says that he had just finished his fried breakfast 2 hours ago and was doing nothing in particular when suddenly, mid-conversation, he became unable to speak. Arthur appears perfectly aware of his surroundings but is unable to understand anything that his wife or the doctor say to him or write down for him. Arthur has difficulty in speaking and when he does speak the speech is unintelligible. On examination, he weighs 108 kg and is hypertensive. Neurological examination reveals increased reflexes and some weakness of his right arm and face; somatosensation on the right side of his face and arm is also absent. His doctor tells his wife that he has just had a stroke and he is immediately prescribed a drug called alteplase (t-PA). Ten days later, there has been some improvement in his condition. All sensation has returned and he is now able to understand verbal and written commands. However, he is still unable to speak properly, and the motor symptoms remain.

This case gives rise to the following questions:

1. What are the main causes of stroke?
2. What is the blood supply to the brain?
3. How does the main arterial blood supply relate to the main functional areas of the cerebral cortex?
4. What are the mechanisms underlying cell injury in stroke and how does this influence treatment?
5. What is the prognosis for this patient?

are approximately 1.2 million stroke survivors in the UK. The cost of stroke to the National Health Service in the UK is estimated to be over £3.4 billion and this is expected to rise over the next 20 years. Stroke is the single largest cause of disability, and a third of people suffering from a stroke have a long-term disability. The proportion of care home residents who have had a stroke is between 25% and 45%.

Head (or traumatic brain) injury accounts for approximately 1% of deaths in developed countries, one third of all trauma deaths and up to one half of road traffic accident-related deaths. Traumatic brain injury is the leading cause of death in young people and it increasingly affects the older population, because of the current demographic shifts that show that the world population is ageing. US studies suggest that the age-adjusted rate of hospitalization for non-fatal traumatic brain injury in the general population is 61/100,000, whereas for those aged 65 years and older this rate is 156/100,000, with falls being responsible for over 50% of cases. In the USA alone, in the 21st century, the elderly population will double to 70 million by 2030, and the costs of caring for older adults with traumatic brain injury, in monetary and human terms will be staggering, as it costs approximately 2.2 billion dollars a year to treat this population. Approximately 50 million people experience traumatic brain injury worldwide in a year and the estimated economic cost of this is approximately US$400 billion. Traumatic brain injury is, like stroke, a common cause of death and disability. The sequelae can be very long-lasting and, in many cases, permanent and life changing. In the USA there were approximately 61,000 traumatic brain injury-related deaths in 2019. In the UK, for every 100 survivors, 60% make a good recovery, 20% have minor psychiatric/psychological problems, 15% are severely disabled and 5% remain in a persistent vegetative state. The mortality rate is approximately 30 people per 100,000. There is considerable overlap in the neurological symptoms presented by patients with head injury and those with cerebrovascular disease.

This chapter describes the vascular supply to the brain and how it is visualized using angiography. Following stroke, it is important to identify the type of stroke, minimize its size and evaluate what treatment options are available to prevent the problem from reoccurring, and to maximize recovery of function after the event. Similarly, acute head injury management aims to control secondary mechanisms of injury: hypoxia, haemorrhage and raised intracranial pressure.

Physiological control of cerebral blood flow

Brain cells are dependent on aerobic metabolism for their survival; if the brain tissue is deprived of oxygen for 20 s (anoxia), an individual lapses into unconsciousness, as the affected neurons cease electrical activity. This can become irreversible if anoxia extends beyond 5 min. It takes longer for this process to occur in the brainstem and spinal cord. The brain represents approximately 2% of body weight but uses 20% of the available oxygen and 15% of the cardiac output. Blood flow is approximately 750 mL/min and this remains constant throughout the day, whether we are asleep, awake, lying down or standing up. The average blood flow is 50–55 mL/100 g of brain tissue/min. If this falls to less than 30 mL/100 g/min, ischaemia (lack of bloodborne oxygen) ensues and infarction (tissue cell death) occurs below 20 mL/100 g/min.

The factors that determine constant blood flow are blood perfusion pressure and the vascular resistance. The cerebral perfusion pressure is defined as the mean arterial pressure minus the intracranial pressure, rather than cerebral venous pressure. This is because the brain is enclosed within the skull; it is the pressure within this 'closed box' that is effectively acting on the arteries and thus is the one that opposes arterial pressure. The cerebral perfusion pressure does not always remain constant, and as mean arterial pressure is closely regulated within a narrow range, changes must occur in the cerebral vascular resistance to compensate for changes in perfusion pressure. This occurs through mechanisms intrinsic to the brain: when perfusion pressure decreases, vascular pressure decreases; if perfusion pressure increases, so does the resistance. Cerebral blood flow is kept relatively constant by several processes. Metabolic mechanisms involve the action of vasodilating agents such as adenosine, K^+, H^+ and nitric oxide (NO), which regulate arteriole size. Autoregulation is a major homeostatic mechanism whose function is to keep blood flow constant over the pressure range 60–150 mmHg. It is closely related to local metabolic processes, and uses chemical and neurogenic mechanisms to control pressure, the most important being the levels of carbon dioxide and oxygen. Hypoxia or hypercarbia cause an increase in cerebral blood flow, whereas hypocarbia causes a decrease in blood flow, by relaxing or constricting the arteriole smooth muscle. These changes are brought about by alterations in the H^+ concentration in the extracellular fluid compartment surrounding the blood vessels. Another source of autoregulation is the level of intraluminal pressure within the arterioles. Any increase in pressure produces a direct, myogenic response that is sufficient to maintain a steady state of perfusion. These processes are not controlled by the sympathetic nervous system, as drugs that affect blood pressure do not, in general, have any effect on cerebral blood flow.

Too much oxygen can also have deleterious effects on brain cells. Increased levels of extracellular oxygen can lead to the formation of free radical ions, such as superoxide (O_2^-), which can damage brain cells by the process of excitotoxicity (see later). Free radicals also destabilize neurotransmission by changing tissue pH and this can increase auto-oxidation, which can further exacerbate the toxicity. In the case of glutamate, increased extracellular accumulation of glutamate depletes antioxidant defences and thus causes oxidative glutamate toxicity.

Not all areas of the brain are equally active at the same time. Oxygen is shunted around to areas (and cells) that need it most for a particular task at a particular time, because they are more metabolically active. For example, there is relatively more blood flow to the motor cortex when someone is performing a motor task. This suggests that blood is shunted around to whichever area needs it. A consequence of this is that areas that are not actively processing information have a decreased blood flow. This observation has led to the development of brain scan techniques that measure regional cerebral blood flow to functionally active areas, following injection of a radioactive isotope of the inert gas xenon (^{133}Xe) into an artery. This was the first method used to provide detailed insight into how various brain areas function in normal and pathological conditions, because of the direct relationship between blood flow and cellular metabolic activity.

Blood supply to the brain

Blood circulation to the brain is via the anterior and posterior circulations. The anterior circulation supplies supratentorial structures (the cortex and diencephalon), whereas the posterior circulation supplies the structures in the posterior fossa (cerebellum and brainstem). Both arterial circulations initially arise from the aortic arch, but the posterior circulation enters the skull cavity through the foramen magnum, while the anterior circulation enters through the foramen lacerum (Fig. 11.1).

The anterior circulation carries 80% of the blood supply to the brain. It is derived from the internal carotid arteries (ICAs), which branch off from the common carotid arteries and enter the brain cavity through the carotid canal (in the skull vault) to emerge on its interior surface via the foramen lacerum (which is only visible in a dried skull, as in life it is filled with cartilage). The arteries make a series of stepwise turns, passing through the cavernous sinus, before emerging, on each side, next to the optic chiasm, where they divide into their major branches, the middle cerebral artery (MCA) and anterior cerebral artery (ACA). The anterior communicating artery connects the two anterior cerebral arteries. The posterior circulation comprises the vertebral, basilar and posterior cerebral arteries (PCAs) and they convey the remaining 20% of the arterial supply to the posterior fossa brain structures and inferior surface of the posterior aspects of the cortex.

The anterior and posterior circulations are connected at the base of the midbrain around the optic chiasm by a network of arteries called the circle of Willis, first described by Thomas Willis, doctor to King James II, in 1664. The arteries that form the circle of Willis are a single anterior communicating artery, a pair of ACAs, ICAs, PCAs and a pair of posterior communicating arteries (Fig. 11.2). There is a substantial amount of anatomical variation between individuals in the arrangement of this circle, due to developmental changes. During embryonic

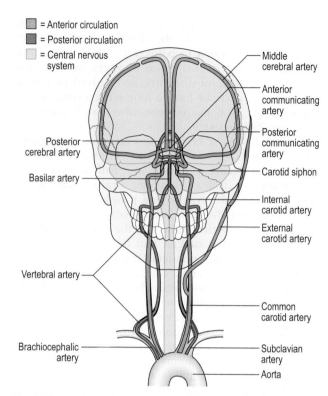

Fig. 11.1 Anterior and posterior circulation to the head. (Adapted from McNeill EM. (1997) Neuroanatomy Primer, Colour to Learn. Lippincott, Williams and Wilkins.)

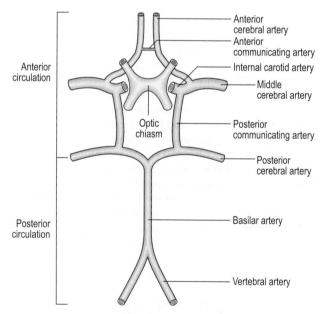

Fig. 11.2 Schematic view of the circle of Willis.

development the ICA supplies the ACA, MCA and PCA, but as the brain develops, the PCA develops from the basilar artery, as the posterior communicating artery atrophies. However, in approximately 20% of people, the embryonic pattern remains and the PCA branches off the anterior circulation. Common variations in the circle of Willis include absence of one or both posterior communicating arteries, origination of the PCAs from an enlarged posterior communicating artery or multiple small anterior communicating arteries. These anastomoses allow for a certain amount of shunting of blood from the anterior to posterior circulation, or from one side to the other in the event of arterial occlusion, but generally the anastomoses are not effective against total occlusion of one of the major supply arteries.

Main terminal branches of the anterior system

The ICA gives rise to several small branches at its proximal portion before dividing into its two main terminal branches—the MCA and ACA. The hypophysial artery forms a plexus around the pituitary stalk. The ophthalmic artery is the most proximal branch of the ICA. It supplies the orbit, the eye muscles and the retina and eventually connects to the external carotid (facial and superficial temporal) arteries through anastomoses with arteries of the forehead and nose (ethmoidal, nasal, supraorbital and supratrochlear). Occlusion of the ophthalmic artery is an important diagnostic sign in transient ischaemic attacks (TIAs) (Box 11.2). Another artery that is important in providing anastomoses between different arterial systems is the posterior communicating artery, which links the carotid and vertebral systems. Clinically, this is one of the most frequent sites for aneurysm formation, at the junction where it leaves the ICA (see later).

The MCA is the largest and most important branch of the ICA and receives 80% of the carotid blood flow (Fig. 11.3). Its proximal part gives off three deep branches. The lateral and medial striate arteries supply the striatum and the internal capsule regions of the brain. Occlusion of these deep arteries is the chief cause of classic stroke, and the most common location is the putamen and internal capsule. The anterior choroidal artery supplies parts of the limbic system, the hippocampus and amygdala in the medial temporal lobe, the posterior part of the internal capsule and the optic radiation and choroid plexus of the inferior horn of the lateral ventricle, which is important in the formation of cerebrospinal fluid (CSF). Occlusion of this artery may cause hemiparesis, hemianaesthesia, hemianopsia and loss of short-term memory.

The more distal part of the MCA travels laterally through the lateral fissure and then separates into superior and inferior branches that supply most of the lateral side of the brain (frontal, parietal, temporal and occipital regions). This ramification is known as the middle cerebral candelabra (from angiographic studies). The branches are named with respect to the cortical region that they supply (see Fig. 11.3).

The ACA supplies the medial side of the frontal and parietal lobes as far back as the parieto-occipital sulcus and overlaps onto the orbital and lateral surfaces of the brain. It winds around the genu of the corpus callosum before dividing into two main terminal branches. The callosomarginal artery supplies the cingulate and fron-

tal gyri and the paracentral lobule (Fig. 11.4). The pericallosal artery supplies the corpus callosum. On the lateral surface of the brain, its branches anastomose with terminal branches of the MCA. The ACA gives off one proximal branch, the recurrent artery of Heubner, which supplies the ventral part of the basal ganglia and the anterior limb of the internal capsule. It anastomoses with the lateral striate arteries of the MCA. Occlusion of this artery is rare but can cause 'clumsy hand' syndrome, with contralateral weakness of the arm and face.

Main terminal branches of the posterior system

The vertebral arteries originate from the subclavian and brachiocephalic arteries and pass through the transverse foraminae of the C1–C6 vertebrae, before entering the skull cavity via the foramen magnum, to travel along the ventral surface of the brainstem. The main branches are the anterior and posterior spinal arteries, which supply the spinal cord (see Chapter 4), and the posterior inferior cerebellar artery, which supplies the medulla and cerebellum. The two vertebral arteries join to form the

---

Box 11.2 Reversible strokes

There are temporary disturbances of blood flow to localized brain areas that can spontaneously resolve and leave no neurological deficits. It is important to recognize these, as they serve notice of impending major illness. Without treatment, one in four people suffer a heart attack within 5 years, and one in six suffer a stroke.

Transient ischaemic attacks (TIAs) cause temporary loss of brain function, lasting less than 30 min, with total recovery within 24 h; there is rarely loss of consciousness. It is possible to have several attacks in one day. Reversible ischaemic neurological defects are lengthy TIAs that continue for more than 12 h before symptoms resolve. It is thought that the majority of these are caused by emboli that break off atherosclerotic plaques. The diagnosis is based on symptoms alone. The symptoms mimic those of true strokes, and severe TIAs cannot be distinguished from real strokes until recovery occurs. They can occur in both the anterior and the posterior circulation. A TIA of the posterior circulation produces symptoms of vertigo, diplopia, ataxia and amnesia, whereas a TIA in the anterior circulation produces symptoms of motor weakness, hemisensory loss, dysphasia, difficulty in reading and writing, and transient monocular blindness (amaurosis fugax). This last symptom is due to occlusion of the ophthalmic artery. It is an important neurological sign, as it reflects proximal blockage of the internal carotid artery.

Ischaemic strokes and TIAs are more likely to occur early in the morning on waking up, as blood pressure is lowered during sleep. When a person gets out of bed, the sudden change in pressure can dislodge an embolism into the arterial circulation.

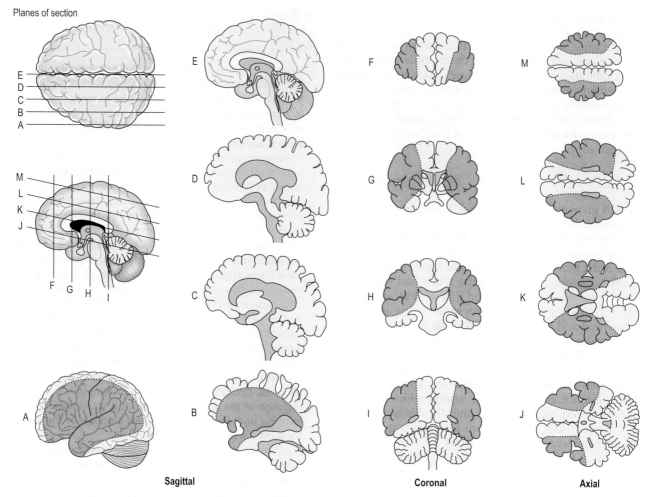

Fig. 11.3 Distribution of the middle cerebral artery in the sagittal (A–E), coronal (F–I) and horizontal (J–M) planes.

basilar artery at the pontomedullary junction. The basilar artery runs in the basilar sulcus on the ventral surface of the pons and ends at the midbrain, where it divides to form the PCA, which travels along the ventral surface of the midbrain, passing around cranial nerve III, to anastomose with the posterior communicating artery. Details of the blood supply to the brainstem are described in Chapter 6. The deep cortical branches of the PCA supply the thalamus and posterior limb of the internal capsule (via the thalamogeniculate and posterior choroidal arteries). Other branches supply the inferior and medial surfaces of the temporal lobe (limbic region) and the occipital lobe. The main terminal branches are the calcarine and parieto-occipital arteries. Terminal branches of the PCA extend onto the lateral surface of the brain to anastomose with terminal branches of the MCA (Fig. 11.5).

Venous system

Cerebral drainage is through valveless superficial and deep veins (Fig. 11.6). The superficial veins are located in the subarachnoid space above each hemisphere; they collect blood from the neocortex and subcortical white matter and empty into the cranial venous sinuses. The upper part of the hemisphere drains via the superior cerebral vein into the superior sagittal sinus, the middle part (via the inferior cerebral veins) into the cavernous sinus and the lower part into the transverse sinus. The deep cerebral veins that drain blood from the caudate nucleus and thalamus (thalamostriate and choroidal veins) join to form the internal cerebral vein on each side and these unite to form the great cerebral vein of Galen. The anterior and deep cerebral veins unite to form the basal vein, which also empties into the great cerebral vein. This pierces the tentorium cerebelli to join with the inferior sagittal sinus, which drains the falx cerebri and then joins with the straight sinus that connects to the transverse sinus. The cavernous sinus drains into the transverse sinuses via the petrosal sinuses. The two transverse, the straight and the superior sagittal sinuses, meet at the confluence of sinuses. Blood drains away 'downhill' through the transverse sinuses to the sigmoid sinus and into the internal jugular vein (at the jugular foramen). The internal jugular vein receives venous drainage from the face, scalp and neck, before draining

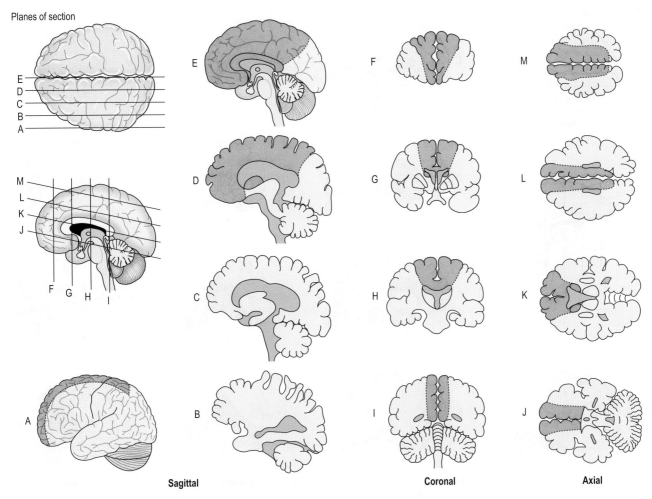

Planes of section

Sagittal   Coronal   Axial

Fig. 11.4 Distribution of the anterior cerebral artery in the sagittal (A–E), coronal (F–I) and horizontal (J–M) planes.

into the subclavian vein and returning to the heart via the brachiocephalic vein and superior vena cava.

Functional anatomy of the cerebral vasculature

Any brain dysfunction of vascular origin will result in specific clinical signs and symptoms. Thus it is essential to have a clear understanding of how the blood supply relates to the functional areas of the brain. This is shown in Fig. 11.7 and Table 11.1. It is essential to be able to distinguish whether a vascular lesion is located within the anterior or the posterior arterial systems.

Angiography

It is not possible to directly examine the cerebral blood vessels in patients (unless it is at post-mortem!). Instead, angiography is used (Fig. 11.8). This method of analysis is generally based on the principle of intravascular injection of a contrast agent, for example, iodine-based, followed by serial, time lapse imaging using X-rays or computed tomography (CT) scans. The analysis can detect three different types of abnormality: structural

abnormality due to stenosis or occlusion, alterations in blood vessel position (due to displacement by a mass lesion) and alterations in flow patterns such as those that occur in arteriovenous malformations or during stenosis or partial vessel occlusion (Figs 11.9, 11.14 and 11.15).

Stroke

Stroke is a generic term which defines neurological deficits associated with a vascular origin. Stroke is a heterogeneous condition that can be associated with a variety of causes. Examples of risk factors for stroke are detailed in Table 11.2. It is notable that many of these factors are modifiable. The genetics of stroke are complex and genetic predisposition is a non-modifiable risk factor. The heritability of stroke is of approximately 30%–40% and a substantial component of this is likely to be linked to known risk factors for stroke. Some Mendelian conditions (e.g. small vessel vasculopathies, sickle cell disease, Marfan syndrome, Fabry's disease and cerebral amyloid angiopathy) have stroke as a primary manifestation. Genome-wide association studies have identified

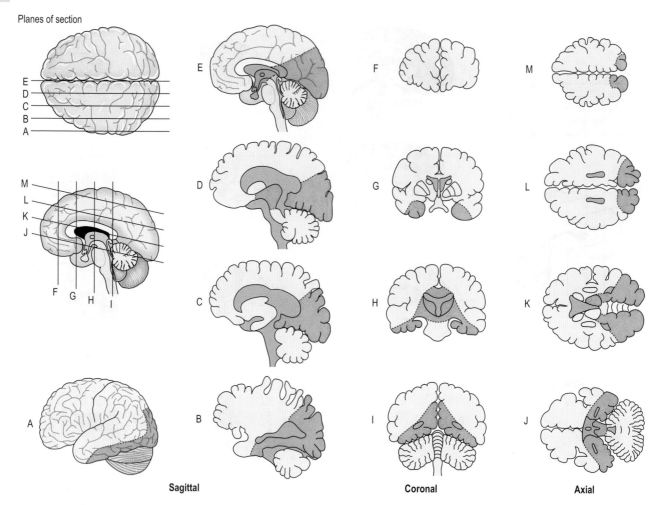

Planes of section

Sagittal   Coronal   Axial

Fig. 11.5 Distribution of the posterior cerebral artery in the sagittal (A–E), coronal (F–I) and horizontal (J–M) planes.

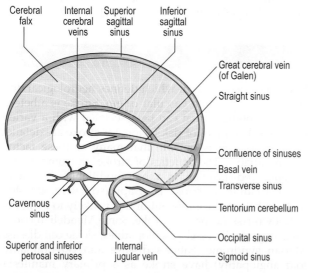

Fig. 11.6 Schematic plane of the cerebral venous circulation.

many common genetic variants associated with stroke; there are more than 35 loci associated with stroke risk. Interestingly, most of these variants occur in non-protein-coding sequences of genes.

There are two main types of stroke: ischaemic and haemorrhagic (Fig. 11.10). Each type has a different cause and both can result in the death of brain tissue. Ischaemic stroke occurs when a blood clot blocks an artery, disrupting the bloodborne supply of oxygen to the brain. It can result from stenosis or thrombosis of large or small arteries or from the presence of thromboemboli in arteries (cardioembolic events). Atrial fibrillation—a disorder of cardiac rhythm associated with atrial cardiopathy—is the leading cause of cardioembolism. Atherosclerosis is the most important cause of ischaemic stroke (Box 11.3).

Stenosis is the narrowing of an artery due to build-up of plaque material, so that blood flow becomes restricted. If 50% of the normal blood pressure is not maintained, then brain damage will occur. Very often, an ischaemic stroke is the result of a build-up of

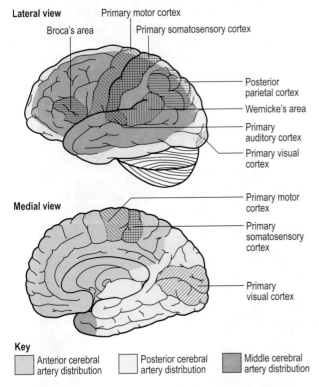

Lateral view

Broca's area
Primary motor cortex
Primary somatosensory cortex

Posterior parietal cortex
Wernicke's area
Primary auditory cortex
Primary visual cortex

Medial view

Primary motor cortex
Primary somatosensory cortex

Primary visual cortex

Key

Anterior cerebral artery distribution

Posterior cerebral artery distribution

Middle cerebral artery distribution

Fig. 11.7 Distribution of the main cerebral arteries with respect to major functional cortical areas.

Table 11.1 Functional areas associated with the main cerebral arteries

Cerebral artery	Cortical area
Anterior cerebral	Paracentral lobule: primary motor cortex and primary somatosensory cortex regions (hip to feet)
	Supplementary motor area (movement)
	Prefrontal and orbitofrontal cortex (cognition and emotion)
	Corpus callosum
	Septal nucleus (pleasure)
Middle cerebral	Frontal lobe: primary motor cortex (hip to head), premotor area, frontal eye field
	Parietal cortex: primary somatosensory cortex (hip to head), primary taste cortex
	Temporal lobe: primary auditory cortex (hearing), primary olfactory cortex (smell)
	Basal ganglia (movement initiation)
	Optic radiation (vision)
	Uncus (emotion)
	Dominant hemisphere: language centres – Wernicke's area (receptive speech) and Broca's area (expressive speech)
	Non-dominant hemisphere: contralateral awareness of self and surroundings
Posterior cerebral	Visual cortex (primary and association)
	Hippocampus (long-term memory)
	Thalamus
	Hypothalamus (autonomic function)

cholesterol and other debris in the arteries over many years. Thrombosis refers to the total blockage of a main brain artery by a blood clot (thrombus), plaque or embolus. A thromboembolism is a piece of plaque that has broken off from a thrombus elsewhere in the body, for example, the heart, and travels through the arterial system until it lodges in a brain artery, cutting off the supply beyond this point. If this occurs in the small blood vessels deep within the brain, the type of stroke is termed a lacunar stroke. The infarcts produced by this type of stroke are small (0.5–10 mm). Lacunar infarcts can also occur in the brainstem.

Classification of stroke

Stroke can be classified as stroke in evolution, where progression of neurological defects occurs over 24–48 hours, suggesting an ongoing infarct, or completed stroke, where infarction is complete and the patient's neurological deficits do not increase further. The latter is the most common type seen. The term stroke is apt because of its distinct temporal profile; for most sufferers, the symptoms come on literally 'at a stroke'. The key symptoms include a sudden numbness, weakness or paralysis on one side of the body. Signs of this may be a drooping arm, leg or eyelid; a dribbling mouth; sudden slurred speech; difficulty in finding words or understanding speech; sudden blurring, disturbance or loss of vision,

especially in one eye; dizziness; confusion; unsteadiness and/or a severe headache.

The effects of a stroke vary enormously, depending on which part of the brain is affected by the disrupted blood supply and the extent of that disruption, which in turn depends on which vessel is affected. Classification of ischaemic stroke is based on artery territory, and there are four main syndromes that correspond to different vascular territories:

1. Total anterior circulation stroke that results from occlusion of the MCA, with or without the ACA

2. Partial anterior circulation stroke that results from occlusion of branches of the MCA or isolated ACA occlusion

3. Posterior circulation stroke affecting the brainstem, cerebellum or occipital lobe

4. Lacunar stroke produced by occlusion of the deep brain (thalamostriate) arteries.

The symptoms associated with each type of stroke are detailed in Table 11.3.

The second main type of stroke is haemorrhagic stroke, when a blood vessel in or around the brain bursts, causing a bleed or haemorrhage within the skull cavity. Long-standing, untreated hypertension is the

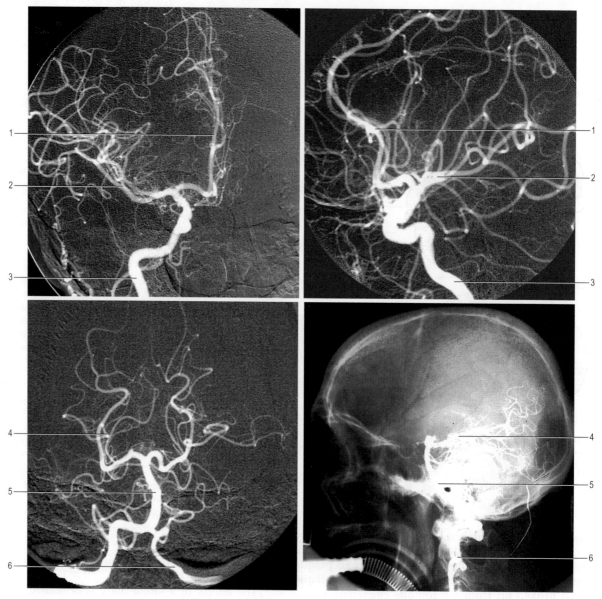

1. Anterior cerebral artery.
2. Middle cerebral artery.
3. Internal carotid artery.
4. Posterior cerebral artery.
5. Basilar artery.
6. Vertebral arteries.

Fig. 11.8 Normal angiogram of anterior (top pair) and posterior (bottom pair) circulations viewed in coronal (left) and sagittal (right) planes.

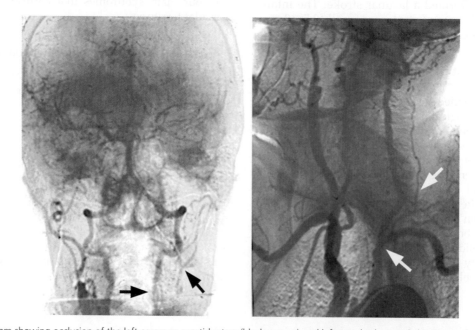

Fig. 11.9 Angiogram showing occlusion of the left common carotid artery (black arrows) and left vertebral artery (white arrows) caused by atheroma.

Table 11.2 Risk factors for stroke

Risk	Consequence
Untreated hypertension	Damages arterial walls
Atrial fibrillation	Increased risk of formation of clots in the heart that may dislodge and travel to the brain (irregular heartbeat)
Smoking	Increases blood pressure and has adverse effects on arterial walls
Diabetes	Increased risk of high blood pressure and atherosclerosis
Diet	Diets high in saturated fat lead to arterial stenosis; high salt levels are associated with raised blood pressure
Heavy drinking	Over time, excessive drinking raises blood pressure; alcohol binges can rapidly increase blood pressure, causing blood vessels to burst
Age	Strokes are more common in people older than 55 years of age, because of the gradual development of atherosclerosis; arteries become less elastic with increasing age
Sex	Men are at greater risk than women, especially if aged less than 65 years
Family history	Having a close relative with a history of stroke increases the risk, as factors such as diabetes and high blood pressure have a genetic component
Contraceptive pills	Make blood more likely to clot and/or raise blood pressure
Genetic	Numerous genetic variants associated with the main subtypes of stroke Complex interactions between predisposing genes and environmental factors
Haematological disorders	Thrombocytosis (platelet disorder that may predispose to cerebral ischaemia) Polycythemia (increases number of blood cells, leading to blood thickening) Haemophilia (blood thinning prevents it from coagulating) Sickle cell disease (causes thrombosis in young black people) Hyperuricaemia (gout; increased uric acid in the blood that may precipitate in blood and block the blood vessel)
Drug abuse	Amphetamine or cocaine abuse induce changes in the vessel tone; this leads to a rapid rise in blood pressure (minutes to hours); amphetamine is associated with haemorrhages (mostly in the subcortical white matter); cocaine is associated with ischaemic and haemorrhagic stroke
Vascular inflammatory disorders	Giant cell arteritis Systemic lupus erythematosus (inflammatory changes stimulate platelet adhesion on damaged surfaces)
Ethnic background	Asians, Africans and Afro-Caribbeans have a higher risk; this is linked to other risk factors such as high blood pressure (Africans) and diabetes (Asians)
Previous transient ischaemic attack (TIA)	20% of patients with TIA will go on to have a full-blown stroke

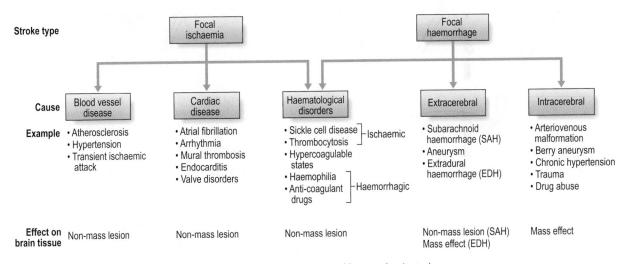

Fig. 11.10 Causes of ischaemic and haemorrhagic stroke.

Atherosclerosis

Atherosclerosis is the most important cause of ischaemic stroke. It is a generalized vascular disease of unknown aetiology, that tends to primarily affect large-calibre blood vessels, such as the carotid arteries (at their bifurcation points), and the circle of Willis at the junction of the internal carotid artery and middle cerebral artery, and vertebral and basilar arteries (Fig. 11.11).

The basic pathological lesion is the atherosclerotic plaque. Damage to the intima layer of the arterial cell wall produces focal desquamation, exposing the underlying connective tissue to circulating platelets. These aggregate and stick to the arterial wall. Aggregation causes platelets to secrete substances that, in conjunction with certain lipids, react to form a fibrous plaque that projects into the arterial lumen. With further arterial damage, this process is repeated, and the plaque enlarges, causing stenosis of the vessel (Fig. 11.12).

Because the plaque slows blood flow, a secondary consequence of this process is a thrombus that may form on the plaque. A thrombus is formed by platelets and fibrin sticking together via interactions with clotting factors that convert soluble fibrinogen to insoluble fibrin. Thrombus formation is particularly likely in veins, where blood flow rate is slower and blood pressure is lower; in addition, the presence of valves provides pockets of stagnant flow. Anything that causes hypercoagulation of the blood, such as inherited protein C or S deficiency or increased amounts of clotting factor VII or fibrinogen (as occurs in pregnancy or after surgery), increases the risk of thrombosis. If an embolus then breaks off a thrombus, it can become lodged in a distal vessel. The combination of changes in the vascular wall, reduced blood flow and increased blood coagulability are known as Virchow's triad.

Drugs such as aspirin or drugs that selectively inhibit the enzyme thromboxane synthase (which converts prostaglandin H_2 to thromboxane A_2, a potent platelet aggregator and vasoconstrictor) or stimulate the production of endothelial prostacyclins (which dilate blood vessels), are useful in preventing thromboembolism complications in atherosclerotic stroke.

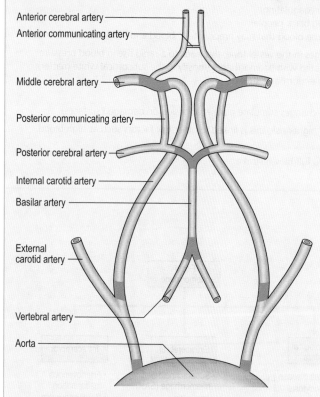

Anterior cerebral artery
Anterior communicating artery
Middle cerebral artery
Posterior communicating artery
Posterior cerebral artery
Internal carotid artery
Basilar artery
External carotid artery
Vertebral artery
Aorta

Fig. 11.11 Locations of severe atherosclerotic blockage of the anterior and posterior circulations.

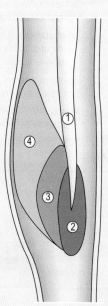

1. Tear in intima wall.
2. Formation of atheromatous plaque by circulating platelets.
3. Emboli settle on the plaque to form a mural thrombus.
4. Blood dams up behind the occlusive thrombus to form a stagnant thrombus.

Fig. 11.12 Formation of an atherosclerotic plaque.

Table 11.3 Neurological signs associated with stroke in the anterior arterial circulation or posterior arterial circulation

Stroke type	Symptoms
Total anterior circulation (high mortality long-term morbidity rates)	Contralateral flaccid hemiplegia (MCA + ACA) Contralateral hemisensory loss (MCA + ACA) Homonymous hemianopsia (MCA – anterior choroidal) Global aphasia (dominant hemisphere, MCA) Sensory neglect (non-dominant hemisphere, MCA) Dysarthria and dysphagia (MCA) Incontinence (ACA) Gait apraxia (ACA) Perception difficulties such as prosopagnosia (recognizing familiar objects or knowing how to use them). There may also be problems with abstract concepts such as telling the time Although vision may not be affected directly, it may be difficult for the brain to interpret what the eyes see Cerebral dementia involving cognitive problems such as thinking, learning, concentrating, remembering, decision-making, reasoning and planning (frontal lobes)
Partial anterior circulation	Different combinations of the above deficits, depending on which area is affected. Some of the more common ones: MCA inferior branches – receptive aphasia, constructional apraxia, expressive aphasia, neglect, perception difficulties; ACA branches – split-brain syndrome (pericallosal artery), dyspraxia
Posterior circulation	Cortical: contralateral homonymous hemianopsia, cortical blindness (visual agnosia), alexia (inability to read), amnesia, disturbances of higher mental function Brainstem: dissociated hemiparesis (ipsilateral face, contralateral body), dissociated hemisensory loss (ipsilateral face, contralateral body), diplopia, dysphagia, dysarthria, vertigo, ataxia
Lacunar	Pure motor hemiparesis (face, arm and leg weakness on one side; no other symptoms except dysarthria; lesion in internal capsule) Pure hemisensory stroke (loss of superficial sensation and paraesthesia of one side of the body; thalamic lesion) Ataxic hemiparesis (distal leg weakness, arm–leg incoordination; Babinski sign and inability to walk unaided; lesion in internal capsule, cerebellum or pons) Dysarthria and clumsy hand syndrome (moderate to severe dysarthria and clumsiness of hand movement and facial weakness on one side; lesion in internal capsule or pons)

ACA, Anterior cerebral artery; MCA, middle cerebral artery.

most common cause of this type of stroke. Intracranial arteries differ from those found elsewhere in the body, in that they are thin-walled and susceptible to blockage or rupture. Thus, untreated hypertension increases the strain on the artery walls, increasing the risk of bursting and bleeding. Onset is sudden, without warning, usually while the patient is awake. Headache is often present but is not a diagnostic feature. Loss of consciousness is also common.

There are several types of haemorrhagic stroke (see Fig. 11.10):

1. A haemorrhagic stroke may be due to an intracerebral haemorrhage, in which a blood vessel bursts within the brain itself. The blood may form a haematoma (a pool of collected blood) within the brain parenchyma (tissue), resulting in a focal mass effect (Fig. 11.13), or in existing spaces such as the subdural or subarachnoid spaces (non-mass effects). Parenchymal haemorrhages occur most frequently in the basal ganglia (50%), thalamus (10%), hindbrain (pons or cerebellum, 20%) or lobular white matter (20%). White matter strokes are often severe and cause extensive neurological deficits by disrupting the passage of axon tracts, such as the internal capsule.

2. A subarachnoid haemorrhage occurs when a blood vessel on the surface of the brain bleeds into the subarachnoid space – the area between the brain and the meninges. The most common cause is head injury (see later).

3. An aneurysm is due to a weakness of the thin-walled intima layer of arteries, that causes a localized dilatation of the artery lumen. Blood collects in these 'berry-like' swellings, called Berry aneurysms. They often occur in the circle of Willis (Fig. 11.14). Eventually, as the pressure builds, the aneurysm bursts and bleeds into the subarachnoid space, causing an increase in intracranial pressure, which can be fatal if not treated. In addition, the filling of the aneurysm balloon can lead to raised intracranial pressure by a mass effect that may cause brain damage. Normally, aneurysms go undetected and they are akin to ticking time-bombs. They may be fortuitously detected in angiograms that are performed for other reasons. If detected, they may be clipped during a neurosurgical

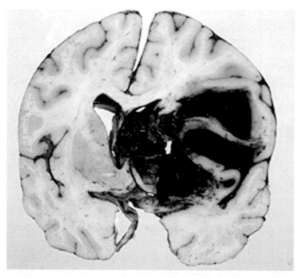
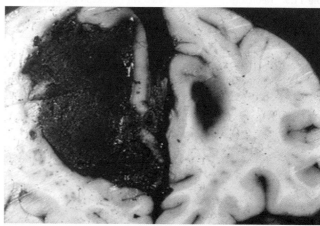

Fig. 11.13 Examples of fatal intracerebral haemorrhage. Left: infarct of the lenticulostriate arteries of the middle cerebral artery. Right: anterior cerebral artery. Both cause death through the consequences of mass effect (see text for details).

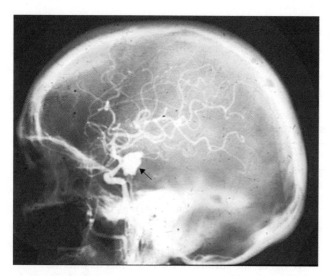

Fig. 11.14 Angiogram revealing an aneurysm (arrow) affecting the posterior cerebral artery.

operation. The classic presentation of a burst aneurysm is a sudden, severe headache, neck stiffness, vomiting and loss of consciousness. Often, there are focal neurological signs.

4. Arteriovenous malformations are congenital abnormalities that result from defective developmental communications between arteries and veins, without the intervening capillaries. They appear in angiograms as a Medusa-like tangle of distorted and contorted blood vessels (Fig. 11.15) that may be atrophied and therefore prone to rupture, or hypertrophic. Often, rapid shunting of blood occurs, producing ischaemia in neighbouring parts of the brain, which may result in tissue infarction or seizure activity.

5. Intraventricular haemorrhage is the most common neurological complication in approximately 40%

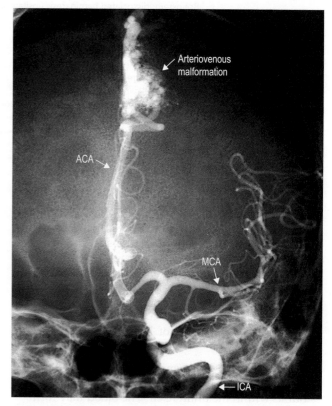

Fig. 11.15 Angiogram showing an arteriovenous malformation located in the anterior cerebral artery (ACA). *ICA*, Internal carotid artery; *MCA*, middle cerebral artery.

of premature babies (<1.5 kg body weight). The hypoxic pressure exerted on the baby's head during delivery can cause haemorrhage. The prognosis for large haemorrhages is poor, but for smaller ones it is good. Children may be left with variable degrees of neurological deficit.

Table 11.4 Clinical features of hypertensive haemorrhage

Location	Coma	Pupil reaction (to light)	Sensorimotor disturbance	Hemianopsia
Basal ganglia (putamen)	Common	Normal	Hemiparesis	Common
Thalamus	Common	Small, sluggish	Hemisensory loss	Transient
Subcortical white matter	Rare	Normal	Hemiparesis and/or hemisensory loss	Common
Cerebellum	Delayed (12–24 h)	Small, reactive	Gait ataxia	No
Pons (often fatal)	Immediate	Pinpoint, non-reactive	Quadriplegia	No

Massive haemorrhages may rupture brain tissue and leak into the ventricles, resulting in blood in the CSF. A fatal outcome occurs when brain herniation occurs, due to the mass effect of the oedema and haematoma. Clinical presentation depends on the site of the haemorrhage. The most common site for hypertensive haemorrhage is in the basal ganglia. The clinical features of hypertensive intracerebral haemorrhage in various brain regions are detailed in Table 11.4.

In the case history presented in Box.11.1, it is likely that Arthur is suffering from atherosclerosis. He has several risk factors that predispose him towards ischaemic stroke: his age, high blood pressure and the fact that he is overweight. His hypertension accelerates the atherosclerotic process and increases the risk of blood vessel damage. Additionally, in older people, the blood vessels have less elasticity, predisposing them to stenosis. The doctor is able to make the diagnosis based on the history (sudden onset) and neurological examination (in this case, it is a partial anterior circulation stroke). Whether the stroke is ischaemic or haemorrhagic cannot be reliably distinguished clinically but, as Arthur did not lose consciousness, it is more likely to be ischaemic. However, several tests and investigations can be performed to confirm the diagnosis. These are detailed in Box 11.4. Neurological impairment can be assessed using the NIH Stroke Scale (NIHSS) (Table 11.5). As a patient gradually recovers some function, the improvement can be assessed using the Barthel Index, which consists of 10 activities that specifically measure a person's daily living and mobility. These include feeding, bathing, moving from wheelchair to bed and return, grooming, transferring to and from a toilet, walking on a level surface, going up and down stairs, dressing and continence of bowels and bladder. They are weighted according to whether the person has received help while doing the task, using scores of 0 (unable), 5, 10 or 15 (independent). Middle scores imply that over 50% of the effort comes from the patient. The scores for each activity are summed to create a total score of up to 100. This is used as a record of what the patient can do independently, without help, but using aids if necessary. The assessment is used to monitor improvement in activities of daily living over time. The higher

Box 11.4 Recognizing and diagnosing stroke

The major signs of stroke can be recognized using the **FAST** system:

F for facial weakness (assessed by asking the person to smile or by observation of a drooping face or eyelid)
A for arm weakness (assessed by asking the person to raise both arms)
S for speech; is the person's speech clear and can they understand what you say?

If the person has failed any of these, then it is:

T time to call the emergency services.

At the hospital, a number of investigations can help identify the type of stroke that has occurred and the best treatment options. The precise tests will differ from person to person, but common tests performed in every stroke patient include:

- Brain scans or angiograms to determine the type and location of the stroke and to look for signs of damage. These are the most definitive diagnostic procedures currently available.
- Doppler ultrasound scans of the carotid arteries to check blood flow to the brain.
- Cerebrospinal fluid examination for diagnosing subarachnoid haemorrhage.
- Blood pressure measurement.
- Blood tests to check blood glucose, blood clotting, cholesterol levels, thyroid function, erythrocyte sedimentation rate, plasma viscosity and the presence of haematological disease.
- Chest X-ray to check for cardiac or respiratory problems.
- An electrocardiogram to measure the rhythm and activity of the heart, or an echocardiogram.

the score, the more 'independent' the person. In the UK, often the 5, 10 and 15 scores are substituted by 1, 2 and 3. This gives a potential maximum of 20 rather than 100. The modified Rankin scale (mRS) is another

Table 11.5   The NIH Stroke Scale (each examination is assessed independently from previous examinations)

Category	Score
1. Level of consciousness	
General response	0 = alert, 1 = drowsy, 2 = stupor, 3 = coma
Response to two questions	0 = both correct, 1 = one correct, 2 = none correct
Response to two commands	0 = both correct, 1 = one correct, 2 = none correct
2. Gaze	0 = normal, 1 = partial gaze palsy, 2 = forced eye deviation
3. Visual fields	0 = normal, 1 = bilateral quadrantonopia, 2 = homonymous hemianopsia, 3 = cortical blindness
4. Facial movement	0 = normal, 1 = minor paresis, 2 = partial paresis, 3 = complete palsy
5. Motor function: arms, legs	0 = no drift, 1 = minor drift, 2 = some effort against gravity, 3 = no effort against gravity, 4 = no movement
6. Limb ataxia	0 = absent, 1 = unilateral presence in arm or leg, 2 = unilateral presence in arm and leg or bilateral, 9 = untestable (no motor function or coma)
7. Sensory	0 = normal, 1 = mild loss, 2 = severe loss (unilateral)
8. Language (aphasia)	0 = none, 1 = expressive or receptive aphasia (mild–moderate), 2 = global aphasia (severe), 3 = mute
9. Dysarthria	0 = normal articulation, 1 = mild–moderate, 2 = unintelligible, 9 = untestable
10. Neglect	0 = none, 1 = partial (can recognize stimuli on right or left but not both), 2 = complete (bilateral neglect)

example of a scoring tool that can also be used to measure disability and functional impairment, and their evolution in time after a stroke.

Mechanisms of cell injury in ischaemic stroke

The brain has a very high rate of oxidative metabolism. Anaerobic metabolism in the brain is negligible and, consequently, the brain is extremely vulnerable to hypoxic damage. Cell death occurs in stroke because of anoxia and the resultant loss of ability of cells to maintain the integrity of the cell membrane and ion gradients, through the activity of the energy-dependent ATPase pumps. The pathophysiological consequences of stroke involve a complex sequence of events. The main mechanisms involved include excitotoxicity, oxidation, inflammation and programmed cell death, and the molecular pathways for these have been extensively studied (Fig. 11.16). These processes evolve over time (Fig. 11.17) and set up several vicious circles that ultimately lead to brain tissue loss. The mechanisms involved are different in different areas of the stroke region: at the site of infarct—the core region—hypoxia is most severe and brain tissue rapidly dies. Surrounding the core is an area called the ischaemic penumbra, where there is residual blood flow and where brain cells undergo potentially reversible injury associated with metabolic failure. These cells have not yet entered signal cascades that lead to cell death. The size of the penumbra is variable. The importance of this penumbra where cell damage may be reversible, is that drugs that target the key players of the pathophysiological cascade may be able to protect the penumbra and so

limit the extent of functional deficit. This is the general principle underlying the concept of neuroprotection.

When the brain becomes hypoxic, ATP levels start to fall and the ATP-dependent Na^+ pumps in the neuronal and glial cell membranes become dysfunctional. The Na^+ that enters the cells, either during action potentials or because of the ongoing leaks in the membrane, cannot be pumped out, causing membrane depolarization. This creates an inward osmotic force, as the influx of Na^+ (and Cl^-) is much greater than the efflux of K^+ and the cells swell due to the passive influx of water, causing oedema. Cells eventually burst, as the cell membrane fails; this is necrotic cell death. The brain is encased in a rigid box—the skull—so if the neurons start to swell, this will increase intracranial pressure, leading to compression of the cerebral blood vessels. Compression of the vessels, especially the veins, reduces the blood flow and hence further decreases the oxygen supply. A vicious circle is set up, that leads to a rapid decline in cerebral perfusion. Brain oedema is one of the earliest events in stroke (or head injury, as discussed later) and its magnitude is one of the major factors that determine whether the patient will survive beyond the first few hours.

The reuptake process that removes glutamate from the synaptic cleft and stabilizes glutamatergic transmission is also energy-intensive and requires ATP. As soon as oxygen levels fall and ATP levels decline, the reuptake process slows down. Consequently, glutamate begins to accumulate in the synaptic cleft and, with the associated rise in extracellular K^+, further depolarization of cells may occur. This leads to more hyperexcitability and more glutamate release, and yet another vicious circle.

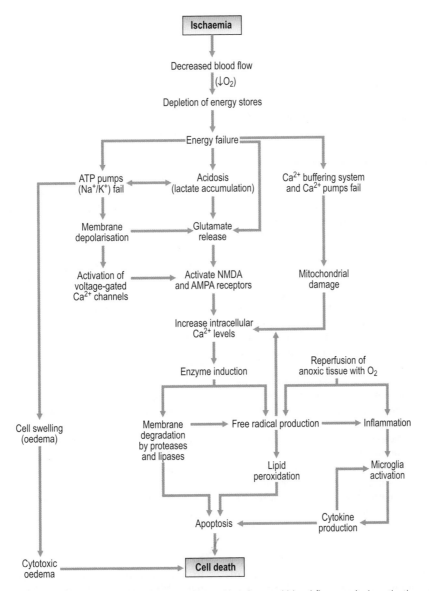

Fig. 11.16 Mechanisms contributing to neurotoxicity in ischaemia. Disruption of normal blood flow results in activation of multiple and complex signal cascades that ultimately result in cell death. The key event is excitotoxicity, leading to increased intracellular Ca^{2+} levels, which result in the generation and activation of free radicals that damage the cells and cause further inflammatory responses. Paradoxically, reperfusion of ischaemic tissue with oxygen can also lead to neuronal damage—reperfusion injury—by causing free radical formation. *AMPA,* 4-amino-3-hydroxy-5-methyl-4-isoxazole propionic acid; *NMDA,* N-methyl-D-aspartate. (Adapted from De Kayser J, et al. (1999) Trends in Neuroscience 22:535–539.)

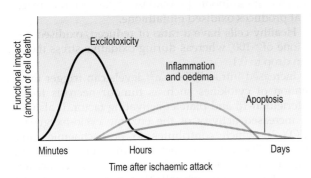

Fig. 11.17 Time course of pathophysiological changes occurring in ischaemic stroke. In the earliest stages, excitotoxic mechanisms damage both neurons and glial cells and contribute to the genesis of inflammation and cell death. (Adapted from Dirnagl U, et al. (1999) Trends in Neuroscience 22:391–397.)

Activation of the N-methyl-D-aspartate (NMDA) glutamate receptor leads to Ca^{2+} influx into neurons. A number of factors normally tightly regulate this receptor, so that Ca^{2+} entry into neurons is closely controlled. Excessive extracellular glutamate levels lead to prolonged neuronal depolarization via 4-amino-3-hydroxy-5-methyl-4-isoxazole propionic acid (AMPA) receptors, which in itself is not harmful. However, the depolarization of the postsynaptic cell also activates the NMDA receptor (which is held inactive at normal resting potentials by the Mg^{2+} block of the receptor) and this in turn leads to further Ca^{2+} entry. This is where critical processes are triggered, due to Ca^{2+} overload, as the Ca^{2+} buffering systems of neurons, mitochondria and the endoplasmic reticulum fail. The rise in internal Ca^{2+} level activates many second messenger systems, which all

Box 11.5   The role of nitric oxide in stroke

Nitric oxide (NO) is produced from arginine via the enzyme nitric oxide synthase (NOS). There are several isoforms of NOS, and NO can also be produced through a NOS-independent mechanism. NO is a gaseous compound with powerful vasodilator properties. The well-known therapeutic actions of nitrates or nitrites given to angina sufferers are likely due to formation of NO and the strong vasodilator action on coronary arteries. NO is also a vasodilator of cerebral blood vessels; NOS is expressed in the endothelial cells lining cerebral blood vessels. Blockade of NO synthesis reduces cerebral blood flow and attenuates the response of cerebral vessels to hypercapnia. However, there are problems with the hypothesis that NO is the intrinsic cerebral vasodilator control substance. If this were the case, NO levels would be expected to increase during cerebral hypoxia, as this is known to be a powerful stimulant of cerebral vasodilatation. However, blockade of NO synthesis does not block hypoxia-induced vasodilatation in the brain. In fact, rather than NO production being part of a protective mechanism against hypoxia, there is considerable evidence that the opposite may be true: release of NO in some cases appears to be a fundamental step in the excitotoxic response. Following cerebral hypoxia, NO reacts with the superoxide anion to form peroxynitrite, which destroys cell membranes. NO also decreases the activity of superoxide dismutase (which inactivates the superoxide anion).

If NO is part of a mechanism that supports oxygen delivery in neurons, why is it also involved in the excitotoxic mechanisms of cell death? There are three different isoforms of NOS—neuronal, endothelial and inducible (found in macrophages)—and they have different functions. Endothelial NOS normally functions as a vasodilator. Increases in endothelial NOS levels that occur in stroke may contribute to reperfusion-induced cell death through production of NO, which can interact with free radical ions.

Neuronal NOS is found in a small proportion of neurons and is upregulated in cells after stroke. Glutamate activates neuronal NOS via Ca^{2+} influx. Here, NOS can act as a death mediator. Interestingly, NOS-expressing neurons appear to be unusually resistant to hypoxic damage, and so the NO released by these cells during extreme hypoxia may cause the death of others. Could the excess NO released during hypoxia act as a selective 'culling' process, so that when life-threatening levels of hypoxia occur, some neurons are actively sacrificed before others? Not all cells in any one brain area may have the same importance to the organism. Cells that have a history of high levels of activity might have high levels of intracellular reducing agents such as vitamin C or glutathione, which would initially protect them from the consequences of NO attack. In contrast, cells that had been relatively inactive before the hypoxia would have less biochemical protection and might be the first to die. In such a way, the brain could attempt a 'damage limitation exercise' to protect the cells that have been most active in the past from the effects of a hypoxic crisis.

NOS inhibitors show neuroprotective effects in animal models of ischaemia, and thus offer a therapeutic option for stroke treatment. However, none of the few clinical trials that have assessed these inhibitors so far has shown a beneficial outcome.

demand energy in the form of ATP or other substrates. However, because of hypoxia, this energy is not available. Disruption of neuronal Ca^{2+}-induced processes leads to the formation of free radicals, such as the superoxide anion (O_2^-), via the activation of NO production (Box 11.5). These free radicals are very reactive and initiate cell damage by reacting with many cell components (e.g. a lipid peroxidation reaction). This eventually damages the cell so badly that it undergoes necrosis (see Fig. 11.17). Thus, glutamate toxicity is a prominent cause of necrotic cell death.

The brain has a number of natural defence molecules to protect against free radical damage. These molecules are reducing agents. They prevent other molecules being oxidized and react with free radicals or oxidizing agents to form inert products. Three of the most important protectors are vitamin C (ascorbic acid), vitamin E (α-tocopherol) and glutathione. Vitamin C is a powerful water-soluble reducing agent that is present in high levels in the CNS, in both neurons and glial cells, and is also found in the CSF. Vitamin C is released into the CSF by neuronal depolarization, and also by increases in neuronal activity. Its CSF levels rise sharply following

ischaemic hypoxia, and this may be a protective measure to 'mop up' free radicals produced by hypoxic metabolism. Vitamin E is a lipid-soluble reducing agent that eliminates free radicals in cell membranes and other lipid-rich structures and acts synergistically with vitamin C. Glutathione is a tripeptide that can exist as a reduced or oxidized form (the latter is a dimer molecule). The enzyme glutathione peroxidase catalyses the reaction that produces oxidised glutathione.

Healthy cells have a ratio of reduced/oxidised glutathione of >100, whereas during oxidative stress the ratio can drop to 0.1.

Increased intracellular Ca^{2+} levels can trigger the formation of cytokines such as tumour necrosis factor-α, interleukin-1β and platelet-activating factor. It also leads to increased activity of the enzyme cyclo-oxygenase 2 (COX-2), which contributes to postischaemic inflammation. The cytokines activate microglia, which then release more cytokines, glutamate and other neurotoxins and attract immune cells that express inducible nitric oxide synthase (iNOS). High intracellular Ca^{2+} levels also damage mitochondria (with subsequent disruption of energy metabolism) and induce apoptosis (cell suicide programmes) via activation of caspases, particularly within the penumbra region. The apoptotic mechanism operates on a slower time scale, occurring over a period of hours to days after the initial focal ischaemic event (see Fig. 11.16). Apoptotic cells do not swell and burst; in this mode of cell death, they shrivel and implode. The initial necrosis and the more delayed apoptosis are only two examples of the various types of cell death associated with injury.

Stroke management: the acute phase, neuroprotection and prevention

There are various dimensions linked to the management of a stroke patient: (1) acute intervention after a stroke and neuroprotection, (2) support during the recovery period and (3) prevention against recurrence of stroke. Prevention can also be implemented from the perspective of reducing the risk of stroke occurring in the first instance, that is, primary prevention.

The acute management of haemorrhagic stroke involves control of the bleeding and limitation of the risk of dangerously high intracranial pressure, because of the pooling of fluid. Surgery may be required to evacuate the blood, control the intracranial pressure and also repair the damaged vessel at the origin of the haemorrhage.

In the acute phase of an ischaemic stroke there are two main approaches: thrombolysis and thrombectomy. Intravenous thrombolysis is the first intervention, based on the use of a recombinant tissue plasminogen activator (alteplase; t-PA), which is the only available compound that can be used at present in the acute phase and that has been shown to improve outcome. The drug cleaves plasminogen and produces plasmin, a fibrinolytic enzyme that breaks down the blood clot. The intravascular infusion of t-PA must start generally within 4.5 h of the stroke onset and presentation of symptoms (although in patients where there is demonstrable evidence of salvageable tissue beyond this time, it could be used up to 9 h after onset). Thrombolysis intervention attempts to reperfuse tissue, as severely compromised tissue in the penumbra, which is still viable, could be rescued by fast reperfusion. However, due to its limited therapeutic time frame, it is only used in a minority of stroke patients, as the majority of stroke patients do not have fast access to a specialist team. Only approximately 15%–60% of acute stroke patients arrive at the hospital within 3 hours after the onset of symptoms. The other approach for acute intervention is thrombectomy, a mechanical removal of the clot. During this procedure, a clot-removing device is inserted through a catheter (usually in the groin) into the affected vessel, to pull out the clot. This procedure is only used to treat patients with clots in large vessels. Most patients are treated within 6 h of symptoms onset, although in some cases thrombectomy can be carried out up to 24 h after onset. Thrombectomy does not significantly reduce overall mortality but reduces disability in stroke survivors. Patients can return home earlier and there are reduced hospital and social care costs. A new interesting development in the stroke field is the introduction of mobile stroke units, which are modified ambulances where a CT scan can be performed and thromboplasty can be implemented. This expedites the process of diagnosis and treatment, improves the triage decision making and increases the overall efficiency of management; it also reduces the pressure on admissions to emergency services.

For both thromboplasty and thrombectomy, it is important to note that reperfusion of the ischaemic tissue may lead to a phenomenon known as 'reperfusion injury' – a paradoxical triggering of processes which can further injure tissue. One of the most critical consequences of introducing oxygen in tissue by restoring blood flow is the enhanced generation of reactive oxygen species (ROS). These can directly damage cells and also activate an inflammatory reaction, increase leucocyte adhesion and activate platelets, which can then aggregate. Neuroprotective drugs are aimed at preventing or reducing secondary cell death in the penumbra region. Such drugs might also be valuable against reperfusion-linked injury. Although much is now known about the molecular pathways of apoptosis, excitotoxicity, neuroinflammation and oxidative stress, clinically effective neuroprotective treatments remain elusive. Numerous drugs that were shown in animal models of stroke to be neuroprotective have failed to achieve their preclinical promise in phase III clinical trials (Box 11.6 and Table 11.6) in terms of improving neurological and functional deficits, therefore no neuroprotective agents are used at present in the acute management of stroke patients. Some of the reasons for the repeated failures are probably that the trials often used drugs to target *one* specific pathway of the pathophysiology cascade, which may be insufficient, and/or the intervention time window was not optimized. It is possible that using combinations of clot-lysing drugs and neuroprotective drugs could achieve synergistic effects in the salvage of the penumbra. Therefore, the search for new drugs that offer neuroprotection acutely after stroke continues.

For prevention, drugs that treat accessory conditions, such as angiotensin-converting enzyme (ACE) inhibitors and diuretics, for the management of hypertension, reduce the risk of stroke. Statins (HMG-CoA reductase inhibitors) are a family of drugs that reduce cholesterol levels by blocking its synthesis. They do have a very rare and important side effect, in that they cause myopathy, resulting in muscle pain and weakness. Statins reduce the risk of stroke by 20%–30%. For people who have already suffered a stroke, secondary prevention measures are required. Individuals are strongly advised to change their lifestyle in order to reduce the relevant risk factors (see Table 11.2). Other preventive measures include administration of agents that prevent platelet aggregation and blood coagulation. Oral anti-coagulation is the therapy of choice for primary and secondary stroke prevention in patients

Box 11.6 Neuroprotection: an elusive goal

Neuroprotection of the penumbra and also of the tissue affected by reperfusion-linked injury, is a worthwhile goal in stroke. However, several decades of work in experimental models of stroke have failed to deliver neuroprotectants that could be used in the clinic in the acute phase of stroke. The question often asked is why? Is it the drug, the trial design or the experimental models used, that led to failure? The answer is probably all three. Animal models of ischaemia generally fall into one of two categories: reversible or permanent. In stroke patients, both types occur, so that animal models never really mimic the clinical situation. Preclinical models use standardized methods to evoke reproducible ischaemic lesions in healthy young animals, whereas the typical stroke patient is usually elderly, with numerous risk factors and complicating diseases such as hypertension or heart disease. Therefore, animal models need to reflect the human condition more accurately. Additionally, in clinical trials, young and old patients are often grouped together, as are the types of stroke that they present with. Thus it is not surprising that no benefit is demonstrated when a drug designed to target a very specific pathophysiological mechanisms is given to such a heterogeneous population of patients. It is becoming increasingly apparent that a drug treatment targeting a single mechanism may not be applicable to all stroke types; the relative weighting of the various components of the pathophysiology cascade may differ between patients. Doses of drugs that are neuroprotective in animal models often have adverse effects in humans. Good examples of these are anti-excitotoxicity drugs such as the NMDA receptor antagonists. These induce psychotomimetic effects such as delirium, hallucinations, paranoia, catatonia and sedation, which preclude their use. In some instances the dose is reduced to suboptimal levels because of overemphasis on safety aspects and this may lead to compromising efficacy. Additionally, the time window for intervention is often very hard to define and extrapolate from animals to humans, therefore it is not known how long neuroprotective therapies should be continued for. Most preclinical observations also indicate that combinations of clot-lysing drugs and neuroprotective drugs have synergistic effects. Thus, drug combinations that promote cell survival and target multiple pathways, in combination with thrombolysis or thrombectomy, may prove to be the way forward in treating stroke in the acute phase. Some of the most promising recent trials with potentially neuroprotective agents in stroke, such as the immunomodulator fingolimod or statins such as atorvastatin, consider the use of thrombolysis and thrombectomy, thus providing a more integrated analysis of efficacy in a real pragmatic clinical context.

It is also important to note that the analysis of outcomes in animal and human studies is different. In animal models, infarct size is most often quantified histologically so that the effect of a drug can be evaluated, usually over a short time span. Behavioural improvement is often not assessed in the chronic phase after experimental stroke. In contrast, in humans, neurological and functional scores are very important. The National Institutes of Health Stroke Scale (NIHSS, Table 11.5) and the Barthel index or the modified Rankin scale, are commonly used at 3 or 6 months after stroke. Recent evidence suggests that the NIHSS score strongly predicts outcome; patients who score 6 or less at 3 months have a good outcome, whilst those that score 16 or more are likely to die or have severe disability. These scores and scales may be less amenable to statistical analysis and may be less sensitive than anatomical markers of infarct size. The latter can be assessed with the use of sophisticated imaging methods such as positron emission tomography and diffusion-weighted and perfusion magnetic resonance imaging, to measure the penumbra and infarct size before and after treatment.

Finally, recent clinical trials which are reporting encouraging results for neuroprotection in stroke are reconsidering old targets, but from a new perspective. For example, the NMDA receptor is targeted not using a classical antagonist approach but using a very specific disruption of the connection of the NMDA receptor subunit GluN2B, to the formation of nitric oxide (NO) (a mechanism which exacerbates toxicity after activation of the NMDA receptor). This disruption, achieved through a small peptide—nerinetide—appears to have beneficial effects, according to the first exploratory clinical trials. Such novel approaches, with more specificity, may lead to much more success in the future.

with atrial fibrillation. Heparin, warfarin or newer drugs such as apixaban (an inhibitor of Factor Xa in the coagulation cascade) can be given to such patients. Aspirin inhibits the enzyme COX and chronic treatment with low dose aspirin (e.g. 75–300 mg/day) reduces the relative risk of stroke by 25% in those who have already had a TIA or stroke. For the prevention of non-cardioembolic ischaemic stroke, antiplatelet agents rather than oral anti-coagulation are recommended to reduce the risk of recurrent stroke. Aspirin monotherapy, the combination of aspirin and extended-release dipyridamole (a nucleoside transport inhibitor and a phosphodiesterase inhibitor) and clopidogrel (a drug that leads to inhibition of the purinergic receptors $P2Y_{12}$ involved in the activation of platelets), used as monotherapy, are acceptable options.

Stroke remains a major public health problem worldwide, and its impact will increase in the decades to come, because of the change in demographics and the increasing ageing population. Better preventive treatment and a much-improved management in the acute phase remain important goals.

Table 11.6 Examples of drugs explored for acute neuroprotection in clinical studies in stroke

Target or Mechanism	Drug
Ca^{2+} channels	Nimodipine (L-type channel blocker)
Glutamate receptors (NMDA type)	Selfotel (competitive receptor antagonist)
GABA$_A$ receptors	Clomethiazole (GABA$_A$ positive allosteric modulator)
Free radical scavenging	Tirilazad Ebselen
Cell membrane stabilisation	Citicholine
Neurotrophic effects	Cerebrolysin (mixture of peptides)
Anti-inflammatory effects	Minocycline Anakinra (IL-1 receptor antagonist)

NMDA, N-methyl-D-aspartate; GABA, γ-aminobutyric acid; IL-1, interleukin-1

Rehabilitation of stroke patients

At least one-third of stroke patients who survive the initial event are left with considerable disability. Recovery from disabling stroke can take at least 3–12 months. The length of time varies widely from person to person. Some of this is due to spontaneous resolution of acute problems such as oedema, compensatory brain plasticity and the effects of drugs that rescue cells in the penumbra. It is now recognized that patients recovering in specialist stroke units, as opposed to general wards, make a better recovery. This is because of the availability of specialist multidisciplinary teams that aim to optimize each patient's recovery and maximize the plasticity of the intact brain.

The purpose of rehabilitation is to help people re-learn skills that they have lost (reablement), learn new skills and find ways to manage any permanent disabilities that they may have been left with.

Medical rehabilitation involves a problem-solving process focused upon disability and handicap by:

1. Assessment, which aims to discover the level of disability, prognostic factors and the patient's goals.

2. Goal planning, which covers the areas of accommodation, personal support and social role of the patient. This is an essential part of the rehabilitation process and should be discussed by the patient, family and carers.

3. Intervention, which tries to reduce the risk of subsequent attacks by addressing potentially treatable risk factors (see Table 11.2).

4. Evaluation by neurological examination.

A rehabilitation programme includes methods designed to help with posture, balance and movement, together with specialist help for specific difficulties such as speech and language. Many different professionals may be involved in this, but the patient's motivation and efforts are equally important. Key experts include doctors and nurses (specialist stroke nurses or community nurses) to oversee medical management; physiotherapists to help with problems of posture and movement; occupational therapists to help with everyday activities at home, leisure and work; speech and language therapists to help with communication problems and clinical psychologists to help with problems affecting mental processes and emotions. As well as reablement, the patient needs resettlement, which may involve adaptation or alteration of their environment (housing and social lifestyles) and involve other professionals such as social workers and dieticians.

Prognosis for recovery

It is imperative that patients receive medical treatment as soon as possible after stroke. Time is of the essence, as the faster the treatment initiation, the better the probability of saving more brain tissue and reducing functional deficits. The initial aim is to stabilize the condition, control blood pressure and prevent the acute complications of stroke, such as aspiration pneumonia or immobility; these account for 35% of acute deaths. The doctor may prescribe drugs designed to prevent a further stroke and to treat any underlying conditions such as high blood pressure or high cholesterol levels.

The brain is capable of great plasticity. In the weeks and months following a stroke, many partially damaged cells recover and start to work again. Meanwhile, other unaffected parts of the brain take over tasks previously performed by the brain cells that are destroyed. This is part of the aim of rehabilitation. The length of time it takes to recover varies widely from person to person. It is common to have an initial spurt of recovery in the first few weeks after the stroke. In general, most of the recovery takes place during the first year to 18 months, but many people continue to improve over a much longer period, especially with sustained rehabilitation.

It is now recognized that patients who suffer small haemorrhagic strokes often make a better recovery than those with ischaemic stroke. Haematomas more often irritate brain tissue rather than physically damage it. The brain absorbs some of the blood from these haemorrhages and, as it does so, the affected area heals and begins to function again, making it possible for normal function to be completely regained after small haemorrhagic strokes.

Head injury

Traumatic head injuries can occur over a wide range of severities. Very severe head injuries involve forces incompatible with life and death is immediate. With most severe head injuries, however, there is a variable

Box
11.7 Brain swelling and raised intracranial pressure

Cerebral swelling after head injury may be caused by either cerebral oedema or vascular haemorrhage. There are three types of cerebral oedema:

1. Vasogenic. This is due to accumulation of water outside cells, as a result of disruption of the blood–brain barrier. After trauma, damaged plasma constituents move into the extracellular space, causing the extracellular compartment to increase in volume, leading to brain swelling.
2. Cytotoxic. As the brain swells due to vasogenic oedema, the tissue becomes ischaemic, cell membranes become damaged and Na^+/K^+ pumps fail to maintain the membrane ionic gradient. Intracellular Na^+ accumulation leads to cell swelling, resulting in cytotoxic oedema.
3. Interstitial. This is a consequence of an increase in the volume of the extracellular fluid in the absence of disruption to the blood–brain barrier, for example, due to insufficient antidiuretic hormone secretion.

In the context of head trauma, vasogenic and cytotoxic oedema are important.

The cranial vault contains the brain and meninges, cerebrospinal fluid and the vascular supply, within a fixed volume. Any increase in volume of one of these must occur at the expense of the others, if the pressure is to remain unchanged. Any uncompensated increase in volume of any of the constituents causes raised intracranial pressure. While raised intracranial pressure is always seen with space-occupying lesions, pressure may rise in the absence of a mass lesion. Brain swelling and hydrocephalus are the two most common generalized causes of raised intracranial pressure.

The brain is only perfused because systemic arterial pressure is higher than intracranial pressure. As intracranial pressure rises, blood flow to the brain decreases, unless the arterial pressure rises in compensation. This compensatory rise does occur when intracranial pressure starts to rise, but cerebral perfusion rapidly falls off as intracranial pressure rises still higher. Tissue ischaemia then leads to cytotoxic oedema and therefore more swelling.

Rising intracranial pressure causes a number of non-specific symptoms, including headache (from stretching and distortion of dura and blood vessels), vomiting (from pressure on the floor of the fourth ventricle), papilloedema (from pressure on the optic nerve sheath) and falling consciousness levels (from pressure on the diencephalon and upper brainstem).

period of survival and the usual cause of death is raised intracranial pressure (Box 11.7) as a result of either brain swelling or a haemorrhage accumulating inside the skull, which distorts the brain and damages vital structures (see Box 11.7). Posttraumatic disability depends on the location and amount of brain damage; the most usual neuropathological causes of long-term disability after a head injury are damage to axons and hypoxic–ischaemic damage sustained at the time of injury.

There are two important mechanisms involved in head injury which have significant consequences for brain tissue: the impact to the head and the movement of the brain, resulting in slightly different patterns of injury. In the human situation, of course, there is almost always impact, with variable amounts of brain movement. Because excessive movement alone can damage the brain, it is important to remember that it is not necessary for the head to hit anything for a severe brain injury to occur.

As a function of the severity of the injury, the patients may present a wide variety of symptoms, for example, nausea and vomiting, headache, confusion, paralysis, dilated pupils, vision changes, dizziness and balance problems, breathing problems, body numbness, seizures and loss of consciousness. The symptoms associated with traumatic brain injury can appear immediately following injury or develop days to weeks later; as a result of the injury, patients can develop a wide range of physical and psychological deficits including major motor impairment, secondary epilepsy, personality change and cognition and memory impairment. It is also now well established that even a single brain injury can significantly increase the risk of developing neurodegenerative diseases later in life, such as Alzheimer's disease. Traumatic brain injury is thus one of the strongest risk factors for dementia.

The severity of head injury is assessed in several ways: by the level of consciousness (Box 11.8), by pupil reactions to light and by neurological and radiological investigations. The Glasgow Coma Scale (GCS) is an important indicator of head injury severity and is used to clinically assess the degree of coma (Table 11.7). This method is easily reproducible and very useful for monitoring changes in the level of consciousness. The GCS score is calculated based on the patient's eye-opening and verbal and best motor responses. Scores in each category range from 1 (no response) to a maximum of between 4 and 6 (for a normal response) and are summed to give a score ranging between 3 and 15. Patients with a score of <8 are in coma and have a severe head injury. A score of 9–12 indicates a moderate head injury and a score >12 indicates a mild head injury. The GCS has prognostic value, as the scores both immediately after the injury and 24 hours later correlate with the degree of long-term impairment.

The brain tissue damage seen in head injury is classified in a number of ways. Clinically, the most useful is as focal or diffuse injury (Table 11.8). Focal injury indicates pathology that can be seen on a CT or magnetic resonance imaging (MRI) scan and which may be neurosurgically treatable. Diffuse brain injury refers to microscopic

Basic mechanisms of consciousness and coma

There are two separate components to consciousness: being awake or alert, and being aware. In order to be fully conscious, a person needs to have both an intact ascending reticular activating system in the brainstem and a functioning cerebral cortex.

Coma is a state of unrousable unresponsiveness, caused by damage to either the diencephalon/midbrain or the hemispheres. After head injury, it may be due to:

- generalized brain swelling causing pressure on the reticular formation
- temporal lobe herniation through the tentorial notch that compresses or distorts the midbrain
- traumatic damage to axons (which effectively leads to deafferentation of the cortex)
- severe hypoxic damage to neurons in the cortex (e.g. from cardiac arrest or impaired cerebral perfusion).

Concussion, in contrast, is a reversible state of unconsciousness of brief duration. Recent research has shown that concussion, as a single episode or repetitive occurrence, although apparently rather innocuous in the acute phase, can have significant consequences in terms of tissue changes and increased risk of developing neurodegenerative disease (see main text).

Table 11.7 The Glasgow Coma Scale

Category	Score
Eye-opening response	
Spontaneous	4
On command	3
In response to pain	2
None	1
Verbal response	
Speaks freely, coherently and purposefully	5
Speaks in a confused, disoriented fashion	4
Uses inappropriate words	3
Makes incomprehensible sounds	2
No response	1
Best motor response	
Obeys commands freely	6
Makes purposeful movements in response to noxious stimuli	5
Withdraws from noxious stimuli	4
Shows flexion after noxious stimuli (decorticate posturing)	3
Shows extension after noxious stimuli (decerebrate posturing)	2
No response	1

damage that cannot be demonstrated with standard imaging techniques, but which clinicians diagnose because they have an unconscious patient whose scan shows very little obvious damage. A CT scan is the gold standard for the first assessment after admission. It is easy to perform and detects fractures and the presence of blood. MRI is not commonly used for acute head injury since it takes longer to perform, is logistically more complicated and more impractical. However, once a patient is stabilized, it can reveal lesions that were not detected on the CT scan.

The response of the brain to injury and the quality of the recovery may be at least partly influenced by certain genetic variations. Genes of interest in traumatic brain injury include genes encoding cytokines such as interleukin (IL)-6, the neurotrophin brain-derived neurotrophic factor (BDNF) or the lipid-binding protein apolipoprotein E (ApoE) and also mitochondrial genes or genes associated with specific neurotransmitter pathways (e.g. dopamine and serotonin). Much attention has been focused on apoE because of its link with Alzheimer's disease. In the nervous system, ApoE acts as a carrier for cholesterol, and it has been reported that the ε4 allele of the gene may confer a less favourable recovery after brain injury. Overall, there is still a clear need for large, adequately powered genome-wide association studies, with appropriate corrections for non-genetic covariates that may influence outcome, before drawing firm conclusions as to the critical role of specific genes.

Table 11.8 Patterns of damage during head injury

Damage	Example
Focal damage	
Scalp	Contusions (bruises) Lacerations
Skull	Fracture
Meninges	Extradural and subdural haemorrhages
Brain	Contusions and lacerations Intracerebral (parenchymal) haemorrhage Axonal damage
Diffuse damage	
Brain	Diffuse axonal injury Hypoxic–ischaemic damage Diffuse brain swelling

Focal pathology in relation to vascular injury

Skull fractures

A skull fracture (Fig. 11.18A) is of relevance because it is an indication of the force of the impact on the head.

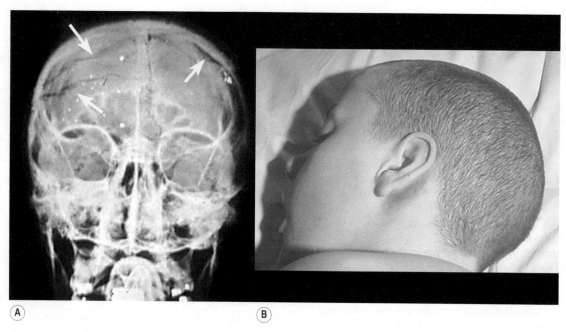

Fig. 11.18 (A) Radiograph showing skull fractures (arrows). (B) Skull base fracture in a baby showing Battle's sign (bruising behind the ear), indicating petrous bone skull fracture.

A depressed fracture, in which an area of skull is driven inwards, needs to be repaired by a neurosurgeon. Depressed fractures may tear arteries or the meninges, leading to haemorrhage. Infection is a possible secondary consequence of skull fractures in which the scalp is torn. Skull base fractures are difficult to see on X-ray images. They are associated with physical signs such as CSF bleeding through the nose (as there is communication with the nasal sinuses), bleeding into the middle ear or Battle's sign (bruising over the mastoid process, Fig. 11.18B). Importantly, Battle's sign takes 1–2 days to appear, so although it is not helpful in acute diagnosis or management of head injury it is useful as a clinical sign for detecting skull base fractures.

Blows around the eyes may fracture the orbit. The medial and inferior walls are paper-thin, and indirect injuries that displace the orbital walls produce 'blow-out fractures', which may involve damage to the air sinuses. Orbital fractures often produce intraorbital bleeding, producing pressure on the eyeball and 'black eyes', as the blood accumulates in the soft tissues around the eye. Orbital fractures may damage the cavernous sinus and thus the blood/nerve supply to the eye. The abducens nerve and ICA run in its substance, and the oculomotor, trochlear, ophthalmic and maxillary nerves run in its lateral wall. Infection can spread to the cavernous sinus via the ophthalmic vein as a result of such fractures.

Meninges

Bleeding in the spaces around the brain is a common feature of closed head injury. In trauma, bleeding may be extradural, subdural or subarachnoid. Extradural and subdural haemorrhages usually need to be evacuated neurosurgically; if left untreated they are important causes of death because they act as mass lesions (Box 11.9).

Extradural haemorrhage

Extradural haemorrhage (EDH) occurs in approximately 10% of severe head injuries and in up to 15% of fatal head injuries. It is important to understand the anatomy and natural history of EDHs, because if an EDH is not diagnosed and treated, it will kill the patient. EDH is an impact phenomenon. It occurs when a blood vessel running between the skull and the dura is torn, in association with a skull fracture. The blood vessel damaged is either an artery or one of the large venous sinuses (the veins are thin walled, with little muscle or elastic tissue and no valves). In many cases, it is the middle meningeal artery that is torn. This artery lies beneath the pterion, where the skull is thinnest, and is relatively easily fractured by a blow to the side of the head. Although the blood flow from the bleed may be rapid, EDHs accumulate slowly, usually over a period of hours, because the dura strongly adheres to the inner aspect of the calvarium, and the enlarging clot slowly strips the dura from the bone. The patient may appear to be lucid immediately after the injury and only becomes unconscious as the haemorrhage enlarges and begins to press on the brain (Fig. 11.20). Because there is so little reserve volume inside the skull, haematomas of more than 75 mL are usually fatal; death is caused by a combination of mass effect and raised intracranial pressure.

On CT or MRI images, EDHs appear convex (Fig. 11.23); the bone sutures limit their spread because the dura mater tightly adheres to the sutures and so they expand inward toward the brain rather than along the skull margin.

Box
11.9   The effects of a mass lesion inside the skull

The cranial cavity is subdivided by the relatively rigid tentorium and falx cerebri into three compartments, with limited capacity to accommodate accumulations of blood or swelling due to oedema without an increase in pressure. Differences in pressure between two adjacent intracranial compartments, or between an intracranial compartment and the spinal canal, cause the brain to be displaced into the lower-pressure compartment (i.e. internal herniation). Raised intracranial pressure can also lead to external herniation of brain tissue through a skull fracture or craniotomy.

There are three sites where herniation tends to occur (Fig. 11.19):

1. subfalcine – herniation of the cingulate gyrus under the falx cerebri
2. tentorial – herniation of the uncus of the temporal lobe through the tentorial notch
3. tonsillar – herniation of the cerebellar tonsils through the foramen magnum and onto the respiratory and cardiac centres of the medulla.

Apart from distorting and causing pressure on the brain, internal herniation compresses blood vessels, leading to secondary ischaemic damage. Cranial nerves are often also compressed, causing focal neurological signs.

With herniation there is downward displacement of diencephalic structures and descent of the brainstem, resulting in buckling of the brainstem, with traction on the external portions of the arterial supply and compression of their internal parts. This creates foci of haemorrhagic necrosis in the midbrain and pons. It is this brainstem damage, along with the rise in intracranial pressure, that leads to death.

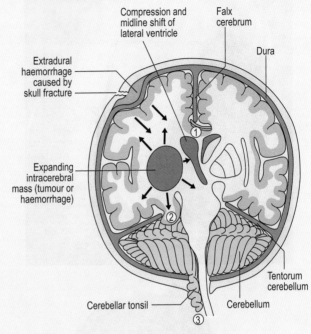

1. Subfalcine herniation.   3. Tonsillar herniation.
2. Uncal herniation.

Fig. 11.19 Schematic showing the neuroanatomical basis for brain herniation syndromes. An increase in the volume of the contents in the skull, such as a brain tumour or intracranial bleed, can cause brain tissue to be displaced at one of the three sites shown.

Subdural haemorrhage

Acute subdural haemorrhage (SDH) is completely different from EDH. It is principally caused by movement of the brain and not by impact. The movement responsible is acceleration, with or without deceleration. When the head undergoes acceleration the inertia of the brain causes its movement to lag behind that of the skull. This leads to traction on bridging veins running between the brain and dura mater, which get torn. Blood from the ruptured vessels spreads slowly and freely through the subdural space (an artificial region within the dura created by the separation of the arachnoid mater from the dura mater and not between the dura mater and arachnoid mater, as its name suggests). SDH can envelop the entire hemisphere (Fig. 11.21, upper image) and may spread into the subarachnoid space below. The bleeding tends to stop spontaneously. Sometimes, the symptoms (headache, drowsiness and confusion) may take days to months to become apparent. Because of the forces involved in producing an SDH, there is very often damage to axons in the underlying brain as well. This is in contrast to an EDH, where the underlying brain tissue is not usually severely damaged. If the blood is not removed, it will compress the brain tissue, leading to infarction.

SDHs are more frequent than EDHs and are common findings in child abuse cases such as 'shaken baby syndrome'. Acute subdural bleeds have a mortality rate of 60%–80% if left untreated. They are also common in chronic alcoholics and the elderly, where cortical atrophy is common, increasing the tension on the bridging veins and thus increasing the likelihood of damage with shearing forces. On CT and MRI images, an SDH often appears crescent shaped, with the concave side facing away from the skull, and may also track along the dural folds (see Fig. 11.23).

Subarachnoid haemorrhage

Subarachnoid bleeding (SAH) is classified into traumatic and non-traumatic (spontaneous) categories; the former is more common than the latter. Traumatic SAH is almost always insignificant and is seen on the surface of the hemispheres in relation to fracture sites or contusions. It most

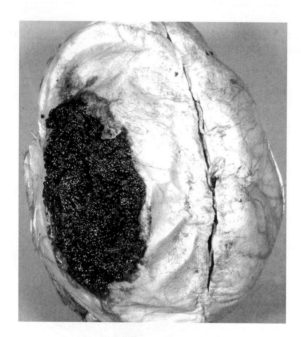

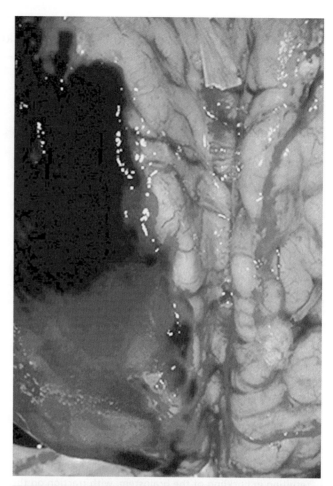

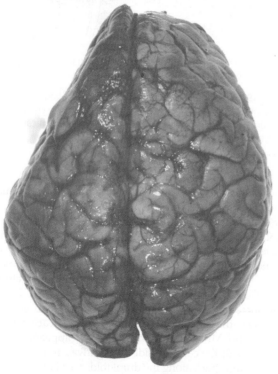

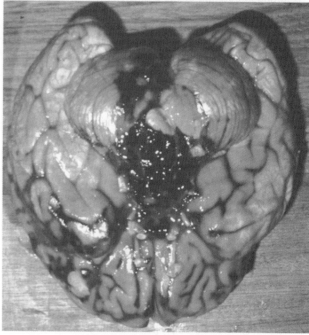

Fig. 11.20 Extradural haematoma (EDH). Top: an example of an EDH caused by rupture of the middle meningeal artery. Bottom: effects of an EDH on the underlying brain tissue, showing severe compression of the left frontal lobe.

Fig. 11.21 Two examples of subdural haemorrhage (SDH), where blood distributes and collects over the surface of the front of the brain (upper figure) or collects at the base of the brain (lower figure).

often results from penetrating brain injury. Occasionally, if a vessel at the base of the brain is damaged, a large amount of blood collects in the subarachnoid space over the base of the brain. On CT or MRI images, fresh blood can be seen invaginating between the cerebral gyri, making the sulci appear white (see Fig. 11.23). Spontaneous SAH is quite different from traumatic SAH, which results from rupture of an aneurysm on a vessel of the circle of Willis (e.g. a Berry aneurysm) (Fig. 11.21, lower image) or an arteriovenous malformation, and is a form of haemorrhagic stroke. Following spontaneous SAH, delayed cerebral vasospasm can occur approximately a week after the event and this can result in cerebral ischaemia or infarction. The vasospasm is treated by 'triple H' therapy consisting of induced hypertension, hypervolemia and haemodilution, in the intensive care unit. This treatment is most effective if started early after diagnosis.

Brain contusions and lacerations

Contusions are caused by impact and can be thought of as brain 'bruises'. They occur on the crests of gyri, particularly where the brain moves over the roughened floor of the skull (Figs 11.22 and 11.23), namely the inferior surface of the frontal lobes, the lateral and inferior surfaces of the temporal lobes, the region adjacent to the lateral fissures or at the orbital poles.

At their mildest, contusions are very small superficial areas of haemorrhagic necrosis confined to the cortex.

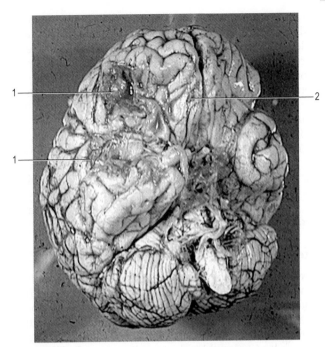

1. Lesion.   2. 'Hollow tooth'.

Fig. 11.22 Traumatic lacerations of right orbital cortex and coup and contrecoup lesions of temporal lobes. The right olfactory bulb is also damaged, as are the crests of the gyri, producing a split hollow tooth appearance.

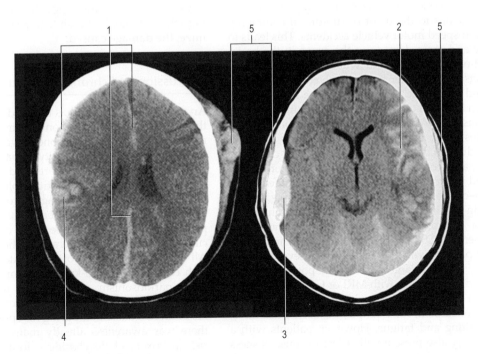

1. Subdural bleed.   4. Contusion.
2. Subarachnoid bleed. 5. Soft tissue injury (extra-cranial).
3. Extradural bleed.

Fig. 11.23 MRI images showing different types of pathology present in head injury. (Left image courtesy of Mr A. Elsmore, right image courtesy of Dr Andrew Downie.)

Larger contusions involve the underlying white matter and may be associated with considerable oedema and a degree of mass effect. Contusions occur at the site of impact ('coup'), and at sites opposite the point of impact ('contrecoup'), depending on the type of blow. The prefrontal cortex and the temporal lobe poles are the parts of the brain most often injured in acceleration–deceleration trauma. These contusions are rarely life-threatening on their own, however, and with increasing survival time, the necrotic brain tissue is resorbed. It is not uncommon to see the remnants of contusional injury as an incidental finding at post-mortem. The term 'laceration' is used when the arachnoid mater and brain are damaged, usually at the site of a fracture, or by a penetrating injury or a large intracerebral haematoma.

Intracerebral (parenchymal) haemorrhage

Bleeding within the brain tissue is usually the result of penetrating head wounds such as those caused by high-velocity impacts, for example, of bullets. Low-velocity focal impact may result in bone fragment penetration from a skull fracture. When parenchymal haemorrhage is the result of a closed head injury, it commonly affects the frontal and temporal lobes.

Diffuse pathology

Diffuse axonal injury (DAI) is the term given to widespread damage to axons in many different brain regions, caused by rapid acceleration/deceleration of the head that stretches the axons to the point of rupture. It commonly occurs in high-speed motor vehicle accidents. This leads to microscopic and gross damage to the axons in the brain, at the junction of the grey and white matter. DAI commonly affects white matter tracts involved in the corpus callosum and brainstem. Interestingly, there is no association between DAI and underlying skull fractures. Another common cause of DAI is 'shaken baby' syndrome, where young babies (often only a few weeks old) are violently shaken by adults. It is a form of child abuse that can occur with as little as 5 s of violent shaking. The anterior temporal lobes and prefrontal cortex region are most affected by acceleration–deceleration injury causing bruising, bleeding and brain swelling; these may lead to brain damage.

DAI is a clinical diagnosis and is often considered when a patient's GCS is <8 for >6 hours. The clinical presentation of patients with DAI relates to the severity of the axonal injury (which is largely assessed at post-mortem, as DAI is very difficult to see with MRI or CT). For example, patients with mild DAI present with signs and symptoms that reflect concussion, for example, headache, dizziness, nausea, vomiting and fatigue. However, patients with a severe DAI may also present with a loss of consciousness and remain in a persistent vegetative state. A patient with severe DAI is usually unconscious from the time of injury, remains in prolonged coma and is severely disabled or vegetative until death, although a very small number will regain consciousness in the first year after the injury.

Hypoxic–ischaemic damage is also very common in head injury. The injured brain is extremely sensitive to hypoxia, and the primary aim of emergency head injury treatment is to maintain oxygenation and cerebral perfusion. Head injuries frequently occur in settings in which there are multiple injuries: injuries to the ribs may interfere with breathing and therefore oxygenation of the blood, while major bleeding will cause shock and hypotension.

Diffuse brain swelling is often seen in head injury, particularly in children, probably partly as a result of failure of cerebral autoregulation (see earlier). Any significant swelling will cause intracranial pressure to rise, and so reduce cerebral perfusion. Diffuse brain injury can impair mental functions such as long-term memory and problem-solving, and result in neglect and prosopagnosia (inability to recognize faces) and an inability to synthesize and analyse information.

Axons are as vulnerable as other intracranial structures to traumatic damage and it is now generally believed that a degree of axonal damage occurs in most head injuries. Experimental work suggests that mild reversible axonal injury is the cause of concussion symptoms, and that scattered irreversible axonal damage may be responsible for a number of the behavioural and cognitive sequelae of mild head injuries, such as the 'punch-drunk syndrome' seen in boxers. With more severe injuries, the amount and distribution of axonal damage often determine the outcome.

With all forms of traumatic axonal injury, whether very mild or very severe, it is clear that the damage does not become irreversible until several hours, possibly days, after injury, providing a 'therapeutic window' during which it may be possible to prevent, or at least minimize, the damage caused.

Concussion and chronic traumatic encephalopathy

An area of research that has received much attention over the last decade is focused on the impact on the brain of repetitive mild injury of a concussive nature, such as that typically seen in high velocity impact sports like rugby, American football, martial arts and boxing. It has been long known that direct repetitive blows to the head can increase the risk of developing neurodegenerative disease later in life. The term 'dementia pugilistica' reflects this particular aspect of increased risk of developing a specific form of neurodegeneration. The boxer Muhammad Ali (Cassius Clay), one of the greatest sportsmen of the 20th century, is a well-known example of this; he developed parkinsonism after retiring from boxing, which many specialists attributed to the repetitive mild injuries his brain had sustained during his sporting life. Therefore, there was awareness already many decades ago of the risk in boxers of developing a form of encephalopathy, characterised by behavioural and mood changes and cognitive dysfunction. A pathologist from Pittsburgh, Dr Bennet Omalu, published a seminal paper in 2005 which described the pathology he found in the brain of a National Football League player, who had died suddenly

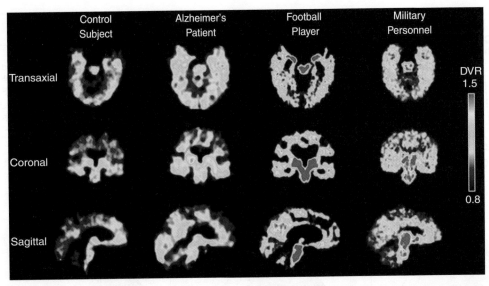

Fig. 11.24 PET imaging using the FDDNP tracer for tau and amyloid deposition. Brain scans of a healthy aged control subject, a person with Alzheimer's disease (AD), a retired football player and a member of the military. The top end of the scale indicates a higher concentration of the tracer, and its binding to protein aggregates. The AD patient shows higher deposits in the parietal, temporal and frontal regions. The football player and the military personnel show high signals for amygdala and midbrain deposition. (From Chen ST, et al. (2018) *Journal of Alzheimer's Disease* 65(1): 79–88.)

following several years of declining cognitive function, depression, disintegration of personal life and destitution, substance abuse and multiple suicide attempts. He clearly showed the presence in tissue of both tau and amyloid pathology, which characterize neurodegeneration (discussed in Chapter 14). This opened up a new research avenue, which led to the realization of a heightened risk of chronic traumatic encephalopathy (CTE) in many sports where the head undergoes numerous episodes of concussion. This created a particular concern about insidious injuries, which may occur while the brain is still developing, for example during contact sports like rugby in school. The head injury assessment (HIA) protocol is now widely used in professional contact sports, in that if a player receives a blow to the head, they are immediately removed and clinically assessed for concussion, using a questionnaire (Cogsport or Impact) to check memory and neurological tests to assess balance. If the player fails the initial test, these are repeated at intervals of 3 and 36–48 hours to monitor recovery.

Research evidence on repetitive concussion and the risk of CTE is now extensive, and there is clear empirical evidence that a wide range of sporting activities, beyond boxing, may expose the players to a significant risk of long-term sequelae. CTE has been extensively confirmed in sportsmen not only through post-mortem analysis but also using *in vivo* imaging tracers. There is significant overlap in neuropathology between CTE and chronic neurodegenerative conditions such as Alzheimer's disease. CTE is predominantly a tauopathy and there has been much effort deployed to identify objective biomarkers (imaging or plasma/CSF measurements) of unresolved brain injury after concussive episodes. These would enable, for example, the development of objective rules guiding the 'return to play' in contact sports. It is also

important to note that repetitive mild brain trauma is also a matter of concern for military personnel. Approximately 20% of military staff returning from combat may suffer long-term from the consequences of mild traumatic brain injury episodes, through concussion and also multiple exposures to blast waves, following detonation of improvised explosive devices. Such acoustic waves can produce forces equivalent to repeated concussive impacts within less than a second in the brain. Positron emission tomography (PET) imaging of neurodegenerative changes allows for comparisons of the specific distribution of protein aggregates between individuals with neurodegenerative disease (e.g. Alzheimer's disease) and CTE, as shown in Fig 11.24.

Treatment of head injury

After a moderate or severe head injury, surgery may be required to remove a hematoma or contusion that is compressing the brain or raising the intracranial pressure. It may be necessary to remove a bone flap. If the brain is very swollen, a decision may be made to delay replacing the bone until the swelling decreases, which may take up to several weeks. An intracranial pressure monitor may be placed intracranially and the patient remains under close observation in intensive care.

The primary injury can induce major tissue disruption, axonal shearing and a compromised blood supply, with subsequent cell loss through necrosis. The injured and dying cells release specialised molecules – 'damage-associated molecular patterns' (DAMPs). These molecules are also known as 'danger-associated molecular patterns' or 'alarmins', as they lead to activation of molecular cascades that characterise the secondary injury

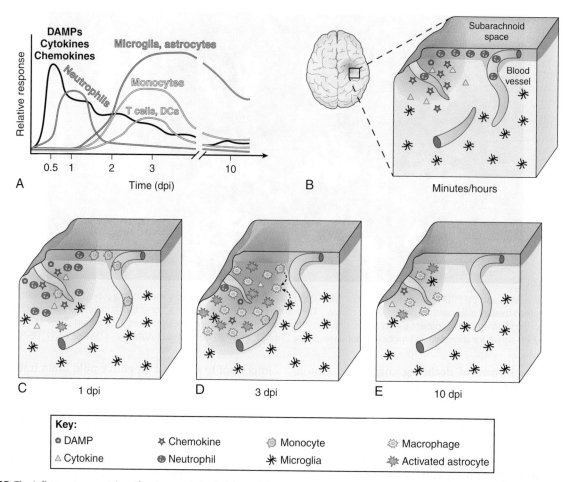

Fig. 11.25 The inflammatory reaction after traumatic brain injury. (A) The timeline of the major components of the response after injury; (B–E) detailed representation of the various players involved in the cellular reactions to injury. *Dpi*, Days post injury. (From GyonevaS and Ransohoff RM. (2015) Trends in Pharmacological Sciences 36:471–480.)

phase in response to the alarm signal represented by the damage incurred by various cell populations. Alarmins include proteins (e.g. heat-shock proteins) and also small molecules (e.g. ATP or uric acid).

The overall aim of treatment after a traumatic brain injury is similar to that of stroke treatment, that is, to prevent secondary brain damage and enlargement of the area of injury. The pathophysiological pathways that underlie the expansion of the injured zone are very similar to those described for stroke. There is a significant role of excessive glutamate release and excitotoxicity, mitochondrial dysfunction, increased oxidation and extensive secondary waves of cell death (e.g. secondary apoptosis). There is delayed axonal degeneration, demyelination and ultimately formation of a glial scar that limits neuroplasticity. There is a very complex inflammatory reaction, with a local component (involving microglia and astrocytes) and a systemic component, involving migration of white blood cells from the periphery into the brain tissue, for example monocytes, T cells and dendritic cells, which are specialised antigen-presenting cells. This complex activation of both the innate and adaptive immune response, cytokines, chemokines (specialised cytokines involved in

chemotaxis, that play a crucial role in the migration of leucocytes) and DAMPs, and also the various cells involved at various stages post-injury, are depicted in Fig. 11.25. The inflammatory response persists for a long time after injury. Studies using PET imaging of brain microglia have revealed that activation of microglia can persist for more than a decade after the brain injury. The persistence of neuroinflammation may play an important role in the increased risk of neurodegeneration that is associated with traumatic brain injury. They may be a critical link in the activation of aggregation processes affecting amyloid and tau proteins after injury.

Acute management is focused on maintaining adequate oxygenation and reducing intracranial pressure. For EDH, surgical aspiration of the clot is a life-saving technique; a ventricular shunt can be placed to reduce hydrocephalus, or drugs such as mannitol (an osmotic diuretic) or dexamethasone (an anti-inflammatory drug) can be used to reduce oedema. Hyperventilation and its consequent hypocapnia also reduce intracranial pressure, as does hypothermia and hyperbaric oxygen or drugs such as phenothiazines.

Even mild head injuries (e.g. concussion) can impair mental processes such as perception, attention and memory. Even though in some cases there may not be anatomical damage, most traumatic head injury patients suffer from long-term complications and disabilities that are physical (pain and headache, epilepsy, hearing, visual or sensory impairment and motor weakness or disequilibrium) and/or mental (memory loss, inability to concentrate, significant personality and emotional changes, language difficulties and depression).

The pharmacological management of head injury is still limited and somewhat empirical. However, encouraging results for the support of cognitive and motor recovery have been obtained in recent years with neurostimulant drugs such as dexamphetamine, methylphenidate, bromocriptine, amantadine, L-DOPA/carbidopa, acetylcholinesterase inhibitors such as donepezil and rivastigmine, which increase attention and heighten arousal levels and selective serotonin reuptake inhibitors (e.g. fluoxetine or sertraline). Neuroprotection in the acute phase, similar to the concept of neuroprotection in the post stroke acute phase, has been extensively explored in experimental animal models of brain injury, but although dozens of compounds have shown clear efficacy in animals, none have made it to the clinic. One of the recent failures was that reported with progesterone, a compound with pleiotropic effects and documented efficacy in numerous experimental studies, which ultimately failed in two large-scale clinical trials in traumatic brain injury, as they did not show improved recovery, as assessed using the Glasgow Outcome Scale (GOS; see later). Thus, the field of neuroprotection is as fraught with failure as the field of neuroprotection in stroke. The mechanism of action of compounds, from dopamine agonists such as bromocriptine, to acetylcholinesterase inhibitors such as donepezil, which appear to exert some beneficial effects in recovery post injury, is still unclear. Protection may be directly related to their known pharmacodynamic characteristics or may result in some cases from some other yet undiscovered property. In the case of head trauma, in a similar manner to stroke, the use of combined medications may have many advantages that are still incompletely explored, because of the intrinsic difficulties associated with therapeutic development of combinatorial strategies. Another strategy explored in several studies has been that of inducing hypothermia post injury, to induce neuroprotection through multiple mechanisms such as reduction in the brain metabolic rate, blockade of excitotoxicity and decreases in oxidative stress and inflammation. Unfortunately, the results of clinical trials testing this strategy have not supported this concept, with the possible exception of a subgroup of patients with increased intracranial pressure, where mild hypothermia could be initiated within 24 hours after traumatic brain injury.

The outcome following head injury is most often assessed with the GOS or the Glasgow Outcome Scale Extended (GOSE). These are simple numerical scoring systems which rate the outcome, from death to good recovery. Patients with mild head injury (usually defined as a GCS score on admission of 13–15) tend to do well. They may experience headaches, dizziness,

The vegetative state of a patient is characterised by lack of awareness, even if a patient has awoken from coma. In this state patients can move their eyelids and have sleep-wake cycles or have permanent apparent wakefulness; they also may have some level of consciousness, and so can respond to some degree to certain types of stimulation. Patients may smile, moan or scream; they may display some eye-tracking movements and sometimes they can swallow. The vegetative state does not totally preclude a possibility of some improvement and some patients may emerge from a vegetative state after a few weeks; however, experience shows that improvement is unlikely after extensive, catastrophic brain injuries, which very likely overwhelm brain compensatory neuroplasticity. If this wakeful, unconscious state persists for more than a few weeks, the patient is considered to have entered a 'continuous' or 'persistent' vegetative state. The use of these terms may vary between countries. In the UK the term 'continuous' is used after more than 4 weeks, whereas the term 'persistent' implies a longer duration (for more than 12 months) and also the increasing probability, based on extensive neurological tests, that the individual will not be able to show any recovery. The existence of a persistent vegetative state also creates the possibility that a request to end life support be made by family and carers. It is important to note that within the last decade, functional neuroimaging studies have provided new information on the residual cerebral function in patients who are in a vegetative state, with some patients clearly displaying some preserved responses. There is no treatment at present for the vegetative state.

irritability or similar symptoms, but these improve in most cases. Patients with moderate head injuries fare less well. Approximately 60% show good recovery, whereas approximately 25% are left with a moderate disability. Death or a persistent vegetative state (Box 11.10) will be the outcome in approximately 7%–10% of cases. The remainder of patients will have a severe degree of disability. Severely head-injured patients have the worst outcomes. Only 25%–33% of these patients have good outcomes. Approximately 35% of these patients do not survive. Some remain in a persistently vegetative state.

Rehabilitation methods are similar to those used in stroke, but often with a special emphasis on cognitive therapy. In general, head injury patients tend to have a better prognosis than stroke patients, partly because head injury patients are in better vascular health and are often younger.

Comments on the case history

Once Arthur's stroke had been diagnosed, immediate treatment was initiated. This should result in a favourable prognosis. Pharmacological treatment was aimed at reducing infarct size and rescuing brain cells in the penumbra region, which would otherwise die from ischaemia. Prompt administration of alteplase—a clot-lysing agent—dissolved the thrombus and restored the cerebral circulation to this region. This resulted in resolution of the sensory loss and language disabilities, suggesting that blood flow was restored to the parietal and temporal lobes. The core region appears to reside in the frontal lobe, and this accounts for the residual motor deficits, including language articulation. It is unlikely that further improvement will occur, and rehabilitation programmes will be needed to allow Arthur to cope with his disabilities. A change of lifestyle is also required, to reduce the risk of subsequent strokes.

Self-assessment case study

A 25-year-old man was involved in a fight outside a pub. According to witnesses, the other man punched him hard on the jaw, causing him to fall against the pavement kerb. He then kicked him in the head for good measure, before running off. The victim lay in the road, not moving. Onlookers in the pub called an ambulance. On arrival at Accident and Emergency, 20 min later, the victim was recorded as having a Glasgow Coma Score (GCS) of 7. A computed tomography scan revealed a right-sided fracture of the pterion, with a small underlying extradural haemorrhage, and a thin subdural haemorrhage on the same side. The brain was swollen and there was some brain shift from right to left. The man's condition deteriorated further and he was placed on a ventilator. Twenty-four hours later, his GCS fell to 3, both pupils became fixed and dilated and, despite full supportive treatment, he remained unconscious and died 2 days later.

After studying this chapter, you should be able to answer the following questions:

1. What are the causes of the different pathologies in this case?

The victim suffered an accelerated fall backwards, followed by rapid deceleration when the impact to the head occurred. Several pathologies are apparent.

- An **extradural haemorrhage** is a complication of a skull fracture, and in this case is over the side of the hemispheres, from damage to the middle meningeal artery.

- **Acute subdural haemorrhage** is caused by movement of the brain.

- **Contusions** are brain 'bruises'; they occur at the site of impact ('coup') and at sites opposite the point of impact ('contrecoup'). Here, impact to the moving head resulted in contrecoup contusions in the frontal and temporal lobes. This would only be seen at post-mortem.

2. What cellular mechanisms may be involved in the pathophysiology of brain injury in this scenario?

The trauma results in a variety of cellular events, including cell death as a result of excitotoxicity due to excess neurotransmitter release, elevated intracellular calcium levels and free radical production, or the production of proinflammatory cytokines by glial cells.

3. What is the pathophysiology of cerebral swelling after head injury?

Cerebral oedema can be divided into three types: a) vasogenic, b) cytotoxic and c) interstitial. The first two are the major types after brain injury. The vasogenic type is due to accumulation of water outside cells, because of the disruption of the blood–brain barrier. The cytotoxic oedema is due to the disruption of cell membranes and the accumulation of Na^+ inside cells, because of the failure of Na^+/K^+ pumps.

4. What are the effects of raised intracranial pressure?

As intracranial pressure rises, blood flow to the brain decreases, unless the arterial pressure rises in compensation. This compensatory rise occurs when intracranial pressure starts rising, but cerebral perfusion rapidly falls off, as intracranial pressure rises further. Tissue ischaemia then leads to cytotoxic oedema, and so more swelling and less perfusion.

In this case, both the EDH and SDH are space-occupying and this raises ICP in addition to generalised brain swelling. The mass lesions cause additional specific neurological signs attributable to the brain shift, by producing cranial nerves and blood vessel compression. Dilatation of the pupil on the side of the lesion is the most consistently reliable sign of an uncus herniation, as the motor fibres of cranial nerve III are compressed by part of the medial temporal lobe. The presence of bilateral unreactive pupils suggests advanced brain herniation, with very high ICP.

INFECTION IN THE CENTRAL NERVOUS SYSTEM

Chapter summary

1. The brain and spinal cord are protected against injury, influx of foreign substances and invasion of pathogens, through a combination of three distinct components: the meninges, the cerebrospinal fluid (CSF) and the blood–brain barrier (BBB).

2. The meninges comprise three distinct membrane layers: the dura mater, the arachnoid mater and the pia mater. The latter two form the leptomeninges and enclose the space where the CSF flows. Dura mater is supplied by meningeal and occipital blood vessels and invaginates to form dural sinuses that compartmentalise various brain regions. The arachnoid layer provides a separation between the systemic circulation and the CSF circulation. The role of the meninges is to limit the movement of the brain within the skull.

3. CSF is produced by the choroid plexuses of each cerebral ventricle chamber. The CSF flows to cisternae at the base of the brain and then around the cerebrum and cerebellum, with final drainage into the dural sinuses and lymphatic vessels. The CSF has a composition similar to plasma and can be analysed by collection of a sample from the subarachnoid space, through lumbar puncture. Importantly, CSF makes the brain essentially weightless within the skull.

4. The BBB is a complex interface between the blood and brain tissue. Its components are specialised endothelial cells, astrocyte endfeet, pericytes and a basement membrane. The BBB is rich in solute transporters and efflux transporters. The former are involved in the traffic of nutrients and other compounds essential for brain metabolism, whereas the latter are involved in the protection against xenobiotics, including therapeutic drugs, thus underlying the development of treatment resistance.

3. Infections of the CNS are caused by a variety of pathogens: bacteria, viruses, protozoa, metazoa, fungi and prions. Infection triggers a

major inflammatory response, which involves several components of the innate immune system. The diagnosis is based on clinical signs and examination of the CSF. Infections include meningitis, encephalitis and abscesses.

4. Bacterial meningitis is a severe and potentially life-threatening condition which requires early management with antibiotics. Therapy includes penicillins and cephalosporins, to which steroids can be added. Individuals at risk require prompt prophylaxis. Vaccines have been developed against various pathogens and they have contributed to a decrease in bacterial meningitis incidence worldwide. Viral meningitis is milder in presentation than the bacterial form and has a better outcome.

Introduction

The central nervous system (CNS) is protected from mechanical injury induced by abrupt movement, or from infection induced by various pathogens, and from the potentially dangerous effects of xenobiotics (including drugs), by three lines of defence: (1) the meninges, a complex system of membranes that surround the brain and spinal cord; (2) the cerebrospinal fluid (CSF), which bathes the nervous tissue and (3) a specialised vascular barrier, the blood–brain barrier (BBB). However, these protections can be breached, unwanted substances can penetrate the CNS and the tissue can be infected by a wide variety of pathogens. Infections lead to various disease presentations which reflect the involvement of the brain and/or its protective layers. They can also lead to the formation of abscesses. The case described in Box 12.1 illustrates the significant neurological consequences of infections.

Types of infection of the central nervous system

There are many different pathogens that can infect the CNS. The causative agents of infections are summarized in Table 12.1. Infections can affect the meninges, the brain tissue, or both, and can therefore be divided into three groups—meningitis, encephalitis and meningo-encephalitis—depending on the tissue affected and the extent of the infection.

The best-known type of generalized brain infection is meningitis, an inflammation of the meninges surrounding the brain. This type of infection is the subject of a large amount of public information and education, concerning both the need for early identification of the condition and rapid treatment (which in many cases is essential), and also raising awareness of the vaccines that are available. The most severe forms of meningitis are caused by bacteria, and if these are suspected to be the causative agents, antibiotics should be given immediately.

When brain tissue (parenchyma) becomes infected, this is called encephalitis, and is most often caused by viruses. In many cases the disease is mild and self-limiting, but some types of encephalitis cause significant mortality.

A number of viruses can cause specific localized infections. One of the most well-known is the polio virus, the causative agent of poliomyelitis, which infects the lower motor neurons of the spinal cord and brainstem, causing paralysis, which may be permanent. Fortunately, this occurs rarely in the UK, because of an extensive vaccination programme, but it still occurs in many less developed countries. Herpes zoster virus, the causative agent of chickenpox, can infect the dorsal root ganglion cells. It remains dormant but can be reactivated later in life, causing shingles. Another virus that infects specific nerve ganglia is herpes simplex virus (HSV). The type 1 virus infects the trigeminal nerve ganglion and can also be reactivated periodically to produce cold sores. The type 2 virus infects the dorsal root ganglion in the sacral region and its reactivation causes genital herpes. Infection with the herpes virus is a common cause of meningoencephalitis.

When the brain infection is due to a localized bacterial infection, a cerebral abscess is produced. The accumulation of pus causes a typical expanding mass in the brain, with many of the signs and symptoms seen in the

Case history

On returning home after attending nursery school, 4-year-old David complains of a headache. Shortly afterwards, he says that he feels sick and is tired. He goes to lie down in his bedroom and asks that the curtains be drawn, even though it is only 2 p.m. After he has actually vomited, his mother notices a rash on his feet while she is changing his clothes. Remembering a leaflet about meningitis she saw in the doctor's surgery, the mother immediately calls an ambulance and David is taken to the local hospital. On examination by the doctor, he is shown to have a fever and neck stiffness, with a positive Kernig's sign. Examining the rash more closely, the doctor notices that it does not go pale when pressed. David is immediately given an intravenous injection of benzylpenicillin and ceftriaxone. The doctor takes blood samples and a throat swab. By this time, David has a deteriorating level of consciousness and he is transferred immediately to the intensive care department. Subsequent culture of the throat sample identifies the presence of *Neisseria meningitidis*. David is very ill for a few days but, because of his mother's prompt action, his illness is not as dangerous as it might have been. The other members of David's family are given antibiotics, as are the other children at the nursery school. Following his successful treatment, David is tested to determine if he has any persisting problems.

This case gives rise to the following questions:

1. What types of infection can occur in the central nervous system?
2. What are the meninges and what is their function?
3. What is the blood–brain barrier and what are its functions?
4. What is meningitis and what are its causes?
5. How is meningitis diagnosed and treated, and what is the likely prognosis?

Table 12.1 Examples of central nervous system infections and their causative agent

Bacteria	*Neisseria meningitidis**, *Streptococcus pneumoniae**, *Haemophilus influenzae*, *Escherichia coli*, *Mycobacterium tuberculosis* (these all cause meningitis), *Mycobacterium leprae* (leprosy), *Treponema pallidum* (syphilis), *Borrelia burgdorferi* (Lyme disease)
Viruses	Herpes simplex (encephalitis), herpes zoster (shingles), poliovirus, rabies, human immunodeficiency virus (HIV), mumps
Protozoa	*Plasmodium falciparum* (malaria), toxoplasmosis, trypanosomiasis (sleeping sickness)
Metazoa	Encysted tapeworm larvae (hydatid disease, cysticercosis)
Fungi	*Cryptococcus neoformans*, *Histoplasma capsulatum*, *Coccidioides immitis*
Prions	Creutzfeldt–Jakob disease (CJD) and new variant CJD

*These two organisms account for approximately 70% of cases of meningitis in the UK.

presence of brain tumours and other space-filling lesions, for example, raised intracranial pressure and risk of herniation. These can be very severe because of the rapid growth of the abscess.

A disease first described in the 1920s that has recently received much attention is Creutzfeldt–Jakob disease (CJD), a degenerative disease of the elderly causing characteristic spongiform changes to the brain. The disease, which is related to bovine spongiform encephalitis (BSE) in cattle and scrapie in sheep, is thought to be due to the presence in the brain and lymphatic tissue of abnormal forms of a protein called prion protein (discussed in Chapter 14). CJD can be transmitted following neurosurgery, as the infective agent is not destroyed by normal sterilization procedures. It has also been transmitted by growth hormone treatment of children of small stature. Interest in this rare disease was stimulated by the appearance of a new form of the disease in 1994, which, unlike classic CJD, occurs in young people. The presence of an epidemic of BSE in British cattle, allied with the suggestion that this new variant CJD (vCJD) is due to the consumption of beef from these infected animals, not only stimulated much research on this subject, but also led to the widespread slaughter of beef herds, and changes in animal feed and slaughter practices in the UK. However, the widely feared vCJD epidemic has not yet occurred; the number of suspected cases per year has been falling and in the period 2017–21 there have been no deaths from vCJD, according to the UK National CJD Surveillance Unit.

A recent example of significant consequences of a viral infection on the CNS is that of the coronavirus SARS-CoV-2, which led to the corona virus disease 19 (COVID-19), a pandemic which emerged in December 2019 in Wuhan, the capital of the Hubei region in China, and rapidly engulfed the world in the following months. As of July 2021, the pandemic had led to more than 4 million deaths worldwide, with clear evidence that the infection is associated with significant neurological manifestations, some of them long-lasting, due to involvement of the peripheral and central nervous system in the response to the pathogen.

The meninges

The meninges are a series of membranes that surround the brain, spinal cord, the optic nerve and the initial segments of the cranial and spinal nerve roots (see Box 12.2). They are separated by CSF, which acts as a cushion, supporting the weight of the brain and protecting it from damage that might be caused by movement. Suspending the brain in fluid reduces the effective brain weight and prevents it from being compressed or bruised by its own

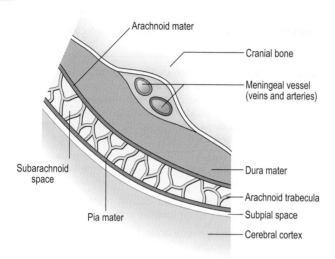

Fig. 12.1 Anatomy of the meninges. The thick dura mater, the arachnoid mater and the pia mater enclose the brain and contain the cerebrospinal fluid.

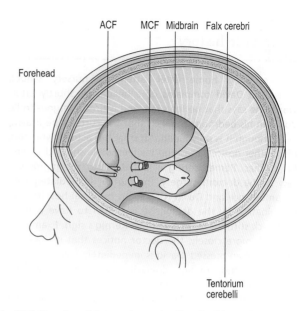

Fig. 12.2 Drawing of the meninges showing the falx cerebri and tentorium cerebelli with the vault of the cranium removed. *ACF*, Anterior cranial fossa; *MCF*, middle cranial fossa.

mass and inertia. The meninges are made up of three distinct layers: the dura mater, the arachnoid mater and the pia mater, each of which has a specific role (Fig. 12.1).

Dura mater

The outermost layer is the dura mater ('dura' means hard or tough). This thick, leathery membrane forms the outer protective layer surrounding the brain. It is composed of two layers: the periosteal layer, which lies close to the periosteum (the inner surface of the skull), and the meningeal layer, which lies closer to the brain. In most areas of the brain, these two layers are fused, but in some regions they enclose blood-filled cavities called dural sinuses, which collect venous blood and eventually drain into the internal jugular vein.

The meningeal layer extends inwards in several places to form septa that partition the brain into separate areas and limit the movement of the brain within the skull (Fig. 12.2). The falx cerebri ('falx' means sickle) is a sickle-shaped sheet that extends into the longitudinal fissure, separating the two cerebral hemispheres. At the front of the brain, it is attached to the crista galli, a projection of the ethmoid bone, and its free edge curves over the corpus callosum to the rear of the skull, above the cerebellum. Here, it attaches to another dural septum, the tentorium cerebelli ('tentorium' means tent). This extends horizontally into the transverse fissure, which extends between the rear of the cerebral cortices and the cerebellum, arching over the posterior cranial fossa. Like the falx cerebri, it does not form a complete sheet; its free edge forms a U-shape, enclosing the midbrain and attaching at the front to the clinoid processes of the sphenoid bone. The cranial region below this is the infratentorial compartment, and the region above is the supratentorial compartment. A third sheet, the falx cerebelli, runs along the midline of the cerebellum, along the vermis. The dura mater of the spi-

nal cord has only a single meningeal layer, which extends from the rim of the foramen magnum to the level of the second sacral vertebra (S2).

The sensory innervation of the dura mater is provided by the trigeminal (to the supra-tentorial region), and vagal and upper cervical spinal nerves (to the posterior cranial fossa). If the dura is inflamed, these nerves are stimulated, giving specific patterns of pain that depend on which areas of the dura are involved (see below).

Blood supply to the dura mater is via three meningeal arteries. The anterior meningeal artery is derived from the anterior pharyngeal artery, supplying the dura around the base of the foramen magnum. The posterior meningeal artery (branches of the vertebral and occipital arteries) supplies the posterior cranial fossa. However, the most important and largest branch is the middle meningeal artery, a branch of the maxillary artery; it supplies the majority of the lateral surface of the meninges and skull and anastomoses with the ophthalmic division of the internal carotid artery. Venous drainage occurs through satellite veins that accompany the arteries and through a network of veins and venous cisterns (lakes) that drain into the venous sinuses. There are also venous connections between the dura mater and skull bones. Diploic veins are large veins with irregular dilatations that connect skull bone marrow pockets to meningeal veins, dural sinuses and peri-cranial veins. Additionally, emissary veins cross the skull bone to make connections between venous sinuses in the dura mater and extra-cranial veins in the scalp.

Arachnoid mater

Lying immediately under the dura mater, separated only by the narrow subdural space, is the arachnoid

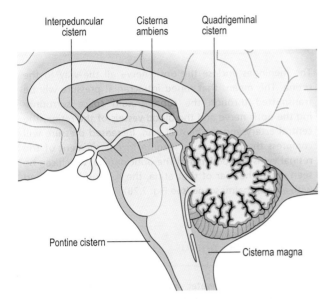

Fig. 12.3 Subarachnoid cisternae. Enlargements of the subarachnoid space form cisternae that contain cerebrospinal fluid.

mater ('arachnoid' means spider-like). This thin membrane, which completely encloses the wide subarachnoid space, is composed of fibrous material and cells connected by tight junctions that seal the space. The arachnoid mater covers the surface of the brain like wrapping paper. However, it does not extend into the individual sulci. Extending from the arachnoid mater across the subarachnoid space to the pia mater are numerous thin extensions, called trabeculae, whose web-like appearance gives the arachnoid mater its name. Together, the (outer) arachnoid mater and (inner) pia mater form the leptomeninges. The subarachnoid space is filled with CSF. Within the fluid are also many major arteries, which then project deep into the brain tissue. In specific areas, particularly around the brainstem, the subarachnoid space enlarges to form cisterns because the arachnoid mater does not dip into the contours of the brain (Fig. 12.3). The largest of these is the cisterna magna, which lies between the cerebellum and the medulla. Folds of the arachnoid mater project through the dura mater into the superior dural sinuses. These are called arachnoid villi or arachnoid granulations, and are involved in the reabsorption of CSF into venous blood (see below). The proliferation of arachnoid cells can lead to the formation of meningiomas.

Pia mater

The third layer of the meninges is the pia mater ('pia' means gentle). This very fine layer of connective tissue follows the contours of the brain, dipping down into the sulci, like shrink-wrap tightly adhering to the CNS surfaces. It is highly vascularised, with small blood vessels, and is permeable to CSF. Where small arteries enter the brain, the pia mater is carried down for short distances into the perivascular space.

Table 12.2 Comparison of blood plasma and cerebrospinal fluid (CSF) composition

	CSF	Plasma
Protein (mg/dL)	35	7000
Glucose (mg/dL)	60	90
Na^+ (mmol/L)	138	138
K^+ (mmol/L)	2.8	4.5
Ca^{2+} (mmol/L)	2.1	4.8
Mg^{2+} (mmol/L)	2.3	1.7
Cl^{--} (mmol/L)	119	102
pH	7.33	7.41

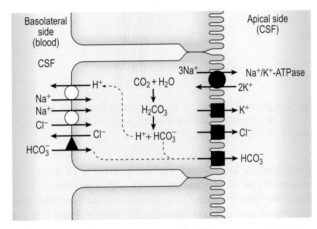

Fig. 12.4 Production of cerebrospinal fluid (CSF) by the epithelial cells of the choroid plexus. Filled circle, primary active transport; open circles, secondary active transport; filled rectangles, facilitated diffusion.

Cerebrospinal fluid production and circulation

The CSF that bathes the brain has an ionic content broadly similar to that of blood plasma, with some small differences (Table 12.2). Under normal conditions, it contains very little protein, no red cells and very few leucocytes. It contains glucose, at about 60% of the level found in plasma, has a total volume of approximately 140 mL and is clear in appearance.

CSF is produced at a rate of approximately 500–600 mL/day. Most of this (60%) is secreted by the choroid plexuses of the lateral, third and fourth ventricles. The remaining 40% is produced from the interstitial fluid. The choroid plexuses consist of loops of capillaries covered by a layer of specialized epithelial cells. These capillaries, unlike brain capillaries which form the BBB (see later), are capillaries that have small openings in their endothelium, known as fenestrae or fenestra, with a diameter of approximately 60–100 nm. The choroid epithelial cells selectively transport ions and glucose into the ventricles, with water following osmotically (Fig. 12.4). The CSF then flows through the ventricles into the subarachnoid

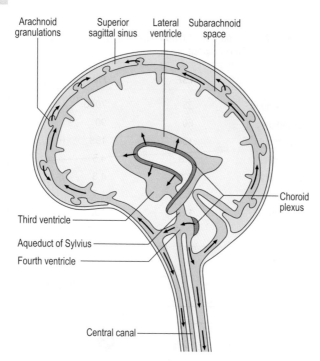

Arachnoid granulations · Superior sagittal sinus · Lateral ventricle · Subarachnoid space

Choroid plexus

Third ventricle

Aqueduct of Sylvius

Fourth ventricle

Central canal

Fig. 12.5 Production and flow of cerebrospinal fluid (CSF). CSF is secreted into the lateral, third and fourth ventricles, and flows into the subarachnoid space. Arrows indicate flow of CSF.

Box
12.2
Papilloedema and fundoscopy

The meninges enclose the optic nerve all the way to the retina. This means that raised intracranial pressure will be transmitted through the subarachnoid space surrounding the optic nerve and the blood vessels of the retina, the central artery and the central vein. Increased pressure will compress the central vein, leading to enlargement of the retinal veins and oedema of the optic papilla, which can be seen when the rear of the retina, the fundus, is examined with an ophthalmoscope (see Fig. 7.2B).

Box
12.3
Hydrocephalus

Hydrocephalus (or 'water on the brain') is the abnormal accumulation of cerebrospinal fluid (CSF). This can occur if the flow of CSF through the ventricles and around the brain is impaired, if there is a reduction in the reabsorption of CSF, and rarely, if there is excess CSF production. The commonest cause of hydrocephalus is the obstruction of the CSF flow from the fourth ventricle into the subarachnoid space, with a consequent enlargement of the ventricles. In babies, whose cranial sutures have not yet fused, this causes enlargement of the head with thinning of the cerebral hemispheres. In adults, because the skull is rigid, the increased pressure compresses blood vessels and damages brain tissue.

space, via the lateral and median apertures of the fourth ventricle. The ventricles are lined with ependymal cells. These are simple epithelial cells with numerous microvilli and one or two cilia on their apical surface. Their basolateral surface is in contact with astrocytic processes. After leaving the ventricles, the CSF flows through the cisternae at the base of the brain, and then travels across the cerebral and cerebellar hemispheres (Fig. 12.5). It is aided by the movement of the microvilli and cilia of the ependymal cells that line the ventricles, and by its reabsorption into the venous sinuses. This reabsorption involves movement of the CSF into the venous blood. Some of the fluid drains into cervical lymph nodes via the sheaths of the cranial nerves and into the spinal veins through arachnoid projections. In some cases, CSF can accumulate and lead to hydrocephalus (Box 12.3). Substances injected into the CSF can travel freely into the brain.

Very little CSF flows through the central canal of the spinal cord, which is not patent in most adults, but some CSF flows within the subarachnoid space through the foramen magnum, towards the lumbar region, reaching the end of the spinal meninges in about 12 hours. The meninges of the spinal cord extend to the S2 but the spinal cord extends only as far as the first or second lumbar vertebral level (L1, L2). The space below L2 forms a large lumbar cistern containing CSF that can be sampled by lumbar puncture (see Box 4.2). There is little danger of damaging the freely floating spinal nerves, as they will drift away from the point of the needle. However, lumbar puncture should not be performed under circumstances of increased intracranial pressure, as this can cause herniation of the brain.

An issue related to the circulation of fluids such as CSF around the brain is that of removal of waste products from brain tissue, which is essential for homeostasis. Research in the last decade has led to the proposal of the existence of a specialised system to carry out this main function: the glymphatic (glia-lymphatic) system. Besides waste elimination, the glymphatic system also facilitates brain-wide distribution of substances including glucose, lipids, amino acids, growth factors and neuromodulators. Another important discovery for the understanding of fluid flow in the brain occurred in 2015, involving meningeal lymphatic vessels. According to data collected in experimental models, the glymphatic flow is initiated by the CSF moving by convection through the periarterial space, driven by arterial pulsatility. The astrocyte endfeet facilitate mixing with the interstitial fluid and waste products therein. The aquaporin-4-4 (AQP4) water channels expressed on astrocytic endfeet play an essential role in this process; AQP4 reduces the hydraulic resistance of cell membranes and facilitates water flow into cells and out of cells. Fluids are then driven towards the perivenous space and along cranial and spinal nerves; ultimately, the fluid is directed towards meningeal lymphatic vessels and the general circulation. Observations in experimental models show that glymphatic efflux of β-amyloid peptides has an important role in the diurnal fluctuation in the levels of these peptides, which suggests that the glymphatic flow

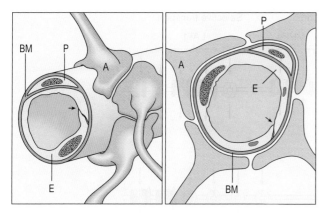

Fig. 12.6 Cells forming the blood–brain barrier. The arrow indicates the inter-endothelial tight junctions. *A*, Astrocyte; *BM*, basement membrane; *E*, endothelial cell; *P*, pericyte.

could be targeted in Alzheimer's disease. The inhibition of the glymphatic-lymphatic waste flow leads to accelerated protein aggregation and cognitive decline in mouse models of Alzheimer's disease, Parkinson's disease and traumatic brain injury. It is interesting to note that glymphatic clearance is turned on during sleep and is largely absent during wakefulness. It has been suggested that the need for sleep, which is seen across species, may be linked to this essential need for efficient and regular brain waste product clearance.

The blood–brain barrier

The BBB is a specialised microvascular structure at the interface between blood and brain tissue; its main role is to control the influx and efflux of substances into and out of the CNS and so has a fundamental homeostatic function. Various conditions that affect the CNS, such as trauma, stroke and multiple sclerosis, can lead to significant disruption of the BBB and impair its function. The existence of a specialised barrier was first proposed following the seminal observations made by Paul Ehrlich, who noticed that a peripherally injected dye did not stain brain tissue. The BBB is extensive; it is the largest interface for blood–brain exchanges and the surface area in an adult is between 12 and 18 m². It is formed from microvascular endothelial cells, which make up the continuous capillaries of the brain. The capillaries are continuous and non-fenestrated. The endothelial cells are surrounded by a layer of basement membrane, which itself is covered by a layer consisting of the endfeet of astrocytes (Fig. 12.6). The maintenance of the barrier function is based on the interaction between the microvascular specialized endothelium, the astrocytic foot processes (which cover close to 99% of the abluminal surface area of the brain capillary), and also pericytes. The astrocytic endfeet do not touch the endothelial cells; together with the pericytes, they are enclosed within the basement membrane that is important in producing factors that induce specific characteristics in the endothelial cells, which form the BBB. These characteristics include high trans-endothelial resistance, which is due

to the length and complexity of the tight junctions and the adherens junctions between the endothelial cells. The tight junctions and adherens junctions lead to polarisation of cells, with an abluminal side (the brain tissue side) and a luminal side (the blood side). Tight junctions involve many specialised proteins. Three major protein types are occludins, claudins and junction adhesion molecule proteins. The adherens junctions are established by homodimers of the transmembrane protein VE-cadherin, across adjacent endothelial cells. There are also very few pores, either small or large, that cross the endothelium. Transcytosis (transcellular transfer of molecules through receptor-mediated capture, internalisation and transfer across a cell soma) is limited. It is this 'tight' barrier that prevents bloodborne compounds from freely entering the brain, unless transported through specific mechanisms.

The brain endothelium is more restrictive, by a factor of 50–100, than other continuous capillaries. The BBB is not an absolute barrier; small non-polar molecules can enter through passive diffusion, but the majority of compounds are subject to specific transport systems. A key BBB characteristic is the presence of specific types of transporters that move molecules into and out of the brain (Fig. 12.7). Thus solutes, such as glucose, lactate, amino acids and fatty acids, are transported through specific transporters: glucose transporter 1 (GLUT1), monocarboxylate transporter 1 (MCT1), L-type amino acid transporter 1 (LAT1) and major facilitator superfamily domain containing 2A transporter (Mfsd2a), respectively. Other transporters provide receptor-mediated vesicular transport, such as the transferrin receptor TRF1 and low-density lipoprotein receptors. Some of the transporters have a key role in removing molecules from the CNS, for example, the lipoprotein receptor-related protein 1 (LRP1) which is linked to the transport of β-amyloid peptides. The BBB also expresses efflux transporters. These transporters are expressed on the luminal side of membranes and use the energy linked to ATP hydrolysis to transport small molecules up their concentration gradient and into the blood. They are also referred to as ATP-binding cassette (ABC) transporters. For example, P-glycoprotein (P-gp), also known as multidrug resistance protein 1 (MDR1), is a multidrug transporter that acts to transport lipophilic molecules out of the brain. The action of this efflux pump, while protecting the brain from many xenobiotics, has the effect of reducing the movement of many therapeutic drugs across the BBB. Another example of a multidrug resistance protein (MRP) efflux transporter is the breast cancer resistance protein (BCRP). The existence of these transporters has important consequences for the treatment of brain-specific illness, as the drugs have to gain access to the brain by travelling across the BBB in some way. Drug transporters can be constitutively expressed or induced, and their presence is a major mechanism underlying treatment resistance.

Several regions of the CNS around the third and fourth ventricles have fenestrated capillaries that lack the properties of the BBB; these are the circumventricular organs (area postrema, subfornical organ, pineal gland and median eminence of the hypothalamus) (Fig. 12.8).

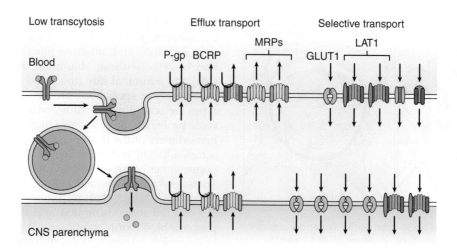

Fig.12.7 Modes of substance transport across the BBB. The diagram shows internalisation through transcytosis and transport through specialised efflux transporters or selective transporters. *BCRP*, breast cancer resistance protein; *GLUT1*, glucose transporter 1; *LAT 1*, L-type amino acid transporter 1; *MRP*, multidrug resistance-associated protein; *P-gp*, P-glycoprotein. (From Profaci C.P. et al (2020). The blood-brain barrier in health and disease: Important unanswered questions. Journal of Experimental Medicine. 217:1-16.).

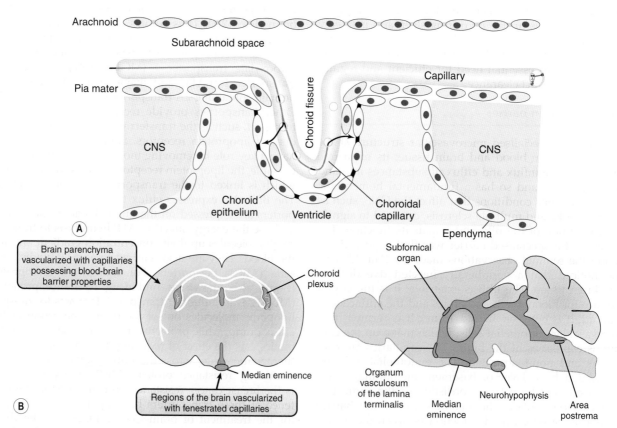

Fig. 12.8 The choroid plexus and brain regions with typical specialised capillaries with BBB properties or with fenestrated capillaries. (A) Composition of choroid plexus. Fenestrations of a choroidal segment of a capillary, showing that substances that escape from the blood into the choroid plexus are stopped by tight junctions (black bars) between choroid epithelial cells. (B) Brain regions with typical specialised capillaries with BBB properties or with fenestrated capillaries. The diagram illustrates the limited areas in the CNS where there are fenestrated capillaries, the circumventricular organs, which lack BBB properties. (From (A) Vanderah TW, Gould DJ. (2016) Nolte's The human brain: an introduction to neuroanatomy, seventhth ed. Elsevier; (B) adapted from Profaci C.P. et al (2020). The blood-brain barrier in health and disease: Important unanswered questions. Journal of Experimental Medicine. 217:1-16.).

They contain receptors which monitor the composition of the extracellular fluid for hormones and other chemical substances.

The choroid plexus is the site of the blood–CSF barrier. It consists of (1) a stroma made of fenestrated capillaries, surrounded by connective tissue containing immune cells and (2) epithelial cells. The epithelial cells are linked through tight junctions, adherens junctions and gap junctions. Certain pathogens can access the CNS through loosening of the tight junctions, leading to paracellular infiltration. The choroid plexuses can also be the site of development of tumours such as choroid plexus papilloma and carcinoma.

Meningitis

Meningitis is an inflammation of the pia and arachnoid mater, often of infectious nature, indicated by an increase in the number of white cells detected in the CSF. Meningitis is most commonly caused by a wide variety of infective agents; however, there are also non-infective causes, such as contrast medium, certain drugs and also tumours. It is normally confined to the subarachnoid space, rather than the subdural space. Infective agents can access the CSF directly via the sinuses or the nasopharynx, through fractures of the skull or, most commonly, from the blood stream.

Meningitis occurs as a result of either organisms crossing the BBB during systemic infection or a breakdown of the barrier due to a skull fracture or neurosurgery. A contiguous infection of the middle ear or paranasal sinuses can lead to infection of the meninges. However, the most common route is through the blood, and subsequent crossing of the BBB. Initially, pathogens colonise and invade epithelial surfaces in the respiratory tract, gastrointestinal tract or lower genital tract. Environmental factors (e.g. smoking or alcohol abuse) and genetic factors contribute to the susceptibility of individuals to blood stream infections. Other host factors include complement system deficiency, immunosuppressive treatment and antibody deficits. Bacteria need to survive the environment of the blood stream, and the polysaccharide capsules of organisms such as *Neisseria meningitidis*, *Streptococcus pneumoniae* and *Haemophilus influenzae* provide protection against attack by opsonins, which are extracellular proteins that act as tags to induce circulating phagocytes to phagocytose the pathogens. How the BBB barrier is breached is not fully understood. It may be that toxins produced by bacteria in the blood stimulate an increase in the permeability of either the BBB or the blood–CSF barrier. A further possibility is that organisms cross into the brain in areas such as the area postrema, a circumventricular organ in the medulla oblongata, devoid of BBB.

Bacterial meningitis

Meningococcal infection is the leading cause of bacterial meningitis in the UK. During 2018–19, Public Health England confirmed 526 cases of invasive meningococcal disease. It should be noted that other bacteria can also be associated with meningitis (Table 12.3). Most cases are sporadic; only approximately 1% of cases are secondary to other known cases.

There are several different serogroups of *N. meningitidis* associated with different risk groups. Most meningitis occurs in children under the age of 4 years, with the greatest age-specific risk at 6–12 months. This is mainly due to serogroup B, but also to serogroup C. There is a second peak in meningitis occurrence in late adolescence, largely due to serogroup C. Serogroup A infection occurs mainly in non-industrialized countries and is associated with epidemics. Certain parts of the world, such as sub-Saharan Africa, have experienced recurring large-scale episodes of meningitis for over a century. There is clear seasonality: outbreaks begin at the beginning of the dry season and end at the beginning of the wet season. This suggests that there are critical specific environmental factors, such as the effect of dry weather on mucous membranes and the impact of weather changes, that affect the transmission of respiratory viruses.

Vaccines against the meningococcal serogroups A, B, C, W and Y are available as single forms or combinations. In the UK, vaccination against serogroup C was implemented in England and Wales in 1998, and serogroup B vaccination in 2015. Vaccination programmes worldwide have resulted in significant decreases in the rate of meningitis caused by the bacterial strains covered by the vaccines.

Meningococci are ubiquitous Gram-negative diplococci. Many people carry meningococci in the nasopharynx and they are passed from person to person by close contact, but most strains are non-pathogenic. However, up to 1% of the population may carry pathogenic strains. The main risk seems to be the recent emergence of a new strain, but it is unknown why a small minority develop meningitis and most people do not.

A particular symptom of meningococcal meningitis is a haemorrhagic rash (Fig. 12.9). This is due to leakage of blood from capillaries into the skin. This can produce petechiae, which are small skin haemorrhages that vary in size from pinpoints to a few millimetres. The rash does not blanch on pressure as can be seen clearly when a glass is pressed on the skin. However, this sign may be sparse and does not occur in all cases, being most common in the more severe forms of the disease. Septicaemia is a dangerous complication of meningitis (Box 12.4).

Table 12.3	Possible causes of bacterial meningitis
Neisseria meningitides (meningococcus)*	
Streptococcus pneumoniae (pneumococcus)*	
Staphylococcus aureus	
Haemophilus influenzae (type b)[†]	
Escherichia coli	
Mycobacterium tuberculosis	
Listeria monocytogenes	

*Major causes of meningitis.
[†]Almost eliminated due to vaccination.

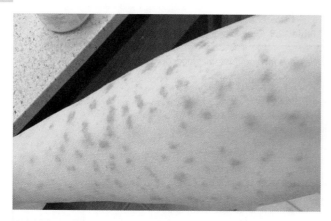

Fig. 12.9 Meningococcal rash. The rash usually manifests itself very early on. It will typically appear as red or purple spots that do not fade upon application of pressure. The spots are caused by bleeding underneath the skin. (From https://www.firstderm.com/life-threatening-skin-rashes/.)

When the infection due to *Neisseria meningitidis* spreads in the blood, a severe form of septicaemia can occur. There is a large drop in blood pressure, due to reduced peripheral resistance. This occurs because of the action of the bacterial endotoxin, which, via increases in nitric oxide synthesis, causes relaxation of vascular smooth muscle. There is increased secretion of a pro-inflammatory cytokine, interleukin-1, which increases capillary permeability. The flow through capillary beds becomes very slow, and eventually clotting factors can accumulate and produce inappropriate clotting in tissues. This is called disseminated intravascular coagulation. As well as reducing blood flow still further and preventing the supply of oxygen and removal of acid products of metabolism from the tissues, this depletes the available clotting factors, allowing blood to haemorrhage from the leaky blood vessels. The severe reduction in blood flow leads to metabolic acidosis, and eventually to skin and limb necrosis.

There are two other main bacterial causes of meningitis. These are *Haemophilus influenzae* type b and *S. pneumoniae*. *H. influenzae* infection usually occurs in young children (<5 years of age), but since the introduction of the Hib vaccine in 1992, this has all but disappeared in the UK. The few cases that still occur mostly affect adults with underlying medical conditions, rather than children. The bacteria can be spread by individuals who are ill with the infection and by healthy people who are carriers. *S. pneumoniae* infection is usually associated with young infants, the elderly with respiratory infections or otitis media (inflammation of the middle ear lining). In neonates the most common causative agents are *Escherichia coli* and group *B Streptococcus*.

A further cause of bacterial meningitis, which is more common in developing countries, is infection with *Mycobacterium tuberculosis*, which causes tuberculous meningitis. This form of meningitis is slow in onset, may occur years after the primary infection and may be preceded by non-specific symptoms.

Other bacteria, such as *Staphylococcus aureus* and *Listeria monocytogenes*, have been associated with meningitis, particularly in immunocompromised patients (see Table 12.3).

Even in the absence of septicaemia, meningitis is still a medical emergency, with the main pathology being cerebral oedema. Once the bacteria survive the passage through the blood stream, they are ready to invade the subarachnoid space; high levels of bacteraemia prompt the entry into this space. It is likely that the weakest point of entry is offered by post-capillary venules. The initial adhesion step involves proteins expressed by the pathogens, such as the bacterial adhesion outer membrane protein porin A (for *Neisseria meningitides*), which interact with laminin receptors expressed by brain endothelial cells, and may also involve other factors such as platelet-activating factor receptor. Ultimately, transcellular and paracellular passage is achieved by the pathogens. In the subarachnoid space there are relatively few phagocytic cells and also low levels of complement. In

normal CSF, the complement system (part of the innate immune system that enhances (complements) the ability of antibodies and phagocytic cells to attack and remove pathogens and damaged cells from an organism, and to promote inflammation) level is too low to have effective anti-bacterial impact. Specialised receptors that detect pathogens—the pathogen recognition receptors (PRR)—are virtually absent and this enables invading bacteria to multiply very rapidly, in a matter of hours after infection. Once the pathogens reach high numbers they begin to die, because of competition for nutrients, and this releases bacterial fragments that are recognised by PRR expressed by immunocompetent cells (e.g. macrophages and dendritic cells) expressed in the tissue in the immediate vicinity of the CSF. An important category of PRR involved in this phase are Toll-like receptors (TLR), which are cell-membrane receptors that are part of the innate immune system defences. Some of the TLR recognise bacterial DNA, lipids and proteins. Other key receptors are the nucleotide-binding and oligomerization domain NOD-like receptors (NLR), which are highly conserved cytosolic PRR that detect the presence of pathogen signals inside host cells. The NLR are key regulators of the inflammatory response and cell death pathways. The concerted action of TLR and NLR leads to activation of transcription factors such as NF-κB, a master regulator of inflammation cascades, and also to activation of the complement system. The latter consists of more than 30 distinct molecular components that synergise and initiate bactericidal attack and thus lead to further enhancement of the inflammation. There is increased production of inflammatory cytokines, such as interleukin-1 and tumour necrosis factor, which increases the permeability of the BBB and attracts large numbers of polymorphonuclear leucocytes. These cells release

Table 12.4 Some non-bacterial causes of meningitis

Type of organism	Examples
Viruses	Enteroviruses (Echovirus, Coxsackie virus types A and B)
	Mumps
	Poliovirus
	Epstein–Barr virus
	Herpes viruses (herpes simplex and herpes zoster)
	Human immunodeficiency virus
Fungi	*Cryptococcus neoformans*
	Candida spp.
Spirochaetes	Leptospirosis, Lyme disease, syphilis

cytotoxic products: reactive oxygen species, reactive nitrogen species and also proteases, which can initiate necrotic cell death. Protein leaks across the endothelium, and water follows, due to the increase in interstitial colloid osmotic pressure, producing cerebral oedema. This raises intracranial pressure and the associated risk of herniation. A poor prognostic feature is the depression of consciousness.

Meningitis can induce significant brain injury, through initiation of cell death processes (necrotic and apoptotic) and pathological changes in the vasculature, for example, vasculitis and vasospasm. Cerebral infarction can be triggered by thrombosis or embolism.

Aseptic and viral meningitis

The term aseptic meningitis is used to describe cases in which there are clinical signs of meningitis, but bacteria cannot be cultured from the CSF. This type of meningitis can have a wide range of causes, including viral and other non-bacterial infections, such as with fungi and protozoa (Table 12.4). Meningitis can also have non-infective, inflammatory causes such as sarcoidosis (a condition characterised by the formation of small collections of inflammatory cells in various organs). Despite recent advancements in molecular diagnosis techniques, aseptic meningitis remains challenging to diagnose and consequently remains underreported worldwide.

Many different viruses can cause meningitis. As the incidence of bacterial meningitis decreases, the proportion of meningitis cases caused by viruses is increasing. In the UK, a study published in 2018 estimated the annual incidence of viral meningitis in adults at 2.73 per 100,000.

Viruses can reach the CNS from the blood stream or through retrograde transmission from nerve terminals at the periphery. They may also emerge after reactivation of a dormant virus already present in the CNS. The majority of viral aetiology of aseptic meningitis

remains unknown. Before the introduction of the measles, mumps and rubella (MMR) vaccine, mumps-related meningitis was the leading cause of viral meningitis. The mumps virus is neurotropic and can directly infect the epithelium of the choroid plexus, whereas enteroviruses are dependent on hematogenous spread. The latter have been found to be the underlying cause of most viral meningitis cases worldwide.

Viral meningitis has a specific seasonality, being common in summer and autumn. Immunocompromised patients have a higher risk of developing this type of meningitis. The penetration of the virus is likely to occur through respiratory secretions or the faecal-oral route. The primary infection of the respiratory and gastrointestinal tracts is followed by secondary infection of the CNS. Viral meningitis has a similar pathophysiology to bacterial meningitis, with the infection triggering a strong inflammatory response. There are increased levels of pro-inflammatory cytokines such as interleukin-1β (IL-1β) and interleukin-6 (IL-6). Viral meningitis is usually less severe than bacterial meningitis and is self-limiting, lasting for 4–10 days. In general, there are few long-lasting major neurological sequelae. However, some patients do report a higher level of depression, anxiety and neurocognitive dysfunction a long time after the infection has cleared. Furthermore, enteroviral meningitis can lead to complications such as meningoencephalitis, myocarditis and pericarditis. Deaths can occur in immunocompromised patients who are vulnerable to infection with opportunistic pathogens and fatal sepsis.

Diagnosis and treatment of meningitis

Meningitis is usually diagnosed by a combination of clinical features and laboratory diagnostic tests. Meningitis usually presents with headache (often of rapid onset), fever, neck stiffness, photophobia and vomiting. In some types of meningitis there is also a rash. There may be altered consciousness, seizures and focal signs (aphasia, hemiparesis or nerve palsies). The headache may be due to inflammation of the supratentorial dura innervated by the trigeminal nerve, while the neck stiffness and reflex neck retraction are due to reflex contraction of the posterior nuchal muscles supplied by the cervical nerves that also innervate the infratentorial dura. Patients may show a positive Kernig's sign: after flexion of the leg at the hip, extension of the knee produces lower back pain, indicating irritation of the meninges.

The progression of bacterial meningitis is so rapid that when meningitis is suspected, treatment should be started before laboratory results are available. Early involvement and advice from a clinical microbiologist can be lifesaving. Intravenous cephalosporin compounds (ceftriaxone or cefotaxime) can be used as emergency treatment. A penicillin compound (e.g. benzylpenicillin, amoxicillin or ampicillin) can also be given immediately, either intravenously or intramuscularly, by the first doctor to suspect meningitis. A broad-spectrum antibiotic can be given for protection against both meningococcal

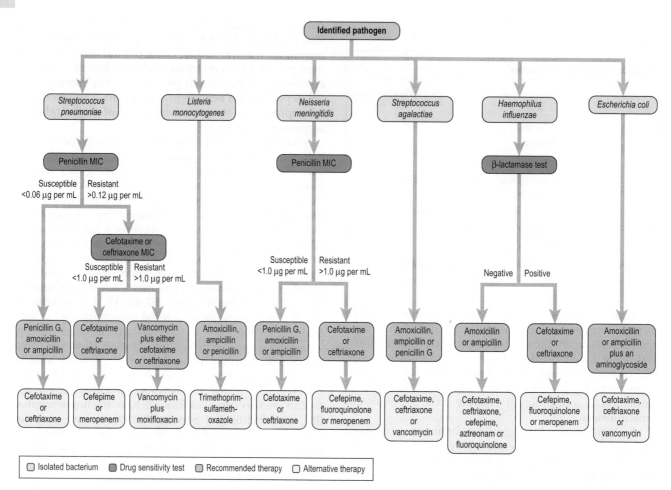

Fig. 12.10 Antibiotic therapy regimes for bacterial meningitis. Examples of therapies based on in vitro sensitivity testing. Alternative therapies are chosen if there are contraindications to the recommended therapy. *MIC*, Minimum inhibitory concentration. (From de Beek D. et al. (2016) Community-acquired bacterial meningitis, *Nature reviews Disease Primers.* 2:1-20.)

and pneumococcal pathogens. Aminoglycosides such as vancomycin can be added to treatment. An overview of the therapeutic algorithm for the treatment of bacterial meningitis, taking into account a determination of bacterial sensitivity in vitro, is shown in Fig. 12.10.

Cerebrospinal fluid sampling and changes in cerebrospinal fluid composition

Meningitis can be diagnosed after sampling the CSF through a lumbar puncture (see Box 4.2, Fig. 4.2). However, if there are any signs of focal intracranial disease or raised intracranial pressure (see Box 7.2), and if subsequent neuroimaging reveals any evidence of impaired CSF circulation, lumbar puncture should not be carried out due to risk of brain herniation. It is also contraindicated in severely ill children, as it may lead to deterioration. Throat swabs can indicate the presence of meningococcal infection.

Normal CSF is clear and contains very few cells. Inflammation of the meninges will increase the number of immune cells present. In bacterial meningitis, these will be predominantly neutrophils, while in other types of meningitis, especially viral, they are mainly lymphocytes (Table 12.5). Approximately 1%–2% of patients with bacterial meningitis will have a normal leucocyte count. The presence of bacteria will make the CSF turbid or even clearly pus-containing and, reflecting the breakdown of the BBB, there will be higher than normal levels of protein. Because of the utilization of CSF glucose by metabolizing bacteria, levels will be abnormally low in bacterial meningitis. CSF pressure is raised, and CSF flow may be impaired due to adhesions of the meninges and the presence of pus.

Culture of CSF (and blood) can reveal the type of bacterial infection present. This is important not only in order to determine the optimal antibiotic combination to use in further treatment, but also to obtain data about the antibiotic sensitivity of the bacteria. While *N. meningitidis* remains sensitive to penicillin, a significant number of *H. influenzae* strains and some *S. pneumoniae* strains show antibiotic resistance (Box 12.5).

Bacteria in cases of meningitis can be identified by examining cultures. Morphology and Gram staining will

Table 12.5 Comparison of cerebrospinal fluid in different types of meningitis compared to normal conditions

Type	Cell count	Cell types	Protein	Glucose
Bacterial	>200/µL	Polymorphs	>1.5 g/L	<40 mg/dL
Viral	50–200/µL	Lymphocytes	<1.0 g/L	Normal (40–70 mg/dL)
Normal	<5/µL	Lymphocytes	<0.45 g/L	Normal (40–70 mg/dL)

Box 12.5 Antibiotic resistance

Both the penicillins and cephalosporins are β-lactam antibiotics (they contain a β-lactam ring in their structure), and act by inhibiting one of the final stages of the synthesis of peptidoglycan, which forms the cell wall of Gram-positive bacteria. More recent broad-spectrum β-lactams are also active against some Gram-negative bacteria. However, some bacterial strains have developed resistance to some of these antibiotics. One of the main mechanisms of this resistance is the production by bacteria of β-lactamases, enzymes which destroy the antibiotics by cleaving the β-lactam ring. This has led to the development of β-lactam antibiotics that are β-lactamase resistant, such as flucloxacillin. β-Lactam antibiotics can induce various adverse effects, including nausea, diarrhoea and rashes. Chloramphenicol acts in a different way from the β-lactams, by inhibiting bacterial protein synthesis. Resistance to chloramphenicol is due to the production by the bacteria of acetyltransferase enzymes, which inactivate the antibiotic by acetylation. Clavulanic acid is a compound that acts as an inhibitor of β-lactamase; it can be co-administered with β-lactam antibiotics, to overcome the impact of β-lactamases.

Methicillin-resistant *Staphylococcus aureus* (MRSA) is a group of Gram-positive bacteria that are associated with infections that are very difficult to treat. The increased resistance of this type of bacterium to antibiotics may have evolved naturally or could be a consequence of horizontal gene transfer (e.g. through transfer of gene material between bacteria through conjugation). MRSA is a common cause of hospital-acquired infections and is a significant risk in patients with a weak immune system, or with open wounds or invasive devices, which provide a route of access and invasion. When MRSA invades the CNS, there can be development of brain or spinal epidural abscesses. Vancomycin and teicoplanin are glycopeptide antibiotics that are effective in most cases, but there are reports of resistance to these drugs. Alternatively, more recent antibiotics such as the streptogramins and oxazolidinones can be tried. Thus second-line therapy may include telavancin, ceftaroline and linezolid. Phage therapy, that is the use of bacteriophages to attack the resistant bacteria, is used in some countries, and is the object of renewed interest in research.

differentiate between the three main bacterial causes and the Ziehl–Neelsen stain identifies acid-fast bacilli such as *Mycobacterium*. However, these are only seen in approximately 20% of cases of tuberculous meningitis. Indian ink can be used to stain fungi.

One of the problems with culturing CSF (and blood) is that it can take some time and, in the case of tuberculosis, may take many weeks. Newer tests enable the causative agents to be identified more quickly. Antigen detection of specific polysaccharides present on the bacterial cell walls, in the CSF or urine, can be used to detect some bacteria. CSF analysis using the technique of DNA amplification by the polymerase chain reaction (PCR) can detect both bacteria and viruses with high sensitivity. PCR is the 'gold standard' for viral meningitis and is increasingly used for bacterial meningitis.

Blood cultures should also be initiated on admission, before lumbar puncture and the beginning of antibiotic treatment. Blood PCR analysis is increasingly important.

Treatment of meningitis

It is very important that antibiotic treatment is initiated immediately on suspicion of bacterial meningitis, as it is still a condition associated with significant mortality. For example, even when meningococcal meningitis is diagnosed early and adequate treatment is started, 8%–15% of patients will die, often within 24–48 hours after the onset of symptoms. The treatments of choice for meningococcal and pneumococcal infection are benzylpenicillin and cephalosporins (cefotaxime or ceftriaxone); previously, ampicillin and chloramphenicol were recommended for the treatment of *H. influenza* meningitis. However, resistance to both these antibiotics has emerged (see Box 12.5). Specifically, strains of this bacterium produce β-lactamase, which degrade the β-lactam antibiotics, and others are resistant through reduced affinity for penicillin-binding proteins. If the causative agent has not yet been identified, a combination of these drugs could be used. The antibiotic treatment should be continued for 7 days after the fever has ceased (14 days for pneumococcal infections). Antibiotics can be combined with steroids.

Other treatment should be aimed at reducing the fever and providing pain relief for headaches. Anticonvulsants should be used for patients with seizures. In cases of septicaemia, fluid balance must be strictly monitored and, if possible, controlled. Septicaemia can lead very rapidly to severe shock, disseminated intravascular coagulation and multi-organ failure.

β-Lactam antibiotics disrupt bacterial cell walls, releasing more of the lipopolysaccharides that cause the inflammatory response. In this way, the treatment can exacerbate the pathology. In cases of infection with *H. influenzae* and *S. pneumoniae* there is evidence that pre-treatment with steroids (e.g. dexamethasone) can reduce the subsequent cerebral oedema and reduce the potential after-effects, such as deafness. However, this has not been shown for *N. meningitidis* and the need for rapid antibiotic therapy would make any delay dangerous.

Bacterial meningitis can progress extremely rapidly and any delay in treatment can increase morbidity and mortality. The most serious form of meningococcal meningitis involves septicaemia and this accounts for most of the significant mortality (up to 57%) associated with this type of meningitis. If septicaemia is not present, the mortality rate drops to 3%, which is lower than that for *H. influenzae* (4%–5%) and *S. pneumoniae* (10%).

There is no specific treatment for viral meningitis. Anti-viral drugs such as acyclovir have only proven to be of benefit in viral encephalitis (see later in the text). Viral meningitis patients can suffer long-term cognitive and psychological sequelae.

Tuberculous meningitis is the most serious extra-pulmonary complication of tuberculosis—an infection caused by the bacterium *M. tuberculosis,* a pathogen discovered more than a century ago by Robert Koch. Tuberculosis continues to be a health problem in many parts of the world. It can affect various organs; the pathogen can persist in the host for a long time and can also develop multi-drug treatment resistance. WHO guidelines for treatment recommend treatment with rifampicin, isoniazid, pyrazinamide and ethambutol for the first 2 months, followed by up to 10 months of rifampicin and isoniazid. Pyridoxine (vitamin B6) is added to avoid isoniazid-induced peripheral neuropathy. Second-line treatments include levofloxacin, moxifloxacin, amikacin, kanamycin and linezolid. There is also focus on the development of new host-directed therapies, which could enhance the protective immune response or regulate the pathological immune response to infection. There is some evidence that dexamethasone used as adjunctive treatment can lead to survival benefits.

Long-term sequelae of meningitis include hydrocephalus, cranial nerve palsies, visual and motor deficits and epilepsy. In children, there may be behavioural disturbances, learning difficulties, hearing loss and epilepsy. Bacterial meningitis during childhood can have a long-lasting effect on educational attainment.

Meningitis and meningococcal septicaemia are statutory notifiable diseases in England, Scotland and Wales and should be reported to the local Consultant in Communicable Disease Control (CCDC). Any immediate contacts and family members of a patient with meningococcal meningitis are at increased risk (800-fold) and should be given antibiotic prophylaxis with rifampicin, ceftriaxone or ciprofloxacin in order to eradicate bacteria.

Table 12.6	Causes of viral encephalitis
Sporadic	
Herpes simplex (HSV)	
Herpes zoster	
Cytomegalovirus	
Epstein–Barr virus	
Adenovirus	
Human immunodeficiency virus	
Epidemic	
Arboviruses	
Eastern equine encephalitis virus	
Japanese B arbovirus	

Despite the progress made in recent decades regarding the management of bacterial meningitis, it remains one of the most dangerous and widespread infections worldwide. Prevention of the disease and early initiation of treatment can limit the morbidity and mortality. Vaccination programmes have made a significant impact, but there is need for sustained vigilance against new strains. Additionally, there is increased concern over the emergence of microbial antibiotic resistance. Apart from improved antibiotics, there is a need for novel treatment strategies based on modulation of the host immune response and regulation of the damage induced by the pathophysiological cascades that lead to production of compounds toxic to host cells during the invasion by pathogens.

Encephalitis

Viral encephalitis is caused by several viruses (Table 12.6), that can be transmitted by animals, resulting in sporadic or epidemic infection. Many sporadic infections cause mild illness with headache and drowsiness, which is self-limiting, but in more severe cases, patients have altered behaviour, seizures, confusion or coma. Brain swelling is common, with its associated risk of brain damage.

In the UK, the most dangerous form of viral encephalitis is that caused by the HSV. While HSV can be identified in CSF with the use of viral antigen immunoassays and amplification of viral DNA using PCR techniques, this is usually too slow to be of clinical use. For this reason, patients with acute encephalitis should be treated with acyclovir immediately, especially if there is evidence of brain swelling on computed tomography (CT) scans (Box 12.6). There are no other specific treatments for encephalitis, except ganciclovir, which is active against cytomegalovirus. Patients may need treatment for seizures and cerebral oedema. Encephalitis may occasionally be caused by other organisms, such as *Mycoplasma*, *Rickettsia* (typhus) and *Histoplasma*.

Acyclovir and anti-viral therapy

While there are many effective anti-bacterial agents that target specific bacterial processes, it is much more challenging to develop drugs that will inhibit viruses without harming the host, because viruses survive by utilizing many of the normal metabolic processes of the host eukaryotic cell. Acyclovir exploits the need of the virus to produce new viral DNA, which it does using a viral DNA polymerase that is different from the mammalian enzyme. Acyclovir is a guanine derivative that is converted to the monophosphate by thymidine kinase. This occurs most rapidly in the virus-infected cells, as the viral kinase is much more effective than the host enzyme. The host cell kinases then convert the monophosphate to acyclovir triphosphate. This compound inhibits the DNA polymerases, thus blocking DNA synthesis. The drug has a poor availability after oral administration, and intravenous administration is required in order to reach high concentrations in target tissues. Acyclovir is effective in encephalitis caused by the herpes simplex virus, herpes zoster virus and the varicella zoster virus. It has no activity against enteroviruses.

Acyclovir is one of the major discoveries in modern medicine, and Gertrude Elion, the pharmacologist involved in its discovery, was awarded the Nobel Prize. The drug was approved in 1981, and its importance is reflected in its inclusion in the World Health Organization List of Essential Medicines, which contains the safest and most effective medicines needed in health systems.

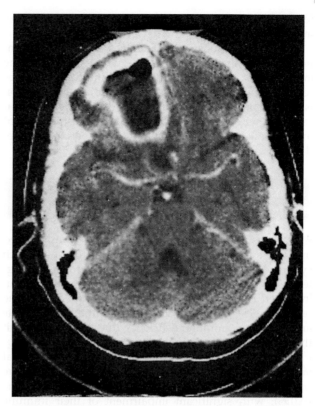

Fig. 12.11 Enhanced axial computed tomography scan showing a right frontal abscess. (From Forbes CD, Jackson WF. (2002) Colour atlas and text of clinical medicine, third ed. Mosby International Ltd.)

As mentioned previously, infection with the SARS-CoV-2 virus, which has caused the COVID-19 pandemic, has shown that this corona virus can trigger long-term neurological consequences: more than 50% of patients can still have neurological symptoms at 3 months after disease onset. The neurological manifestations of the disease are either a consequence of the virus itself or the immune response to the virus. The initial presentation of the infection includes as cardinal symptoms: fever, headaches, loss of smell and taste, and myalgia. Subsequent systemic complications, such as coagulopathy, the intense proinflammatory cytokine storm and multiple organ dysfunction, also contribute to neuronal damage. Finally, the long stay in intensive care of severely ill patients, under invasive ventilation, leads to the usual complications seen in critical care units, such as confusion and weakness. There is prolonged cognitive impairment and also a significant level of persistent anxiety and depression.

Cerebral abscesses

Brain abscesses may be a consequence of trauma or surgical interventions, or can develop after spread of an infection in adjacent structures such as the middle ear or certain paranasal sinuses, or systemic infection. A range of bacteria, fungi and protozoa (e.g. *Streptococcus*, *Staphylococcus*, *Bacteroides* and *Proteus*) can cause focal areas of infection, leading to abscesses in the brain and spinal cord. As the infection could reach the brain from infectious sites elsewhere in the body (e.g. endocarditis or pulmonary infections), or from a contiguous location (dental, sinus or ear infections), identification and treatment of the primary source of the infection should form part of the overall treatment.

The majority of cases occur between the third and fifth decade of life. The patient usually has a combination of progressive headache, focal neurological signs, altered mental status, seizures and fever. The investigation of choice is a CT or magnetic resonance imaging scan. Lumbar puncture should not be performed because of the risk of herniation, but could be considered when there is evidence of a limited mass effect. CSF analysis may reveal pleocytosis (high number of lymphocytes), high levels of protein and decreased glucose. A few weeks after infection, an abscess becomes encapsulated and can be clearly seen (Fig. 12.11). The central area of the abscess will have a low-density appearance, there will be prominent ring enhancement of the lesion, which appears bright, and there will be an oedematous surrounding area of low density. Because of the mass effect of the abscess, there may also be a shift in the midline and compression of the ventricles. Aerobic organisms (e.g. streptococci), more so than anaerobic organisms, are involved in abscesses.

Treatment in most cases involves surgical intervention. This involves excision or CT-guided aspiration. The latter is also preferred when there are multiple abscesses requiring drainage. Abscess recurrence after aspiration is not uncommon. Antibiotics are required (e.g. cephalosporins with added metronidazole) and also treatment for cerebral oedema (e.g. mannitol or hypertonic saline) if there is a risk of herniation.

Brain infections in the immunocompromised patient

An increasing number of patients have compromised immune systems. This may result from treatment with cytotoxic drugs or immunosuppressant steroids, or long-term severe general illness. In these patients, there is an increased risk of infection with bacteria and fungi. One of the largest groups of immunocompromised patients are those with immune deficiency due to infection with the human immunodeficiency virus (HIV).

Infection with HIV can cause neurological disease at any stage, but most problems occur when patients have progressed to acquired immune deficiency syndrome (AIDS), with significant impairment of their immune systems. A few weeks or months after HIV infection, a patient can develop meningoencephalitis, when the infection involves both the meninges and the brain parenchyma. Like other immunocompromised patients, HIV patients are prone to a wide range of infections, both with organisms that are normally pathogenic but cause more severe infections in these patients, and with organisms that are not normally pathogenic (i.e. opportunistic infections). HIV infection and AIDS remain leading causes of years of life lost to disability.

HIV can infect and replicate in the microglial cells of the brain, which can act as a reservoir of infection. The active replication of HIV in the brain leads to increased permeability of the BBB, allowing easier access to infecting organisms and, as a consequence, 80% of HIV-positive patients develop neurological disease. Any treatment aiming to eradicate HIV must also be able to eradicate the virus present in the brain, because the movement of macrophages across the BBB could result in re-infection.

The neurological condition specific to HIV infection is HIV-associated dementia. This slowly developing dementia is thought to be due to a direct effect of HIV infection of the brain (see Chapter 14 for more details). Anti-retroviral therapy has evolved significantly in recent decades and suppresses viral replication, decreases viral load, reconstructs the immune system, reduces the risk of transmission, improves the quality of life and prolongs life expectancy. Therapy consists of various classes of drugs: (1) nucleoside reverse transcriptase inhibitors (NRTI), (2) non-nucleoside reverse transcriptase inhibitors (NNRTI), (3) fusion inhibitors, (4) protease inhibitors, (5) integrase strand transfer inhibitors and (6) C-C chemokine receptor type 5 (CCR5) inhibitors. The

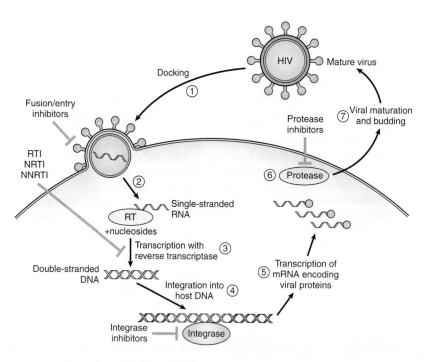

Fig. 12.12 The life cycle of HIV and therapeutic targets. The diagram illustrates the mode of action of major anti-viral strategies. The numbers indicate the targets and mechanisms. *NNRTI*, Non-nucleoside reverse transcription inhibitors; *NRTI*, nucleoside reverse transcription inhibitors; *RT*, reverse transcription; *RTI*, reverse transcription inhibitors. (From Atta M.G. et al, (2019). Clinical Pharmacology in HIV Therapy. *Clinical Journal of the American Society of Nephrology*. 14:435-44.

first five classes target various steps in the viral life cycle (shown in Fig. 12.12), whereas the CCR5 inhibitors—more recently developed drugs—have as a rationale the role of the CCR5 receptor in the process by which HIV enters cells and then spreads. Hence, antagonists of this receptor are entry inhibitors. Drugs can be used as monotherapy or in combination, and evidence suggests that combinatorial treatments are more effective. Present recommendations favour the use of triple combination therapy as first-line treatment, for example, two NRTIs plus one NNRTI, protease inhibitor, fusion inhibitor or integrase strand transfer inhibitor. Pharmaco-enhancers (e.g. cobicistat, which inhibits liver microsomal enzymes and thus enhances the effect of anti-retroviral drugs), can also be added. Finally, preventive treatment with neutralising HIV antibodies is also a growing area of interest.

Self-assessment case study

A young woman aged 24 years is admitted to hospital complaining of severe headache, neck stiffness, fever and photophobia. On examination, she has no signs of papilloedema, and a lumbar puncture is performed. This shows clear cerebrospinal fluid (CSF) with an increased number of lymphocytes, a slightly raised protein level and a normal CSF glucose level. The woman is admitted and given acyclovir. However, subsequent analysis of the CSF shows no evidence of herpes simplex virus infection. After 4 days, the patient is sent home and, although she continues to have headaches for a couple of weeks, she has no other sequelae.

After studying this chapter you should be able to answer the following questions:

1. What do the presenting symptoms suggest about her condition?

The presenting symptoms suggest that she is suffering from meningitis. This may be due to many possible causes but it is very likely that this patient has a viral meningitis.

2. What is the clinical significance of the lack of papilloedema?

This suggests that there is a lack of raised intracranial pressure, therefore carrying out a lumbar puncture was safe.

3. What do the CSF results indicate?

The CSF results confirm the possibility that this patient suffers from viral, not bacterial, meningitis.

4. Why was she given acyclovir?

Acyclovir is an efficacious anti-viral drug, which prevents the replication of the virus by blocking DNA synthesis. It was given as a precautionary measure, while waiting for the results of the exploration of the CSF and the identification of the virus type.

EPILEPSY

Chapter summary

1. Epilepsy is a generic term for a type of brain disorder characterized by recurrent unprovoked seizures, which result from abnormalities in the electrical activity of the brain. Focal seizures generally involve limited brain areas, and sometimes spread to affect larger areas. Generalized seizures start in both brain hemispheres and are associated with a loss of awareness. Status epilepticus is a specific type of epilepsy characterized by prolonged seizures and is a life-threatening medical emergency. Epilepsy can be associated with many co-morbidities and it increases the risk of premature death.

2. The aetiology of epilepsy is diverse: structural, genetic, immune, infectious or metabolic. In some cases the cause is unknown. Analysis of the electrical activity of the brain (electroencephalogram) and structural imaging can help diagnose the epilepsy type and identify brain areas likely to be the cause of epilepsy.

3. The abnormal activity of the brain leading to emergence of seizures can involve changes in glutamatergic or GABAergic transmission, thereby changing the balance excitation/inhibition in the brain, or can also be a consequence of alterations in ion channels, which change intrinsically neuronal excitability. Many types of juvenile-onset epilepsies are channelopathies, as they are underlied by specific mutations in ion channels such as the sodium channel. Mutations in pathways involved in cell growth and development are also associated with epilepsy.

4. The pharmacological treatment of epilepsy is based on the use of a variety of anticonvulsant drugs. First generation drugs include phenytoin, carbamazepine, sodium valproate and ethosuximide, while more recent drugs include lamotrigine, topiramate, tiagabine, levetiracetam, stiripentol and perampanel. These drugs act through

a variety of mechanisms: voltage-dependent ion channel blockers, ligand-gated ion channel antagonists or allosteric modulators, or inhibitors of neurotransmitter uptake or neurotransmitter-metabolizing enzymes. Approximately one-third of epileptic patients are treatment-resistant.

5. Non-pharmacological approaches to the management of epilepsy, to address the issue of treatment-resistance, include surgery (to remove an identified epileptogenic focus), corpus callosotomy (to abolish the spread of seizures) and vagus nerve stimulation. A ketogenic dietary approach based on a high fat/protein to carbohydrate ratio is very effective in some forms of epilepsy in children.

Introduction

In adults, once the brain has reached maturation, control over sensorimotor and autonomic functions is expected, as well as complete awareness of one's behaviour and reactions under various social circumstances. One of the commonest neurological diseases, epilepsy, often deprives an individual of this control and can lead to a dramatic loss of contact with reality, through loss of consciousness. This is illustrated in the case history in Box 13.1. As will be discussed, epilepsy is a major medical problem that poses a therapeutic challenge, can significantly disrupt the course of normal life and its quality and may bring social stigma to the sufferer.

General description of epilepsy

Epilepsy is the name given to a heterogeneous group of conditions characterized by the occurrence of spontaneous, unprovoked seizures. A seizure is a sudden, abnormal, paroxysmal change in the electrical activity of the brain; it reflects large-scale synchronous discharges of groups of neurons and can cause changes in behaviour, movement, mood, sensation and levels of consciousness. Epilepsy exists in all mammals. It is an ancient disorder that can be traced back to the first medical records in the history of humanity. In ancient times, it was considered a condition due to the control exerted on individuals by 'evil spirits'. This was associated with significant stigma, which could culminate in the individual being sacrificed for the perceived benefit of the community. In the 5th century BCE Hippocrates clearly stated his belief that 'the brain is the seat of this disease'. Significant progress has been made in the neurobiology of epilepsy and its clinical management, in recent decades, but the stigma associated with this condition, at least in some societies, is still significant.

For a diagnosis of epilepsy there must be evidence that there have been at least two seizures on separate occasions. The types of seizure that occur in epilepsy are very varied. They range from generalized seizures, with loss of consciousness and body muscle spasms (commonly known as 'grand mal'), to the much less overwhelming absence seizure (also known as 'petit mal'), the only sign of which is that the person stops what they are doing and appears to be staring into the distance. Seizures are generally self-limiting phenomena. However, in some cases, generalized seizures are not self-limiting, and the patient may have recurrent seizures for 10–20 min, without regaining consciousness. This is status epilepticus and is a serious, life-threatening medical emergency.

There are three levels of diagnosis in epilepsy: seizure type, epilepsy type and epilepsy syndrome. From the perspective of onset of a seizure, there are *focal seizures* (the term used previously was 'partial seizures'), which begin focally, in a limited brain area and sometimes may spread to both hemispheres; *generalized seizures*, which involve both hemispheres of the brain from the onset; and seizures of *unknown onset*. This leads to several epilepsy categories: focal, focal/generalized, generalized and unknown. Finally, epilepsy syndrome refers to a cluster of specific seizure features, brain electrical activity profile and brain imaging changes. An epilepsy syndrome could include associated psychiatric and cognitive abnormalities, sometimes mental retardation, and the definition of a syndrome has significant prognosis and management implications.

Overall, there are still ambiguities even using this system based on several diagnostic levels, and the clinical presentation is often very complex. This complexity is reflected in the extended classification, which is regularly reviewed and updated, to incorporate new knowledge and insights. This detailed classification system was devised by the International League Against Epilepsy (ILAE). The latest ILAE classification is shown in Fig. 13.1.

Gaby is a 22-year-old student who is studying to become a teacher. She has no previous serious medical history. One day, as she relaxes with her fellow students after an examination, she feels strange, with butterflies in her stomach and a sensation of fear and anxiety. She then collapses rigidly onto the floor. She has strong convulsions for about 2 min, during which she knocks against a chair. Her body then relaxes and, for the next 3 min, she is unarousable. When she wakes up she is confused and tired, and also bruised from hitting the chair. She is taken to hospital by her colleagues, where the doctor tells her she has had a seizure. There is no family history of seizures. She undergoes a series of tests, including an electroencephalogram (EEG) and a brain scan. A few weeks later, she has a second seizure at home. Following a consultation with the hospital specialist, she starts taking sodium valproate. Gaby is also advised to change her type of contraceptive pill. She is very concerned about the implications of having this disease for her career choice as a teacher.

This case gives rise to the following questions:

1. What is epilepsy?
2. What does an EEG measure and how is it used in the diagnosis of epilepsy?
3. What are the mechanisms of excitation and inhibition in the brain and how are seizures produced?
4. What types of epilepsy are there?
5. How is epilepsy treated?
6. What restrictions are there for patients with epilepsy?

The different types of seizure associated with various types of epilepsy are associated with different patterns of muscular activity. Myoclonic seizures involve either localized or widespread, rapid, irregular jerking of muscles, while in tonic seizures there is a sudden rigidity of muscles, either extended or flexed. Clonic seizures involve the rhythmic jerking of many muscles, and in tonic–clonic seizures, there is clonic jerking after initial tonic rigidity. Atonic seizures involve sudden generalized muscle relaxation.

A presentation of seizures is not uncommon in emergency medicine. Patients presenting with seizures may have a history of a seizure disorder. If possible, obtaining a history will establish if there is any alcohol or substance abuse or recent traumatic injuries. The individual may carry a card identifying them as an epilepsy patient. The first steps in emergency management are: protect the person against injury by cushioning their head, remove glasses, keep them comfortable and do not restrain them, and make sure there are no harmful objects nearby; when the seizure stops, place the individual in the recovery position until they recover consciousness, and request hospital admission.

Epidemiology and causes of epilepsy

Epilepsy is a common neurological disorder. The prevalence of the various types is 0.5%–1% worldwide and the lifetime incidence is 1%–3%. Epilepsy is the third biggest contributor to the global burden of neurological disease. A majority of epileptic patients live in resource-limited, developing countries, which has implications for

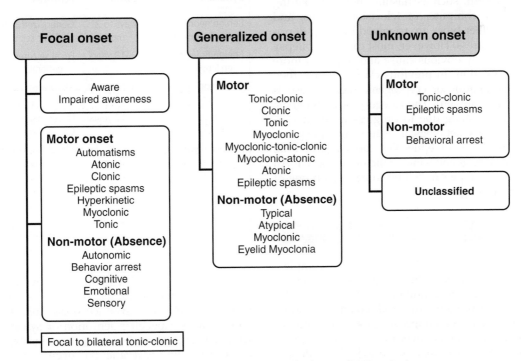

Fig. 13.1 Classification of seizure types by the ILAE (2017 version).

the correct diagnosis and management of the condition. The World Health Organization estimates that up to 70% of people living with epilepsy could live seizure-free, if they were properly diagnosed and treated. In poor countries, epilepsy is often associated with infectious diseases such as malaria and neurocysticercosis.

Epileptic seizures generally have three phases: a prodromal phase where the person is aware that a seizure is coming and this can be associated with auras or other specific signs. This is followed by the ictal phase (ictal is a term derived from the Latin word 'ictus' meaning 'blow' or 'stroke', and refers to the seizure event), which is the time from the first symptom to the end of the seizure, and lastly the postictal (recovery) phase. People who suffer from epilepsy have a predisposition to recurrent seizures, and epilepsy can have significant cognitive and psychological consequences. Epileptic patients can have a high frequency of depression and have a higher risk of suicide than the general population. Certain patterns of psychosis are associated with epilepsy. Psychotic disorders are classified as ictal, if they are an expression of the seizure activity; postictal, when they occur within a week of a seizure; and interictal, when they occur independently of seizures. Interictal psychosis may also be an unwanted effect of the anti-epileptic therapy. Epilepsy can be associated with lethality, direct effects (e.g. falls, road traffic accidents, drowning) or indirect effects (psychiatric complications, adverse effects of medication). Sudden unexpected death in epilepsy (SUDEP) affects ~1:1000 epilepsy patients.

Epilepsy can be linked to a variety of primary causes, such as brain tumours or meningitis, and metabolic abnormalities such as hypoglycaemia and uraemia (Table 13.1). Some types of seizure are induced by very ordinary sensory stimuli, such as flashing lights, flickering fluorescent lights, computer or television screens, and strobe lighting. Other types are triggered by sleep deprivation or intense stress. However, most cases of epilepsy have no immediately obvious cause and require a more extensive investigation. In previous classifications, they were termed idiopathic or cryptogenic (i.e. a cause is suspected but not proven). The category of cryptogenic epilepsies is diminishing due to progress in the understanding of various aetiological aspects of epilepsies. Overall, the aetiology of epilepsies can be structural, infectious, immune, genetic, metabolic or unknown. An epilepsy or seizure type can belong to more than one of these aetiological subgroups.

Diagnostic investigations of epilepsy

A patient with suspected epilepsy requires a complete neurological examination. The diagnosis of epilepsy is primarily clinical. The definition of epilepsy is: (1) a patient with two or more unprovoked seizures >24 hours apart, (2) a patient with an unprovoked seizure who has >60% risk of another seizure over the following 10 years or (3) a patient with one or more seizures in the context of a specific epilepsy syndrome.

Table 13.1 Some causes and predisposing factors of epilepsy

Metabolic disturbances (especially electrolyte imbalances and uraemia)

Hypoxia

Chronic alcohol abuse (seizures either during heavy drinking or during withdrawal)

Some neuroactive drugs (either in overdose or at normal levels in susceptible patients)

Drug withdrawal states (especially phenobarbitone and benzodiazepines)

Strokes (haemorrhagic or ischaemic)

Aneurysms

Perinatal trauma and anoxia

Central nervous system infection (meningitis, encephalitis, cerebral abscess)

Traumatic brain injury

Family history

Intrauterine infections (e.g. rubella)

Developmental abnormalities

Craniotomy

Degenerative brain disorders

Brain tumours

Table 13.2 Examples of childhood epileptic syndromes

Syndrome	Age of onset	Features
Benign neonatal familial convulsions	Days to 2 months	Generalized or focal, tonic or clonic seizures
Benign Rolandic epilepsy	3–13 years	Focal seizures with secondary generalization
Childhood absence epilepsy (CAE)	3–12 years	Many absences Convulsions rare
Juvenile absence epilepsy	7–17 years	Fewer absences than with CAE Convulsions common
Juvenile myoclonic epilepsy (Janz syndrome)	10–20 years	Myoclonic jerks on waking Generalized tonic–clonic seizures Occasional absences
Infantile spasms (West's syndrome)	3–7 months	Flexor spasms, tonic and atonic seizures, progressive mental handicap

A detailed history is essential, and eyewitness reports on the presentation of the seizure are very valuable. Some patients may experience an aura before a seizure, that is, a peculiar sensation or symptom, such as strange smells or unpleasant taste, epigastric pressure or a general feeling of *déjà vu* (i.e. even if the environment is new, it feels familiar, as though they have been there before). If an aura precedes the attack, its description can help identify a possible focus of functional or structural abnormality in the brain.

When diagnosing epilepsy, it is important to first make sure that there is no confusion with conditions that produce similar clinical signs such as syncope, transient ischaemic attacks (TIAs), hypoglycaemia, migraine or pseudoseizures (also called psychogenic non-epileptic seizures, where there is no objective evidence of brain electrical abnormalities). Once the diagnosis of epilepsy is confirmed, it is important to obtain additional information and determine possible causes. In an adult with no previous history of epilepsy, it is important to carry out brain imaging to exclude the possibility of a tumour or other mass-filling lesion as the cause of the seizures. Establishing whether there is a family history of epilepsy is also important, for its link to a possible genetic cause (Box 13.2).

Electroencephalography and magnetoencephalography

Electroencephalography and magnetoencephalography are based on the generation of electrical and magnetic fields as a consequence of the electrical activity of neurons. An electroencephalogram (EEG) is a non-invasive method of measuring the surface electrical activity of the brain. When cortical neurons are active, the electrical currents that flow across the neuronal cell membranes also set up extracellular currents that flow through the extracellular space. Recordings of these currents can be made at sites distant from where the currents are generated. In the case of an EEG, these currents are measured by electrodes placed on the scalp. The changes in electrical potential measured by the EEG are the summated ionic currents produced by the large numbers of neurons found under the electrodes in the cortex (Box 13.3). These scalp electrodes are positioned using a conductive gel or paste according to a standard pattern specified by an international system, and the potential difference is measured between pairs of electrodes. The major sites of placement of electrodes on the scalp are shown in Fig. 13.2. Electrodes can also be embedded in a mesh, forming a cap, which can be fitted on the patient's head. Most commercially available array head nets are equipped with 64, 128 or 256 electrodes. Some are customizable, hence the optimal number of electrodes can be chosen for a particular clinical or research aim.

While the largest signal generated by neurons is the action potential, it is a very short-lasting event and,

---

Box 13.2 Genetics of epilepsy

There is a strong correlation between epilepsy and family history, with approximately 30% of patients having a close relative with epilepsy. At present, there are more than 500 genes associated with epilepsy, and this list is likely to grow. The genetic abnormalities seen in epilepsy include single mutations, copy number variations, microdeletions and microduplications. Mutations can occur in protein-coding exons and also in non-coding regions. For most epileptic syndromes, the mode of inheritance is complex. For example, common forms of idiopathic epilepsy, such as juvenile myoclonic epilepsy or juvenile and childhood absence epilepsy (see Table 13.2), do not follow a simple Mendelian mode of inheritance. Identification of the genes mutated in idiopathic epilepsies shows that these forms of epilepsy are most often channelopathies; that is, they are due to mutations in voltage- or ligand-gated ion channels (e.g. cholinergic nicotinic receptors, Na^+, K^+ and Ca^{2+} channels, and $GABA_A$ receptors). These mutations ultimately lead to altered neuronal excitability.

The strongest example that illustrates the importance of genetics in epilepsy is represented by the developmental and epileptic encephalopathies (DEE), which are complex conditions associated with mutations in more than 60 genes. DEE are a heterogeneous group of rare neurodevelopmental disorders characterized by (1) early-onset seizures that are often intractable, (2) EEG abnormalities, (3) developmental delay or regression and (4) in some cases, early death. An example of DEE is Dravet syndrome (DS). DS is characterized by febrile seizures within the first year of life in an otherwise healthy child, evolving into a combination of intractable febrile and afebrile seizures, with developmental arrest or regression in the following years. More than 80% of DS patients carry a de novo mutation of the SCN1A gene, encoding $Na_V1.1$ (the voltage-gated sodium channel type I α subunit). Other clinical epilepsy presentations associated with mutations in SNC1A include: generalized epilepsy with febrile seizures plus (GEFS+), severe myoclonic epilepsy borderline (SMEB), intractable childhood epilepsy with generalized tonic-clonic seizures (ICE-GTC) and infantile partial seizures with variable foci. It has been hypothesized that $Na_V1.1$ mutations lead to reduced sodium currents and subsequent hyperexcitability in neural networks, that are linked to a GABAergic deficit.

Focal epilepsy (more than 60% of all epilepsy presentations), which is common in adults, is associated with a variety of mutations in genes encoding ion channels and also genes involved in cell growth pathways such as the mechanistic target of rapamycin (mTOR) -linked pathways. mTOR regulates cell proliferation, autophagy and apoptosis, and is involved in multiple signalling pathways. Brain somatic mutations in the genes encoding mTOR components have been linked to focal cortical dysplasia, which is often seen in focal epilepsies.

Determining a genetic cause in an individual with epilepsy may be a key step towards a better and more personalized clinical management of the patient. It may lead to the avoidance of therapeutic errors, such as using sodium channel blockers in DS, and the consideration to use stiripentol—a compound which enhances GABAergic activity.

Cerebral cortical neurons and the generation of electrical signals

The cerebral neocortex has six distinct layers, with layer 1 lying just beneath the pia mater, and layer 6 just above the white matter (see Fig 15.6). Within these layers, there is a relatively similar arrangement of the different cell types throughout the brain, although the thickness of the layers varies in the different functional regions of the cortex. Cortical networks are composed of glutamatergic excitatory projection neurons and local GABAergic inhibitory interneurons that modulate signal flow. Although they represent a minority of the total neocortical neuronal population, GABAergic interneurons are highly heterogeneous, forming functional classes based on their morphological, electrophysiological and molecular features, as well as connectivity and in vivo patterns of activity. The cells with the largest cell bodies in the cortex are the pyramidal cells, which are found in layers 2, 3 and 5, oriented with the apex of their long dendrites running upwards towards the brain surface. From their base, long axons descend through deeper layers and leave the cortex. Areas rich in pyramidal cells are mainly output layers. The cortex also contains non-pyramidal cells, which are usually smaller and have no specific orientation of their dendrites. Their axons terminate locally, in the same layer or immediate vicinity. Non-pyramidal cells are involved primarily in receiving inputs from thalamic and other afferents, and in the local processing of information. As pyramidal cells are orientated with their dendrites at right angles to the cortical surface, when they are active, the potentials generated in the extracellular fluid give the largest signal at the brain surface.

unless action potentials occur simultaneously, they cannot summate to produce a large enough extracellular electrical potential to be measured by the scalp electrodes. Therefore, most of the electrical activity measured in an EEG comes from the summation of postsynaptic potentials. Although these are smaller than action potentials, they are much slower in their development and can therefore summate. Electrical activity recorded by electrodes placed on the scalp or surface of the brain mostly reflects summation of excitatory and inhibitory postsynaptic potentials in apical dendrites of pyramidal neurons in the superficial layers of the cortex. Quite large areas of cortex, in the order of a few square centimetres, have to be activated synchronously to generate enough potential for changes to be registered by scalp electrodes. The direction of the waves recorded by the EEG electrodes depends both on whether the postsynaptic potential is excitatory or inhibitory and on the depth of the activity within the cortex. Within the cortex, much of the activity is usually contained within individual local areas, with outputs to distant areas, allowing for extensive parallel and serial processing of sensory and motor information. When the activity of several groups of neurons is synchronized, a seizure can occur.

Invasive EEG can be used in selected cases. It might be offered to a patient with no underlying structural pathology identified on neuroimaging, but in whom other investigations have generated a suspicion as to the location of an epileptogenic region. It utilizes cortical depth electrodes (inserted surgically under stereotactic magnetic resonance imaging [MRI] guidance) and subdural electrodes (strips or grids, which require craniotomy for placement). Cortical stimulation can be performed with either type of electrode. Electrode selection and placement is determined by the location of the epileptogenic zone. In general, wider areas of cortex are covered by subdural electrodes, whereas depth electrodes are more suitable for suspected deep lying foci.

Normal EEG patterns

A clinician uses an EEG to obtain information about electrical brain activity. Although the EEG pattern of every individual is unique, there are several common patterns that can be related to specific brain states. The EEG shows characteristic patterns when a person is alert, drowsy or asleep. The amplitude of the EEG waves depends on the synchronicity in the activity of the underlying neuronal circuits. A frequency that is too high or too low, is indicative of impaired cortical function. In addition, the presence of unusual waveforms, such as sharp spikes, spike-and-wave potentials or unusually slow waves, indicates a brain lesion and may explain the emergence of seizures.

Fig. 13.3A shows the normal EEG in the awake state. It consists of a set of parallel recordings obtained from

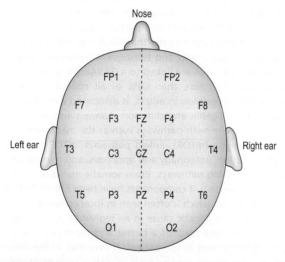

Fig. 13.2 Standard placement of EEG leads. The letters and numbers correspond to specific anatomical positions. *C*, Central; *F*, frontal; *O*, occipital; *P*, parietal; *T*, temporal.

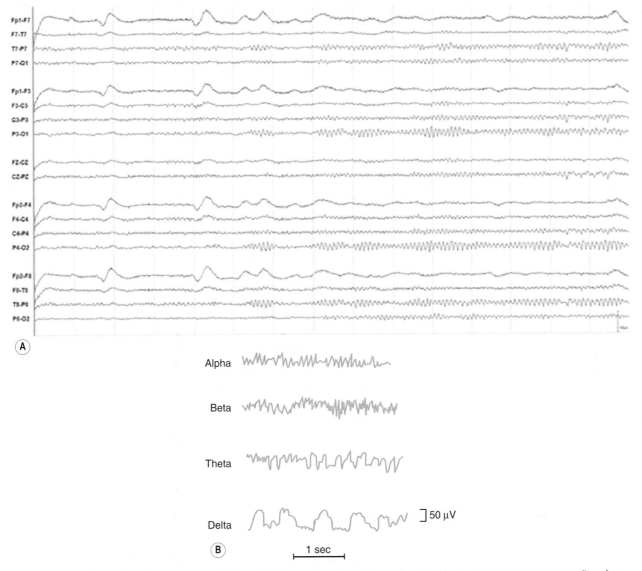

Fig. 13.3 EEG recording and major wave types. (A) Normal EEG recording during the awake state. The traces represent wave recordings from various electrode combinations. (B) Major wave types. *C,* Central; *F,* frontal; *Fp,* frontoparietal; *O,* occipital; *P,* parietal; *T,* temporal. (A, From Shin et al. (2014) Review of epilepsy—aetiology, diagnostic evaluation and treatment. Int. Journal of Neurorehabilitation. 1:130. B, From Guyton AC, Hall JE. (2006) Textbook of medical physiology, 11th ed. Philadelphia: Elsevier Saunders.)

multiple electrode combinations, reflecting various wave patterns. The major types of EEG waves are shown in Fig. 13.3B. EEG waves are also described in Chapter 16 (Box 16.8, Fig. 16.4), with reference to their link to sleep and wakefulness. In general, an EEG wave that is of low amplitude and high frequency, with no obvious pattern, indicates an alert or awake state. Healthy adults typically manifest relatively low-amplitude, mixed-frequency background rhythms, also termed desynchronized. These are *beta* waves and have a frequency of 13–30 Hz. This type of desynchronized activity occurs because the brain neurons are all working independently so that many of the different frequencies of activity cancel out each other. However, when a person is relaxed, especially with their eyes closed as in sleep or quiet contemplation, the amplitude increases

but the frequency is low. This rhythm of activity is the *alpha* rhythm and occurs because neurons are now firing synchronously. These slow synchronous waves are of relatively low amplitude and have a frequency of 8–12 Hz. They are largest in the parieto-occipital region, but if a relaxed person is disturbed, opens their eyes or become anxious, the *alpha* rhythms abruptly stop. Occasional slower *theta* (4–7 Hz) or even *delta* (1–3 Hz) frequencies transiently may be seen during normal wakefulness, but usually these slower activities only become prominent during drowsiness. Therefore, *theta* and *delta* waves are not normally seen in awake adults. Irregular *theta* waves (4–7 Hz) are common in children and are seen in adults during rapid eye movement (REM) sleep. Low-frequency (4 Hz or less), high-amplitude *delta* waves are only seen in sleep or during anaesthesia or coma. Other characteristic EEG patterns can occur, such as the sudden high amplitude bursts called 'sleep spindles', which happen during stage 4 sleep. Sleep is characterized by very specific EEG profiles for each sleep stage (Fig. 16.4). When the brain ceases activity (i.e. death), the EEG pattern becomes a flat line.

Electroencephalogram patterns in epilepsy

The EEG is an essential element in the diagnosis of epilepsy. It provides important information about background activity and epileptiform discharges, and is required for the diagnosis of specific syndromes. This guides the selection of anti-epileptic medication and prognosis. There are often dramatic and very characteristic changes in the EEG patterns of patients with epilepsy, as shown in the example EEG recording of a young patient with Lennox-Gastaut syndrome, which is a severe form of childhood-onset epilepsy characterized by multiple seizure types (Fig. 13.4), but unless the recording is prolonged, the patient may not have a seizure during the EEG procedure.

Around 50%–70% of patients with epilepsy will show characteristic epileptiform activity between seizures; this is the interictal activity. In some cases, it is also possible to induce abnormal activity by forced hyperventilation (3 min) or flashing lights (stroboscopic photic stimulation). As noted in Fig 13.4, EEG changes may take the form of 'spikes and waves', which reflect the underlying depolarization of the cortical neurons. Certain patients with epilepsy show no abnormal interictal activity, while a significant number (0.5%–2%) of randomly selected individuals without epilepsy show similar interictal EEG patterns. These false positive results rise to 5%–10% in first-degree relatives of patients with confirmed epilepsy.

During a seizure, the large-amplitude spikes and waves may be generalized, occurring in all electrodes or they may only occur in a subset of the recordings. The region of focal epilepsy origin can be determined by the pattern of the EEG abnormalities. This is necessary for the surgical treatment of epilepsy.

In absence seizures (Fig 13.5), the EEG shows a rhythmic 3–4 Hz spike-and-wave potential from most scalp electrodes, whereas in 'grand mal' seizures, the EEG shows higher-frequency, irregular, large-amplitude waves from most recording sites. In some cases the EEG may show the focal discharges spreading across the brain to give a generalized pattern. Fig. 13.6 shows the EEG typical of a 'grand mal' seizure. There is an abrupt onset of generalized rapid spikes at the start of the tonic phase, and as the spike firing frequency decreases, the individual spikes become far enough apart that each spike can generate a separate clonic jerk, representing the clonic phase.

A development in the management of epilepsy, based on EEG recording is the potential prediction of seizures. There is accumulating evidence that seizures often have a specific circadian pattern, and that they develop minutes to hours before their clinical expression. In the future, it may be possible to define the exact characteristics of the

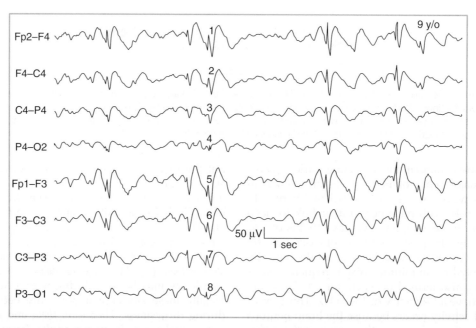

Fig. 13.4 EEG recording in Lennox-Gastaut syndrome. The traces show generalized sharp spike and slow-wave discharges on the EEG of a 9-year-old child with intellectual disability and uncontrolled typical absence, tonic, and atonic generalized seizures. This combination of clinical and EEG features constitutes Lennox-Gastaut syndrome. (From Emerson RG, Hahn CD (2022) Bradley and Daroff's neurology in clinical practice. 8th edn. Edited by J Jankovic, NJ Newman, JC Mazziotta, SL Pomeroy. Philadelphia: Elsevier Inc.)

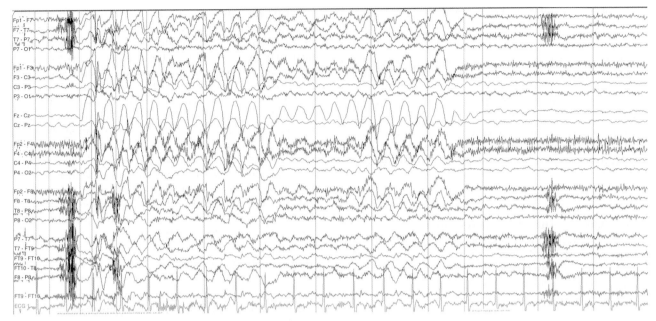

Fig. 13.5 EEG recording in absence seizure. The traces show an EEG in a 2-year-old boy presenting with absence seizures at only 23 months of age. High voltage, generalized 3–4 Hz paroxysmal slow waves superimposed upon a normal background, accompany staring spells. The lowest trace shows the electrocardiogram (ECG). (From DiBacco ML, Gibson KM, Pearl PL (2022) Bradley and Daroff's neurology in clinical practice. 8th edn. Edited by J Jankovic, NJ Newman, JC Mazziotta, SL Pomeroy. Philadelphia: Elsevier Inc.)

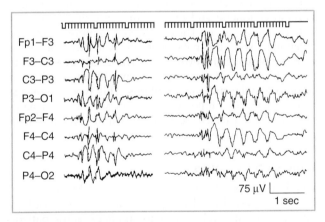

Fig. 13.6 EEG characteristics of tonic–clonic seizure. Example of generalized spike-wave patterns in primary generalied (idiopathic) epilepsy. This patient had mainly tonic–clonic seizures with occasional absence attacks. (From Emerson RG, Hahn CD (2022) Bradley and Daroff's neurology in clinical practice. 8th edn. Edited by J Jankovic, NJ Newman, JC Mazziotta, SL Pomeroy. Philadelphia: Elsevier Inc.)

EEG changes that precede a seizure, and devise a therapeutic strategy to prevent the onset of the clinical seizure. There is some evidence that seizures can be predicted from changes in the EEG at least 20 min before they occur, with some more subtle changes occurring up to 90 min before seizure onset. An implantable device could warn of the impending seizure and intervene with focal stimulation (closed-loop stimulation) or focal application of drugs, so that the seizure can be prevented.

Other diagnostic techniques

Structural changes in the brain that lead to epileptic foci can be studied by MRI and computed tomography (CT). An MRI can reveal previously undetected structural abnormalities that may play a causal role. Therefore, it is used for investigating aetiology and also for selecting patients for surgical treatment. The technique can reveal several types of cerebral abnormality such as hippocampal sclerosis, small lesions (invisible on CT scans) and cortical dysgenesis.

Magnetic resonance spectroscopy (MRS) can detect changes in the biochemistry of the brain. The analysis of nervous tissue proton MRS spectra shows three major peaks: N-acetylaspartate (NAA), creatine and phosphocreatine, and also a peak for choline-containing compounds. A reduction in the NAA peak is generally viewed as reflecting neuronal loss or dysfunction. A reduction in the NAA peak and a concomitant increase in the other two major peaks may indicate neuronal loss accompanied by gliosis. MRS spectra can also provide information on tissue inositol, lactate, gamma-aminobutyric acid (GABA) and glutamate concentrations. Also, MRS can help in the detection of hippocampal sclerosis and abnormal cortical foci. Positron emission tomography (PET) and single photon emission computed tomography (SPECT) can be used to investigate brain metabolism and also the presence of neuroinflammation, using specific markers; they may enable the detection of seizure foci. Especially when several of these investigations are used in combination, they can be of help in refining the diagnosis and devising the best therapeutic strategy.

Examples of types of seizure

Fig. 13.1 details that there are three main types of seizure onset: focal onset, generalized onset and unknown onset. The type of onset is determined based on clinical characteristics, EEG and imaging data. Examples of characteristic features of various types of seizures are given below.

Focal onset seizures

These seizures occur when the seizure activity starts in a focal brain area. In a large proportion of cases, the seizures are limited and there is full awareness. In some cases, awareness may be lost and the seizures may generalize, as described below.

Focal seizures

In the simplest type of focal seizures, there is no loss of consciousness. The origin of focal seizures leads to symptoms that depend on the area involved. For example, convulsive limb movements on one side of the body indicate an epileptic focus in the motor cortex of the contralateral side. The patient may experience weakness in the affected muscles after the seizure. Other focal symptoms may include tingling, hallucinations (visual, olfactory or gustatory) and swallowing or chewing movements. The latter are indicative of temporal lobe epilepsy, which is the commonest form of focal epilepsy. Because of the temporal lobe involvement in memory, it is not surprising that the focal symptoms can include a feeling of 'déjà vu', a feeling of a rush of memories, or memory loss. The patient may appear detached and slow, and may have repetitive movements such as lip-smacking and chewing movements and make unusual noises. Sometimes this behaviour is more complex and may be aggressive. The other area commonly affected in focal seizures is the frontal lobe. Focal epilepsies are often associated with structural changes, which can include developmental abnormalities in the young, and trauma-induced damage or tumours in older patients.

Some focal seizures can be associated with impaired consciousness. They are often more severe forms of temporal lobe epilepsies and may last for between 30 s and 1–2 min. Although the patient may be unable to communicate or respond to commands, consciousness may not be completely impaired. During the seizure patients may be able to continue simple motor behaviour. Usually there is no loss of postural control. In general, patients are amnesic of the seizure.

Focal seizures with secondary generalization

Focal epilepsy may sometimes spread over the cerebral cortex, first on the side of the initial focus, and then to the opposite hemisphere. This can be seen in the EEG by a gradual increase in the ictal activity, starting with the focal area and gradually including all the traces. A particular example of this type of seizure is known as Jacksonian epilepsy, in which the focal signs start either in the face or at the extremities of a limb. Movements then rapidly spread across the face or ascend the limb, leading to a generalized seizure (see below). As the focal seizure may spread very rapidly, the patient may not remember the focal start of the seizure. The only indication that this is not a primary generalized seizure (apart from an EEG, which may be hard to obtain) is the evidence of focal movements (as reported by an observer) and unilateral postictal motor weakness (known as 'Todd's paralysis'), which may be seen if the initial focus of the seizure is in the motor cortex.

Generalized onset seizures

Generalized seizures involve both hemispheres of the brain and abnormalities can be seen simultaneously in all the EEG traces. Seizures of this type are thought to originate from midline structures such as the thalamus, which diffusely innervate the entire cortex, thus triggering a generalized seizure.

Absence seizures

This type of seizure, also known as 'petit mal', usually starts in childhood and may occur many times each day, lasting for only 5–15 s. The condition is reminiscent of 'daydreaming', with the patient staring vacantly, sometimes with eye-blinking and eye-rolling. The EEG shows a characteristic bilateral 3-Hz waveform, seen in all traces, with synchronized spike-and-wave patterns. This type of epilepsy is often diagnosed following the poor school performance of an inattentive child. It is thought that this type of seizure results from abnormalities in T-type Ca^{2+} channels.

Tonic–clonic seizures

This is the type of seizure suffered by Gaby (Box 13.1). These seizures, also called 'grand mal', are the most typical type seen in adults. Prior to an attack, some patients may experience vague symptoms, called an 'aura'. This may be a smell or a taste, or just 'feeling strange'. It may last for a few seconds, which may be enough for the patient to be able to lie down, thus preventing injury due to falling during the seizure. However, many patients have no warning. The typical seizure of this type has three phases. The first is the tonic phase, which lasts for about 10–40 s. The patient becomes very rigid, as all the muscles in the body undergo tonic, sustained contraction. The patient falls rigidly and, as the respiratory and laryngeal muscles are also contracted, may let out a cry or grunt as air is forced out of the chest through the taut vocal cords. During this time there is no respiration, so the patient becomes cyanotic. This is followed by the clonic phase, during which the muscles go into strong, random contractions. This limb-jerking may be accompanied by urinary and faecal incontinence, and there may be tongue-biting and frothing at the mouth. Breathing is jerky and inefficient, and there is tachycardia. This phase usually lasts for 2–3 min, although it can last for longer. The third phase is a coma (the patient is unconscious and the muscles are flaccid) in which the patient's breathing becomes regular and their colour returns to normal. The length of this period is related to the duration of the previous tonic–clonic phases. When patients wake they may be confused and have a headache.

During a seizure of this type the levels of neuronal activity are very high but, because of the reduction (or lack) of respiration, blood oxygenation is poor. During this time there is an accumulation of lactic acid in the brain, and it is this hypoxia and acidosis which is probably the cause of the coma. Blood tests show a low pH and low $pO2$. There are increases in creatine phosphokinase and serum prolactin levels.

Repeated seizures can lead to neuronal degeneration, which is thought to be due to the excessive release of glutamate during the seizure. This can cause cell death through the mechanism known as excitotoxicity, which is also implicated in cell death due to stroke (see Chapter 11).

Febrile seizures

Also known as febrile convulsions, this type of seizure, which may be generalized or focal, occurs commonly in young children under the age of 5 years and is triggered by fever. Comparison of the EEGs of children and adults shows that the electrical activity of the adult brain is more stable than that of children, and this instability of the immature brain seems to be increased by fever. These seizures cause anxiety in parents, who may be worried about the future development of epilepsy. However, these seizures usually occur only once, and in the small proportion of cases where epilepsy does develop later, there are other associated risk factors (Table 13.1).

Table 13.3 Examples of anticonvulsant drugs

First generation drugs	New drugs
Phenytoin	Lamotrigine
Sodium valproate	Vigabatrin
Carbamazepine	Topiramate
Phenobarbitone	Tiagabine
Acetazolamide	Gabapentin
Clobazam	Levetiracetam
Ethosuximide	Perampanel
Clonazepam	Stiripentol
Primidone	Zonisamide

Status epilepticus

Usually, epileptic seizures are self-limiting, but sometimes the seizures continue without the patient regaining consciousness. Status epilepticus is defined as a convulsive seizure that continues for a prolonged period (> 5 min), or convulsive seizures that occur one after the other (e.g. more than 2 seizures within 5 min), with no recovery between seizures. Status epilepticus is an emergency and requires immediate medical attention. Convulsive status epilepticus is associated with a mortality of 10%–15% and is one of the reasons why the mortality of patients with epilepsy is three times that of age-matched controls. Deaths during convulsive status epilepticus are due to the hypoxia and intense acidosis that occur during a seizure. If there is no time for recovery between seizures, this condition worsens and can lead to cerebral oedema, brain damage and cardiorespiratory failure. A non-convulsive form of status epilepticus can also occur and may follow convulsive status epilepticus. It is characterized by continuous seizure activity, as detected by EEG.

Neurobiology of epilepsy

The cellular basis of epilepsy is still incompletely understood, but from a fundamental neurophysiology perspective it is believed that epilepsy may be due to intrinsic neuronal hyperexcitability (e.g. due to dysfunctional voltage-gated ion channels), increased activity at excitatory synapses or insufficient activity of inhibitory circuits. As mentioned elsewhere in this book, the major neurotransmitters mediating fast neurotransmission in the brain are the amino acids glutamate and GABA. These neurotransmitters play a large part in controlling the excitation–inhibition balance in the central nervous system (CNS). In addition, many other ligand-gated and voltage-gated ion channels contribute to the modulation of the excitability of neuronal networks.

Glutamate transmission

Glutamate receptors are of two main types: ionotropic and metabotropic (see Chapter 15). The fast, ionotropic receptors are divided into N-methyl-D-aspartate (NMDA) and non-NMDA receptors. NMDA receptors are permeable to both Na^+ and Ca^{2+} and are blocked at normal resting potential by Mg^{2+}. This blockade is removed by depolarization, so NMDA receptors can only be activated in a neuron that is already partially depolarized. NMDA receptors are involved in a process called long-term potentiation (LTP; see Chapter 14). During LTP, the simultaneous activity of multiple inputs to a neuron will activate NMDA receptors, which consequently strengthens the connection between the active neurons, which is why the indiscriminate blockade of NMDA receptors may have very unfavourable effects on cognition (as LTP is critical for learning and memory).

The non-NMDA receptors are AMPA receptors (named after the preferred agonist 4-amino-3-hydroxy-5-methyl-4-isoxazolepropionic acid [AMPA]) and kainate receptors (named after kainic acid, which is an agonist). These non-NMDA receptors can be activated at normal resting potentials, and their activation leads to depolarization. When activity levels are high, the neuron will be sufficiently depolarized for both NMDA and non-NMDA receptors to be activated. This will allow Ca^{2+} to enter the cell, where it acts as a second messenger. Glutamate receptor agonists, such as kainic acid and ibotenic acid, can induce various types of seizure in animals. Furthermore, structural changes in glutamate receptors have been found in surgical specimens from epileptic patients. The pyramidal cells of the cortex are glutamatergic and there is some evidence that glutamatergic dysfunction may be associated with certain types of epilepsy. However, NMDA receptor antagonists have limited antiepileptic activity and induce unacceptable adverse effect; therefore they cannot be used clinically. However, in recent years, it has become apparent that AMPA receptors can be successfully targeted for the treatment of epilepsy. The involvement of AMPA receptors in epilepsies is also supported by the existence of genes associated with epilepsy that encode for AMPA receptor subunits, and also proteins involved in the anchorage of AMPA receptors to membranes.

GABA transmission

There are two main types of GABA receptor: $GABA_A$ receptors, which are ionotropic receptors, and $GABA_B$ receptors, which are metabotropic and G-protein-coupled receptors. When activated, $GABA_A$ receptors, which are multimeric proteins composed of several different subunits, open an integral Cl$^-$ channel. This tends to clamp the neuronal potential closer to the resting potential. $GABA_A$ receptors are postsynaptic, whereas $GABA_B$ receptors are found both post- and presynaptically. There are many different types of inhibitory non-pyramidal cell in the cortex. Many of these cells do not have dendritic spines and are termed non-spiny neurons. Some of these inhibitory cells have synapses on the pyramidal cells that are close to the cell body, while excitatory inputs tend to arrive on the pyramidal cell dendrites. This means that activity in inhibitory synapses that use GABA will have a powerful influence on the firing patterns of the excitatory pyramidal cells. Inhibitory postsynaptic potentials are the mechanism by which neurons

are prevented from firing. Some theories of the genesis of epilepsy postulate that a reduction in GABAergic activity allows the uncontrolled discharge of large numbers of neurons. Lower than normal numbers of GABAergic neurons have been found in tissue from patients with epilepsy refractory to treatment. Furthermore, increasing GABAergic activity is the mechanism of action for several of the drugs used to treat epilepsy.

Ion channels and neuronal excitability

Neuronal membrane excitability is controlled by complex mechanisms, which depend on the coordinated activity of multiple ion channels. A wide range of loss-of-function mutations in Na$^+$ channels are associated with epilepsy. It has been suggested that fast firing inhibitory neurons are particularly affected by these mutations. The rising phase of the action potential is caused by a current that flows through fast-inactivated Na$^+$ channels. This current is also associated with a slow-inactivation component. The blockade of this component can lead to a switch in the firing of neurons from regular spiking to burst firing. Certain types of genetically determined epilepsies, such as the familial generalized epilepsies with febrile seizures, are associated with changes in the molecular structure of Na$^+$ channels; such mutations decrease the rate of inactivation of Na$^+$ channels (Fig. 13.7).

K$^+$ channels also have a role in excitability; in particular, they are critically involved in the repolarization of the membrane. The blockade of the K$^+$ M-current (which is inhibited by the activation of muscarinic acetylcholine receptors) leads to a shift towards greater depolarization of the membrane. The K$^+$ channel subunits KCN2 and KCN3 contribute to this current, and mutations in the genes that encode these subunits are associated with the phenotype of benign neonatal familial convulsions.

Finally, Ca^{2+} currents are also an important element in the control of neuronal excitability, and converging evidence suggests that dysfunctional Ca^{2+} channels may be associated with epileptogenesis. Absence epilepsies have been associated with changes in a low-threshold Ca^{2+} current in neurons of the reticular nucleus in the thalamus.

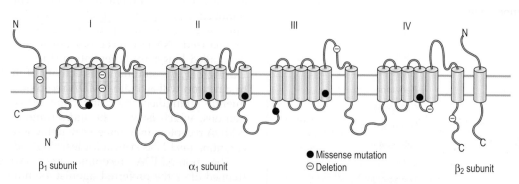

Fig. 13.7 Mutations in Na$^+$ channel subunits associated with idiopathic epilepsy.

Mechanisms underlying seizures and epileptogenesis

There is ample evidence that changes in excitatory and inhibitory signalling, and also in the intrinsic excitability of neurons, play a significant role in epilepsy. This is supported by the genetics of epilepsy (Box 13.2). Nonetheless, it is also important to note that the majority of mutations in epilepsy are not linked to ion channels. The reason why seizures start and how they are maintained remains incompletely understood in most cases. The timing of the development of secondary, acquired epilepsy is also enigmatic; for example, more than 50% of individuals who suffer a traumatic brain injury are at risk of developing a seizure disorder, but this may take months or years. This silent period suggests that there is a very gradual transformation in the neural networks, which leads to a new abnormal set point.

Experiments carried out in animal models of epilepsy, using various protocols that induce seizures, have investigated the events underlying interictal and ictal electrical activity. Recently developed genetic mouse models recapitulate many of the features of human epilepsy resulting from a specific genetic defect in a particular receptor or voltage-gated ion channel. One of the key challenges is to understand the development of epileptogenesis, that is, the process by which normal brain activity progresses towards the generation of abnormal electrical activity. This is a key process for the evolution of the acquired epilepsy that follows a traumatic brain injury, a stroke or an episode of status epilepticus. Furthermore, the present view on epileptogenesis is that it does not cover just the period between the initial stimulus and the first secondary seizure, it may also characterize a new state of the brain, which is long lasting, and possibly irreversible, with ongoing epileptogenesis as a form of aberrant neuroplasticity across a lifetime.

There are several different ways of producing epileptiform activity in animals. Some of these involve drugs that either inhibit GABA or increase glutamate activities. $GABA_A$ antagonists such as bicuculline and picrotoxin, and glutamate agonists such as kainic acid can all produce seizure activity. A well-established model in epilepsy research is called 'kindling', in which repeated high-frequency stimulation of parts of the limbic system can produce long-term changes in excitability, so that seizures can be produced by quite low levels of stimulation for months after the initial stimulation period. Some models analyse changes in brain tissue slices, where the layered structure of the brain and local electrical circuits can be maintained. Intracellular and extracellular recordings from these preparations reveal some common underlying patterns.

Neurons in a region with epileptogenic activity fire bursts of action potentials. This is thought to be due to a slow depolarizing shift, called a 'paroxysmal depolarization shift'. This induces action potentials from a group of neurons, and these are superimposed on the shift (Fig. 13.8). This is followed by a period of hyperpolarization, during

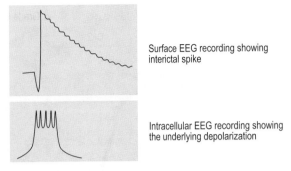

Surface EEG recording showing interictal spike

Intracellular EEG recording showing the underlying depolarization

Fig. 13.8 An interictal spike produced by slow depolarization underlies the burst firing of neurons.

which the activation of both voltage- and Ca^{2+}-sensitive K^+ channels stops the spiking activity.

When the interval between interictal spikes shortens, the period of hyperpolarization is reduced. As a result of increased neuronal firing, there is an increase in extracellular K^+ levels, which depolarizes neurons and puts them closer to the firing threshold. However, the mechanism by which local inhibition is sufficiently reduced to allow the synchronous discharge of large numbers of neurons, is not known.

Another aspect of the pathophysiology of epilepsy is linked to the structural changes that may underlie epilepsy. In one common type of epilepsy in adults—mesial temporal sclerosis (MTS)—seizures originate in the hippocampus and sometimes progress to secondarily generalized seizures. Possibly due to neuronal damage in infancy, there are losses of neurons in specific hippocampal areas (Fig. 13.9). In response to the cell loss, there is sprouting of the axons of excitatory glutamatergic granule cells (also known as mossy fibres) (Fig. 13.10). These form connections with other granule cells of the dentate gyrus, which are not inhibited by the normal inhibitory connections. This leads to a set of excitatory loops that have a high propensity to produce seizures.

Another theory of epileptogenesis involves deficits in specific inhibitory neurons, for example, the chandelier cells of the cortex. They are a subset of GABAergic inhibitory interneurons that release GABA via axoaxonal contacts onto the initial segment of pyramidal cells (Fig. 13.11). Histologically, they appear as cartridges or 'chandelier' profiles. These cells express high levels of the GABA transporter GAT1, which can be used as a marker for their presence. In some forms of epilepsy there is a loss of chandelier cells, as shown by a detectable loss of GAT1 in brain tissue. It is suggested that loss of just a few of these cells would have a significant effect on the excitability of the pyramidal cells. This is because a single chandelier cell innervates a few hundred pyramidal cells. The theory also suggests that, because of the normal individual variation in the number of GABAergic neurons, loss of chandelier cells would be sufficient to produce epilepsy in an individual with lower than average numbers of inhibitory neurons.

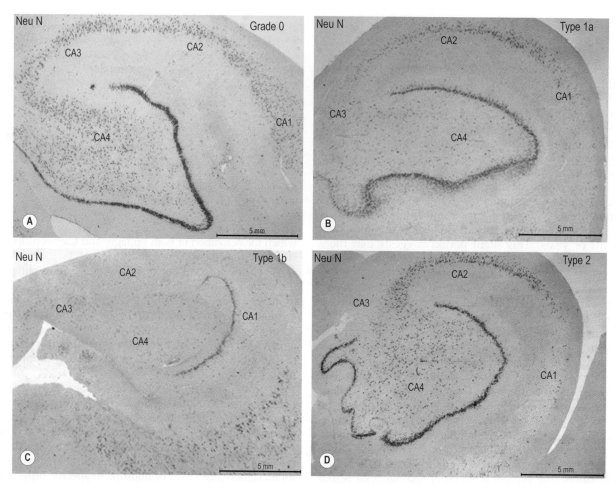

Fig. 13.9 Sclerosis of the hippocampus in epilepsy. Neuronal immunoperoxidase staining for the NeuN antigen shows in (A) normal cell distribution and density and in (B), (C) and (D) significant loss of neurons in various fields of the Cornu Ammonis (CA). 0, no loss of pyramidal neurons in the CA; 1A, loss in CA1, CA3, CA4; 1b, severe loss in all subfields; type 2, loss in CA1. (From Savitr Sastri, B.V., Arivazhagan, A., Sinha, S., et al. 2014, 'Clinico-pathological factors influencing surgical outcome in drug resistant epilepsy secondary to mesial temporal sclerosis', *Journal of the Neurological Sciences,* vol. 340, no. 1-2, pp. 183–190.)

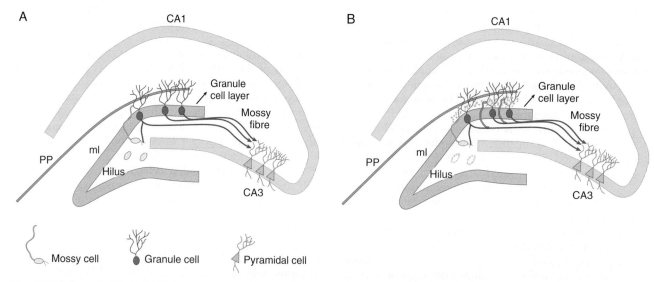

Fig. 13.10 Fibre sprouting in the hippocampus in epilepsy. (A) Shows the hippocampus circuitry in a normal brain and (B) shows the sprouting of mossy fibres into the dentate inner molecular layer in an epileptic brain, following the loss of hilar cells. *ml,* Molecular layer, *PP,* perforant path. (From Cavarsan, C. F., Malheiros, J., Hamani, C., et al. 2018, 'Is Mossy Fiber Sprouting a Potential Therapeutic Target for Epilepsy?', *Frontiers in Neurology,* vol 9, article 1023.)

EPILEPSY

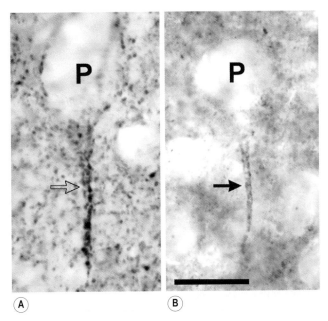

Fig. 13.11 Pre- and postsynaptic markers for GABAergic neurotransmission. Chandelier cells labelled with GAT1 (A) synapse onto pyramidal neurons (P) labelled with an antibody against the GABA$_A$ receptor (B). (From Volk, Lewis. Physiology and Behaviour 2002; 77: 501–505.)

Neuroinflammation (involving microglia and astrocytes) and changes in energy metabolism (in particular mitochondrial deficits) have also been linked to the pathophysiology of epilepsy. Mitochondria are essential organelles involved in cellular energy-generating processes. Compromise of the mitochondrial ability to produce energy in the form of ATP can disrupt multiple functions, and the deficit in energy production alters the balance of neuronal excitation and inhibition, which can lead to seizures. Microglial activation is one of the earliest cellular events described in epileptogenesis models. Activated microglia can release a host of chemokines and cytokines. Inflammatory cytokines, such as interleukin-1β (IL-1β), tumour necrosis factor-α (TNF-α) and interleukin-6 (IL-6), can contribute to both acute neuronal excitability and chronic molecular changes that could play a part in the development of epilepsy. There may be increases in the activity of tissue proteases, which remodel the brain extracellular matrix. Astrocytes can downregulate glutamate transporters and potassium channels, acquire a pro-inflammatory phenotype and proliferate. Neuroinflammation is also linked to disruption of the blood-brain barrier which is a consequence of the direct action of cytokines and chemokines released by activated glia.

There is evidence that epileptogenesis is also associated with epigenetic changes such as alterations in DNA methylation, histone acetylation and changes in the expression of non-coding RNAs.

Pharmacological treatment of epilepsy

There is a wide range of anticonvulsant drugs available for the treatment of epilepsy (Table 13.3). The term 'anticonvulsant' or 'anti-epileptic' are used interchangeably, but it could be argued that the present drugs only act symptomatically and do not change the process of epileptogenesis, therefore the term 'anticonvulsant' is more appropriate. Because patients already have epilepsy when they are diagnosed, the drugs used at present are, strictly speaking, anticonvulsants, that is, they prevent or reduce the established seizure activity. In the past decade many new drugs have been introduced, as well as improved formulations of older anticonvulsant drugs. In cases where epilepsy is likely to develop, for example, following head trauma or perinatal hypoxia, drugs that could prevent the future development of seizures—true anti-epileptics—would be useful, but no such compounds have yet been developed for clinical use. Active attempts are being made in animal models of epilepsy to understand the mechanisms that underlie epileptogenesis, that may open up new therapeutic avenues. However, evidence suggests so far that even when drugs are introduced early, and they at least partly control the seizures, they do not affect the progression of epilepsy.

It is important to note that primary generalized seizures are usually more easily controlled than focal epilepsies. Many patients can, after a period of remission, stop their treatment but there may be a recurrence of seizures, which may have consequences for employment and activities such as driving (see below).

Mode of action of anticonvulsant drugs

Ion channel inhibitors

Several different anticonvulsant drugs, from first generation drugs to more recent drugs, inhibit voltage-sensitive channels, thus reducing neuronal excitability.

Phenytoin—one of the oldest anticonvulsant drugs—blocks voltage-sensitive Na$^+$ channels preferentially in their inactive state. This occurs just after the channel opens, which means that the blockade is use-dependent. This therefore tends to block activity in those pathways showing high-frequency repetitive discharges. Phenytoin blocks the spread of seizures, but has little effect against the epileptic focus. The pharmacokinetics of this drug is complex and can change over the therapeutic range. At higher doses, it can show saturation (or zero-order) kinetics, so called because of enzyme saturation. At that point, small increases in the dose can lead to significant increases in plasma concentration, so monitoring of the plasma concentration is required. Phenytoin is an inducer of hepatic microsomal enzymes and therefore can interfere with the metabolism of other drugs. It has a number of side effects, including gum hypertrophy, acne and hirsutism, and it is teratogenic. It is used in all forms

THE NERVOUS SYSTEM   287

Table 13.4   Efficacy of anti-epileptic drugs against common seizure types

Drug	Focal seizures	Focal—Secondary generalized seizures	Tonic–clonic seizures	Absence seizures	Myoclonic seizures
			Seizure type		
Phenytoin	1	1	1	2	2
Carbamazepine	1	1	1	2	2
Valproate	1	1	1	1	1
Lamotrigine	1	1	1	1	2
Gabapentin	1	1	?1	?	2
Topiramate	1	1	1	?	1
Clobazam	1	1	1	1	1
Phenobarbitone	1	1	1	0	?1
Tiagabine	1	1	?1	2	2

0, ineffective; ?1, probably effective; 1, proven efficacy; ?, unknown; 2, precipitate or worsens seizures.

of epilepsy, with the exception of absence seizures, which it can aggravate (Table 13.4).

Carbamazepine has a mode of action on Na^+ channels similar to that of phenytoin. It can induce rash, hepatotoxicity and blood dyscrasia. It is also an enzyme inducer and has teratogenic effects. It can be used for simple and complex partial seizures and tonic–clonic generalized seizures.

Ethosuximide, which is effective specifically in preventing absence seizures, acts by blocking the T-type Ca^{2+} channels found in thalamic neurons, which are thought to generate this type of seizure activity.

Sodium valproate has a complex pharmacology, but one of its mechanisms of action is the inhibition of Na^+ channels. The drug can also block L-type Ca^{2+} channels. Furthermore, it may increase GABAergic transmission by stimulating GABA synthesis and inhibiting its metabolism. It is effective in patients with all types of seizure, easy to use and generally well tolerated, although it can induce unwanted effects such as tremor and weight gain.

Some of the newer anti-epileptic drugs also affect the function of ion channels. Lamotrigine induces use-dependent blockade of Na^+ channels and reduces Ca^{2+} currents. Gabapentin is also associated with a reduction in voltage-dependent Ca^{2+} currents. Topiramate has a complex pharmacology, but part of its mechanism of action is also the blockade of Na^+ channels. Levetiracetam has no effect on voltage-dependent Na^+ or L-, P-, Q- or T-type Ca^{2+} channels, but selectively inhibits N-type Ca^{2+} channels, with no effects on other channels. Zonisamide blocks both Na^+ and Ca^{2+} channels.

GABA receptor modulators

Benzodiazepines such as clonazepam and clobazam, and barbiturates such as phenobarbitone, act by binding to the $GABA_A$ receptor. $GABA_A$ receptors are pentameric proteins, made up of five subunits surrounding a Cl^- channel. The majority of $GABA_A$ receptors in the brain contain α-, β- and γ-subunits, each of which can be transcribed from a family of genes (for more detail see Chapter 16). On the $GABA_A$ receptor complex there are binding sites for GABA and also modulatory binding sites for a number of other compounds. There are sites for both benzodiazepines and barbiturates, and these compounds act as positive allosteric modulators at the $GABA_A$ receptor, that is, they amplify the response to GABA. Benzodiazepines increase the frequency of Cl^- channel opening, whereas barbiturates increase the duration of channel opening. At high concentrations, barbiturates can have intrinsic effects, independent of the presence of GABA. They commonly induce sedation and their therapeutic window is much narrower than that of benzodiazepines. Clobazam is used as adjunctive therapy, whereas clonazepam is used for generalized seizures and absence seizures (if ethosuximide fails) and can also be used for status epilepticus. Both compounds suppress the spread of seizures, but have little effect at the epileptic focus. In contrast, phenobarbitone can suppress activity at the epileptic focus. Primidone is metabolized in the body to phenobarbitone. Stiripentol is a drug recently introduced for the treatment of Dravet syndrome (see Box 13.2). It enhances GABA signalling through an effect similar to that of barbiturates, by enhancing the duration of the channel opening. It can also modulate GABA uptake and metabolism. Felbamate is a drug that can act as a positive modulator of $GABA_A$ receptors and as a blocker of NMDA receptors; its use is restricted for severe forms of epilepsy, such as Lennox-Gastaut syndrome.

Agents that increase the levels of GABA

The metabolism of GABA is a cycle, involving glutamate and glutamine, occurring between neurons and glial cells.

Figure 13.11, after its release into the synaptic cleft, GABA is transported into surrounding neurons and glial cells by high-affinity transporters such as GAT1. It is then broken down by GABA transaminase (GABA-T) to produce glutamate. Glutamate is metabolized to glutamine, which is then transported back into the neuron or glia. GABA is synthesized in neurons from glutamate, by the action of glutamic acid decarboxylase (GAD). This shunt enables the carbon skeleton of GABA to be returned to the neuron via glutamine, which has no neurotransmitter action.

Two anticonvulsant drugs act on elements of this cycle to increase GABA concentrations. Tiagabine blocks the reuptake of GABA by the GABA transporter GAT1, while vigabatrin is a selective irreversible inhibitor of GABA-T (Fig.13.12). Sodium valproate can also inhibit GABA-T. Both vigabatrin and tiagabine are used as adjunctive therapy in partial seizures.

Other drugs

As illustrated above, the pharmacology of epilepsy is complex and some of the compounds in present use may have efficacy because of the multiple targets they affect. For example, the same drug can inhibit voltage-gated ion channels, act at the benzodiazepine site of the $GABA_A$ receptor and suppress the release of monoamines! Which component of such a spectrum is the most important is not always clear and it may be that synergism is an important concept in the design of new drugs. Some other new drugs affect entirely new targets, for example, levetiracetam (and more recently, brivaracetam), which targets the presynaptic vesicle protein SV2A (blockade of this protein may reduce the recycling of vesicles during vesicle endocytosis), and perampanel, which acts as an antagonist at AMPA receptors. Topiramate is a carbonic anhydrase inhibitor. Zonisamide is a drug that blocks sodium channels and also calcium T-type channels but it may also have modulatory effects on GABAergic and glutamatergic signalling. Fig. 13.12 summarizes the various types of drugs that modulate excitatory and inhibitory synapses and are used as anti-epileptic medication. However, many of the diverse new second-generation anti-epileptic drugs, although in general are better tolerated, have so far failed to show significantly more efficacy than the established first-generation drugs. This may be because new drugs are tested preclinically on the same animal models as the old drugs, and such models may be inadequate and fail to reveal new targets with entirely new mechanisms of action. Furthermore, in some cases, although the rationale for the new target is sound, the drugs may induce unacceptable side effects.

General comments on anticonvulsant medication

The unwanted effects induced by anticonvulsant drugs are numerous, and some of the drugs used to treat epilepsy can have significant drug interactions with other drugs. Some do this by inducing metabolizing liver enzymes, thus increasing the metabolism of other medications, including warfarin and the contraceptive pill, as well as other anti-epileptics. Sodium valproate, used in the case history given in Box 13.1, inhibits the liver metabolism of some drugs, increasing their half-life.

Many of the drugs used to treat epilepsy are teratogenic, and this may determine the treatment given to women patients who wish to become pregnant. A lower dose of a safer drug and, in some cases, folate supplements and early screening for foetal abnormalities, are of benefit.

Anticonvulsant drug concentrations can be measured in the blood, and this is particularly useful in optimizing the dose of drugs such as phenytoin, which have a relatively narrow therapeutic window before reaching saturation kinetics. Knowledge of drug levels may also be useful in assessing compliance, particularly in cases where a patient is brought into hospital unconscious.

To conclude, different drugs are recommended for use in patients with generalized or focal epilepsies (Table 13.4) and some drugs are preferred in different age groups.

Characteristics of the ideal drug and strategy for the treatment of epilepsy

The choice of a drug usually depends upon the patient's seizure type (see Table 13.4). The pharmacokinetic characteristics, including absorption, elimination and potential for drug interactions (e.g. through potentiation or inhibition of common metabolic pathways), are of critical importance for patients who also take medication for other conditions, and for patients with impaired renal or hepatic function. The ideal drug would have a rapid absorption rate, low plasma protein binding, rapid CNS penetration and be eliminated predominantly by the kidneys. The new anticonvulsant drugs do not prompt the same concerns about interactions, because they have much better pharmacokinetic profiles than the older drugs (such as phenytoin and carbamazepine) and therefore require less monitoring for potential interactions. The potential interaction of anticonvulsant therapy with the contraceptive medication used by a young woman with epilepsy is illustrated in the case history given in Box 13.1. The new anti-epileptic drugs, such as vigabatrin, gabapentin, lamotrigine, tiagabine and levetiracetam, do not affect the metabolism of the contraceptive pill. However, caution is warranted concerning the effects of these new drugs on the foetus, as there is insufficient information to determine whether they are teratogenic or not.

The goal of anti-epileptic therapy is to keep the patient free of seizures, with no adverse effects on brain function. However, many of the drugs used to treat epilepsy have considerable side effects, both on the CNS and on other organs. In order to ensure patient compliance over what will probably be an extended period of time (sometimes a lifetime), it is important to test different drugs until a satisfactory drug regimen is established. Usually, a patient will be given a single

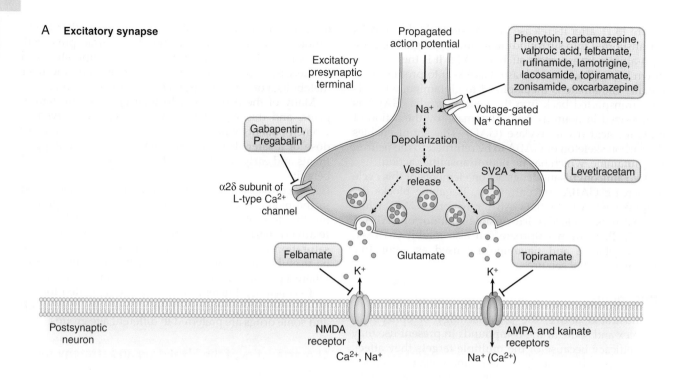

A **Excitatory synapse**

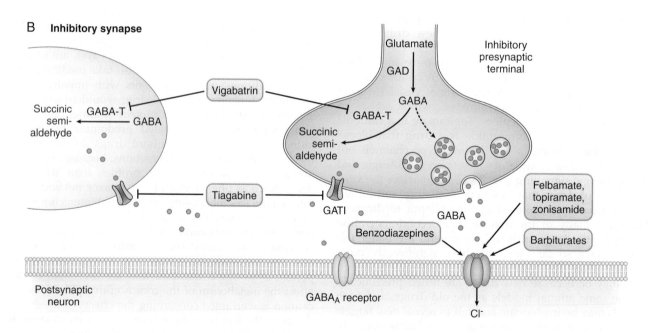

B **Inhibitory synapse**

Fig. 13.12 Overview of the A) Excitatory synapse and B) Inhibitory synapse, indicating the mode of action of several major anticonvulsant drugs. *GAT1*, GABA transporter; *GABA-T*, GABA transaminase; *GAD*, glutamic acid dehydrogenase; *SV2A*, presynaptic vesicle protein SV2A. (From Bialer M, White HS. (2010) Key factors in the discovery and development of new anti-epileptic drugs. *Nature Reviews Drug Discovery* 9:68–82.)

drug (monotherapy) and the dosage varied until either seizure activity is stopped or there are adverse effects. Additional drugs should also be tried on a monotherapy basis, before they are added (if monotherapy is ineffective). It is unusual to give more than three drugs simultaneously. Approximately 60% of patients are controlled with a single drug. In other patients better results are obtained by adding a second and even a third drug. If a patient still suffers seizures after the addition of multiple drugs, this is referred to as refractory epilepsy. Unfortunately, up to 40% of individuals suffer from this intractable, pharmaco-resistant epilepsy (Box 13.4).

Other treatments for epilepsy

Surgery

In patients with focal epilepsy that cannot be adequately controlled by drugs, surgical removal of the epileptic focus may be possible if it is in an area of the brain that can be removed without leaving a major neurological

> **Box 13.4** Pharmaco-resistance in epilepsy
>
> The phenomenon of pharmaco-resistance in epilepsy is significant. There are at least four different types of drug resistance: (1) resistance de novo or ab initio, where the patient never experiences seizure relief, from the beginning of pharmacological management; (2) delayed resistance, when the patient experiences seizure reduction at the beginning but then the treatment loses efficacy; (3) a fluctuating pattern, where the treatment efficacy waxes and wanes; and (4) the epilepsy is initially drug-resistant but improves with time. More than 30% of patients with epilepsy are pharmacological treatment-resistant. Fewer than 5% of patients who are refractory to first-generation anticonvulsant drugs are free of seizures with the newer drugs. Intractability of seizures is associated with various factors, such as onset of seizures in the first year of life, structural brain lesions (e.g. hippocampal sclerosis), brain tumours and neurodevelopmental abnormalities. Pharmaco-resistance is frequent in patients with focal seizures. Pharmaco-resistance may be due to genetic factors, disease-related factors or drug-related factors. Genetic polymorphisms in the drug target may underlie lack of response to a drug. On the other hand, the resistance may be due to the ongoing reorganization of neuronal networks triggered by the seizures. Disruption of the blood–brain barrier and persistent neuroinflammation may play a role. Last, but not least, drug uptake into the brain may be drastically reduced by the overexpression of multidrug transporters in the blood–brain barrier, whose activity leads to significant drug efflux. One such transporter is the P-glycoprotein, encoded by the MDR1/ABCB1 gene. If this is the case, inhibitors of these transporters, or drugs that are not substrates of these transporters, might be the answer to the problem of resistance. Pharmaco-resistance has been recently shown in experimental models to be associated with changes in certain non-coding RNAs such as specific microRNAs, which indirectly control protein synthesis. Novel oligonucleotide inhibitors targeting microRNAs (antagomirs) might become an innovative therapeutic option in drug-resistant epilepsy.

deficit. The area to be removed can be pinpointed using MRI and EEG recordings. The aim of the surgery is to obtain either complete freedom from seizures or amelioration of the seizure frequency. The types of epilepsy most amenable to this type of treatment are epilepsy due to MTS or tumours. Other rare surgical interventions include separating the two hemispheres of the brain by sectioning of the corpus callosum (callosotomy), in order to prevent seizures becoming generalized to both hemispheres.

Nerve stimulation

Vagus nerve stimulation is currently the most widely used adjunctive therapy in pharmaco-resistant partial epilepsy. Since its introduction in the late 1990s, it has been used on thousands of patients worldwide. The left vagus nerve is stimulated with electrodes that are connected to a pulse generator in the left part of the chest. Intermittent stimulation of the nerve reduces seizure frequency by 50% in up to 43% of patients with pharmacologically refractory partial-onset seizures. However, in some patients there is a delay of several months before a beneficial effect can be seen. Transcranial magnetic stimulation or stimulation through scalp depth electrodes has also been attempted with some success. A possible mode of action is disruption of the neural patterns required to initiate seizure activity, altering neurotransmitter levels or increasing blood flow to key brain areas.

Closed-loop neurostimulation is a form of neuromodulation that provides therapeutic stimulation only when necessary. An early application of closed-loop neurostimulation was for the treatment of refractory epilepsy, when seizures were not adequately controlled by medication alone. Much like a pacemaker stops abnormal heart rhythms, a closed-loop device aims to halt epileptic seizures by delivering stimulation when it detects the beginnings of seizure activity. A programmable responsive neurostimulation brain implant for the treatment of certain types of epilepsy received approval from the FDA in November 2013. Studies have demonstrated favourable outcomes, with 53% median seizure reduction after 2 years and 70% median seizure reduction after 5 years.

Dietary approaches

The ketogenic diet is one of the oldest available treatments for epilepsy, and one of the most successful treatments for medically intractable epilepsy in children. It is also effective in adult epileptic patients, but compliance is less than that seen in children. The principle is based on the physiology of starvation (fasting). The brain usually uses glucose as its preferred energy source but can metabolize ketones under starvation. During extended periods of fasting, ketones cover up to 60% of the human brain's energy consumption. In the ketogenic diet, carbohydrate intake is very limited and most of the calorie intake is in the form of fat. The metabolism of fat leads to production of ketone bodies (ketogenesis): β-hydroxybutyrate (>85% of circulating ketones), aceto-acetate and acetone (not circulating, only found inside cells). While on the diet children also receive vitamins and minerals, in particular, calcium supplementation. This diet was proposed more than 80 years ago and was based on observations on the effect of fasting on epilepsy that date back to the Middle Ages. Prospective and retrospective studies have repeatedly confirmed the efficacy, tolerability and safety of this diet, but its mechanism of action remains incompletely understood. Several potential mechanisms may underlie the efficacy of ketones in epilepsy. Ketones reduce neuronal electrical hyperactivity through various mechanisms that ultimately stabilize the resting neuronal membrane potential. They increase ATP production, therefore they support the Na^+/K^+ ATPase activity and clearance of glutamate from the synaptic cleft. The increased production of ATP leads to a concurrent increase in adenosine as a breakdown product, which has an inhibitory effect. β-Hydroxybutyrate can activate certain voltage-gated K^+ channels. In addition, acetoacetate can block vesicular glutamate transporters, thus ultimately depleting the presynaptic stores of glutamate and reducing excitation. There is also some evidence that ketones could increase the production of GABA.

Treatment of status epilepticus

Treatment of this medical emergency is in three parts. First, the patient must be given immediate resuscitation (ABC: Airway, Breathing and Circulation). Drugs are then given to control the seizures and, finally, identification and possible treatment of the underlying cause of the status epilepticus are required. Drugs given initially are usually diazepam (or other benzodiazepines such as lorazepam). If these are ineffective at suppressing seizure activity, the barbiturate phenobarbitone or the anticonvulsant phenytoin can be used in large intravenous doses. If seizures continue, general anaesthesia using thiopentone should be applied, with ventilation and intensive care treatment.

Some patients will have a previous diagnosis of epilepsy. Their condition may be caused by a failure to take their medication, which can be determined by measuring drug blood levels. If this is the case, their normal medication should be resumed; otherwise, treatment should be as for new cases. In patients with no previous history of epilepsy, status epilepticus may be caused by several factors, such as trauma, alcohol abuse, drug overdose, tumours or stroke. Status epilepticus is a major risk factor for developing secondary epilepsy.

Social consequences of epilepsy

There is still a significant social stigma associated with a diagnosis of epilepsy. Social stigma is the term given when a person's social, physical or mental condition influences other people's views of them or their behaviour towards them. Members of the general public may be uneasy with someone with epilepsy. This may possibly be overcome by informing them exactly what the seizures entail, but, because of fears of rejection, many epileptics try to hide their condition.

A diagnosis of epilepsy may have severe consequences for a person's present or future employment prospects. Some jobs are completely inaccessible to people with epilepsy, such as the police and fire services, or the armed forces. They also cannot fly aircraft or drive trains.

There are strict regulations governing whether a person with epilepsy can hold a driving licence. For example, in the UK, if you have had epileptic seizures with loss of consciousness, you will lose the right to drive and the licence will be revoked. You can reapply if you have not had a seizure for at least a year. Further restrictions apply with regard to heavy goods vehicles and passenger service vehicles. This directly limits the type of occupation available to someone with epilepsy, and depending on where they live and their need for a car as a means of transport, it may limit their choice to jobs not requiring a driving licence.

There are occupations that may be difficult for someone with poorly controlled epilepsy, such as teaching young children or working at height. There may be reluctance among employers to employ someone with epilepsy, because of fears that their customers or other employees might be upset by someone having a seizure, or that they may be held responsible if the epileptic person injures themselves during a seizure.

A person with epilepsy may be advised about the dangers of certain leisure activities. Water sports and climbing should not be done unsupervised, and riding a bicycle, particularly on the public highway, may be dangerous. Simple measures, such as not locking the bathroom door, may be advisable. Patients with photosensitive epilepsy may be advised to sit further away from the television than normal and avoid computer games with flashing lights. Stroboscopic disco lights usually operate at too low a frequency to induce seizures, but highly sensitive individuals may be affected by striped objects or Venetian window blinds.

A better future for epilepsy patients will depend on an improvement in patient stratification and the ability to offer personalized seizure management based on complex algorithms derived from accurate characterization of the cellular and molecular signature of the individual's seizures. This remains an overarching goal for this complex disease.

Self-assessment case study

A 6-year-old girl has been observed by both her parents and her teacher to have frequent 'vacant' spells during class, when she stares into space and does not respond to her name. Her parents take her to the general practitioner, who immediately refers them to a local paediatrician.

At the hospital, EEG is performed, during which the doctor asks the girl to hyperventilate for 3 min. This provokes one of the 'spells'. She is initially prescribed sodium valproate but this is changed to ethosuximide, which prevents further seizures. Every few years she stops the medication, but this provokes a return of her vacant spells until she is 17 years old, when there is no recurrence.

After studying this chapter you should be able to answer the following questions:

1. What type of epilepsy does she have?

She is likely to suffer from childhood absence seizures.

2. Why is she asked to hyperventilate during the EEG procedure, and what will the EEG show?

Hyperventilation can act as a trigger of seizures in more than 90% of cases of childhood absence seizures. The EEG can show typical spike-and-wave pattern of discharges.

3. What are the possible reasons for changing her medication?

She may have shown an incomplete response to valproate. Ethosuximide is a highly specific drug used for the management of absence seizures.

4. Why does she periodically stop taking her medication?

In most cases, childhood absence seizures spontaneously disappear, often by adolescence. This also proves the case in this patient. Stopping the medication every now and then helps to assess whether the condition has resolved on its own.

DEMENTIA

Chapter summary

1. Dementia is a term used to describe several conditions that are associated with major impairment in cognitive function, in the ability to interact with others and to plan and execute daily activities. Most forms of dementia are progressive and have some genetic determinant. This group of diseases includes Alzheimer's disease (AD), vascular dementia, dementia with Lewy bodies, frontotemporal dementia, HIV-related dementia and Creutzfeldt–Jakob disease.

2. Memory is a key cognitive domain impaired in dementia. The cellular mechanisms underlying learning and memory involve processes such as long-term potentiation and long-term depression. These have been characterized in structures such as the hippocampus, cerebellum and amygdala. They are adaptations in the strength of synapses, which are linked to significant changes in glutamatergic signalling involving N-methyl-D-aspartate (NMDA) and 4-amino-3-hydroxy-5-methyl-4-isoxazole propionic acid receptors. They underlie neuronal plasticity.

3. AD is the most common form of dementia and is characterized by major brain atrophy, a decline in brain metabolism and cholinergic signalling and specific pathological features such as amyloid plaques and neurofibrillary tau tangles. Symptomatic treatment is based on acetylcholinesterase inhibitors such as donepezil, and memantine, an NMDA receptor antagonist. There is intense focus on the development of disease-modifying treatments that could directly target amyloid and tau pathology. Such treatments could be based on the use of vaccines against amyloid and tau aggregates.

4. Biomarkers of dementia have the potential to significantly change the way conditions such as AD can be managed in the future. Biomarkers can be based on measurements of specific compounds in cerebrospinal

fluid or plasma and can also be based on imaging, using ligands that bind to markers of processes such as those involved with amyloid and tau pathology. Biomarkers can help monitor disease progression and response to treatment. As pathological processes in dementias such as AD may be active for many years before clinical presentation, biomarkers would enable more effective intervention at earlier stages of the disease.

Introduction

Dementia is a generic term (from the Latin '*demens*', meaning 'without mind, out of one's mind') for a range of conditions that are characterized by a progressive and irreversible loss of higher mental functions, general cognitive abilities and, in particular, memory, as reflected in the presented case (see Box 14.1). As dementia is not a single disease per se and can be a symptom of various diseases, the DSM-5 has replaced the term 'dementia' with the category 'major neurocognitive disorder'. Cognitive decline in dementia is associated with other significant alterations in mood and behaviour that lead to complete disintegration of the personality. Dementia progression can become a terrifying experience for both patients and carers, although in many cases the patients may not be as aware of their condition as their carers.

Dementia occurs mainly in the elderly, and patients become progressively more dependent; it is the main cause of disability among older adults and affects approximately 50 million people worldwide. Dementia was a relatively rare occurrence before the 20th century, as fewer people lived to old age in the preindustrial society. Changes may be slow and insidious, and may be ignored initially, so dementia may be at an advanced stage at the time of diagnosis. There are several major types of dementia. Alzheimer's disease (AD) is the commonest form of dementia in the elderly, followed by dementia with Lewy bodies, frontotemporal dementia and vascular dementia. Dementia may also occur in younger patients, for example, secondary to other conditions such as in patients infected with the human immunodeficiency virus (HIV).

Causes and diagnosis of dementia

Dementia leads to a gradual loss of cognitive function, without impairment of consciousness. Pseudo-dementia is a form of impaired thinking that occurs in some patients with severe depression. Certain types of dementia are also associated with very specific behavioural and personality changes (e.g. moral disinhibition in frontotemporal dementia).

Dementia is distinguished from acute confusion by several criteria (Table 14.1). In acute confusional states the patient responds to some stimuli in a purposeful manner but is often disoriented, sleepy, inattentive or agitated (delirium). Furthermore, there are often

---

Box 14.1 Case history

Seventy-eight-year-old Gary P. is seen by his general practitioner after his wife expresses concern about his condition. He has gradually become very forgetful over the last 1–2 years. She says that he recently got lost when out shopping, even though they had lived in the same place for years, and that at a recent family gathering he had not been able to remember the names of some of the younger family members. He has always managed the household bills but recently she has taken over, as he complains that 'things are getting too complicated'. He complains that he cannot find things around the house because his wife keeps moving them, which she denies.

Gary has had no significant medical problems in the past and his physical examination is normal. He looks fit and he takes no medication. He speaks fluently but makes frequent errors, either using incorrect words or substituting made-up words instead. He can name three objects but cannot recall them later. When asked the name of the current Prime Minister, he says 'I've never met him'.

Gary's wife is very anxious and asks the doctor whether her husband is developing Alzheimer's disease, as his mother died 'senile' 20 years ago. She wants to know about any treatment that could help him and slow down his mental decline.

This case gives rise to the following questions:

1. How do you test for dementia?
2. Does this man suffer from dementia?
3. How are memories formed and maintained?
4. What is Alzheimer's disease and what are its causes?
5. What is the treatment for dementia and can its progression be stopped?

Table 14.1 Differences between acute confusional states and dementia

Criteria	Acute confusion	Dementia
Level of consciousness	Impaired	Normal
Course	Acute/fluctuating	Chronic/progressive
Autonomic dysfunction	Present	Absent
Prognosis	Usually reversible	Generally irreversible

Table 14.2 Conditions associated with dementia

Degenerative/ inherited diseases	Alzheimer's disease
	Frontotemporal dementia (Pick's disease)
	Dementia with Lewy bodies
	Huntington's disease
	Wilson's disease
	Parkinson's disease
Autoimmune disease	Multiple sclerosis
Vascular causes	Vascular dementia
	Cerebral vasculitis
Space-occupying lesions	Chronic hydrocephalus
	Normal pressure hydrocephalus
	Tumour
	Chronic subdural haematoma
Infection	HIV-associated dementia
	Creutzfeldt–Jakob disease
	Abscess
	Syphilis (now rare)
	Postmeningitis
	Postencephalitis
Traumatic	Post head trauma
	Punch-drunk syndrome (dementia pugilistica)
Toxic	Cerebral anoxia (due to cardiac arrest, respiratory failure or carbon monoxide poisoning)
	Alcohol and drugs (e.g. barbiturates)
	Occupational exposure to toxins
	Heavy metal poisoning
Metabolic or nutritional causes	Hypothyroidism
	Hypocalcaemia
	Vitamin B12/folic acid/niacin deficiency
	Thiamine deficiency (often in alcoholics) leading to Korsakoff's syndrome and Wernicke's encephalopathy

autonomic disturbances (fever, tachycardia and sweating) and motor abnormalities (tremor and myoclonus). A presentation of dementia may emerge in a variety of diseases and syndromes with very diverse causes (Table 14.2). The degenerative/inherited types of dementia are non-reversible. Other causes are either reversible or can be partially reversed or halted with treatment. Dementia can range in severity from mild, when a patient may still be independent in a few activities, to severe, when total dependence occurs. Mild cognitive impairment is the term that describes the earlier phase of symptomatic cognitive impairment that precedes mild dementia, and is described in DSM-5 as a 'minor neurocognitive disorder'.

Irrespective of dementia being of a primary or secondary nature, a key element in the diagnosis is the psychological testing of the patient. The criteria for dementia, as defined by DSM-5, include: (1) evidence of significant cognitive decline from a previous level of performance in one or more cognitive domains (learning and memory, language, executive function, complex attention, perceptual-motor and social cognition); (2) the cognitive deficits interfere with independence in everyday activities (at a minimum, assistance should be required with complex instrumental activities of daily living, such as paying bills or managing medications); (3) the cognitive deficits do not occur exclusively in the context of a delirium; (4) the cognitive deficits are not better explained by another mental disorder (e.g. major depressive disorder, schizophrenia). Testing of the higher mental functions of a patient involves examining their speech abilities and requires appropriate attention, although some aspects can be tested without speech. Patients also need to be able to hear or read instructions.

Cognition is a generic term that defines all mental processes that allow us to perceive and form a concept of the world surrounding us. Cognition includes global consciousness, orientation and attention, various aspects of memory, executive function, execution of motor sequences, perception and language. Cognitive function can be examined initially using standard tests such as the Mini Mental State Examination (MMSE) (Table 14.3). This test is a simple method of scoring mental performance and the maximum score is 30. However, this test cannot detect small degrees of impairment and results depend on the patient's initial intrinsic cognitive abilities. The MMSE is also weighted towards aspects of memory and attention. Addenbrooke's Cognitive Examination (ACE) is a more recent test that addresses some of the weaknesses of the MMSE. ACE is composed of tests of attention, orientation, memory, language, visual perception and visuospatial skills. The Montreal Cognitive Assessment (MoCA) is another screening method for the detection of cognition abnormalities. It assesses short-term memory recall, visuospatial abilities, executive function, attention, concentration and working memory, orientation to time and place, language and

Table 14.3 Mini Mental State Examination

Test	Maximum score
Orientation	
What is the year, month, day, date, season?	5 (1 mark per item)
Where are you (country, county, town, hospital, ward)?	5 (1 mark per item)
Retention	
Name three objects and then repeat these named objects	3 (1 mark for each object)
Calculation and attention	
Count up in 7s five times or spell 'world' backwards	5 (1 mark for each correct addition or correct letter)
Recall	
Recall the three objects named earlier	3 (1 mark per object)
Language	
Show the patients simple objects (e.g. a pencil and a watch) and ask the patient to name them	2 (1 mark for each object named)
Repeat the phrase 'No ifs, ands, or buts'	1
Give a three-stage command, e.g. 'Take the paper in your right hand, fold it in half and put it on the floor.'	3 (1 mark for each stage)
Read and obey the written command 'Close your eyes'	1
Write a sensible sentence, with a subject and a verb	1
Copy a picture (two intersecting pentagons)	1

Box 14.2 Mild cognitive impairment—a prodrome to Alzheimer's disease

Mild cognitive impairment (MCI) is an age-related syndrome that may be the precursor to Alzheimer's disease (AD). MCI is characterized by significant memory impairment in the absence of dementia. Patients with MCI have memory deficits that are at least one and a half standard deviations below the mean of the population. It is important to look for verbal memory impairment, since this is one of the primary deficits in patients who progress to AD. Impaired delayed recall is also a good predictor of progression to AD. MCI as a clinical entity is heterogeneous: some patients with MCI may have very early AD, whereas others may never progress to AD. However, in many cases, MCI is a transitional stage between normal ageing and AD, the annual conversion rate reaching 15%. It is important to identify which MCI patients will progress to AD. At present, there is no reliable clinical method to determine which patients will progress to AD and which patients will not. In the future, the choice of appropriate AD biomarkers (Box 14.3) will help to identify such patients, who may already have significant pathological changes in the brain. MCI patients represent the most promising population of patients for whom prophylactic treatment could be initiated very early on in order to delay the onset of AD.

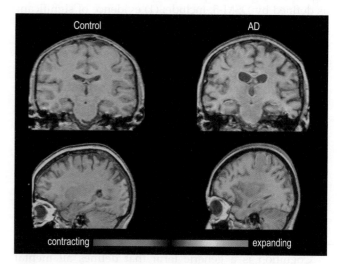

Fig. 14.1 Neuroimage showing brain atrophy and ventricular enlargement in a patient with Alzheimer's disease (AD) compared with an age-matched control. These are fluid-registered volumetric MRI scans from a 60-year-old patient with AD (right) and a normal age-matched control. (From Johns P. (2014) Clinical neuroscience, Churchill Livingstone, Elsevier Ltd., Oxford.)

---

abstract reasoning. It is valuable for the detection of mild cognitive impairment, a state that may represent a transition state between normal brain ageing and the development of dementia (Box 14.2).

Dementia is associated with structural changes, for example, cortical atrophy, enlarged ventricles and widening of the sulci, which can all be detected using computed tomography (CT) and magnetic resonance imaging (MRI) scans (Fig. 14.1)—the former being less sensitive than the latter. Imaging can add to the specificity of diagnosis of certain subtypes of dementia. At the same time, these techniques can also show the significant overlap between dementias: for example, AD can be associated with white matter lesions revealed by MRI, whereas vascular dementia can be associated with temporal lobe atrophy revealed by CT and MRI. Functional MRI (fMRI) is a more recent technique that provides information on blood flow and cerebral metabolism. It provides better identification rates than MRI, and used in conjunction with psychological testing it can enable the location of function in the brain, monitor deficiencies and evaluate the effects of treatment. Both resting-state fMRI and task-related fMRI can reveal significant changes in dementia at an early stage. CT and MRI scans can also identify tumours, haematomas and hydrocephalus, which can present with dementia. Dementia subtype-specific pathological changes can be detected postmortem (e.g. spongiform changes in Creutzfeldt–Jakob disease (CJD) or amyloid plaques and neurofibrillary tau tangles in AD). Pathological markers can also be detected *in vivo* using positron emission tomography (PET) imaging with specific ligands. However, such changes may occur rather late in the evolution of the disease (see later). Blood tests can identify reversible causes of dementia, such as hypothyroidism and vitamin deficiencies. They can also identify the presence of infection, for example, HIV status. Analysis of the cerebrospinal fluid (CSF) can be used to assess specific biomarkers of disease or identify infectious causes, for example, neurosyphilis and meningitis. Liver function tests can identify Wilson's disease (rare genetic disorder associated with copper accumulation in key organs such as the brain and the liver, which can lead to cognitive impairment and dementia features).

Neurobiology of learning and memory

Although specific types of dementia have distinct characteristic features, impairment of learning and memory is the major cross-cutting feature, hence it is essential to review our present understanding of the cellular and molecular basis of these cognitive processes. Learning is the acquisition of new facts and behaviours through experience, and memory is the storage and recall of those facts and behaviours. In order to learn, the brain must be able to change in response to experience, that is, it must show plasticity.

Learning can be divided into two types:

1. Declarative learning is acquiring information about facts, events or rules. It is learning 'why'. This is linked to the formation of two types of memory: episodic memory (remembering events such as last year's holiday) and semantic memory (remembering facts such as Ulaanbaatar is the capital of Mongolia).

2. Procedural (motor) learning is learning complex actions such as how to ride a bicycle (or walk!). It is learning 'how'.

Damage to specific areas of the brain shows that episodic memories are stored in areas of the frontal cortex, whereas semantic memories are distributed across a number of areas, each dealing with a characteristic of the memory, such as its appearance or sound. Semantic knowledge uses categories such as 'fruit' or 'animals'. This is shown by very particular lesions, which lead, for example, to patients being unable to name all types of fruit.

Declarative learning is relatively easy to acquire; many memories need only a single exposure. They require conscious recall and may be forgotten. In contrast, procedural learning is slow, in that for many skills repeated practice is required. Its recall is unconscious

and it is not easily lost. Although there are differences in the cellular mechanisms underlying these forms of learning and memory, they all involve a selective strengthening of specific neural connections.

Short-term and long-term memory

Short-term memory, such as remembering a new telephone number, is easily disrupted until it has been stored in long-term memory, a process called consolidation. After consolidation, it can remain stored permanently, although the ability to retrieve it from the long-term store depends on factors such as how often it is retrieved. Only a small number of short-term memories are consolidated, and this depends on the level of arousal and attention, which will depend on the personal significance of the information.

Short- and long-term memory are separate processes, and items do not have to pass through short-term memory in order to reach long-term memory. This is shown in the few patients whose short-term memory is damaged but who can still consolidate memories into long-term memory.

Amnesia

Memory impairment (amnesia) occurs in two ways. The classification reflects the pattern of loss with reference to the time when the incident triggering amnesia occurred. The inability to form new memories is *anterograde amnesia* and this is linked to a defect in the memory storage process that creates memories. Long-term memories are intact. In most cases of this type of amnesia, patients lose declarative memory—the recollection of facts—but they retain procedural memory. For instance, they are able to remember how to ride a bicycle or a horse, and may be able to learn certain new skills, but they may not remember what they had for breakfast earlier in the day. A failure in recall leads to the inability to retrieve previously stored memories (that preceded the time of the event that led to amnesia), producing *retrograde amnesia*. This type of amnesia may be progressive, with more recent memories being lost first. The patient is left with memories that reach further back into the past.

Models of learning and memory

Learning and memory have been studied in several experimental model systems. Simple invertebrates, such as the marine mollusc *Aplysia californica*, have been used to elucidate possible changes in ion channel activity and intracellular signalling underlying simple learning patterns. The fruit fly, *Drosophila melanogaster*, has been used to probe genetic aspects of learning. However, in mammals, it is the extensive study of changing patterns of synaptic activity in the hippocampus and the cerebellum (mostly in rodents) that forms the basis of current theories regarding memory, as discussed below.

Involvement of the hippocampus in memory formation

Central to our understanding of the role of the hippocampus is the famous patient H.M., described by Scoville and Milner in 1957, who had a bilateral resection of the medial structures of the temporal lobe, including the anterior two-thirds of the hippocampus, to control seizures; following the operation, the patient became unable to form new memories. Additional, more recent evidence, particularly from clinical cases, shows that the hippocampus is central in the consolidation of newly acquired memories, particularly declarative memory. Patients with either accidental lesions of the hippocampus, surgical removal of the hippocampus (for intractable temporal lobe epilepsy) or who have suffered transient hypoxia that is sufficient to destroy neurons in the hippocampus, suffer from severe anterograde amnesia. They retain short-term memory and can recall previously stored long-term memories, but are unable to consolidate new memories.

Central to the present theories of memory formation is the idea that there are long-term changes in synaptic connectivity, either by acquisition of new connections or by strengthening of existing synapses. This is known as Hebb's rule, after Donald Hebb, who carried out influential work on the subject. It states that if two neurons are excited simultaneously, active synapses between them will be strengthened, that is, cells that 'fire together, wire together'. This means that Hebbian synapses can act as coincidence detectors, measuring the correlation between pre- and postsynaptic firing. This property would seem to be a requirement for any sort of associative learning, in which the stimulus and the response are closely paired.

Long-term potentiation in the hippocampus

The hippocampus, a part of the limbic system that lies in the medial temporal lobe, has a trilaminar structure and relatively simple circuitry. This means that thin brain tissue slices, which can be maintained *in vitro*, can be used to study changes in connectivity. It is possible to stimulate inputs to neurons in the slices and record the responses of other neurons in the circuits.

Information processed by the sensory neocortex provides input to the hippocampus via the entorhinal cortex (Brodmann's area 28). This projects through the perforant path to the granule cells of the dentate gyrus (Fig. 14.2). The granule cell axons, called mossy fibres, synapse on large pyramidal cells in the CA3 hippocampal region. CA stands for Cornu Ammonis (or ram's horn), referring to the shape of this area. There are two outputs from CA3 neurons. First, fibres leave the hippocampus via the fornix and travel to the hypothalamus, which then connects with the thalamus. Outputs from the anterior nucleus of the thalamus project to the cingulate cortex and entorhinal cortex. This is known as the Papez circuit (see Chapter 1) and it functionally links the

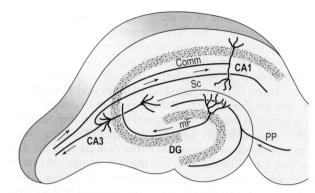

Fig. 14.2 Circuitry of the hippocampus. Stippled areas represent granule cell bodies in the dentate gyrus and pyramidal cells in CA3 and CA1. *Comm*, Commissural fibres; *DG*, dentate gyrus; *mF*, mossy fibres; *PP*, perforant path; *Sc*, Schaffer collaterals.

hippocampus to cortical regions. Second, the CA3 axonal projections to the CA1 region, called Schaffer collaterals, synapse on large numbers of neurons in this region. Some CA3 fibres cross in the ventral commissure of the hippocampus and innervate the contralateral septal nucleus, forming a highly interconnected network. The CA1 outputs convey the results of hippocampal processing, via the subiculum, back to the entorhinal cortex and the sensory neocortex. The hippocampus also receives diffuse innervation, via the fornix, from a number of other brain regions, particularly a cholinergic input from the septal nucleus.

Stimulation of Schaffer collaterals results in an excitatory postsynaptic potential (EPSP) in the CA1 neurons. The phenomenon of long-term potentiation (LTP), discovered in 1973, is the long-lasting increase in synaptic strength, as measured by the size of the EPSP that is observed after high-frequency stimulation of the Schaffer collaterals (typically 100 stimuli at 100 Hz). This potentiation is input-specific, in that LTP is not induced at all synapses but only at those with high-frequency input. It is also state-dependent; if the CA1 neurons are already depolarized when stimulated, the degree of stimulation necessary to produce LTP is less but only if the activity is closely linked in time. In this way, LTP has many of the properties required of a Hebbian synapse. LTP has also been shown to occur in the neocortex, the amygdala and other structures such as the spinal cord.

Molecular mechanisms of long-term potentiation

The mechanisms underlying the increased responsiveness of postsynaptic neurons involve two populations of ionotropic glutamate receptors on the CA1 cells: the 4-amino-3-hydroxy-5-methyl-4-isoxazole propionic acid (AMPA) and N-methyl-D-aspartate (NMDA) receptor types (Fig. 14.3). AMPA receptors can open in response to released glutamate and allow influx of Na^+, which depolarizes the neuron, producing an EPSP. However, there are also NMDA receptors, which at normal resting membrane potentials are blocked by Mg^{2+}. This

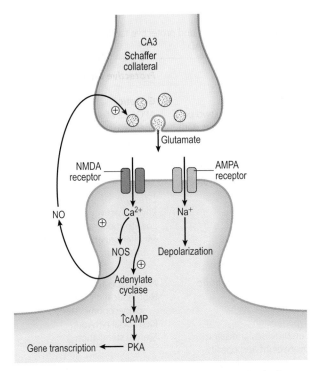

Fig. 14.3 Molecular mechanisms of long-term potentiation in the hippocampus. *AMPA*, 4-amino-3-hydroxy-5-methyl-4-isoxazole propionic acid; *cAMP*, cyclic adenosine monophosphate; *NMDA*, N-methyl-D-aspartate; *NOS*, nitric oxide synthase; *PKA*, protein kinase A.

blockade is released by depolarization (e.g. linked to the activation of AMPA receptors). Therefore, during high-frequency input, or if the neuron has already been depolarized, both AMPA and NMDA receptors can be activated. Activation of NMDA receptors allows the influx of both Na$^+$ and Ca^{2+}, and it is the Ca^{2+} influx that is critical for the development of LTP. The influx of Ca^{2+} can lead to activation of enzymes such as calcium calmodulin-dependent kinase II (CaMKII). This enzyme can engage the actin cytoskeleton, and this can lead to dendritic spine enlargement. In the absence of extracellular Ca^{2+}, or if the intracellular Ca^{2+} is buffered, LTP does not occur.

There are two phases in LTP. If the high-frequency input only occurs once, LTP lasts for approximately 3 hours and decays. This transient, early LTP is not dependent on protein synthesis, as it cannot be prevented by protein synthesis inhibitors. It involves mainly recruitment of extra-synaptic AMPA receptors. In some cases additional recruitment may involve intracellular receptors. However, if the high-frequency input is repeated a few times, a second phase occurs—a form of late LTP that lasts for at least 24 hours and is dependent on protein synthesis. Late LTP requires Ca^{2+} to activate, via the second messenger cyclic adenosine monophosphate (cAMP), a cascade of enzymes (such as protein kinase A (PKA)) that culminates in the activation of genes and changes in gene activity. Additional factors involved in the transition from early LTP to late LTP include brain-derived neurotrophic factor (BDNF) and transforming

growth factor β1 (TGF-β1). By activating complex gene transcription programmes, LTP can change the long-term structure of synapses.

To summarize key features of these processes:

- Postsynaptically, in early LTP, there are increases in the numbers and sensitivity of AMPA receptors. In late LTP new synapses are formed.

- Presynaptically, in early LTP, there is an increase in the release of glutamate. This requires the presence of a chemical messenger, a retrograde transmitter, which travels across the synaptic cleft to trigger increased release. It has been suggested that gaseous transmitters such as nitric oxide (NO) or carbon monoxide (CO) are possible candidates. In late LTP an increased number of release sites increases the amount of glutamate released.

Long-term depression

If LTP were the only mechanism acting to encode memories, there would be very limited fine-tuning of signal strengths in the central nervous system (CNS), as all active synapses would eventually end up being strong. As a necessary balance to learning-enhanced activity, there is also activity-dependent long-term depression (LTD). This can be observed in the hippocampus, where low-frequency, long-period stimulation (1 Hz, 10–15 min) depresses the EPSP for several hours. LTD and LTP are mutually exclusive, suggesting that they act via similar mechanisms.

A completely different form of LTD is observed in the cerebellum, where it is thought to be involved in procedural (motor) learning (see Chapter 9). Purkinje cells in the cerebellum receive inputs from climbing fibres and parallel fibres. Parallel fibre firing results in activation of both AMPA receptors and metabotropic glutamate receptors (mGluRs) on Purkinje cells. These mGluRs are linked to phospholipase C and the production of the second messengers inositol 1,4,5-tris-phosphate and diacylglycerol, and subsequent rises in intracellular Ca^{2+}. Climbing fibres activate AMPA receptors, the depolarization of which results in the opening of voltage-dependent Ca^{2+} channels and a large rise in intracellular Ca^{2+}. The final outcome of the simultaneous activation of both the climbing and parallel fibres is a cascade involving cyclic GMP, a number of protein kinases and, possibly, NO. This eventually decreases the responsiveness of the AMPA receptors and reduces Purkinje cell firing.

Learning and the amygdala

Aversive learning is a form of associative learning in which a noxious stimulus (unconditional stimulus) is associated with a neutral stimulus (conditional stimulus) until the neutral stimulus can evoke the same response (conditional response) as the normal response (unconditional response) to the noxious stimulus.

Aversive learning involves neurons in the amygdala. The amygdala activates pathways that are involved in the response of the sympathetic nervous system to stress: the 'fright, flight or fight' response. Aversive learning underlies the process of fear conditioning and also involves LTP-like mechanisms, in particular in the lateral nucleus of the amygdala. Neurons in the amygdala fire in patterns that correlate with the development of the conditioned response. Lesions of the amygdala prevent this from occurring and prevent expression of the acquired responses. Antagonists of the NMDA glutamate receptor block both fear conditioning and amygdala LTP induction.

Alzheimer's disease

In 1906 the German psychiatrist and neuroanatomist Alois Alzheimer reported to a regional meeting of psychiatrists in Tübingen 'a peculiar severe disease process of the cerebral cortex'. He described a 50-year-old woman who had presented with paranoia, progressive sleep disturbance and memory impairment, aggression and confusion, and that he had followed her until her death, 5 years later. He noted at postmortem the presence in brain tissue of distinctive amyloid plaques (that he called 'miliary foci') and neurofibrillary tangles (NFTs). This was the first case of the disease that was to be named after him. AD is the most common form of dementia and manifests as a progressive loss of memory, particularly recent memories, and a profound alteration of other cognitive functions. In the last stages of the disease, patients require round-the-clock care, which puts a tremendous strain on carers. Hallucinations and confusion are common, and aggression, depression and parkinsonism also occur in some patients. The average life expectancy after diagnosis is 8–12 years. However, individuals can live with this condition for as long as 20 years. More than 40 million people are affected worldwide by AD. Age is the major risk factor for developing AD, and as many countries have ageing populations, a worldwide healthcare crisis is very likely if no treatment is found to protect against the disease, or at least delay or stop its progression.

AD is predominantly a disease of the elderly. The prevalence of late-onset AD is approximately 5% in 70-year-olds and over 20% in people aged over 80 years. By 80 years of age, nursing home admission is expected for 75% of people with AD, compared with only 4% of the general population. However, the disease can also be found in younger people and in some cases from the age of 30 years onwards. Early-onset AD represents less than 5% of cases of AD, and represents a familial, inherited form of the condition.

A variety of factors can be protective or, on the contrary, increase the risk of developing AD and this knowledge is of particular value especially for late-onset, sporadic AD (Table 14.4), as this may lead to implementation of measures that would decrease the risk on a

Table 14.4 Risk factors and protective factors associated with late-onset AD

Risk factors	Protective factors
Genetic Familial aggregation (two or more family members with the disease) APOE ε4 allele Other genes (e.g. CR1, PICALM TREM2, CLU, TOMM40)	*Genetic* APOE ε2 allele Specific mutations in the APP gene
Lifestyle Sedentary life Smoking Heavy alcohol intake Diet rich in saturated fats High blood pressure	*Lifestyle* Physical activity Low-to-moderate alcohol intake Mediterranean diet rich in unsaturated fats
Vascular and metabolic Atherosclerosis Diabetes Hypertension Cerebrovascular disease Overweight and obesity High serum cholesterol	*Psychosocial* High education and high socioeconomic status Rich social network Mental stimulation
Other Traumatic brain injury Depression Infections	*Drugs* Anti-hypertensive drugs Statins Hormone replacement therapy Nonsteroidal anti-inflammatory drugs (NSAIDs)

population scale. Risk factors for developing AD include a genetic predisposition (i.e. increased risk if there are already cases of AD in the family). Environmental factors are also important. For example, there is a significant association between traumatic brain injury and the risk of later developing AD. Similarly, there is a link between the repeated, subchronic damage suffered, for example, by boxers due to repeated brain concussion, which is associated with punching, and the development of *dementia pugilistica* ('punch-drunk syndrome'), which is a form of dementia (see Table 14.2). Dementia pugilistica is considered today as a form of *chronic traumatic encephalopathy*, a condition characterized by brain damage subsequent to multiple concussion episodes, such as those that can occur in professional athletes and also military personnel in the context of war. Present concern is also raised around the mild repeated concussions incurred by a juvenile brain during school sports.

When making a diagnosis of AD it is important to exclude other possible causes of dementia, some of which may be treatable (see Table 14.2).

Historically, dementia was only definitively attributed to AD after the patient had died, with confirmatory pathological evidence at autopsy. However, with the discovery and validation of new imaging tools, *in vivo* confirmation of diagnoses has become possible, at least in clinical research settings, even if not in routine clinical practice. The clinical assessment of patients involves simple scoring systems such as the MMSE (see Table 14.3). More comprehensive tests can also be used, such as the AD Assessment Scale (cognitive subscale) (ADAS-Cog), AD Cooperative Scale (activities of daily living) (ADCS-ADL), AD Cooperative Scale-Clinical Global Impression of change (ADCS-CGIC) and the Neuropsychiatric Inventory (NPI).

The early diagnosis of AD is an area of much interest, especially from the perspective of prevention. It is likely that it would be much easier to slow down the pathogenic process if the treatment were started at a very early stage of the disease, such as that represented by the mild cognitive impairment presentation seen in certain individuals (see Box 14.2).

Genetics of Alzheimer's disease

In a small percentage of patients (<5%), AD is characterized by an early onset (<65 years). Within this group, there are familial autosomal dominant forms of AD (possible onset as early as 20 years old and an average onset age of 46 years). Genetic linkage analysis has shown that these are associated with mutations in one of three identified genes: APP, PSEN1 and PSEN2, encoding the amyloid-beta precursor, presenilin 1 (PS1) and presenilin 2 (PS2) proteins, respectively. The existence of mutations in these genes on chromosomes 21, 14 and 1, respectively, has lent much support to the 'amyloid cascade hypothesis' of AD, which is still a major hypothesis in the present understanding of this disease. Interestingly, AD can occur with a very early onset (30–40 years) in people with Down's syndrome. Almost all individuals with Down's syndrome who live beyond the age of 30 years have dementia by the age of 65 years, and neuritic plaques are detected in the brain much earlier. Down's syndrome is caused by the presence of an extra chromosome 21 (hence the name trisomy 21), and this led to the early suggestion of a link between chromosome 21 and AD. Amyloid peptide, which is the core constituent of plaques, is derived from the amyloid precursor protein (APP) and it was subsequently discovered that the gene encoding APP resides on chromosome 21. In Down's syndrome it is likely that excess production of APP leads to AD. Several other mutations in the APP gene are also associated with early-onset, familial forms of AD. Linkages found between genes located on chromosomes 14 and 1 and early-onset familial AD have led to the identification of the PSEN1 and PSEN2 genes. The PSEN1 gene is associated with approximately 2% of all AD cases (and 30%–40% of all early-onset cases), while the PSEN2 gene is linked to the disease developing in families of Volga German descent (~1% of early-onset cases). The PSEN1 gene is fully penetrant, whereas the PSEN2 gene shows incomplete penetrance, as individuals can live to an old age and not show symptoms of the disease. PS1 and PS2 are proteins associated with the γ-secretase enzyme complex (see below).

However, the majority of AD cases are sporadic and occur in aged individuals. There is a faster progression of the disease in the early onset familial autosomal dominant AD forms in comparison with the sporadic form with late onset (>65 years). For the sporadic form, the genetic basis is much more complex, with susceptibility likely conferred by a variety of more common but less penetrant genetic factors, interacting with environmental and epigenetic influences. AD is certainly multifactorial, with high heritability (~70%). Over the last decade, more than 40 genes/loci have been linked to AD risk and their discovery has enriched biological knowledge of the disease beyond the amyloid-centred hypothesis. In 1993 it was reported that the ε4 allele of the apolipoprotein E (APOE) gene (on chromosome 19) substantially increases the risk for sporadic AD, an association which has been confirmed in most ethnic groups with the exception of some African populations. Age, family history in a first-degree relative, and APOE4 genotype confer the greatest risks of developing AD. APOE encodes apolipoprotein E (apoE), a protein involved in the storage, transport and metabolism of cholesterol. The APOE locus has three alleles: ε2, ε3 and ε4. Susceptibility to AD depends on the combination of alleles inherited from both parents, not on any mutation in the genes themselves. The risk of developing AD increases and the mean age of onset decreases with each copy of the ε4 allele inherited. Conversely, inheritance of the ε2 allele decreases the risk and increases the mean age of onset, which indicates a protective role for this allele. The presence of ε4 does not cause AD but does increase the likelihood of the disease developing at an earlier age. As well as being applicable to late-onset, sporadic AD, this correlation also has validity in early-onset familial cases. Although exact allelic frequencies vary between racial and ethnic groups, the most common allele in the US population as a whole is ε3 (74%), followed by ε4 (16%) and ε2 (10%). This means that the rarest combination is ε2/ε2, which is present in less than 1% of the population, and the most deleterious combination, ε4/ε4, is present in approximately 2.5%. When APOE genotypes were compared in two US groups of 176 AD patients and 91 non-AD controls, 17% of AD patients had the ε4/ε4 genotype, compared with 2% of the controls. The ε3/ε4 genotype was also more prevalent in the AD patients: 43% compared with 21% in the controls. Similar results were shown in a study of Japanese AD patients, although the frequency of ε4 alleles is lower (9%) in Japan. This leads to a predicted lower number of ε4/ε4 and ε3/ε4 individuals in the population, and correlates with a lower prevalence of AD, with a higher mean age of disease onset in Japan.

Another gene associated with an increased risk for sporadic AD is TREM2, encoding a transmembrane protein expressed in cells of the myeloid lineage, including microglia and macrophages. Some of the rare variants of this gene increase the risk to a level comparable with the ε4 allele of APOE. There are many other genetic risk factors associated with sporadic AD that have less

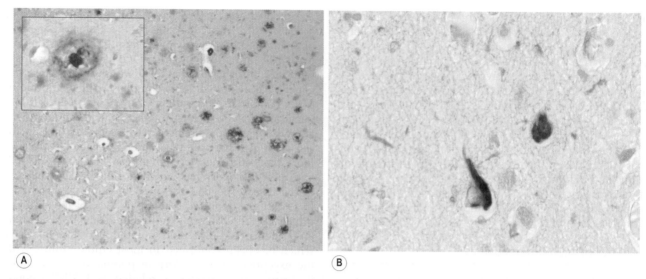

Fig. 14.4 Alzheimer's disease pathology. (A) Amyloid plaques; multiple extracellular plaques in the brain parenchyma and the inset shows a plaque with its dense amyloid core in detail. (B) Neurofibrillary tangles; the tangles fill the neurons and have either an almost spherical appearance or an elongated appearance, reflecting the shape of the neuronal soma in which they are deposited. (From Johns P. (2014) Clinical neuroscience, Churchill Livingstone, Elsevier Ltd., Oxford.)

impact than APOE or TREM2 mutations. Examples include: CLU (encoding the glycoprotein clusterin, also known as apolipoprotein J), CR1 (complement receptor 1), PICALM (phosphatidyl inositol binding clathrin assembly protein), ABCA2 (ATP-binding cassette transporter A2) and SORL1 (sortilin-related receptor 1). They are linked to diverse cellular pathways and mechanisms such as amyloid aggregation, trafficking and clearance, lipid transport, synaptic vesicle dynamics, neuroinflammation and the immune system.

Pathology of Alzheimer's disease

AD is associated with a complex pattern of neuronal degeneration. Brain weight can be reduced by 30%–40%. MRI scans show loss of cortical grey and white matter, dramatically enlarged ventricles, cortical thinning and widened sulci (see Fig. 14.1). Atrophy is also present in subcortical regions. Neuronal loss is significant in the hippocampus; frontal, parietal and anterior temporal lobes; amygdala and olfactory system. There is wide inter-individual variation in the degree of cell loss. There is a large reduction in the marker for cholinergic neurons—choline acetyltransferase (CAT)—which reflects the major loss of neurons in the basal forebrain cholinergic nuclei. There is significant microglia activation and astrocyte activation. AD evokes changes in astrocytes that reduce their neuroprotective homoeostatic role, and there is some experimental evidence that astrocytes exhibit aberrant Ca^{2+} signalling, which may contribute to cognitive dysfunction.

There are also significant losses in other neurotransmitter systems, such as the noradrenergic (e.g. losses in the locus coeruleus), serotonergic and glutamatergic systems. In particular, there are losses in the glutamatergic pathways projecting to and from the hippocampus.

This leads to functional isolation of the hippocampus and very likely underlies the inability to form long-term memories, that is common in AD.

Although the exact pattern of neuronal loss varies from patient to patient, the appearance of the brain at postmortem examination shows two characteristic features in AD: neuritic plaques and NFTs (Fig. 14.4). In fact, until relatively recently, the only certain way of confirming a provisional diagnosis of AD was the identification of these histopathological features. The patient in the case history given in Box 14.1 is likely to be suffering from AD, at an early stage. Progress with the development of biomarkers for AD will increase the confidence by which living patients are diagnosed early in the future (Box 14.3).

Neuritic plaques: amyloid pathology

Neuritic plaques are extracellular structures that consist predominantly of insoluble aggregates of β-amyloid (Aβ) peptides, hence their alternative name, amyloid plaques. There are also other proteins associated with plaques, including apoE, components of the complement cascade (part of the immune system that increases the ability of antibodies and phagocytic cells to clear debris and pathogens) and cytokines such as midkine, which may modulate the formation of fibrillar amyloid. The plaques are surrounded by dystrophic neurites and reactive astroglia and microglia. While neuritic plaques are particularly prevalent in areas of the AD brain showing substantial neuronal loss, neuritic plaques are found, albeit usually at a lower frequency, in normal elderly people without AD. Thus, the number of plaques is not invariably related to AD, as there are normal elderly people with large numbers of plaques, and some AD patients who have few, if any, plaques. Deposits of amyloid peptides can also occur in vessels, giving rise to cerebral amyloid angiopathy.

Biomarkers in Alzheimer's disease

It is becoming increasingly important to define disease bio-markers for Alzheimer's disease (AD) that would consolidate the diagnosis and also allow us to follow the evolution of the disease and the success of treatment regimens.

There are two biomarkers in the cerebrospinal fluid (CSF) of AD patients that reflect amyloid and tau pathology in the brain parenchyma: (1) the 42 amino acid form of Aβ amyloid peptide ($A\beta_{1-42}$) or the ratio ($A\beta_{1-42}/A\beta_{1-40}$); and (2) tau pro-tein (total tau and phosphorylated tau). The concentration of $A\beta_{1-42}$ is decreased in the CSF of AD patients, by approxi-mately 40%–50%. There is a significant correlation between the decrease in $A\beta_{1-42}$ concentration and the increased num-ber of amyloid plaques in areas such as the neocortex and hippocampus. More recently, it has become apparent that reduced plasma levels of this peptide (or the reduced 42/40 peptide ratio) are also indicative of the central changes in amyloid aggregation, although the reduction is less than that measured in CSF: only around 15%. In contrast, tau levels increase in CSF. The level of soluble tau protein in the frontal cortex is highly predictive of the degree of cogni-tive impairment, and CSF levels of total and phosphorylated tau are increased in AD patients. This reflects the increased hyperphosphorylated state of the protein in the brain paren-chyma, and the increased secretion of tau from neurons.

Neuroimaging is used as a biomarker source. Major advances in imaging of AD pathology have come from the development of positron emission tomography (PET) ligands, which bind to amyloid aggregates and tau tan-gles, allowing longitudinal monitoring of the disease evo-lution and response to treatment. Present PET ligands for amyloid include ^{18}F-florbetabir, ^{18}F-flutemetamol and ^{18}F-florbetaben. Amyloid PET imaging is the most used bio-marker in current clinical trials. There is also active research focused on developing selective tau pathology ligands that show good brain penetrance. Neurodegeneration can be followed using volumetric MRI and also meas-urement of neurofilament L (a structural component of axons) in CSF and plasma. Cerebral hypometabolism can be followed using ^{18}F-fluorodeoxyglucose PET analysis. Neuroinflammation can be detected using ligands for trans-locator protein (TSPO), which is expressed in activated micro-glia. Therefore, this wide variety of biomarkers could enable us to follow in detail the complex timeline of AD pathology mechanisms and help characterize the optimum timing of therapeutic interventions targeting specific key components of the pathology.

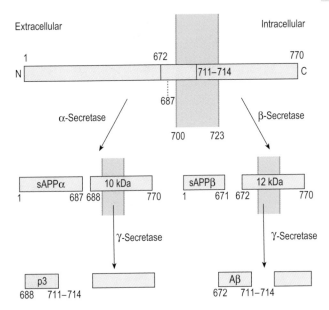

Fig. 14.5 Structure of amyloid precursor protein (*APP*) and its processing by α-, β- and γ-secretase enzymes. β-Amyloid (*Aβ*) represents the amyloid peptides.

Pathogenic APP mutations are clustered around the cleavage sites of β- and γ-secretases. α-Secretase cleaves membrane-associated APP at a site (residue 687) just out-side the membrane; under physiological conditions, this cleavage affects more than 90% of APP. The N-terminal fragment is secreted (sAPPα) and there is some evidence that it is neuroprotective. This leaves an 83-amino acid C-terminal fragment, which is cleaved by the γ-secretase enzyme complex, to produce a smaller peptide, p3. APP can also be cleaved by β-secretase at residue 671. This results in a smaller fragment, sAPPβ. The remaining 99-amino acid fragment is then further cleaved by γ-secretase, in the region 711–714, to produce the Aβ peptide (672–711 to 714). Although Aβ occurs in a range of lengths, some forms, particularly the longer ones such as $A\beta_{1-42}$, are more prone to aggregation and, ultimately, the forma-tion of plaques. As the α- and β-secretases cleave the same precursor in different positions, cleavage of APP by the α-pathway cannot produce Aβ, and the p3 peptide does not appear to form plaques. Thus, processing of APP via the α-secretase pathway is also called the 'non-amyloidogenic pathway'. However, processing of APP via the alterna-tive pathway involving the β-secretase (in particular the BACE1 form of the enzyme) and γ-secretase pathways leads to production of Aβ peptides which form aggregates of insoluble β-pleated sheets of fibrillar Aβ peptide (hence the name β-amyloid). The importance of this pathway is also supported by the discovery in 2012, in an Icelandic study, of a mutation in APP that *reduces* this amyloidogenic cleavage and is associated with decreased risk of AD.

Aβ monomers are produced intracellularly and once they are released from cells aggregation can be initiated. Aggregation proceeds gradually and there is evidence that the intermediate, oligomeric forms of Aβ are synaptotoxic and disrupt LTP and synaptic plasticity. Thus, they may be

The Aβ peptides present in plaques contain between 39 and 42 amino acids. Aβ peptides are the product of cleav-age by proteases of APP, an integral membrane protein with a single transmembrane segment, a C-terminal cyto-plasmic domain and an N-terminal extracellular domain. APP is a protein associated with neuronal development, neurite outgrowth and axonal transport. APP is pro-cessed by three proteases: α-, β- and γ-secretases (Fig. 14.5).

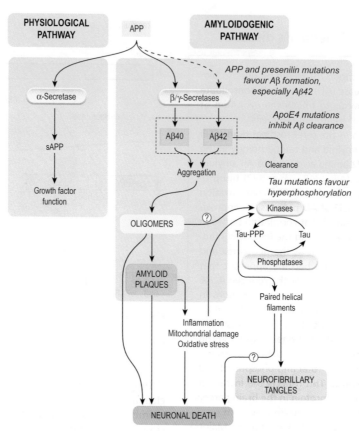

Fig. 14.6 The amyloid cascade. Amyloid precursor protein (*APP*) can be cleaved following the non-amyloidogenic pathway or the amyloidogenic pathway. Copy number variations or mutations in APP can lead to increased levels of amyloid peptides and subsequent aggregation into oligomers and plaques. This aggregation leads to activation of kinases and phosphorylation of tau, which ultimately leads to neurofibrillary tangles and neuronal death. There are mechanisms within this cascade that are still incompletely understood. *Aβ*, β-amyloid. (After Ritter JM, Flower R, Henderson G, Loke Y-K, MacEwan D, Rang HP (2019) Rang and Dale's pharmacology, 9th edition, Elsevier Ltd., Oxford.)

the key forms of aggregates to target for early disruption of the aggregation process and disruption of the pathological cascade. Fibrillization is increased with higher concentrations of Aβ, in particular the longer forms such as $Aβ_{1-42}$; thus any production of larger amounts of Aβ than normal or production of the larger, less soluble forms of Aβ will tend to ultimately increase plaque formation. Once the Aβ plaque has started to form, other molecules interact with the nascent plaque to eventually produce the mature plaque, with associated areas of cell death. The formation of amyloid aggregates can also trigger other processes, such as phosphorylation of the tau protein, which is a major event in the pathology (Fig. 14.6).

Neurofibrillary tangles—tau pathology

Neurofibrillary tangles (NFTs) are dense aggregates of long, unbranched filaments that are found in the cytoplasm of neurons, in particular cortical pyramidal cells. Electron microscopy shows that they consist of two 10-nm filaments that are twisted in a helix, with a period of about 80 nm, to form paired helical filaments (PHFs). These filaments are composed of the microtubule-associated protein tau, in an abnormally phosphorylated form that self-assembles to form PHFs. They are referred to as 'threads' when present in neurites. NFTs are also seen in other neurodegenerative diseases and the number of NFTs correlates well with the severity of dementia. Remnants of dead cells that once contained NFTs are seen as extracellular 'ghost' tangles. In AD, neurons in the entorhinal cortex are often very enriched in tangles. Although tangles contain many different proteins, the core of the tangle is made up of tau protein. Physiologically, the tau protein binds to microtubules and may form cross-bridges between microtubules that stabilize the microtubules, promoting tubulin polymerization and microtubule bundling, which are essential for axon elongation and maintenance. Tau is a phosphoprotein; its biological activity is regulated by phosphorylation, carried out by various kinases, such as glycogen synthase kinase 3 (GSK-3), cyclin-dependent kinase-5 (cdk-5) and PKA. Tau is a negative regulator of protein translation and experimental evidence indicates that it is involved in long-term memory and associative learning. It is encoded by a gene localized on chromosome 17. Six tau isoforms are expressed in the adult human brain, as a result of mRNA alternative splicing. Tau isolated from PHFs is hyperphosphorylated when compared with normal tau and this greatly reduces its ability to bind to microtubules. Phosphorylation appears to inhibit both tau–tau

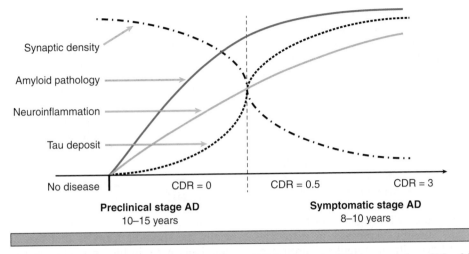

Fig. 14.7 The timeline of key pathological processes in Alzheimer's disease (*AD*) in relation to clinical presentation. CDR = 0 indicates normal cognition and CDR = 3 indicates severe dementia. (After Long and Holtzman, Alzheimer Disease: An Update on Pathobiology and Treatment Strategies, Cell, 179(2): 312–339, 2019.)

interactions and tau–tubulin binding. Tau–tau (and tau–tubulin) binding occurs at a site that is masked by phosphorylation of tau. It has been suggested that normal tau can self-aggregate by undergoing a critical conformational change that allows self-association, and that it is an autocatalytic event in which the presence of altered tau can promote the alteration of other tau molecules. Tau is also released from neurons, therefore tau pathology can spread along trans-neuronal routes, in a stereotyped fashion, along neuroanatomically connected regions. This has been compared to the action of prion proteins (PrP) (see the discussion of Creutzfeldt–Jakob disease), in which the normal α-helical form is thought to be converted to the pathogenic β-sheet form of the protein by the presence of the β-form, which induces the switch. Tau pathology appears first in the trans-entorhinal region, then spreads to the limbic region and neocortical areas. This spreading of tau pathology strongly correlates with the extent of cognitive and clinical symptoms.

The amyloid cascade hypothesis

As reviewed above, extracellular plaques and intracellular tangles are key AD features, and, historically, the 'amyloid hypothesis' and the 'tau hypothesis' postulated these to be distinct phenomena of the pathology. The tau-focused hypothesis proposed that it is the formation of fibrillary tangles and the subsequent disruption of axonal transport that is the key pathological event and the reason for cell death and cognitive impairment. This idea is supported by the good correlation between the severity of dementia and the frequency of tangles. Accumulated evidence shows that these two aspects of the pathology are very closely interconnected. For example, inhibition of the enzyme GSK-3, which phosphorylates tau, results in reduced production of Aβ peptides. It has also become clear that amyloid pathology is a very early event, detectable even in the absence of symptoms, and amyloid aggregates can trigger hyperphosphorylation

of tau. Therefore, in our present understanding of the timeline, amyloid changes precede tau pathology and so it has been suggested that AD pathological processes are initiated by amyloid but propagated by tau. Thus AD could be described as an amyloid-triggered tauopathy. Longitudinal CSF and imaging biomarker studies indicate that global amyloid accumulation is required for the spread of tau. Interestingly, *in vitro* data in human neurons indicate that increased amyloid peptide levels are sufficient to drive tau pathology.

However, there are still several unknowns in the pathology cascade as it is presented today (see Fig. 14.6), and the proposed timeline of key processes (see Fig. 14.7). The manner in which the formation of plaques and tangles is linked to cell death is still incompletely understood. For example, it has been shown that aggregates of Aβ can disrupt Ca^{2+} homeostasis in neurons. Even a relatively small reduction in the ability of cells to regulate intracellular Ca^{2+} could leave them vulnerable to damage by excitotoxicity, ischaemia and free radicals. Finally, parallel processes, such as increased oxidation, neuroinflammation (strong activation of astrocytes and microglia) and mitochondrial dysfunction (with subsequent disrupted energy metabolism), also exacerbate amyloid and tau pathology and are likely to contribute to neuronal demise.

The role of apoE

The important risk associated with the APOE gene has stimulated research on the functions of the ApoE protein. It is involved in the recycling of cholesterol during membrane repair and remodelling and it binds to both lipoproteins and the low-density lipoprotein (LDL) receptor. The affinity of binding to the different types of lipoprotein and the LDL receptor varies with the different apoE isoforms (ε1–4), but the significance of these different interactions is unclear. It has been suggested that the ε4 isoform is less effective than ε2 and ε3 at repairing membrane damage. Neurons may be particularly susceptible to this reduced effectiveness of apoE, as the other apolipoproteins—apoB and apoA1—are not found in the brain. The ε4 isoform also reduces the clearance of amyloid peptides.

ApoE can bind to both Aβ and tau proteins, both *in vivo* and *in vitro*. After a long period of incubation (days) apoE and Aβ form fibrils, but these are not the same as the types of fibril seen with Aβ alone or *in vivo* plaques. ApoE binding to plaques is extracellular, but apoE can enter the neuronal cytoplasm, which is a necessary property for interaction with tau proteins *in vivo*. ApoE4 may have direct pathological effects on neurons, independent of interaction with amyloid peptides and tau. It can reduce neurite growth, induce hyperactivation of neuronal networks and weaken blood–brain barrier integrity. It should be noted that dementia susceptibility genes, such as APOE (and also CLU), are strongly expressed in astrocytes. ApoE4 exacerbates Aβ deposition, promotes neuroinflammation and also impairs neurovascular coupling.

Alzheimer's disease and neuroinflammation

Neuroinflammation is a key factor considered to play a critical role in the development of AD. Microglia are activated and proliferate locally at the sites of amyloid aggregates. Microglia can produce proinflammatory cytokines and free radicals, which could maintain a chronic inflammatory response. In both head injury and cerebral ischaemia, activation of microglia and increases in APP expression appear very rapidly. Aβ is known to activate microglia. The complement protein C1q—a key component of the classical complement pathway—binds to Aβ, triggering the complement cascade. In this way the inflammatory process may be both initiated and potentiated by Aβ. Proinflammatory cytokines possibly play a critical role in AD. Interestingly, chronic use of nonsteroidal anti-inflammatory drugs (NSAIDs) has been associated with a decreased risk of AD.

Another interesting concept that has received interest in the last decade is the possibility of an association between AD and an infectious cause. Aβ peptides can inhibit the growth of Gram-positive and Gram-negative bacteria and herpes virus, and also prevent entry of the virus into cells. Therefore they may act as protective antimicrobial/antiviral peptides in the brain. Foci of infection in the brain could trigger aggregation phenomena and neuroinflammation. There is also evidence that such infectious particle-linked processes that enhance neuroinflammation could be triggered by rather common, periodontal infections.

Other pathological processes

With increasing age, there is an accumulation of abnormally glycated proteins, called advanced glycosylation end-products (AGEs), and an increase in the production of free radicals, consistent with a permanent state of oxidative stress. Owing to the reduced rate of protein turnover with age, this leads to an increased accumulation of damaged proteins and lipids. Several features have suggested that these mechanisms are exacerbated

in AD, leading to abnormal modifications of proteins, including Aβ and tau, which can stimulate their aggregation. It has been shown that AGE-modified Aβ can act as a template for further deposition of soluble Aβ. Tau protein from AD brains, but not from normal brains, is also AGE-modified and undergoes oxidation-induced cross-linking. For example, in brain injury-related AD it is possible that an increase in oxidative stress due to high levels of cell damage, both acute and chronic, could act as a triggering factor for the development of AD.

Treatment of Alzheimer's disease

Our integrated view of the pathoaetiology of AD, especially the sporadic form, is that this disease may begin relatively early in life, much before its clinical presentation in old age, and that it is linked to genetic risk factors and also various environmental stressors which amplify the genetic risk. Regardless of the major primary cause, a cascade of irreversible events is triggered that compromises neurotransmission and leads to major synaptic loss, neuronal loss and compromised brain connectivity.

The existing treatments for AD are symptomatic. They address the disruption of neurotransmission, which is a consequence of neurodegeneration, as discussed in detail below. However, emerging therapies are attempting to address the primary cause of the disease, and thus not only reverse the symptoms, but also modify the disease process. A summary of various therapeutic interventions is shown in Table 14.5.

Cholinesterase inhibitors

In AD there is a significant loss of forebrain cholinergic projection neurons. These represent an important part of the cholinergic neuron population in the CNS (Box 14.4).

Table 14.5 Selected therapeutic strategies in Alzheimer's disease

Target	Therapeutic agent
Cholinergic	Cholinesterase inhibitors
Glutamatergic	Memantine
Antioxidants	Vitamin E
	Selegiline
Anti-inflammatory	Nonsteroidal anti-inflammatory drugs (NSAIDs)
Reduction of risk factors	Statins
	Vitamins B_6 and B_{12}
	Folic acid
Anti-amyloid	Secretase inhibitors
	Immunization
Anti-tau	Kinase inhibitors
	Immunization

The cholinergic system in the forebrain

Acetylcholine (ACh) is a neurotransmitter present in several large clusters of projection neurons in the central nervous system (Fig. 14.8), as well as in numerous interneurons. The human cholinergic systems in the basal forebrain include neurons in the septal and diagonal complex and in the basal nucleus (nucleus basalis) of Meynert.

Several subgroups can be distinguished:

- Group Ch1 of the medial septum comprises 10% of the cells in this area.
- The diagonal band of Broca comprises groups Ch2 and Ch3.
- The largest group of cholinergic cells in the basal forebrain (~90 %)—Ch4—is represented by the basal nucleus of Meynert. The number of cholinergic cells in Ch4 is approximately 210,000 per hemisphere.

Groups Ch1 and Ch2 provide cholinergic input to the hippocampus, the Ch3 cells provide innervation to olfactory areas and the Ch4 cells innervate the cortex and amygdala. All cholinergic cells in the basal forebrain express high- and low-affinity receptors for the neurotrophin nerve growth factor (NGF). This suggests that this neurotrophin is critical for their survival. However, attempts to use NGF therapeutically to protect cholinergic cells in Alzheimer's disease (AD) have not had much success.

ACh is synthesized from acetyl coenzyme A (acetyl-CoA) and choline. Choline is present in extracellular fluid and is taken up into the terminal through an active uptake system. Dietary supplements of choline have been used in an attempt to boost the falling levels of ACh in the brain in AD, but this strategy has had very limited success.

ACh can bind and activate both nicotinic and muscarinic receptors. The former are ligand-gated ion channels, whereas the latter are metabotropic receptors, coupled to G proteins. Positron emission tomography (PET) studies suggest that nicotinic receptor deficits are an early phenomenon in AD. Interestingly, it has been shown that Aβ peptides can block the interaction of nicotinic agonists with their receptors, suggesting a direct link between amyloid pathology and impaired neurotransmission.

The muscarinic receptors M1 to M5 have a widespread distribution in the body. M1 and M2, and to a lesser extent M3, M4 and M5, are present in the CNS. M1 receptors mediate excitatory effects, whereas M2 receptors have mainly inhibitory effects and a predominantly presynaptic location. Using non-selective muscarinic ligands, PET studies have shown that age and AD lead to decreased muscarinic receptor binding in the cortex. It has been reported that M1 agonists may decrease the levels of Aβ amyloid by shifting processing of APP towards the non-amyloidogenic pathway. Thus, a therapeutic strategy based on muscarinic agonists might not only improve cognition but might also have a disease-modifying effect by interfering with plaque formation.

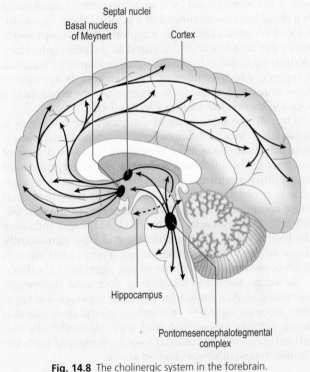

Fig. 14.8 The cholinergic system in the forebrain.

The role of acetylcholine (ACh) in cognition is well established in experimental models. For example, cholinergic receptor antagonists, such as the muscarinic antagonist scopolamine, impair learning and memory. Therefore the cognitive deficit seen in AD is at least partly due to the deficit in ACh. A deficit in cholinergic transmission is also supported by a significant decrease in choline acetyltransferase (ChAT) activity in the cortex and hippocampus of patients with AD. It has been shown that there is a correlation between the loss of cortical cholinergic receptors and synapses and cognitive decline.

Inhibiting the cholinesterase activity that inactivates ACh would lead to potentiation of the failing cholinergic signal. There are two types of cholinesterase: acetylcholinesterase (AChE) and butyrylcholinesterase (BuChE). The two types are related structurally but their distribution in the body, substrate specificity and functional roles differ. AChE is present in the brain and its main function is to hydrolyse the released acetylcholine. BuChE is present in the brain but also in the skin, gastrointestinal tract, liver and plasma, and has a broader substrate specificity than AChE. Tacrine was the first cholinesterase inhibitor to be approved for the treatment of AD, at the beginning of the 1990s. This drug inhibits both AChE and BuChE and was shown to improve the MMSE score. However, it is associated with a high incidence of gastrointestinal side effects, such as diarrhoea, nausea and vomiting, and can induce hepatotoxicity. It was withdrawn in 2013, and replaced by second-generation inhibitors such as donepezil, rivastigmine and galantamine.

Donepezil is a non-competitive, non-selective, reversible inhibitor of AChE, whose long half-life makes once-daily dosing possible. In clinical trials it has been shown that the administration of donepezil to patients with moderate-to-severe AD leads to improved cognition and daily functioning compared with patients who receive a placebo. However, when treatment is stopped there is an immediate and accelerated deterioration in all measures and, by the time drug washout is complete, the scores of patients receiving the drug and those receiving the placebo become the same. Therefore it is unlikely that cholinesterase inhibitors modify, even in a minor way, the disease process. Rivastigmine is another example of a cholinesterase inhibitor. It is a pseudo-irreversible inhibitor of AChE and is not metabolized by liver microsomes. Galantamine is a cholinesterase inhibitor and a positive allosteric modulator of nicotinic cholinergic receptors. The latter property may offer an advantage compared to the other inhibitors, as the drug could enhance the signal mediated by nicotinic receptors, which is relevant for cognition. It appears to have fewer and milder side effects than the other inhibitors and there is less tolerance to its effects.

Overall, the tolerability of cholinesterase inhibitors is reasonable. Most inhibitors have unwanted gastrointestinal effects that are more prominent in the first year of treatment. The inhibitors induce a global improvement in cognitive performance, although the response is variable between patients. It is still unclear how beneficial these compounds are in the severe forms of the disease. Starting therapy early, at the mild AD stage, increases the likelihood of a better outcome and may significantly delay admission to nursing homes. There is not enough evidence to prove superiority of one agent over another.

Based on the same rationale of decreased cholinergic signalling in AD, muscarinic receptor agonists and nicotinic receptor agonists or allosteric modulators are also being actively researched, and they may offer distinct advantages, such as reduced toxicity compared with the cholinesterase inhibitors named above.

Glutamatergic agents

Glutamate is a key excitatory transmitter both in corticosubcortical projections and in corticocortical fibres. It is likely that the physiopathology of AD involves an excitotoxic component, which may be due to dysregulated glutamatergic transmission. Furthermore, the toxicity of glutamate is enhanced by amyloid peptides. In addition, the increased activation of glutamatergic transmission through NMDA receptors could enhance the production of phosphorylated tau.

Memantine is an uncompetitive NMDA receptor antagonist that has relatively strong voltage dependence and rapid unblocking kinetics. The interaction of memantine with the NMDA receptor channel is reminiscent of the action of Mg^{2+}, which blocks the channel under resting conditions. Because of its voltage dependence and fast kinetics, it has been suggested that memantine does not interfere with normal glutamatergic transmission, but blocks increased transmission under chronic conditions of hyperactivity. It has been shown that memantine significantly slows down the rate of cognitive and functional decline and has a positive synergistic effect with cholinesterase inhibitors such as donepezil, without adding to the burden of unwanted effects. It is used in the moderate-to-severe stages of AD.

Antioxidants

Like other neurodegenerative diseases, AD has been associated with increased levels of oxidative stress and free radical-induced damage. Both the monoamine oxidase type B (MAO_B) inhibitor selegiline and vitamin E have been shown to have mild beneficial effects in AD. Similarly, the herbal extract of *Ginkgo biloba* may provide some neuroprotection; this would be a consequence of a postulated improvement in blood flow and reduced oxidation and neuroinflammation. This extract is approved in some countries for use in dementia, but its effectiveness remains controversial.

Nonsteroidal anti-inflammatory drugs

Epidemiological evidence shows that the use of certain NSAIDs, such as ibuprofen, reduces the risk of developing AD. However, preventive or interventional clinical trials designed to confirm and further investigate such observations have failed to show an overall significant neuroprotective effect of NSAIDs. However, it is not contested that AD physiopathology involves an inflammatory component; thus, a better understanding of this component may help in the elucidation of the exact role of anti-inflammatory therapies in the management or prophylactic treatment of AD.

Reduction of risk factors

There is a possible link between cholesterol and AD, and several epidemiological studies have shown that the use of statins, which decrease the production of cholesterol, leads to a decreased risk of developing AD. Cholesterol reduction leads to a reduction in the activity of β-secretase and possibly γ-secretase, and an increase in α-secretase activity. Large-scale prospective studies are required to confirm these observations and clarify the role of cholesterol in the middle or late stage of the disease.

Similarly, a strong link between hypertension and cognitive impairment is well recognized, and hypertension has been linked to AD. Thus, although midlife hypertension is a risk factor for late-life dementia, hypertension may also promote the neurodegenerative pathology underlying AD by producing microinfarcts/bleeds and white matter lesions, resulting in CNS ischaemia. Poor vascular health reduces Aβ and tau clearance and increases levels of γ-secretase. Randomized control trials of anti-hypertensive drugs, especially if started during midlife, show reduction in the risk of dementia.

A link has been suggested between increased circulating homocysteine levels and AD. Present trials are investigating the possible neuroprotective role of a combination of vitamin B_6, vitamin B_{12} and folic acid to decrease homocysteine levels.

In terms of potential modifiable factors, attention is also being given to the monitoring of good quality sleep in elderly individuals, as there is some evidence that sleep impairment can influence the development of AD, possibly by affecting amyloid peptide clearance through the glymphatic system. Interestingly, sleep deprivation in healthy humans leads to an increase in CSF tau levels.

A critical issue is how the genetic and lifestyle factors interact, that is, whether the genetic risk for dementia can be modified by a healthy lifestyle. Recent epidemiological studies showed that modifiable lifestyle risk factors were able to decrease dementia risk only in people who did not have an APOE4 allele (i.e. have a low genetic risk), suggesting genetic susceptibility trumps lifestyle factors in terms of cognitive decline.

Anti-amyloid strategies

Inhibition of secretases

The amyloid cascade starts with production of amyloid peptides, in particular the $Aβ_{1-42}$ form, through proteolysis of APP by secretases. Inhibition of β- or γ-secretase could lead to decreased production of amyloid peptides and a reduced risk of aggregation and subsequent formation of plaques. There have been substantial efforts to develop inhibitors of β-secretase (especially the BACE1 isoform of the enzyme) and also inhibitors of modulators of γ-secretase activity, although nothing has moved successfully to the clinic so far.

Vaccines against amyloid peptides

The principle of targeting neurotoxic protein aggregates by developing vaccines is, in principle, applicable not only in AD but also other types of neurodegenerative diseases (Box 14.5). Much hope was generated when it was shown that transgenic mice made to overproduce amyloid peptides showed a reduced plaque burden when vaccinated with $Aβ_{1-42}$. This beneficial effect could also be obtained by direct administration of anti-amyloid antibodies. It was thought that this effect may be linked to mechanisms such as: (1) antibodies bind to the plaque and activate the surrounding microglia to phagocytose the plaque and (2) antibodies act as a peripheral 'sink' and pull out the peptides from the brain into the circulation. Although the first trials

Box 14.5 Immunization against neurodegeneration—new therapeutic hope

The use of vaccinations is historically associated with the treatment of infectious diseases. Therefore, its possible relevance in neurodegenerative disease was ignored for a long time. Another reason for this was that the central nervous system (CNS) was considered to be a place where primary immune responses do not occur. Any involvement of the CNS in immune reactions was rather considered to be harmful.

In 1999 Schenk and collaborators showed that experimental immunization with β-amyloid (Aβ) peptide can reduce amyloid load, and this turned public and scientific attention to vaccination as a treatment approach in neurodegeneration. This report was followed by the observation in preclinical models that the administration of antibodies, that is, passive immunization, could reduce the amyloid burden. It was shown that antibodies 'coated' amyloid plaques in the brain and could trigger a classic immune response, culminating with the removal of the labelled plaques by activated microglia. Immunization also reversed the cognitive impairment, which was confirmed in two different transgenic mouse models.

These studies also noted that the cognitive improvement was likely to be due to a reduction in a pool of non-deposited Aβ, likely the oligomeric form, as the reduction was seen in diffuse deposits but not in fibrillar deposits. Subsequent work also led to the suggestion that the beneficial effect of immunization is not necessarily associated with penetration of the antibody into the CNS. What was seen after passive immunization was a large increase in plasma Aβ concentration. Hence, the antibodies could trigger a 'sink effect' that promotes the clearance of amyloid from the brain parenchyma into the peripheral compartment.

A third possibility was that the antibodies prevent the formation of oligomers and protofibrils, thus ultimately protecting against the formation of large insoluble plaques. Whatever the mechanisms involved in the effects of vaccination, when the experimental studies were transferred to the clinic for the first time, several patients developed brain inflammation, which led to the cessation of the clinical trial. This reaction was likely to be due to a stimulation of T-cell-mediated immunity. It was hoped that slight modifications of the immunization strategy would avoid the activation of T-cells and its potentially fatal consequences. Recent progress in the production of a variety of vaccines against amyloid pathology has shown that it is possible to develop agents which are safe, although the various vaccines tested in the last two decades have disappointed in terms of efficacy. However, with a better understanding of the mechanisms involved in antibody-mediated clearance of abnormal proteins, this strategy could be extended to other types of neurodegenerative disease characterized by abnormal peptide aggregates which are neurotoxic.

in patients using an amyloid vaccination strategy were stopped due to development of brain inflammation in a number of patients, much research has been focused over the last two decades on various types of vaccines, targeting various amyloid epitopes, amyloid species and aggregation stages, and with improved brain penetrability. There have been some very encouraging results using antibodies such as aducanumab, and this approach still holds promise.

Anti-tau strategies

In parallel with efforts to develop an improved and efficacious vaccine against amyloid pathology, there are parallel efforts to develop a vaccination approach (passive or active) against tau. There is also much interest in targeting tau kinases. Inhibition of the activity of kinases that hyperphosphorylate tau can be achieved with various existing compounds, including drugs such as lithium and sodium valproate, whose strong inhibitory effect on kinases such as GSK-3β is rather unexpected. Lithium can reduce amyloid peptide levels in an experimental mouse transgenic model, so this therapeutic principle has considerable potential and is currently under study.

Other types of dementia

Vascular dementia

After AD, vascular dementia is the second most common type of dementia in the elderly. AD and vascular dementia may often coexist, as confirmed at postmortem. It is caused by reoccurring thromboemboli from either extracranial sources or, more commonly, small vessels in the brain. Patients often have vascular disease such as coronary heart disease or peripheral vascular disease. The pathological presentation is heterogeneous and complex. It includes infarcts, microhaemorrhages and global hypoxic ischaemic injury. White matter injury, with or without axonal loss, is common. Unlike with AD, onset is rapid and progression of the disease is stepwise, with focal neurological defects, which is consistent with multiple, small infarcts (Fig. 14.9). These infarcts may be accompanied by brief periods of impaired consciousness and visual or sensory loss. As the disease evolves there is significant impairment of cognition, for example, in executive function (planning, decision making, flexibility) and processing speed. At present there is no disease-modifying treatment; the symptomatic treatment of the cognitive dysfunction includes cholinesterase inhibitors (galantamine, donepezil, rivastigmine) and memantine. The progression of the disease could be halted if further strokes can be prevented, so management of this condition needs to focus on the reduction of cardiovascular risk factors. Observational studies suggest that targeting risk factors may decrease the risk of vascular dementia. As a prevention strategy, for example, the American Heart Association/American

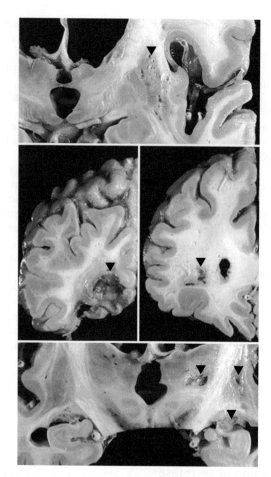

Fig. 14.9 Vascular (multiinfarct) dementia. Infarcts of variable size and location are indicated (arrowheads) in four pathological specimen examples. (From Klatt EC. (2021) In: Robbins and Cotran, Atlas of Pathology, 4th edition, Elsevier Ltd., Oxford.)

Stroke Association recommend monitoring health status using a score based on assessing the components of the 'Life's Simple 7 Rule': smoking status, level of physical activity, healthy diet score, body mass index (ideally <25 kg/m^2), blood pressure (<120/<80 mm Hg, untreated), total cholesterol level (<200 mg/dL, untreated) and fasting blood glucose level (<100 mg/dL, untreated). Increases in life expectancy, a worldwide trend, are associated with an increased risk of ischaemic events and stroke, so an increase in this type of neuropathology is likely in the future. There is a significant need for biomarkers of early diagnosis and the monitoring of disease progression.

Dementia with Lewy bodies

In western populations dementia with Lewy bodies comprises 5%–6% of cases of dementia diagnosed in primary and secondary care settings. This type of dementia is pathologically characterized by Lewy bodies, which are intraneuronal, proteinaceous structures with radiating filaments, which can also be detected in neurites (Lewy neurites). The major protein detected in Lewy bodies is α-synuclein, present in an aggregated form. These protein aggregates can also be found in the brain of parkinsonian patients, in nigrostriatal neurons and in neurites (see Chapter 10). However, in dementia with Lewy bodies the aggregates are more widely distributed in the CNS, as well as the peripheral autonomic nervous system. Autonomic dysfunction is reflected by symptoms such as orthostatic hypotension, sexual dysfunction, delayed gastric emptying and constipation. There is significant dopaminergic and cholinergic dysfunction. Patients with Lewy body dementia have major sleep impairment (in particular, REM sleep behavioural disorder during which patients act out their dreams or produce vocalizations and other abnormal movements), visual hallucinations, fluctuations in cognitive function and some evidence of parkinsonism. Diagnosis is difficult and definitive diagnosis is only obtained at autopsy. Pure AD, by definition, has no Lewy bodies, but modern sensitive techniques have shown that Lewy bodies do occur in AD. The presence of α-synuclein in Lewy bodies has led to the suggestion that dementia with Lewy bodies and PD both be considered synucleinopathies. Thus, new treatments addressing this common pathogenesis, for example, vaccines targeting the aggregation of α-synuclein, may be effective in the two diseases. There are no specific treatments for this type of dementia, and management of this dementia is difficult because of the need to control a variety of symptoms—medication for one type of symptoms may worsen another. A worsening of the condition can be caused by even small amounts of antipsychotic drugs, which will exacerbate the parkinsonism, whereas dopamine agonists will exacerbate the neuropsychiatric problems. Cholinesterase inhibitors such as rivastigmine and donepezil can improve attention and processing speed and alleviate apathy. When these inhibitors are not tolerated, the NMDA receptor antagonist memantine can be used with some benefit. The individual disease evolution may differ but all patients will gradually develop increased disability and death will ensue. Average survival after onset of the disease is approximately 8 years, although some patients may live longer.

Frontotemporal dementia

Frontotemporal dementia is an umbrella term for a range of complex and heterogeneous forms of dementia that affect the frontal and temporal lobes. The onset of this condition occurs at an earlier age than AD, commonly between 40 and 65 years of age, affecting both sexes approximately equally. Patients with this type of dementia have dramatic changes in their personality and behave in a socially inappropriate manner. They can be impulsive or emotionally indifferent and lose the ability to use language in both receptive and expressive aspects. They show apathy and decreased personal hygiene. Frontotemporal dementia is classified into two main types: the behavioural subtype (previously known as Pick's disease) and the language subtype, the latter being subclassified into non-fluent and semantic variants of primary progressive aphasia. There is also a form of frontotemporal dementia with amyotrophic lateral sclerosis. The behavioural variant is characterized by symptoms such as loss of behavioural inhibition, decreased social cognition, inertia, loss of empathy and perseverative or compulsive behaviours. The semantic variant patients have difficulty in naming or recognizing objects or drawings, limited speech production and inability to recognize words. The non-fluent variant leads to impaired speech production and difficulty in the comprehension of complex sentences.

Frontotemporal dementia is a highly inheritable disorder, and variants have been linked to a range of specific genetic mutations, some of which are shared with amyotrophic lateral sclerosis. Examples are mutations in the following genes: MAPT (on chromosome 17, encoding the tau protein), GRN (also on chromosome 17, encoding the protein granulin), C9orf72 (chromosome 9 open reading frame 72, expansion mutation) and TARDBP (on chromosome 1, encoding transactive response DNA binding protein 43 (TDP-43)). Frontotemporal dementia is difficult to diagnose; structural MRI can reveal atrophy of the frontal and/or temporal lobes but not at an early stage of the disease. Neurofilament light (neurofilament L)—a structural component of axons—is a promising biomarker; it is increased in CSF and plasma and its levels are associated with severity of disease, brain atrophy and survival duration. There are no specific treatments at present. Pharmacological management can be attempted: selective serotonin reuptake inhibitors have been used to control impulsivity and disinhibition, and antipsychotic drugs have been used to control agitation. Other supportive management includes physiotherapy, occupational therapy and speech and language therapy.

HIV-associated dementia

More than three decades ago, after the onset of the human immunodeficiency virus/acquired immunodeficiency syndrome (HIV/AIDS) epidemic, it became apparent that there was a very clear neurovirulence associated with HIV. Infection with HIV can lead to neurological symptoms in both the early phase and the later stages. The infection causes cognitive and motor dysfunction, and prior to the introduction of effective antiretroviral therapies, large numbers of infected adults (one-third) and even more children (one-half) ultimately developed HIV-1-associated dementia (HAD). Worldwide, although advances in the treatment of HIV have dramatically improved survival rates, the infection continues to be a cause of neurological impairment, ranging from a mild cognitive dysfunction to severe dementia, collectively designated as 'HIV-associated neurocognitive disorder'. Two-thirds of the cases affected by this disorder occur in sub-Saharan Africa. The symptoms of HAD include apathy, depression, poor concentration and memory, tremor, hyperreflexia, seizures and myoclonus. HIV enters the CNS through infected monocytes and leads to the activation of resident microglia. Pathological changes are detected in the basal ganglia, neocortical grey matter, cerebellum and brainstem.

The intensity of the HAD symptoms correlates with the degree of monocyte infiltration and microglial activation. The neurological dysfunction is a consequence of the damage sustained before initiation of antiretroviral therapy and also the persistent immune activation associated with the residual presence of the virus. Many of the drugs used to treat HIV infection do not penetrate well into the brain; therefore, CNS infection of macrophages and microglia creates a reservoir that is not affected by peripheral treatments. Patients with advanced HAD show cerebral atrophy, with losses of up to 30% of neocortical neurons. Neurons may be either damaged directly by HIV proteins or killed by compounds released from infected cells. Neurons themselves are not infected with HIV, but it is thought that infected macrophages and microglia release neurotoxic compounds, such as glutamate, which can trigger excitotoxicity (see Chapter 11) and inflammatory cytokines. Large neurons seem to be more susceptible than small neurons and the infection leads to free radical production, metabolic compromise and oxidative stress, which lead to neuronal death. Antiretroviral therapy can improve cognitive impairment but the effect is both limited and variable. Impairment can persist even in those with an undetectable plasma viral load.

Creutzfeldt–Jakob disease

Creutzfeldt-Jakob disease (CJD) is a rare disease that affects approximately 1/1,000,000 of the population annually and is characterized by rapidly progressing dementia, personality changes, psychosis, involuntary movements, speech impairment, myoclonus and ataxia. Most patients die within a year after disease onset. CJD belongs to the larger family of transmissible spongiform encephalopathies. The name of these conditions arises from the appearance of vacuoles within the brain, as observed postmortem. The disease is associated with widespread neuronal loss, astrocytic gliosis and spongiform changes. Clinical diagnostic criteria use a combination of characteristic neuropsychiatric symptoms, CSF levels of protein 14-3-3 (a protein involved in phosphorylation processes), MRI using fluid-attenuated inversion recovery (FLAIR) and diffusion-weighted (DW) analysis to detect changes in tissue intensities, and EEG (patients may present a characteristic pattern of periodic sharp waves). There are three types of CJD: sporadic (the most common), inherited (linked to specific mutations) and acquired (e.g. transmitted by exposure to specific medical procedures). Medical procedures that are associated with the spread of this form of CJD include transfusion of blood from an infected individual, use of human-derived pituitary growth hormones for gonadotropin hormone therapy, and some transplants (e.g. corneal transplants or dura mater grafts). Variant CJD is a form of acquired CJD believed to be due to ingestion of beef from cattle affected by bovine spongiform encephalopathy ('mad cow disease'). The transmissible agent responsible for CJD is a prion protein (see Chapter 12). Stanley Prusiner, who was awarded the 1997 Nobel Prize

for his work on prions, coined the term 'prion', which was derived from 'proteinaceous infectious particle', a unique type of infectious agent. Prions are misfolded proteins that can multiply in the host latently for many years and ultimately lead to large-scale neurodegeneration. The PrP is encoded by a gene that is present and expressed to the same extent in the cells of normal and affected individuals. The functions of the normal variant of PrP (named PrP^c) are not fully understood; the protein may have roles in intercellular signalling and innate immunity. Prions are composed of an abnormal, protease-resistant form of PrP, designated PrPS^c, which differs from PrP^c by its β-sheet structure (in contrast to the α-helices that characterize the structure of PrP^c). The increased presence of β-sheets leads to the formation of fibrils, which ultimately deposit in the brain. It is unknown how PrP^c converts into PrPS^c (possibly a spontaneous conversion or triggered by a mutation in the prion gene PRNP) or how the fibrillary deposits are responsible for generalized neurodegeneration. PRNP mutations account for 10%–15% of sporadic forms of CJD.

A CSF-based sensitive test has recently been developed for the detection of pathogenic prions. It is important to note that infectious prions may not be inactivated by routine surgical instrument sterilization procedures; therefore the WHO has recommended the destruction of instrumentation as required. There is at present no treatment for this disease and there is evidence that the incidence of sporadic CJD is increasing, with potential incubation times longer than four decades. Symptomatic treatment includes opioids for pain management, benzodiazepines for myoclonus, and antidepressant drugs.

General considerations in the management of Alzheimer's disease and other types of dementia

A review of the AD drug development pipeline in 2020 shows 121 agents being explored in clinical trials for use in AD, most of them disease-modifying agents and targeting a variety of pathological mechanisms such as amyloid, tau, neuroinflammation, neurogenesis, energy metabolism and synaptic and vascular protection. There is much hope that progress will be made in the following decades, possibly using combinatorial approaches. However, the pharmacological and non-pharmacological management of dementia sufferers at present poses numerous challenges. Patients and their carers are affected not only by the cognitive loss, but also by all the other symptoms that may be comorbid with dementia such as psychosis, aggression, depression and the generalized change in personality. Such neuropsychiatric disorders occur in up to 90% of dementia patients and are one of the main causes of admission to residential homes.

Depression in dementia is widely studied because of the difficulties of differential diagnosis between a depressive syndrome and the early stage (or prodromal stage) of dementia. Often, depression is reactive at the beginning (as a consequence of the psychological impact of the diagnosis) but later on may increase in severity and result from changes in the corticolimbic circuitry. Preference is given to treatment with antidepressant drugs, such as selective serotonin reuptake inhibitors, as these are generally better tolerated than other antidepressant drugs and they have no anticholinergic effects that may accelerate cognitive decline.

Psychosis is treated with antipsychotic drugs. Newer antipsychotics, such as risperidone and quetiapine, are preferable because of the reduced anticholinergic component and also because they are better tolerated overall. The use of antipsychotics should be limited because of the increased risk of mortality in this population.

It is also important to make sure that pain and infection, or any other cause of distress, are kept under control and that the patient is placed in a supportive environment as the disease progresses.

Care strategies must also take into account what has long been neglected: care-giving to a patient with dementia can itself lead to pathology in the carer. Therefore, preventive healthcare strategies must be developed for carers and respite care must be made more available. The move from care at home to institutional care must be better planned and should not only be a reaction to a crisis or the consequence of carer burnout.

Self-assessment case study

Sheila B. was a 74-year-old woman admitted to hospital with a history of rapid decline in mental status. She had started deteriorating 4–5 months before admission. She had cared for her terminally ill husband for 2 years and began showing signs of depression after his death. The family assumed that this was a natural reaction to grief and that it would subside. However, the antidepressants prescribed by her general practitioner (GP) had no effect and, 3 weeks before admission to hospital, her confusional state became significant and she started having auditory and visual hallucinations, for which the GP prescribed haloperidol.

On admission, her pupils were reactive and equal. She had very brisk symmetrical reflexes, myoclonus and limited verbal communication. The computed tomography scan was normal and a magnetic resonance imaging scan showed mild, chronic ischaemia of the white matter. The electroencephalogram showed repetitive sharp waveforms and a high level of protein 14-3-3 was detected when the cerebrospinal fluid was analysed. The status of the patient continued to deteriorate and a brain biopsy showed early spongiform change, neuronal loss and reactive astrogliosis. Her mental status continued to decline further, with akinetic mutism and onset of seizures. She was discharged to a hospice, where she died after 2 months.

After studying this chapter, you should be able to answer the following questions:

1. What is a 'spongiform change' and how can the symptoms of this patient's disease be explained?

The typical spongiform aspect at pathological examination suggests that this patient suffered from Creutzfeldt–Jakob disease (CJD). The symptoms and other test results are supportive of this diagnosis.

2. What caused the disease that affects this patient?

There are several types of CJD: sporadic (the most common), inherited (linked to specific genetic mutations) and acquired (transmitted by exposure to specific medical procedures or by ingestion of food infected with prions, which are the pathological substrate of this disease). It is unclear what the most likely cause was in this patient.

3. What are the treatment options available?

There are no disease-modifying treatments at present for CJD. The only treatment is symptomatic, for example, the use of benzodiazepines to control motor problems, or antidepressant drugs.

SCHIZOPHRENIA AND NEURODEVELOPMENTAL DISORDERS

15

Chapter summary

1. Schizophrenia is a complex chronic psychiatric disorder that is accompanied by significant impairment in cognition, awareness, affect and social behaviour. Evidence indicates that schizophrenia is linked to abnormalities in neurodevelopment. Other conditions that are strongly linked to altered neurodevelopment and are characterised by disrupted communication and socialisation patterns include autism-spectrum disorders (autism, Asperger's syndrome).

2. Schizophrenia and autism-spectrum disorders have a significant heritable component. The genetic alterations include mutations and copy number variations that cover the whole genome. Environmental factors also influence the risk of developing these disorders. Such factors include prenatal and perinatal injury and infections, the parents' age, maternal metabolic disorders such as gestational diabetes and obesity, adverse socio-economic circumstances and misuse of drugs during the critical period of central nervous system maturation.

3. The pathophysiology of schizophrenia and autism-spectrum disorders is reflected in a wide range of structural abnormalities, which affect regions such as the prefrontal cortex, hippocampus, thalamus and cerebellum. There is an indication of impairment in the maturation of cerebral circuits and the stabilisation of synapses, and this leads to complex changes in brain connectivity.

4. The pharmacological management of schizophrenia is based on the use of antipsychotic drugs. A common characteristic of all classes of antipsychotics is the blockade of dopaminergic receptors. Treatment-resistant patients may respond to the drug clozapine. Antipsychotics improve positive symptoms but have limited impact on negative

symptoms and cognitive dysfunction. They also induce a wide range of adverse effects that decrease patient compliance.

5. Non-pharmacological management of schizophrenia and autism-spectrum disorders involves multidisciplinary approaches and is aimed at improving the integration of patients in the community and thus increasing their socialisation.

Introduction

One of the most complex aspects of human brain function concerns the processes of cognitive control, development of appropriate patterns of behaviour within a social context and congruent emotional reactions. Psychosis is a term that defines a state of mind characterised by a loss of contact with reality. Short episodes of psychosis can be associated with a wide variety of conditions, for example, neurodegenerative diseases such as Alzheimer's disease or Parkinson's disease, brain tumours, drug misuse or malaria. In patients who present with psychosis, behaviour is profoundly altered and the symptoms that emerge are diverse, bizarre and disturbing, often leading to a gradual and irreversible alienation. Psychoses challenge our understanding of higher brain functions and their pathophysiology is much more complex than that associated with sensory or motor dysfunction. Schizophrenia is a complex, chronic psychiatric disorder that has psychosis at its core. Schizophrenia is illustrated in the case history presented in Box 15.1. In order to understand the pathology of major psychotic disorders, such as schizophrenia, it is important to identify the cerebral circuits and neurotransmitters that play key roles in consciousness, cognition, emotions and moral reasoning.

Schizophrenia: the clinical diagnosis

The patient described in Box 15.1 was previously diagnosed with schizophrenia and the analysis of this case starts with a brief mental state examination in order to assess the following: (1) appearance and behaviour, (2) speech, (3) affect, (4) thoughts, (5) perceptions, (6) cognitive state and (7) insight.

The examination of the patient (Box 15.2) confirms the abnormal behaviour, deficits and distorted mental perceptions that are indicative of major psychosis, in the absence of an organic cause. Furthermore, the mood of the patient is depressed and there is a clear risk of suicide.

Schizophrenia is characterised by three major symptom clusters: positive symptoms, negative symptoms and cognitive symptoms. Patients present with abnormal ideas, abnormal perceptions, motor, volitional and behavioural disorders, formal thought disorder and emotional disorders. These are described below. The diagnosis

Box 15.1 Case history

Jane was a 22-year-old Physics undergraduate. She also used to work in the evenings as a proofreader. Two years ago, in her final year at university, she visited her doctor accompanied by her parents, who were very concerned about changes in her behaviour and communication at home. She had become withdrawn and rather obsessed with religion. Finally, she confessed to her parents that she had a mission to save the country from a nuclear disaster and said that her 'internal voices' would guide her. Jane was diagnosed with schizophrenia and was prescribed an antipsychotic. However, although the medication helped a little and 'the voices' became less persistent, she complained that she felt rather dizzy and tired for most of the time, and that she put on weight. The drugs made her feel so strange that at times she did not take them. She could not continue her studies, and she started drinking immoderately. She claimed that she felt 'mentally numb'.

You see Jane as a specialist, after a recent suicide attempt. Following this, an antidepressant drug was added to her antipsychotic medication. Her family continue to wonder what may have caused this disease and want to know if their daughter will ever recover. They are distraught and ask if you can prescribe a better treatment.

This case gives rise to the following questions:

1. What is the explanation for the symptoms presented by this patient?
2. What are the neurobiological mechanisms underlying this type of mental dysfunction?
3. What has triggered this major disruption of normal behaviour?

Case history (continued)

The patient's appearance is striking: she is dishevelled and her clothes are untidy and unsuitable for the season. This suggests little interest in personal grooming, which is confirmed by the inappropriate choice of clothes. She is quiet during the interview and needs prompting to answer questions. Her face lacks expression. She tells you that the voices are still visiting her but are much kinder now. They come mostly during the night, and she thinks they know that she cannot sleep, especially since she started taking the new drug alongside her old medication. The cognitive assessment reveals that Jane has a significant attention deficit. Towards the end of the interview, she says abruptly that she hates her life.

The questions that need to be addressed are as follows:

1. Is this patient receiving the most appropriate treatment?
2. Is this patient still at risk of taking her own life?
3. What is the long-term prognosis?
4. Is there a role for the family in the successful management of this patient?

according to DSM-5 is based on the presence of two or more characteristic symptoms—delusions, hallucinations, disorganized speech, grossly abnormal psychomotor behaviour (such as catatonia) or negative symptoms (e.g. blunted affect, lack of interest in socializing)—for a significant portion of time during a 1 month period, with signs of the disturbance persisting for at least 6 months. At least one of these two symptoms should include delusions, hallucinations or disorganized speech.

Positive, negative and cognitive symptoms

It is important to note that these three main categories of schizophrenia symptoms may evolve in terms of relative intensity during the disease.

Positive symptoms are characterized by the existence of an abnormal behavioural pattern; they include delusions, hallucinations, thought disorder, bizarre behaviour and catatonia (a psychomotor syndrome marked by a significant decrease in an individual's reactivity to their environment, and presenting with stupor, mutism, motor rigidity or paradoxical and purposeless excitement and agitation).

Negative symptoms are characterized by the absence or diminution of normal function and reactions. Examples of negative symptoms include apathy, affective blunting, incongruity of emotions, lack of insight, social withdrawal, impaired judgement, poor initiative and lack of motivation, drive and interest in personal hygiene.

Cognitive symptoms are characterised by decreased executive function and attention, and impaired language, memory and processing speed. Patients have difficulty in planning and have impaired problem solving.

Positive symptoms are particularly associated with acute episodes, whereas negative symptoms underlie the severe disability associated with chronic schizophrenia. There is evidence that positive and negative symptoms respond differently to treatment, and that the relative balance between the two has prognostic implications. Furthermore, cognitive symptoms are strong predictors of long-term outcome.

Abnormal ideas

The main abnormal idea in schizophrenia is delusion, that is, a belief that is erroneous and out of keeping with the individual's background, and is held by the patient with intense conviction. Patients may present with various types of delusion: delusions of persecution (e.g. external forces are trying to harm the patient or damage his or her reputation), grandiose delusions (e.g. patients may believe that they have a divine purpose or supernatural powers), hypochondriacal delusions (e.g. a belief that the body is rotten and diseased) and delusional mood (e.g. everything seems strange or full of a hidden intricate meaning).

Abnormal perceptions

The cardinal symptom in this class is the hallucination, which is perception without an object. Hallucinations may occur in any sensory modality: auditory, visual, somatic, olfactory and gustatory. Auditory hallucinations (hearing voices) are by far the most prominent and are considered to be the commonest symptom of schizophrenia. They can be the first sign of schizophrenia or may appear at a later stage of the disease. The source of the voices can be difficult to locate: voices can surround the patient, come from a particular point in space or originate within the patient's head or body. They can be menacing, encouraging, mocking or simply neutral and observing (Box 15.3). The importance of auditory hallucinations in schizophrenia has led certain specialists to consider them as typical 'first-rank symptoms', that is, of particular relevance for the diagnosis of schizophrenia.

Motor, volitional and behavioural disorders

Bleuler (1911) provided the first description of 'peculiar forms of motility, stupor, mutism, stereotypy, mannerism, negativism, spontaneous automatism and impulsivity'. Stereotypies are purposeless acts that are carried out repetitively, such as rocking or rubbing of the hands. Patients may also present with strange mannerisms (e.g. when they eat they put the hand round the back of the head to bring the food to the mouth) or bizarre postures. Facial expressions may be altered by grimacing. In states of catatonia the patient sits or lies expressionless, motionless and mute, sometimes in very uncomfortable and contorted postures. Sometimes, the catatonic patient shows paradoxical agitation. In contrast, in states of catalepsy (waxy flexibility), the patient's limbs can be manipulated by the observer and the patient may maintain the final position for a long time.

Patients may present with bouts of extreme hyperactivity, which may be associated with destructiveness: they may destroy furniture and crockery or take off their clothes and run around naked. The impulsive behaviour may lead, in rare instances, to very violent acts, such as homicide, for which the patient cannot give any explanation.

Formal thought disorder

This refers to disturbances in thinking that may lead to unintelligible speech. Speech may suffer from derailment and loosening of associations (a tendency to be deflected from the main point of the discussion and a failure to follow a train of thought through to its conclusion) and may also abound in neologisms (new words invented by patients). There is poverty of content of speech and, although speech may be abundant, it fails to convey any information (Box 15.4).

Emotional disorders

One of the most typical examples of emotional dysfunction in schizophrenia is affective flattening. Patients lose natural reactions to usual social cues. Facial expression is reduced and there is an apparent indifference to emotive topics. Patients may come across as cold and detached, and unable to establish a rapport. Schizophrenics may also display inappropriate affect (e.g. smiling or laughing when discussing death or attending a funeral) and shallowness of emotions.

Presentation and epidemiology of schizophrenia

Schizophrenia is a very broad diagnosis and includes a multitude of clinical presentations. This significant clinical heterogeneity suggests differences in the underlying mechanisms. Apart from the criteria defined by DSM-5 and described above, diagnosis also requires evidence of gradual and sustained deterioration in work, interpersonal relationships, communication and self-care. The patient in the case history presents with auditory hallucinations (hearing 'voices') and delusions of influence, social withdrawal and decreased personal grooming. The general low mood and previous suicide attempt, as well as the loss of interest in personal appearance, reflect the coexistence of significant depression. The depressive symptoms may be part of the illness or a secondary psychological reaction. The natural evolution of the disease is complex and variable (Fig. 15.1). There are cases in which several acute episodes are followed by what

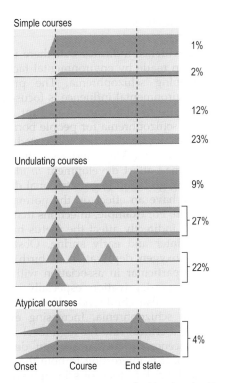

Simple courses

1%

2%

12%

23%

Undulating courses

9%

27%

22%

Atypical courses

4%

Onset   Course   End state

Fig. 15.1 Examples of disease courses of schizophrenia. The diagram illustrates various possible courses of schizophrenia and the relative percentage of patients affected within a subtype. (From Bleuler M. (1978) In: PJ McKenna (ed) Schizophrenia and related syndromes. Oxford: Oxford University Press, p. 55.)

appears to be full recovery. The intensity of the episodes may vary. Other cases are characterized by gradual deterioration and resistance to treatment. Finally, other cases stabilize at a moderate level of disability. A diagnosis of schizophrenia has lifelong consequences for affected individuals and their families.

Schizophrenia is associated with an increased risk of premature mortality, including deaths from suicide and metabolic and cardiovascular disease. Schizophrenia has a consistent prevalence worldwide (~1%) with apparently no significant influence of culture, ethnic background or socio-economic group. There is a slightly increased prevalence in urban areas. No overall difference exists between the sexes. However, the average age of onset appears to be earlier in men (between 15 and 25 years) than in women (between 25 and 35 years). Men also have a poorer response to treatment than women and a worse long-term outcome.

Aetiology of schizophrenia

Genetic aspects

Family, twin and adoption studies suggest that schizophrenia has a significant genetic component, with heritability up to 80%. Relatives of schizophrenic patients have a higher risk for developing the illness. Risk is positively correlated with the degree of genetic relatedness (Fig. 15.2). However, schizophrenia does not follow

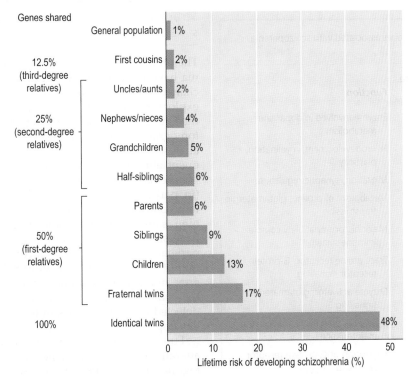

Fig. 15.2 Correlation between genetic relatedness and lifetime risk of developing schizophrenia. (From Barondes SH. (1993) Molecules and mental illness. New York: Scientific American Library, p. 150.)

a classic genetic Mendelian model. Monozygotic twins have a concordance rate of 50% for schizophrenia but this falls to 15%–18% in dizygotic twins. Schizophrenia is not associated with a single major locus but with multiple genetic loci of modest effect which are epistatic (i.e. interactive), thus leading to a high cumulative risk. Nevertheless, 89% of patients have parents who are not schizophrenic, 81% of patients have no affected first-degree relatives and 63% of patients have no family history of the disease.

Research on the genetics of schizophrenia has identified a wide range of mutations and gene copy number variations, scattered across the genome, in this complex polygenic psychiatric disorder. Large scale genome-wide association studies have identified more than 100 associated regions. There is significant overlap in common risk variants between schizophrenia and bipolar disorder, and schizophrenia and major depressive disorder.

The genes affected are associated with a multitude of targets and processes that can impact brain structure and function. They include neurodevelopment, myelination, signalling (e.g. glutamatergic and dopaminergic transmission), receptors and ion channels, receptor scaffolding proteins, synaptic formation, maintenance and plasticity, and the immune system. A few examples are shown in Table 15.1. There is increasing evidence that the numerous and various implicated genes converge upon common biochemical pathways and signalling networks. This is particularly relevant both for a better understanding of the pathophysiology of the disorder, and also for new and improved therapeutics.

Table 15.1 Examples of genes associated with schizophrenia

Gene	Chromosome locus	Function
COMT	22q11	Enzyme involved in dopamine metabolism
NRG1	8p21-p12	Neurodevelopment, myelination, plasticity
DISC1	1q42.2	Migration, synaptic regulation
PRODH2	22q11.21	Metabolism of proline; glutamatergic transmission
MHC	6p22.1	Major histocompatibility complex; immune system
TAAR6	6q23.2	Trace amine receptor; G-protein receptor signalling
G72	13q32-34	Enzyme activator; glutamatergic signalling
DNTBP1	6p22.3	Dysbrevin; synaptic formation and maintenance
RGS-4	1q21-q22	Regulation of G-protein receptor signalling
DRD3	3q13.3	Dopamine receptor signalling

Environmental factors

Accumulating evidence indicates that there is a significant contribution made by environmental factors to the risk of developing schizophrenia. The predominant model of an environmental influence is focused on neurodevelopment and factors that can disrupt it. There is a higher risk of schizophrenia for people born in winter months (i.e. a 5% increase in risk associated with birth between December and May) and also after viral epidemics, which may affect development *in utero*. Events that occur during gestation (e.g. nutritional deficiencies, infections) may have an effect on the normal development of the brain. For example, infections that will affect the mother and indirectly affect the foetus have a peak incidence in winter and early spring. Obstetric complications (e.g. oxygen deprivation at birth) may also be relevant, in particular in association with a genetic risk. Socioeconomic deprivation, especially in an urban environment, and also childhood adversity have been associated with schizophrenia. Increasing evidence is also supporting a critical role for high-level use of cannabis in adolescence, in the subsequent development of schizophrenia. It is interesting to note that several of the environmental risk factors for schizophrenia are also associated with other neurodevelopmental problems including intellectual disability, autism and attention deficit-hyperactivity disorder.

Neurobiology of schizophrenia

Structural, functional and neuropathological studies

The profound behavioural alterations seen in schizophrenia have led to extensive studies on the structural brain changes that may characterize this disease. The detailed exploration of structural changes became possible with the development of imaging techniques. Computed tomography and magnetic resonance imaging (MRI) analyses during the last 30 years show that one of the frequent abnormalities in schizophrenic patients is lateral ventricular enlargement (Fig. 15.3). Striatal and thalamic (in particular the medial nuclei) shrinkage are important contributors to this enlargement, and cortical thinning is also observed. Studies using high-resolution MRI have shown a gradual loss of grey matter, affecting the parietal, temporal and frontal cortices, during the evolution of schizophrenia. Longitudinal studies suggest that grey and also white matter changes are progressive and they continue after the disease onset. They can also be detected in ultra-high risk individuals who subsequently develop the disease.

Functional analysis of the brain has also revealed alterations in schizophrenia. Although electroencephalogram abnormalities are reported to be present in up to 80% of schizophrenic patients, the changes are relatively non-specific and may be encountered, although

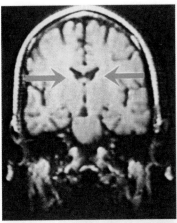
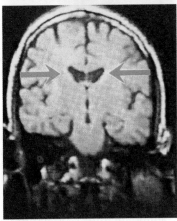

Fig. 15.3 Magnetic resonance imaging (MRI) analysis of schizophrenic brain. The images show the MRI scans of the brains of a pair of identical twins, only one of whom suffers from schizophrenia (bottom). Note that the twin with schizophrenia has much larger ventricles. (From Barondes SH. (1993) Molecules and mental illness. New York: Scientific American Library, p. 153.)

at a lower frequency, in normal individuals. Increased delta and decreased alpha waves are apparent in individuals with psychosis, and they indicate an altered arousal state, which leads to reduced ability to attend to relevant stimuli. Studies analysing cerebral blood flow and metabolism support the concept of 'hypofrontality' in schizophrenia. Cerebral blood flow can be monitored while schizophrenic patients and controls are performing the Wisconsin Card Sorting Test (Box 15.5). The schizophrenic patients' performance is worse than that of controls on this test. This impairment is accompanied by smaller increases in blood flow to the prefrontal cortex during the task. Such differences are not found when a control psychological task is used. Therefore, schizophrenia is clearly associated with dysfunction in prefrontal cortical circuits. This conclusion corroborates the observations on the marked reduction in cortical thickness in the dorsal prefrontal cortex of schizophrenic patients. This reduction appears to be associated not with a decrease in neuron numbers but with a decrease in the number of distal dendrites, dendritic spines and axon terminals. Altered packing of neurons can also lead

to significant differences in laminar cell density in the schizophrenic brain. Recent positron emission tomography studies also document a clear reduction in synapses in corticolimbic circuits (see below). This can be revealed using a specific marker for synapses (Fig. 15.4). Overall, all these changes profoundly alter the dynamics of cortical circuits and their activity.

Psychophysiological changes and information processing

One of the reproducible findings in schizophrenia is that of event-related potential (ERP) abnormalities. ERPs reflect different stages of information processing in the brain. ERP abnormalities reflect a deficit in the processing of sensory information, which is associated in particular with medial temporal lobe dysfunction. Eye-tracking (i.e. ability to follow a moving target with the eyes) changes are also reported in approximately 50% of schizophrenic patients. The changes are likely to reflect dysfunction in the connections between the frontal eye fields (i.e. regions of the frontal lobe that show increased activity during execution of eye movements) and the temporal and parietal cortices. Eye-tracking deficits are particularly robust phenotypic markers of familial risk for schizophrenia.

Schizophrenia and corticolimbic circuits

The results of structural and functional imaging studies suggest critical involvement of cortical and limbic structures in schizophrenia. The term 'limbic' was coined by the French neurologist Paul Broca in 1878 and referred initially to the medial surface of the brain, in particular structures that form a ring around the ventricles and the brainstem. According to this definition, the limbic system includes the cingulate gyrus and the cortex on the medial surface of the temporal lobe, in particular the hippocampus (Fig. 15.5). Broca's anatomical concept of a 'limbic lobe' was

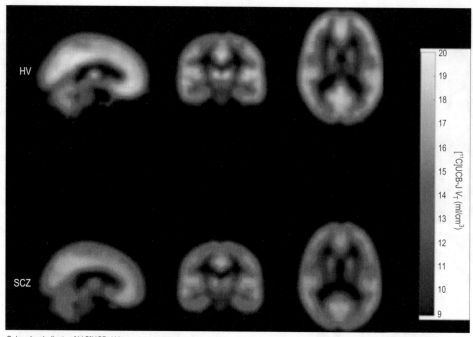

Fig. 15.4 Positron emission tomography (PET) study using the protein SV2A as a marker of synapses. The images indicate a marked reduction in synapses in the frontal and cingulate cortex of schizophrenia patients (SCZ) versus healthy volunteers (HV). (From Onwordi EC, Halff EF, Whitehurst T, et al. (2020) Synaptic density marker SV2A is reduced in schizophrenia patients and unaffected by antipsychotics in rats. Nature Communications 11:246.)

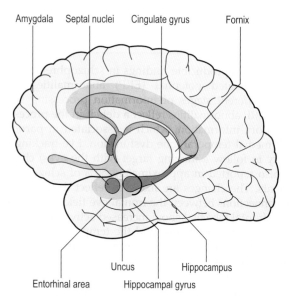

Fig. 15.5 Limbic structures. The diagram represents the right hemisphere (medial aspect). (From Brodal P. (1998) The central nervous system – structure and function. Oxford: Oxford University Press, p. 556.)

subsequently expanded and given a functional dimension by the American neurologist James Papez. He suggested that limbic structures are interconnected and that the cingulate cortex plays a major role in emotional behaviour.

The view put forward by Papez was essentially correct inasmuch as the limbic system and its connections are important in the control of emotions (see Chapter 1,

Figs 1.17 and 1.18). However, the limbic system must be seen in the context of the other cortical areas, with which it has abundant direct or indirect connections. A brief overview of cortical organisation is provided in Box 15.6 and Fig. 15.6. In recent years particular attention has been given to the study of the connections between limbic structures and the prefrontal cortex (including the premotor and supplementary motor areas and the frontal eye field). The prefrontal cortex receives information from the cingulate gyrus and also from the parietal, occipital and temporal lobes. Fibres connect it reciprocally with the mediodorsal nucleus of the thalamus. The thalamus is connected with the globus pallidum and amygdala. Therefore the prefrontal cortex integrates information about all sensory modalities and the motivational state of the individual. Much has been learned about the roles of the prefrontal cortex from cases of lesions (Box 15.7). Changes observed in limbic structures and in the prefrontal cortex in the brain of schizophrenic patients suggest that some of the circuits involving these brain areas become dysfunctional in schizophrenia. In particular, there is evidence of thalamocortical dysconnectivity: a decrease in connections between the thalamus and prefrontal cortex, while there is an increase in motor/somatosensory-thalamic connections.

The neurodevelopmental hypothesis of schizophrenia

Despite the onset of the disease in early adulthood, it is now acknowledged that abnormalities in the brain of

Cortical organization

The cerebral cortex contains billions of neurons and, in mammals (particularly primates and humans), it quantitatively dominates the rest of the nervous system. The activity of cortical neurons is involved in higher mental functions such as the determination of personality, memory, cognition and emotions. Phylogenetically, the cerebral cortex developed from a more primitive and evolutionarily old, three-layered structure, called the allocortex, to a six-layered structure termed the neocortex (isocortex). The allocortex includes the hippocampus, a three-layered structure termed the archicortex, and the olfactory area, which is the oldest cortex and is termed the paleocortex. Other parts of the limbic system such as the cingulate and parahippocampal gyri and anterior insula region have a transitional four-layered structure (termed the mesocortex). Together, the allo- and mesocortex comprise much of the limbic system. More than 95% of the human cortex is neocortex and has the same basic six-layer structure, with cells of similar morphological characteristics defining distinct layers. There are two main types of cells in the neocortex: granule cells which are largely inhibitory interneurons that modulate the function of the pyramidal cells, and glutamatergic projection neurons that form the majority of neurons in the cortex. Granule cells predominate in layers II and IV, whereas pyramidal cells are located in layers III and V. Pyramidal cells are distinguished by an axon that arises from their base, and an apical dendrite that can cross several layers situated above the layer in which the neuronal cell body lies. Layer I is the molecular layer and contains largely intracortical dendrites and very few cells. Layers II and IV contain cells with small bodies that are densely packed. Layer III contains medium-sized pyramidal cells and layer V contains large pyramidal cells. Layer VI contains cells that have heterogeneous shapes. From a functional point of view, layers II and IV predominantly receive input, whereas pyramidal cells in layers III and V are the source of cortical output, either directed at other cortical areas (layer III) or directed subcortically (layer V). Layer VI is also largely efferent (see Fig. 15.6).

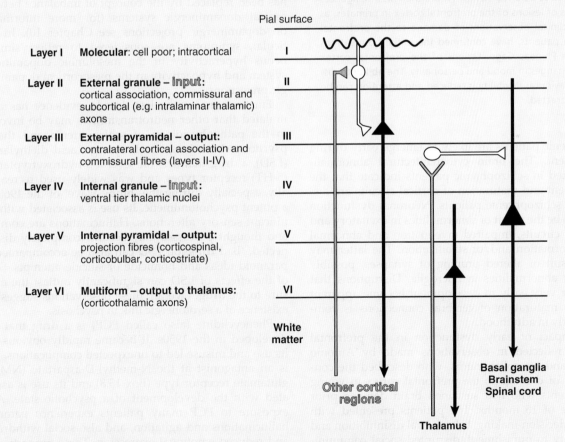

Layer I	**Molecular**: cell poor; intracortical	I
Layer II	**External granule – Input:** cortical association, commissural and subcortical (e.g. intralaminar thalamic) axons	II
Layer III	**External pyramidal – output:** contralateral cortical association and commissural fibres (layers II-IV)	III
Layer IV	**Internal granule – Input:** ventral tier thalamic nuclei	IV
Layer V	**Internal pyramidal – output:** projection fibres (corticospinal, corticobulbar, corticostriate)	V
Layer VI	**Multiform – output to thalamus:** (corticothalamic axons)	VI

Pial surface

White matter

Other cortical regions

Thalamus

Basal ganglia
Brainstem
Spinal cord

Fig. 15.6 Schematic diagram showing neuronal connections within the layers of the neocortex.

<table>
<tr><td>**Box 15.7**</td><td>**The prefrontal cortex and its role in cognitive function and emotional expression**</td></tr>
</table>

The first insight into the importance of the prefrontal cortex was offered by the case of Phineas Gage in 1848. This 25-year-old foreman had a tamping iron pushed through his skull, through the accidental blasting of explosives used on the construction site where he was working. The metre-long iron rod entered his head below the left eye and, after passing through the left frontal lobe, exited through the top of the head. The hole through the skull was more than 9 cm in diameter and significant damage was caused to both hemispheres, in particular the frontal lobes. After extraction of the rod, the patient overcame the infection that developed and made a full recovery. However, his personality was profoundly altered. The doctor who had taken care of him described how Gage became impatient, impulsive, unpredictable and undecided, and described him 'indulging at times in the grossest profanity—which was not previously his custom'. His personality was changed so profoundly that his friends considered that 'he was no longer Gage'. His emotional behaviour and moral reasoning seemed to be affected much more than his intelligence.

Studies of lesions of the prefrontal cortex in primates, as well as clinical observations of damage to the prefrontal cortex in patients, have confirmed the initial observations made on Phineas Gage. Lesions of the prefrontal cortex lead to changes in mood and personality. The ability to display behavioural flexibility is reduced and attention can be easily distracted.

schizophrenic patients are likely to emerge early during development. The brain cytoarchitectural abnormalities reported in schizophrenic patients indicate that the development and maturation of cortical circuits are disrupted in schizophrenic patients. Neuronal dysfunction is likely to be the result of abnormalities in excitatory and inhibitory circuits, impaired myelination and abnormal synapse formation and/or stabilization. The latter may be the result of altered pruning of synapses, possibly driven by abnormalities in microglia. Disruptions that may occur very early in development become apparent when the maturation of cerebral connections is completed, early in adulthood.

The impact of early dysfunction in the prefrontal cortex is reflected in observations made by Antonio Damasio and his collaborators, who described the consequences of damage to the prefrontal cortex in young adult patients who had sustained brain damage prior to the age of 16 months. The patients presented with impaired decision-making, behavioural disinhibition and insensitivity to punishment, disrupted social communication and abnormal emotion. The patients had defective social and moral reasoning, which suggests that the acquisition of complex social conventions and moral

rules (a 'sense of right and wrong') had been impaired. However, the patients were relatively normal in terms of intellect, memory, language and academic achievement.

Neurotransmitters in schizophrenia

The complex alterations that affect the behaviour and mood of schizophrenic patients have led to a quest to define the critical transmitter(s) involved in this disease. For more than six decades dopamine has been considered to be a key neurotransmitter in schizophrenia. The hypothesis that dopaminergic systems are involved in the pathophysiology of this disease was based primarily on pharmacological evidence. Chlorpromazine, a dopamine receptor antagonist discovered by serendipity, was the first drug that provided significant improvement in schizophrenic patients. In contrast, direct and indirect dopaminergic agonists, such as amphetamine, can induce psychotic symptoms in normal individuals and exacerbate psychosis in schizophrenic patients. All the drugs currently used to treat schizophrenia are dopamine receptor antagonists. Studies in drug-free or drug-naive schizophrenic patients suggest a mild elevation in dopamine receptors. However, the initial emphasis on generalized dopaminergic hyperactivity has been replaced by the concept of imbalance between central dopaminergic systems (for more information on dopaminergic projections see Chapter 10). In particular, symptoms are considered to reflect simultaneous hyperactivity in the mesolimbic dopaminergic system and hypoactivity in the mesocortical dopaminergic projections.

Furthermore, in the last decade, evidence has accumulated that other neurotransmitters may be involved in the pathophysiology of schizophrenia and that of psychotic states in general. Lysergic acid diethylamide (LSD), a drug that acts on several 5-hydroxytryptamine (5-HT) receptor types and was widely used recreationally, especially during the 'hippy wave' of the 1960s, is a potent psychotomimetic. Its use is associated with significant sensory alterations. Hallucinations are common and thought processes may become completely disconnected. 'Bad trips' on LSD can also be accompanied by paranoid ideas and homicide or suicide attempts. Some of the effects of LSD can significantly outlast the exposure to the drug. Overall, these observations suggest the existence of a serotonergic link in psychosis.

Phencyclidine (also called PCP) is a drug that was developed in the 1950s. It became rapidly obvious that its use and misuse led to unexpected complications. PCP is an antagonist at the N-methyl-D-aspartate (NMDA) glutamate receptor type (Box 15.8) and its use is associated with the development of a psychotic state. After exposure to PCP many patients experience paranoia, hallucinations and agitation, and also social withdrawal and reduced emotional expression. These properties are shared by ketamine, a drug used in general anaesthesia and pain management and, more recently, treatment-resistant depression. PCP and ketamine can precipitate

Box 15.8 — Glutamate and its receptors

Glutamate is the main excitatory amino acid in the brain. In the cortex it either originates in cortical afferents or is present in corticocortical fibres. After release from nerve terminals, glutamate can bind to two categories of receptor: ionotropic and metabotropic.

Ionotropic receptors

These are ligand-gated ion channels that are divided into three main types, named after their prototype ligand: (1) the NMDA type (after N-methyl-D-aspartate), (2) the AMPA type (after 4-amino-3-hydroxy-5-methyl-4-isoxazole propionate) and (3) the kainate type (after kainic acid). The AMPA receptor is associated mainly with Na^+ and K^+ conductance, whereas the NMDA receptor is also significantly associated with Ca^{2+} permeability. Another interesting characteristic of the NMDA receptor is its blockade by Mg^{2+} under resting membrane potential conditions. Thus, it is only when the neuronal membrane is depolarized that the channel allows passage of ions after binding of glutamate. The NMDA receptor type also requires glycine as a coagonist for stimulation of the receptor. This complex receptor also has various other modulatory sites. Phencyclidine and ketamine are NMDA channel blockers. Glutamate receptors are involved in learning and memory (see Chapter 14).

Metabotropic receptors

Metabotropic receptors for glutamate (mGluRs) are receptors coupled to G-proteins. On the basis of sequence homology, transduction mechanisms and pharmacological profile, they can be divided into three families: the mGluR I family (coupled to activation of phospholipase C activity), and the mGluR II and mGluR III receptors (coupled to inhibition of adenylate cyclase).

Table 15.2 Classification and examples of antipsychotic drugs

First generation—typical antipsychotics

Phenothiazines: chlorpromazine, thioridazine, fluphenazine, trifluoperazine

Butyrophenones: haloperidol, benperidol

Thioxanthenes: flupenthixol, clopenthixol, thiothixene

Second generation—atypical antipsychotics

Substituted benzamides: sulpiride, amisulpride

Clozapine, olanzapine, risperidone, quetiapine

Third generation antipsychotics

Aripiprazole, brexpiprazole, cariprazine

---

cortical GABAergic cells—the parvalbumin-expressing neurons—have been reported in schizophrenic patients.

Therefore, what is gradually emerging is a new understanding of the pathophysiology of psychoses and a more integrated view of the alterations in schizophrenia that involve several important transmitters that we are currently aware of, such as dopamine, 5-HT, glutamate and γ-aminobutyric acid (GABA).

Treatment of schizophrenia

Despite the still incompletely understood aetiology and neuropathology of schizophrenia, existing treatments can improve the condition of a significant number of patients. Current treatments are still dominated by 'the dopamine theory of schizophrenia' (as discussed above). Antipsychotic drugs (also known as 'neuroleptics' or 'major tranquillizers', although these terms are rather obsolete) consist of a wide range of dopaminergic antagonists, which belong to various chemical classes (Table 15.2). These drugs can also be divided into 'typical' neuroleptics, which are the oldest compounds, and 'atypical' neuroleptics, which have been developed more recently. The oldest class of antipsychotic drug is the phenothiazine class, with its prototype drug chlorpromazine (Box 15.9).

All antipsychotic drugs act as dopamine receptor blockers, with significant affinity for the D_2 type, not the D_1 type, receptor. One of the most elegant studies in support of the importance of the blockade of dopamine receptors was published by Johnstone and her collaborators in 1978. This study compared the efficacy of the α- and β-isomers of the neuroleptic drug flupenthixol in acute schizophrenia. Only α-flupenthixol has dopamine receptor antagonist properties and the study showed that only this isomer had antipsychotic efficacy (Fig. 15.7).

The general blockade of dopamine receptors by antipsychotic drugs leads inevitably to extrapyramidal motor symptoms due to disruption of nigrostriatal dopaminergic transmission, and endocrine dysfunction (hyperprolactinaemia) due to blockade of dopaminergic

---

psychotic episodes (e.g. in schizophrenic patients in remission). PCP is no longer used clinically but it is still widely abused (snorted or smoked), especially in the USA. Chronic PCP users can develop violent criminal behaviour. The effects of PCP suggest that deficits in glutamatergic transmission may be associated with schizophrenia. Such deficits may significantly affect thalamocortical projections, which are glutamatergic. Postmortem analysis of the brains of schizophrenic patients shows loss of neurons in the mediodorsal thalamus. The analysis of changes in cortical layers shows a loss of thalamic axon terminals in layer III and a loss of dopaminergic innervation in layer VI of the prefrontal cortex. Thus, these observations suggest a dual cortical deficit in dopaminergic and glutamatergic input, which is likely to affect the activity of pyramidal neurons. Finally, alterations in glutamatergic signalling may also lead to impairment of GABAergic cortical transmission. Significant alterations in a subpopulation of

SCHIZOPHRENIA AND NEURODEVELOPMENTAL DISORDERS

Chlorpromazine: a milestone in the history of psychiatry

Before the advent of modern medical treatments, psychosis—also known as 'madness'—was the main reason for the existence of asylums. These institutions were full of patients with varied types of psychosis, which often made them dangerous to themselves and society. Many moving accounts exist of the lives of the 'insane' in such institutions. A young psychiatrist, newly appointed to Fulbourn Mental Hospital in Cambridgeshire, wrote these notes in 1953: 'I was taken in by someone who had a key to lock the door and lock it behind you. The crashing of the keys in the lock was an essential part of asylum life then just as it is today in jail… Some wards were full of tousled, apathetic people just sitting in a row because for 20 years the nurses had been saying, "sit down, shut up". Others were noisy. The disturbed women's ward was a phantasmagoric place. The women were in "strong clothes", shapeless garments made of reinforced cotton that couldn't be torn. Many of them were "in locked boots" which couldn't be taken off and thrown.'

Prior to the 1950s, medicine had nothing to offer apart from heavy sedation and custodial care. The enthusiasm of the medical profession for various rather crude treatments waxed and waned: the induction of insulin coma, prolonged narcosis with barbiturate drugs or massive severing of fibres in the frontal lobe through lobotomy. Everything changed when the drug chlorpromazine was introduced. Preliminary experimental observations showed that chlorpromazine had a significant sedative effect. As described by Henry Laborit, the French doctor involved in its development, the drug produced 'not any loss in consciousness, not any change in the patient's mentality, but a slight tendency to sleep, and above all "disinterest" for all that goes on around him'. When the drug was tried in the clinic, aggressive psychotic patients were controlled for the first time without recourse to force. The French psychiatrists Delay and Deniker, who were involved in the first studies, coined the term 'neuroleptic'. By the mid-1950s, it became clear that chlorpromazine was going to radically change the management of schizophrenia.

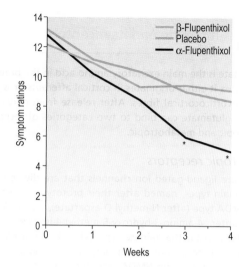

Fig. 15.7 Clinical improvement in acute schizophrenic patients treated with the two isomers of flupenthixol or placebo. (From Johnstone et al. (1994) In: McKenna PJ, (ed) Schizophrenia and related syndromes. Oxford: Oxford University Press, p. 144.)

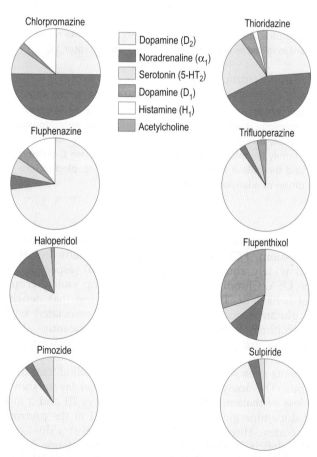

Fig. 15.8 Pharmacodynamic profiles of antipsychotic drugs. The pie charts represent the relative receptor-blocking activities of antipsychotic drugs. (From McKenna PJ (ed). (1994) Schizophrenia and related syndromes. Oxford: Oxford University Press, p. 138.)

transmission in the tubero-infundibular pathway. Apart from the blockade of dopamine receptors, antipsychotic drugs also act as antagonists at other receptors, such as the cholinergic muscarinic, H_1 histamine, α_2-adrenergic and 5-HT_2 receptors (Fig. 15.8). This pharmacological lack of selectivity of action was well reflected from the beginning in the commercial name of chlorpromazine: 'Largactil!' The inevitable consequence of this lack of selectivity is the occurrence of unwanted effects, which decrease compliance.

Table 15.3 gives an overview of the main unwanted effects of antipsychotic drugs, which affect a range of systems and physiological processes. The intensity of

Table 15.3 Unwanted effects of antipsychotic drugs

Psychomotor performance

The effects on cognition and psychomotor performance are complex and depend on the subject and the task assessed. Phenothiazines, in particular, tend to induce drowsiness and fatigue. The sedation is related to the anti-histaminergic action and the α_1-adrenergic receptor blockade.

Extrapyramidal effects

Parkinsonian symptoms are the most common: tremor, rigidity, bradykinesia.

Akathisia (continuous motor restlessness) can be misinterpreted as incomplete control of psychotic symptoms.

Acute dyskinesia and dystonia: tonic contractions of muscles in the face, tongue and neck, and also of the truncal muscles, which may lead to abnormal postures.

Seizures

Many neuroleptics can lower the seizure threshold and should be used with caution in untreated epileptic patients.

Endocrine effects

The disrupted dopamine control over pituitary function leads to increased prolactin release and swelling of the breasts (gynaecomastia) and lactation (galactorrhoea).

Cutaneous effects

Chronic exposure to neuroleptics may lead to pigmentation and also photosensitivity.

Hepatotoxicity

Chlopromazine, in particular, may induce obstructive jaundice.

Haematological effects

Agranulocytosis occurs rarely with typical neuroleptics but its incidence is much higher with clozapine. It is the most serious haematological abnormality induced by antipsychotics. It presents with fever, fatigue and prostration, and ulceration of the mouth, throat, nose, rectum or vagina. The mortality rate can reach approximately 30%.

Cardiovascular effects

Neuroleptics can induce significant postural hypotension with tachycardia. This is largely due to α-adrenergic receptor blockade.

Metabolic effects

Weight gain induced by neuroleptics may be related to a stimulation of appetite and/or a reduction in basal metabolic rate. Excessive weight is associated with additional health risks such as hypertension and diabetes mellitus.

Anticholinergic effects

These effects are due to blockade of muscarinic receptors. They include decreased salivary flow, blurred vision and impaired accommodation, constipation and urinary hesitancy or retention.

Sexual dysfunction

Antipsychotics can significantly affect sexual function. They can lead to loss of sexual drive, erectile and ejaculatory dysfunction, priapism and menstrual irregularities.

these unwanted effects can be very significant. For example, obesity may occur in about one-third of patients who receive fluphenazine or flupenthixol. This prevalence is four times higher than that in the general population. The host of anticholinergic effects induced by antipsychotic drugs (constipation, difficulty in urinating, dry mouth and blurred vision) is of particular concern in elderly patients. Furthermore, the postural hypotension induced by neuroleptics, and also the interference with temperature control (hypothermia or hyperthermia), are particularly troublesome in the elderly. The choice of neuroleptic is, even today, often determined by its unwanted effects and their acceptability. For example, the sedation induced by chlorpromazine may be very useful in an agitated schizophrenic, whereas its antimuscarinic effects may make it quite unacceptable in an elderly patient with micturition problems. Haloperidol is less hypotensive than chlorpromazine but has significant extrapyramidal motor effects.

Neuroleptic malignant syndrome is an idiosyncratic response to antipsychotic medication and consists of hyperthermia (sometimes with profuse sweating), tachycardia, muscular rigidity and fluctuating levels of consciousness. It is a rare but potentially lethal complication of antipsychotic drugs. The mortality rate can reach 20%–30%. Dantrolene and dopaminergic agonists such as bromocriptine, and cooling and rehydration, have been used to treat this syndrome, which may last for several days. No particular class of antipsychotic is more or less likely to induce this syndrome. Patients may be at greater risk at the beginning of treatment or after a dose increase. Atypical neuroleptics such as clozapine may be used to manage patients who have already had an episode of neuroleptic malignant syndrome.

Some complications of treatment with antipsychotic drugs emerge after a specific duration of exposure to these drugs. One such example is tardive dyskinesia. This includes orofacial, trunk and limb dyskinesias. The orofacial movements include protrusion of the tongue, lip-smacking, pursing and sucking movements, puffing of the cheeks and chewing. The involuntary limb movements are purposeless and jerky. The condition is both socially and physically disabling. Spontaneous fluctuations in the severity of movements may occur from day to day or even within hours or minutes. Most often, tardive dyskinesia does not disappear upon reduction of the dose or withdrawal of the drugs. However, the dyskinesia may slightly improve or stabilize over a number of years. Newer drugs, the 'atypical neuroleptics' such as clozapine, olanzapine, risperidone and quetiapine, have fewer unwanted effects. In particular, the incidence of extrapyramidal effects is much lower than with the 'typical' neuroleptics and they have higher efficacy than the old neuroleptics in treating negative symptoms. Clozapine shows unique efficacy in treatment-resistant patients. Unfortunately, it is associated with an increased risk of leukopenia and agranulocytosis (1%–2%). Its use requires regular blood cell counts. A common characteristic of second generation, atypical antipsychotics such as risperidone, is their high affinity for $5-HT_2$ receptors. Therefore the new antipsychotics are better described as dopamine and 5-HT receptor antagonists. The lower potential for induction of extrapyramidal symptoms could be due to complex interactions between 5-HT and dopaminergic systems in the brain, and also to a reduced degree of occupancy of dopaminergic receptors. In the case history it is not unlikely that Jane was initially prescribed an old type of antipsychotic drug, so the choice of a better, atypical compound may improve her compliance.

Some antipsychotic drugs (e.g. haloperidol and flupenthixol) can be given as a depot slow-release preparation, which is useful when compliance with treatment is unpredictable. This approach makes chronic schizophrenia more manageable in the community, provided that adequate structures and support are available. The drugs are administered as fatty acid esters (e.g. haloperidol decanoate, fluphenazine decanoate and pipotiazine palmitate) by deep intramuscular injection at intervals of 1–4 weeks. It is less easy to control the dose administered, especially when a reduction of the dose is required. It may take several weeks to decrease plasma concentration or to control the severity of unwanted effects.

A third generation of antipsychotic drugs is represented by drugs with more complex profiles such as aripiprazole (a partial agonist at D_2 receptors), brexpiprazole (an agonist at D_2 receptors and a partial agonist at the $5-HT_{1A}$ receptor) and cariprazine (a partial agonist at D_3/D_2 receptors).

Apart from medical treatment, schizophrenic patients may benefit from cognitive therapy and occupational therapy. Cognitive improvement, through social skill development and cognitive behavioural treatments, hold much promise but more research is required to maximize the potential of these approaches, which are complementary to medical treatment. It is also important to note that families and carers of schizophrenic patients require long-term support because of the distressing and unpredictable nature of this chronic disease.

Comments on the management of schizophrenia and the long-term prognosis

Schizophrenia is a complex mental illness that still poses a therapeutic challenge in a significant number of patients. It must be remembered that schizophrenia is not a homogeneous disease, and recent research has reinforced this concept of extreme heterogeneity. There are numerous phenotypes and each poses its own problems during long-term management. In many patients schizophrenia presents a chronic course, which is particularly disabling, especially because of the social isolation associated with negative symptoms. The evolution of schizophrenia is sometimes complicated by the use of addictive substances. Jane's use (and abuse?) of alcohol illustrates this tendency. The prognosis for each patient depends on the balance between positive and negative symptoms, the cognitive impairment, their response to treatment, and also the lack of complicating factors such as the development of drug addiction or other circumstances involving high levels of stress. In some patients the response to treatment (especially the positive symptoms) is good and they may return to an almost normal level of functioning – at least between episodes of relapse. The risk of suicide will not disappear during the course of the disease and may be exacerbated by the presence of depression. Of patients with schizophrenia, 10%–15% commit suicide. The long-term outcome in schizophrenia is variable. Schizophrenia consists in many cases of a sequence of exacerbations followed by improvements, throughout lifetime. About one-third of patients have one or a limited number of acute episodes, with full or partial remission between episodes. Another one-third of patients develop a chronic condition that is stable and controlled to a variable extent by antipsychotic medication. Patients who relapse after cessation of treatment require constant, long-term medication on a type and dose of antipsychotic drug that they tolerate reasonably well (in terms of unwanted effects). The value of maintenance antipsychotic drug treatment in schizophrenia is supported by numerous studies. Research suggests that these drugs may have effects that are far more complex than the blockade of neurotransmitter receptors. Their chronic use may alter the expression of genes critically involved in the generation and maintenance of synapses. Therefore, if a deficit in synapse stabilization that is partly developmental is at the core of the pathophysiology of schizophrenia, some antipsychotic drugs may affect, at least partly, the primary cause of the disease. Future studies will be required to consolidate these observations. Finally, the remaining one-third of patients has a progressive debilitating psychosis with increasing impairment and no return to baseline. It is important to bear in mind that this core group of chronic schizophrenic patients have only very moderate improvement, even if treated with newer drugs, and remain the most challenging patients of all.

Other psychoses and neurodevelopmental disorders

Psychotic states can be induced by exposure to a variety of psychoactive compounds, some of which have been mentioned already. The differential diagnosis of schizophrenia must take into account psychoses that may occur in the context of disorders such as temporal lobe epilepsy, multiple sclerosis, alcoholism or delirium and dementia in elderly people.

Neurodevelopmental disorders are a complex family of disorders. Examples of such disorders are autism and Asperger's syndrome.

Autism, also known as autism-spectrum disorder (ASD), was defined as a syndrome and introduced to the medical world by the Austrian child psychiatrist Leo Kanner in 1943. The term reflects withdrawal from others and marked self-centredness. Kanner described a distinctive syndrome in children, characterized by a solitary nature and an inability to relate to people and to situations. Other features included the performance of repetitive activities, mutism or abnormal language. The abnormalities of speech in autistic children include echolalia (repeating, like a parrot, words or sentences without any understanding) and avoidance or confusion of personal pronouns (e.g. 'he' for 'she', or 'you' for 'we'). Autistic children can have variable degrees of intellectual disability. It is a common, highly heritable (estimates ranging from 40% to 90%) and heterogeneous disorder. More than 100 genes and genomic regions have been associated with autism, and genetic variations include point mutations and copy number variations. Environmental risk factors associated with autism include preterm birth or neonatal hypoxia, gestational diabetes mellitus, maternal obesity and paternal age >50 years. Most recently, altered zinc levels in developing neurons have been linked to developmental abnormalities in synapse maturation. During synaptic neurotransmission zinc enters the target neuron to bind to the Shank2 and Shank3 proteins, to accelerate the maturation of ionotropic glutamate AMPA receptors. Zinc shapes the properties of developing synapses via Shank proteins. A lack of zinc during early development might contribute to autism through impaired synaptic maturation and neuronal circuit formation. It has been suggested that the fundamental failure in autism is the lack of development of a 'theory of the mind': autistic children have no concept of what other people think or feel, and this leads to a lack of empathy and no, or very little, attachment to other people. Humans, animals and objects seem to be treated alike, more like 'tools' to satisfy the child's needs. Such children sometimes display unusual features of memory or skill. The worldwide prevalence of autism is approximately 1% and it is more common in males. The typical patterns of autistic behaviour usually emerge after up to 18–20 months of apparently normal development. The diagnosis is based on a developmental history provided by parents and the observation of how the child interacts with parents and other individuals. The aetiology of autism is unknown and there is evidence for genetic factors. It is likely that autism is a disorder with a major neurodevelopmental component: a disruption in brain formation *in utero* emerges in childhood when the brain is growing rapidly and its connectivity evolves towards maturation. Although autism and schizophrenia are clearly different disorders, there are strong resemblances in terms of the existence of motor, speech and behavioural abnormalities. Neuropathological abnormalities have been described in the hippocampus, mamillary nuclei, amygdala and anterior cingulate cortex. Imaging studies have revealed smaller volumes of the putamen, pallidum, nucleus accumbens and amygdala, increased thickness in the frontal cortex and decreased thickness in the temporal cortex. Cerebellar abnormalities (such as loss of Purkinje cells) are a constant feature. The degree of cerebellar grey matter reduction is correlated with autism symptom severity. There is evidence of disruption in white mater integrity and also whole-brain altered connectivity, with evidence of both hypo- and hyperconnectivity in various cerebral circuits. Some of these changes are reported before the emergence of behavioural symptoms. Autism is also associated with epilepsy. Various types of epilepsy (e.g. absences, generalized tonic–clonic seizures and complex partial seizures) affect 35%–45% of autistic children and adults. No definitive neurochemical abnormality has yet been defined as pathognomonic for autism, but there is converging evidence in support of dopaminergic dysfunction.

Various drug treatments have been tried in autism and have mostly symptomatic value. For example, antipsychotic drugs such as risperidone and aripiprazole can be used for irritability, agitation and aggression. Other medications can target frequent comorbidities, such as anxiety or epilepsy. Dietary interventions (e.g. supplementation with vitamin B6 or magnesium) have been attempted and can provide some improvement. More recently, there has been interest in the therapeutic exploration of the neurohormonal oxytocin and vasopressin systems, which can act as modulators of social behaviour. Therapy mostly focuses on behavioural interventions, delivered by parents or therapists, and the development of structured education programmes. The various therapies are focused on the aim of promoting independence in adulthood and improved social functioning. Only a very small proportion of children with autism develop into normal adults. The majority of autistic children will show psychiatric impairments throughout life. In other cases there is some improvement and it is possible for the patient to lead an almost independent adult life.

Asperger's syndrome has broadly similar features to autism but is milder and does not become apparent until after 3 years of age. DSM-5 has included this disorder in the ASD category but this classification remains controversial. It is much more common in boys than girls. Language is affected (e.g. atypical syntax, idiosyncratic vocabulary) and features stereotyped repetition of phrases. Unlike with autism, intelligence may be normal or above average. Patients affected by the syndrome may display exceptional abilities in very narrowly defined fields. However, they fail to develop peer relationships, show little reciprocity and have very poor social communication skills. Overall, social skills are very limited. Outcome is variable between patients. A proportion of patients with Asperger's syndrome may develop mild schizophrenia. They may display obsessive behaviour and forms of bizarre violence.

There is still much debate about whether autism and Asperger's syndrome should be viewed as part of a continuum or as two distinct conditions. Irrespective of the best classification, it is likely that these represent two related conditions characterized by major disruption of social contact and abnormalities of affect.

Self-assessment case study

Richard was a rather quiet baby who gave no particular concern to his parents in his first 16 months of life. They had noticed that Richard's peers at the nursery were much livelier than their son and seemed to take more pleasure in interacting with adults, but they assumed that their child was just shy and that he would develop later. However, he gradually showed clear lack of progress in the acquisition of even rudimentary language. He also developed a strong aversion to strangers and a tendency to violent temper tantrums if his daily routines were upset. Otherwise, he was a healthy, nice-looking child and physically rather energetic.

When Richard was 3 years old, he was diagnosed with autism. His parents have already consulted several specialists before they come to see you. They ask you to give them your opinion and prognosis and indicate the best treatment available.

After studying this chapter you should be able to answer the following questions:

1) Is the evolution of the condition described in this child compatible with a diagnosis of autism?

Yes, autism can emerge after 1–2 years of apparently normal development, so this is a typical presentation.

2) What is the neurobiological substrate of this disease?

The cause of autism remains unknown. Structural abnormalities have been described in a variety of structures including the amygdala, cerebellum and cerebral cortex. There is evidence of widespread alterations in cerebral connectivity.

3) What are the treatment choices available?

There is no optimum pharmacological management. Symptomatic treatment may be focused on alleviating comorbidities such as anxiety or seizures. Therapy focuses mostly on behavioural approaches and structured education programmes aimed at improving the socialisation of the autistic individual.

DEPRESSION AND ANXIETY

16

Chapter summary

1. Depressive disorders are common mental disorders that are characterized by depressed mood, loss of interest or pleasure, feelings of guilt or low self-worth, disturbed sleep and appetite, low energy and poor concentration. Bipolar disorders are characterized by altered episodes of mania and depressed mood. These disorders can become lifelong disabling conditions and are associated with an increased risk of suicide.

2. As a function of their severity, depressive disorders can be managed with various pharmacological and non-pharmacological treatments, such as psychotherapy, which could also be combined. Treatment can lead to remission, but relapses may occur. Some patients may have treatment resistance, which could be managed with electroconvulsive therapy.

3. Antidepressant drugs belong to a variety of pharmacological classes, and most of them modulate serotonergic and noradrenergic (monoaminergic) transmission, which may become dysfunctional in depression. There is a time lag between initiation of treatment and onset of clinical efficacy, and treatment may need to be maintained after apparent remission.

4. Anxiety disorders are the most common mental health disorders and include phobic and non-phobic disorders. Relapses may occur after remission. Non-pharmacological treatments include a variety of psychotherapy approaches, such as cognitive behavioural therapy and interpersonal therapy, and are recommended as the first line of treatment. Pharmacological management includes selective serotonin reuptake inhibitors and serotonin and noradrenaline reuptake inhibitors. Anxiolytic drugs such as benzodiazepines, which modulate GABA transmission, could also be prescribed, but for a limited time, because of the higher risk of dependence.

5. Sleep is a vital physiological process that occurs in cycles and is controlled by several neurotransmitter systems, including monoamines and peptides. Insomnia is a disruption of normal sleep patterns, which can be associated with environmental factors, stress and various medical conditions. Sleep problems are common in anxiety disorders, and it is well established that lack of sleep can worsen anxiety and increase the risk of developing an anxiety disorder. Hypnotics such as the 'z-drugs', which are short-acting non-benzodiazepine compounds, can be used in insomnia management.

Introduction

Depression and anxiety represent, in a broad sense, transient states experienced by almost all individuals at some point in their life. In contrast, neurological dysfunction caused by acute trauma or neuronal degeneration is reflected in specific impairment, where no confusion exists between the diseased state and the normal state. In some individuals, depression and anxiety reach an intensity and duration that totally disrupt normal life activities. The classification of these disorders and their diagnostic criteria are regularly reviewed. The efficacy of most drugs used for these conditions is moderate. It may still be believed, erroneously by some, that depression and anxiety are not major medical problems but rather transient states that resolve, sooner or later, with full remission. However, as the case history in Box 16.1 indicates, this is not so, and the disease burden they represent for the patient, the family and society is significantly underestimated.

Classification of mood disorders

'If sorrow persists, then it is melancholia.'

Hippocrates (460–370 BC)

Descriptions of depressed states date back to Sumerian and Egyptian documents. Later, Hippocrates, Galen and other medical authors of antiquity continued to describe depression and its possible causes and treatments. The term 'melancholia' was used until the late 19th century, when Kraepelin introduced the term 'manic depression', to differentiate this severely disturbed mental state from schizophrenia.

Depression is a general term that defines a family of diseases. Table 16.1 gives the present classification of these disorders according to the American Psychiatric Association Diagnostic and Statistical Manual of Mental Disorders 5 (DSM-5). Most of this chapter is dedicated to the discussion of major depression disorder and bipolar disorder. The classification of depressive states is complex and evolving, because the classification relies on clinical phenotypes and not stringent aetiologically linked criteria. Furthermore, currently, there are no clear biological markers or objective diagnostic tests that would allow for a reliable biology-based classification.

Clinical features of mood disorders

Depression is characterized by a series of changes that gradually cause significant impairment of the activity of the individual concerned. Table 16.2 shows typical core symptoms of depression. These are psychological and somatic.

Psychological symptoms include feelings of misery, guilt, hopelessness and general pessimism. Some patients may become irritable or aggressive. Enjoyment of various activities is lost (i.e. there is anhedonia, which means 'loss of pleasure'), and energy is low. Interest, concentration and the ability to function efficiently and make decisions are significantly impaired. Some patients show very severe mental and physical slow-down (retarded depression). Other patients present with a paradoxical reaction characterized by increased activity and restlessness (agitated depression). Delusions and hallucinations may develop in some patients (depression with psychotic features). These have the same negative and destructive tone as the other symptoms.

Somatic symptoms are very common and often dominate the presentation of the case when patients consult a doctor. Sleep is almost always disturbed, with early-morning waking or difficulty in falling asleep. Most patients lose weight, but in some patients, the opposite is seen: they eat more and gain weight. Patients may also suffer from nausea, constipation and headaches. Often, patients find it easier to talk about the somatic symptoms and feel rather embarrassed about revealing their psychological problems.

Depression can be rated using a variety of scales. Examples of such include the Hamilton Depression Scale, the Beck Depression Inventory and the Zung Self-Rating Depression Scale. For example, in the Hamilton

Box 16.1 Case history

William is a scientist who shares his time between work at the university and writing about science. Over several weeks, around his 45th birthday, he feels increasing fatigue and has trouble sleeping. He has started going to bed early because he feels tired all the time and because he tends to be awake at dawn, unable to go to sleep again. His wife notices that he no longer enjoys his hobbies. He is often irritable and impatient with his children. Things take a turn for the worse when William cancels a series of lectures and meetings because he feels that he can no longer cope with his work. His insomnia is getting worse, and he is losing weight. He consults his doctor, who diagnoses depression and prescribes venlafaxine. William is sceptical about treatment and is reluctant to take the medication. He explains to his doctor that he knows that antidepressant drugs can make you feel unwell. He remembers from his childhood that his mother had been suffering from periods of depression and had to take drugs. She had never fully recovered, up to her accidental death a few years ago. William asks his doctor whether other approaches could be used instead of drugs. He is worried about 'getting addicted' to drugs and not being able to have a normal life without them. William's doctor explains that cognitive behavioural therapy is another option, and that it may be possible to consider using this therapy.

William starts taking the medication and, although he sees no major change in the first 2 weeks, after 3 months of treatment, he feels well and fully resumes his activities. His mood is much improved, and while on a holiday, he decides to stop taking the medication. Unfortunately, less than 2 years after this first episode, William feels unwell again, and he needs to stop work and start a new course of venlafaxine. The drug is less efficacious this time, and the doctor is very concerned about the feelings of guilt that William now experiences and his heightened level of anxiety. He arranges with William to start regular psychotherapy sessions with a therapist, in parallel with the medication.

This case gives rise to the following questions:

1. What triggers the depressive symptoms?
2. What is the cause of depression?
3. How can drugs help, and what other non-pharmacological alternatives are there?
4. Why do patients relapse?
5. What is the long-term management of depression?

Table 16.1 DSM-5 classification of depressive disorders

Disruptive mood dysregulation disorder

Major depressive disorder

Persistent depressive disorder (dysthymia)

Premenstrual dysphoric disorder

Substance/medication-induced depressive disorder

Depressive disorder due to another medical condition

Other specified depressive disorder

Unspecified depressive disorder

Table 16.2 Symptoms of depression

Psychomotor retardation or psychomotor agitation

Fatigue or loss of energy

Diminished ability to concentrate

Diminished interest in social activity

Depressed mood

Feelings of guilt and worthlessness

Suicidal ideation

Insomnia

Weight loss and decreased appetite

Lack of interest and anhedonia

include three entities: bipolar disorder I, bipolar disorder II and cyclothymia. These conditions are characterised by alternating episodes of depression and mania. The frequency of the episodes and their severity may increase as the disease evolves. The manic attack is characterized by symptoms that are the opposite of those seen in depression. Patients are overactive, disinhibited, unfocused and extravagant. They can become completely irresponsible and display unlimited confidence in themselves. They may engage in unrealistic business ventures, reckless driving, incredible buying sprees and numerous sexual liaisons. They appear to need little food or sleep. Thought and speech are intense, with a dominating flight of ideas. Thought content can be grandiose, and delusions and hallucinations with a paranoid content may develop. In extreme cases, hospital admission is required (under the provisions of national mental health acts such as the UK Mental Health Act 2007) because of the patient's loss of insight into their illness.

Epidemiology of depressive and bipolar disorders and their natural evolution

According to the World Health Organisation, depressive disorders are among the top 20 medical conditions associated with a significant burden of disease. Prevalence and incidence are in similar ranges worldwide. Women

Depression Scale, 21 questions cover the various symptoms and their intensity. The total score reflects the severity of depression (Box 16.2). Depression is diagnosed according to the DSM-5 classification by the presence of at least five out of nine key symptoms, present for at least 2 weeks and of sufficient severity to cause significant distress or impairment in social, occupational or other areas of functioning.

Bipolar disorders (commonly called manic-depression syndromes) are classified separately in DSM-5, and they

Box 16.2 The Hamilton Rating Scale for Depression (to be administered by a healthcare professional)

Patient's name

_____

Date of assessment

_____

To rate the severity of depression in patients who are already diagnosed as depressed, administer this questionnaire. The higher the score, the more severe the depression.

For each item, write the correct number on the line next to the item (only one response per item).

1. **DEPRESSED MOOD** (Sadness, hopeless, helpless, worthless)
    0 = Absent
    1 = These feeling states are indicated only on questioning
    2 = These feeling states are spontaneously reported verbally
    3 = Communicates feeling states non-verbally—i.e. through facial expression, posture, voice and tendency to weep
    4 = Patient reports these feeling states VIRTUALLY ONLY in his spontaneous verbal and non-verbal communication

2. **FEELINGS OF GUILT**
    0 = Absent
    1 = Self-reproach, feels he has let people down
    2 = Ideas of guilt or rumination over past errors or sinful deeds
    3 = Present illness is a punishment. Delusions of guilt
    4 = Hears accusatory or denunciatory voices and/or experiences threatening visual hallucinations

3. **SUICIDE**
    0 = Absent
    1 = Feels life is not worth living
    2 = Wishes he were dead or any thoughts of possible death to self
    3 = Suicidal ideas or gesture
    4 = Attempts at suicide (any serious attempt rates 4)

4. **INSOMNIA EARLY**
    0 = No difficulty falling asleep
    1 = Complains of occasional difficulty falling asleep—i.e. more than ½ hour
    2 = Complains of nightly difficulty falling asleep

5. **INSOMNIA MIDDLE**
    0 = No difficulty
    1 = Patient complains of being restless and disturbed during the night
    2 = Waking during the night—any getting out of bed rates 2 (except for purposes of voiding)

6. **INSOMNIA LATE**
    0 = No difficulty
    1 = Waking in early hours of the morning but goes back to sleep
    2 = Unable to fall asleep again if he gets out of bed

7. **WORK AND ACTIVITIES**
    0 = No difficulty
    1 = Thoughts and feelings of incapacity, fatigue or weakness related to activities, work or hobbies
    2 = Loss of interest in activity, hobbies or work—either directly reported by patient, or indirect in listlessness, indecision and vacillation (feels he has to push self to work or activities)
    3 = Decrease in actual time spent in activities or decrease in productivity
    4 = Stopped working because of present illness

8. **RETARDATION (PSYCHOMOTOR)** (Slowness of thought and speech; impaired ability to concentrate; decreased motor activity)
    0 = Normal speech and thought
    1 = Slight retardation at interview
    2 = Obvious retardation at interview
    3 = Interview difficult
    4 = Complete stupor

9. **AGITATION**
    0 = None
    1 = Fidgetiness
    2 = Playing with hands, hair, etc.
    3 = Moving about, can't sit still
    4 = Hand wringing, nail biting, hair-pulling, biting of lips

10. **ANXIETY (PSYCHOLOGICAL)**
    0 = No difficulty
    1 = Subjective tension and irritability
    2 = Worrying about minor matters
    3 = Apprehensive attitude apparent in face or speech
    4 = Fears expressed without questioning

11. **ANXIETY (SOMATIC)** Physiological concomitants of anxiety (i.e. effects of autonomic overactivity, 'butterflies', indigestion, stomach cramps, belching, diarrhoea, palpitations, hyperventilation, paraesthesia, sweating, flushing, tremor, headache, urinary frequency). Avoid asking about possible medication side effects (i.e. dry mouth, constipation)
    0 = Absent
    1 = Mild
    2 = Moderate
    3 = Severe
    4 = Incapacitating

12. **SOMATIC SYMPTOMS (GASTROINTESTINAL)**
    0 = None
    1 = Loss of appetite, but eating without encouragement from others. Food intake about normal
    2 = Difficulty eating without urging from others. Marked reduction of appetite and food intake

13. **SOMATIC SYMPTOMS GENERAL**
    0 = None
    1 = Heaviness in limbs, back or head. Backaches, headache, muscle aches. Loss of energy and fatigability
    2 = Any clear-cut symptom rates 2

14. **GENITAL SYMPTOMS** (Symptoms such as loss of libido, impaired sexual performance, menstrual disturbances)
    0 = Absent
    1 = Mild
    2 = Severe

15. **HYPOCHONDRIASIS**
    0 = Not present
    1 = Self-absorption (bodily)
    2 = Preoccupation with health
    3 = Frequent complaints, requests for help, etc.
    4 = Hypochondriacal delusions

Continued

Box 16.2 The Hamilton Rating Scale for Depression (to be administered by a healthcare professional)—cont'd

16. **LOSS OF WEIGHT**
_____
A. When rating by history:
0 = No weight loss
1 = Probably weight loss associated with present illness
2 = Definite (according to patient) weight loss
3 = Not assessed

17. **INSIGHT**
_____
0 = Acknowledges being depressed and ill
1 = Acknowledges illness but attributes cause to bad food, climate, overwork, virus, need for rest, etc.
2 = Denies being ill at all

18. **DIURNAL VARIATION**
_____
A. Note whether symptoms are worse in morning or evening. If NO diurnal variation, mark none
0 = No variation
1 = Worse in A.M.
2 = Worse in P.M.
B. When present, mark the severity of the variation. Mark 'None' if NO variation
0 = None
1 = Mild
2 = Severe

19. **DEPERSONALIZATION AND DEREALIZATION** (Such as feelings of unreality and nihilistic ideas)
_____
0 = Absent
1 = Mild
2 = Moderate
3 = Severe
4 = Incapacitating

20. **PARANOID SYMPTOMS**
_____
0 = None
1 = Suspicious
2 = Ideas of reference
3 = Delusions of reference and persecution

21. **OBSESSIONAL AND COMPULSIVE SYMPTOMS**
_____
0 = Absent
1 = Mild
2 = Severe

Total Score_____

are almost twice as likely to be diagnosed with depression as men. For example, estimates of the prevalence rates of a major depressive episode in 2017 in the USA were 8.7% in females compared with 5.3% in males. A cross-sectional survey of 11 countries, published in 2011, found that the lifetime prevalence of bipolar spectrum disorders was 2.4%.

Depression can occur at any age; it affects children, adolescents, adults and the elderly. For many patients, major depression is a lifelong disorder that consists of episodes of relapse separated by remission intervals. Bipolar disorders are also highly recurrent, and full recovery is rare. The mean age of onset of depression has decreased gradually from the 40- to 50-year age range to the 25- to 35-year

age range. Stress is considered one of the main risk factors for the development of depression. Evidence suggests that negative psychosocial factors (e.g. bereavement or loss of a job or social status) may trigger the first depression episode. However, this is more likely to happen in susceptible individuals (i.e. against a predisposing genetic background). Depression is associated with an increased mortality rate compared with the rest of the population, due to an increased suicide rate. Accumulating evidence indicates that major depressive disorder may confer a higher risk for several non-communicable diseases such as diabetes, obesity, coronary heart disease, stroke and dementia. The converse is also true, in that these chronic health conditions appear to increase the likelihood of developing depression.

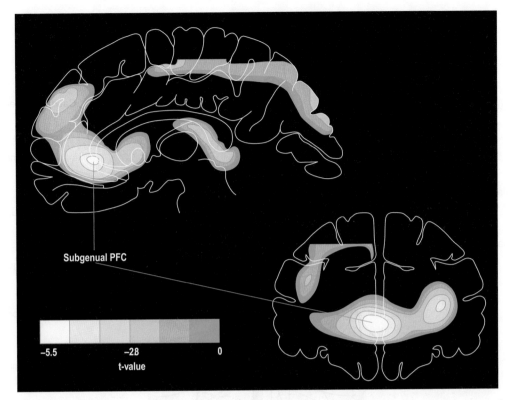

Subgenual PFC

-5.5   -28   0
t-value

Fig. 16.1 Hypometabolism in the subgenual prefrontal cortex (PFC) in major depression. Positron emission tomography image showing an area of decreased glucose metabolism and cerebral blood flow in the subgenual prefrontal cortex in unmedicated depressed patients. (From Drevets et al. Subgenual prefrontal cortex abnormalities in mood disorders (1997) *Nature*. 386:824-827.)

Depression can occur in association with other medical conditions, for example, Parkinson's disease, head trauma, cancer, diabetes, or endocrine dysfunctions such as hypercortisolaemia or hypothyroidism.

Genetics of mood disorders

Twin and adoption studies support a genetic link in depression, and it is well established that first-degree relatives (parents, siblings and children) of individuals with major depressive disorder are at high risk of developing the disease. Approximately 40%–50% of the risk of developing depression is genetic. Twin studies show that genetic factors may have a far greater aetiological role in bipolar depression than in non-bipolar major depression.

The lifetime risk of developing the illness in relatives of patients with major depression is as follows:

- first-degree relatives: 10%–20%
- dizygotic twins: 15%–30%.
- monozygotic twins: 50%–70%.

There is also evidence for a shared genetic susceptibility between major depression and bipolar disorder.

Genome-wide association studies (GWAS) have identified more than 80 risk loci for major depression. The analysis of the genetic risk data shows an association with several markers of monoamine transmission, for example, the 5-hydroxytryptamine (5-HT) transporter, 5-HT receptor genes and dopamine receptor genes, genes encoding inactivating enzymes such as monoamine oxidase A and also genes associated with GABAergic and glutamatergic transmission.

Neurobiology of depression

Structures involved

The anatomical and physiological basis of depression remains incompletely understood. However, imaging and postmortem analyses are now providing information about the structures and circuits involved, and clearly indicate that depression is associated with functional and structural changes. Positron emission tomography (PET) studies of cerebral blood flow and glucose metabolism showed abnormal activity in structures involved in emotional behaviour. They support the involvement of limbic, cortical and subcortical structures such as the cingulate cortex, hippocampus, thalamus, amygdala and the hypothalamus. In particular, studies in unmedicated patients with depression show changes in glucose metabolism in the dorso-anterolateral and dorsomedial prefrontal cortices and in the anterior cingulate cortex ventral to the genu corpus callosum (Fig. 16.1). In contrast, metabolic activity is increased

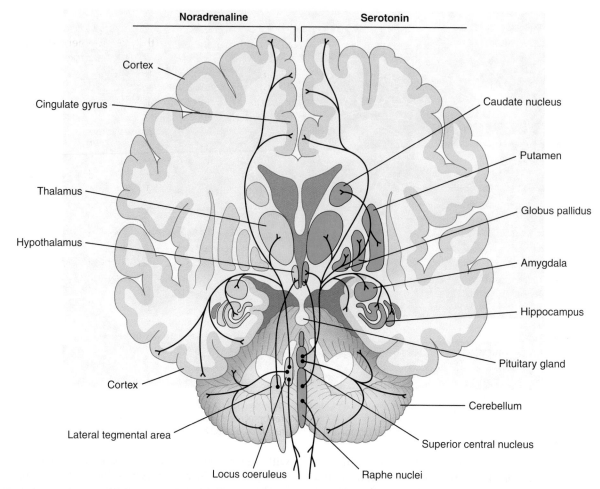

Noradrenaline   **Serotonin**

Cortex

Cingulate gyrus

Thalamus

Hypothalamus

Cortex

Lateral tegmental area

Locus coeruleus

Caudate nucleus

Putamen

Globus pallidus

Amygdala

Hippocampus

Pituitary gland

Cerebellum

Superior central nucleus

Raphe nuclei

Fig. 16.2 The ascending noradrenergic and serotonergic pathways. The diagram shows the origin of noradrenergic and serotonergic projections and the various structures innervated by these monoamines.

in the left and right orbital/ventrolateral prefrontal cortex, the posterior cingulate cortex, the anterior insula and the left amygdala. Antidepressant treatment reverses some of these changes, for example, the increased metabolism in the amygdala. The amygdala is involved in autonomic, emotional and neuroendocrine responses to stress; there is a positive correlation between its activation and the severity of depression ratings. Furthermore, the degree of activation of the amygdala correlates with the levels of circulating cortisol under stress conditions. Brain connectivity studies indicate that depression may be associated with alterations in the 'default mode network' (a circuit which includes the posterior cingulate cortex, the precuneus, the medial prefrontal cortex, the ventral anterior cingulate cortex and the lateral and inferior parietal cortex), which is involved in self-reflective thinking and social cognition. These circuit alterations may be linked to a serotonin deficit.

Postmortem studies show reductions in the density and size of neurons and glia in the prefrontal cortex of individuals with major depression. Interestingly, these structural changes occur in areas where there was previously increased glucose metabolism. The latter is closely correlated with activation of glutamatergic transmission.

Therefore, it is conceivable that chronic hyperactive glutamatergic transmission leads to alterations, in particular atrophy, of the neuropil. The amygdala and prefrontal cortex are linked by excitatory amino acid projections, and it has been shown that surgical lesions that interrupt these projections can relieve depressive symptoms that are resistant to pharmacological treatment. Finally, another correlate of depression is decreased hippocampal neurogenesis, that is the process that continues to generate new neurons into adulthood.

Neurochemistry

Since the introduction of the first antidepressant drugs in the mid-20th century, the theory on the causality of depression that has dominated the field has been 'the monoamine theory of depression'. This postulates that in the brain of depressed individuals there is hypoactivity of monoaminergic systems. The emphasis has been on the noradrenergic and serotonergic ascending systems, which extensively innervate the forebrain (Fig. 16.2). Noradrenergic cells located in the locus coeruleus and serotonergic cells located in the raphe nuclei provide

Table 16.3 Abnormalities of the hypothalamus–pituitary–adrenal axis in depression

Increased plasma cortisol

Increased urinary free cortisol

Abnormal cortisol circadian rhythm

Increased CRF in the cerebrospinal fluid

Decreased response of ACTH after CRF stimulation

Decreased glucocorticoid receptor sensitivity

Increased circulating ACTH

Increased adrenal gland size

ACTH, Adrenocorticotrophin; CRF, corticotrophin-releasing factor.

extensive innervation of subcortical structures and cortical areas, which are part of a complex network whose abnormal connectivity underlies the depressed state. However, the monoamine deficiency theory is now considered a rather simplistic model of the pathophysiology of depression. Patients with major depression do not consistently demonstrate alterations in monoamine function, although reductions in the activity of the 5-HT and noradrenaline systems can be seen in some patients. The role of monoamines in the pathophysiology of depression cannot be contested, as drugs that are effective in the clinic act on monoaminergic systems.

The cholinergic system may also be involved in depression; cholinomimetics have depressogenic and anti-manic effects, and in depression, there is enhanced sensitivity to cholinergic stimulation. Reduced cerebrospinal fluid (CSF) and plasma gamma-aminobutyric acid (GABA) levels have also been reported in depression, and there is evidence that antidepressant treatment may enhance GABA signalling. Finally, the existence of a glutamatergic link is strongly supported by various observations: antidepressants reduce the expression of N-methyl-D-aspartate (NMDA) receptor subunits, and ketamine (an NMDA receptor antagonist) has antidepressant effects. Furthermore, it is known that stress increases glutamate release, whereas antidepressant drugs may decrease the release and/or increase the reuptake of the excitatory amino acid.

Many depressed patients also present with neuroendocrine changes, in particular, a series of abnormalities in the hypothalamus–pituitary–adrenal (HPA) axis (Table 16.3). Notable among these are the increased level of plasma cortisol and the absence of response to dexamethasone challenge. In the dexamethasone suppression test, depressed patients cannot suppress cortisol secretion when the synthetic glucocorticoid dexamethasone is administered. The secretion of cortisol is under the control of the hypothalamus and the hormone corticotrophin-releasing factor (CRF), also known as corticotrophin-releasing hormone (CRH). Hypersecretion of CRF has been reported in some depressed patients. CRF binds to two receptor subtypes: CRF_1 and CRF_2.

CRF_1 receptor antagonists have shown antidepressant potential. The excess release of cortisol is being considered as a risk factor for the development of hippocampal atrophy (which has been described after intense stress). Thus there is a possible link between stress as a triggering factor in depression, HPA abnormalities in patients with depression and the brain structural changes reported in depression.

A possible link between depression and neuroinflammation has also gained attention. PET studies indicate microglial activation in patients with depression. This activation is correlated with the duration of depression, and it is decreased when therapeutic interventions lead to improvement of symptoms. There are also reports of high levels of proinflammatory cytokines in plasma in patients with treatment-resistant depression. Neuroinflammation may be linked to abnormalities in serotonin transmission and a metabolic shift that leads to an increased production of kynurenine from tryptophan (instead of production of serotonin), which ultimately may increase glutamatergic signalling. The decreased neurogenesis associated with depression may also be linked to neuroinflammation.

Treatment of depression

The management of depression can involve pharmacological and non-pharmacological approaches. There is evidence of synergism between these approaches, therefore, optimum results could be reached by therapeutic combination strategies.

Pharmacological management

The pharmacological treatment of depression is based on the use of drugs belonging to several classes, as shown in Table 16.4. Drugs are classified according to their structure (e.g. tricyclic antidepressants [TCAs]) or their mechanism of action (e.g. monoamine reuptake inhibition vs. monoamine oxidase inhibition). Most drugs currently prescribed act on monoaminergic transmission. For all antidepressant medications, the onset of full clinical efficacy occurs at least 2–3 weeks after initiation of treatment. This indicates that it is not the immediate changes that follow the acute administration of these compounds that are responsible for their therapeutic effect but the delayed secondary effects. For example, with many antidepressant drugs, chronic treatment leads to downregulation of β- and α_2-adrenoceptors and 5-HT_2 receptors. Antidepressant drugs also activate neural plasticity mechanisms, for example, upregulation of factors such as brain-derived neurotrophic factor (BDNF), which could counter the structural alterations seen in depression, such as synaptic loss, network changes and decreased neurogenesis.

TCAs were the first-line medication for several decades before the development of selective serotonin

Table 16.4   Major classes of antidepressant drugs

Tricyclic antidepressants

Amitriptyline, clomipramine, desipramine, doxepine, imipramine, nortriptyline, protriptyline

Monoamine oxidase inhibitors (irreversible)

Phenelzine, tranylcypromine, isocarboxazid

Monoamine oxidase A inhibitors (reversible)

Moclobemide

Atypical antidepressants

Mirtazapine, bupropion, trazodone, tianeptine

Selective serotonin reuptake inhibitors

Citalopram, fluoxetine, fluvoxamine, paroxetine, sertraline

Serotonin and noradrenaline reuptake inhibitors

Venlafaxine, duloxetine

Noradenaline reuptake inhibitors

Reboxetine

reuptake inhibitors (SSRIs). Drugs in the TCA class, such as amitriptyline and imipramine, inhibit the noradrenaline and 5-HT uptake systems with variable affinities (Box 16.3, Fig. 16.3). However, at clinically relevant concentrations, they also have significant affinity for various receptors (e.g. α_1-adrenergic, H_1 histaminergic and muscarinic), where they act as antagonists. This property is responsible for their numerous side effects. For example, they induce anticholinergic antimuscarinic effects such as dry mouth, constipation, blurred vision and difficult micturition. They induce postural hypotension and sedation (consequences of adrenergic and histaminergic blockade). At high doses, they have cardiac toxicity, and overdoses are lethal. They induce strong potentiation of the effects of alcohol; combining drinking with antidepressant drugs may lead to severe respiratory depression.

Monoamine oxidase inhibitors (MAOIs) are irreversible inhibitors of monoamine oxidases. Monoamine oxidases A and B (MAO_A and MAO_B) are the enzymes primarily responsible for the breakdown of monoamines, such as dopamine, noradrenaline and serotonin. The MAO_A and MAO_B genes are next to each other on the human X chromosome. Monoamine oxidases are located

Box 16.3   Monoamine transporters

A monoaminergic neuron releases amine by exocytosis, triggered by depolarization of the nerve terminal. Release is followed by diffusion of the transmitter away from the synaptic cleft, activation of pre- and postsynaptic receptors and reuptake of the released amine into the presynaptic nerve terminal. The process of reuptake of monoamines is carried out by specialized plasma membrane transporters. The transporters for noradrenaline, 5-hydroxytryptamine (5-HT) and dopamine are termed NET, SERT and DAT, respectively, and they control the half-life of monoamines in the extracellular space (see Fig. 16.3). Psychoactive substances (e.g. cocaine and amphetamine) or therapeutic drugs (e.g. antidepressants) modify the activity of monoamine transporters. Transporters use the energy from the Na^+ transmembrane gradient to transport the transmitter inside the terminal. NET limits the availability of noradrenaline for diffusion. It can transport molecules that are structurally similar to noradrenaline such as dopamine, cocaine and amphetamine. DAT is located around the active zone of the synapse and is considered to play a major role in the regulation of extracellular levels of dopamine. DAT is also a target for cocaine and amphetamine. It has been shown that the motor stimulant effects of these drugs are absent in DAT knockout mice (i.e. animals that do not express the transporter). The 5-HT transporter is part of the same transporter family, and it is the target for selective serotonin reuptake inhibitors (SSRIs). At clinically relevant doses of SSRIs, there is 70%–80% occupancy of the 5-HT transporter.

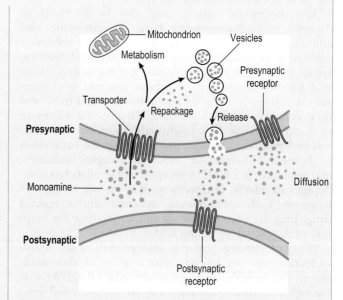

Fig. 16.3 Schematic representation of plasma membrane monoamine transporters. NET, DAT and SERT are localized in the presynaptic plasma membrane. Uptake of the neurotransmitter from the extracellular space takes place via a process that is coupled to ion transport and can also occur in the reverse direction. The neurotransmitter can then be repackaged in vesicles for subsequent release and/or can be inactivated, e.g. by the monoamine oxidase enzymes.

in the presynaptic terminal and are associated with mitochondria. The inhibition of these enzymes increases the cytoplasmic concentration of amines. MAOIs do not differentiate between the two enzyme types. They were the first drugs introduced clinically for the treatment of depression but were replaced by TCAs, which had higher efficacy. There is a risk of dangerous interaction of MAOIs with tyramine-containing food (e.g. red wine, mature cheese and broad beans). Tyramine is an amine substrate of MAO_A and MAO_B and is normally metabolized by these enzymes in the gut and liver. Tyramine can displace noradrenaline from its storage vesicles and ultimately increase its level in the synaptic cleft. Inhibition of monoamine oxidases leads to high levels of tyramine and an increase in the release of noradrenaline. The result can be a massive hypertensive crisis, with possible intracranial haemorrhage. This chain of effects is called the 'cheese effect' (because tyramine is found in mature cheese and other types of food). Indirectly acting sympathomimetic amines such as ephedrine and amphetamine can also cause hypertension in patients who are taking MAOIs. Apart from these specific unwanted complications of treatment, MAOIs can also induce postural hypotension, weight gain, antimuscarinic effects and hepatotoxicity. They also interact dangerously with the opiate analgesic pethidine: the syndrome is characterized by hypotension, restlessness and coma.

The drug moclobemide represents an example of a second generation of MAOI and acts as a reversible inhibitor. This compound is specific for MAO_A and has an efficacy comparable to that of other MAOIs, but there is a significantly decreased risk of a 'cheese effect', due to the reversible nature of enzyme inhibition. It is expected that this type of drug could gradually replace the first generation MAOIs.

MAOIs are more effective drugs than TCAs or SSRIs in atypical depression, for example, depression characterized by weight gain and hypersomnia or in patients who do not respond to other antidepressants.

SSRIs, such as citalopram, fluoxetine, paroxetine and sertraline, have largely replaced other antidepressants, in particular TCAs, in the treatment of most types of depression. These compounds have a higher selectivity for the 5-HT reuptake system than TCAs (Table 16.5). The most selective is citalopram (and its S-stereoisomer, escitalopram). SSRIs have a much more acceptable profile of side effects and are safer than TCAs in overdose. The unwanted effects of SSRIs include nausea, headache, insomnia and sexual dysfunction. It is important to note that although SSRI antidepressants offer significant advantages over TCAs in tolerability and safety, they are not more efficacious in severe, life-threatening depression.

Atypical antidepressants include drugs such as trazodone (5-HT reuptake inhibitor and $5-HT_2$ receptor antagonist), mirtazapine (an α_2, $5-HT_2$ and $5-HT_3$ receptor antagonist), bupropion (an inhibitor of dopamine and noradrenaline reuptake) and tianeptine (a 5-HT reuptake enhancer and agonist at μ-opioid receptors). These compounds have complex mechanisms of action. Overall, they have fewer side effects than TCAs and are less toxic in overdose.

Serotonin and noradrenaline reuptake inhibitors (SNRIs), such as venlafaxine and duloxetine, appear to have some advantages over SSRIs. This may be due to the synergism of blockade of 5-HT and noradrenaline uptake. In contrast with TCAs, these drugs do not have significant activity at other targets, which may explain their much milder profile of unwanted effects. Venlafaxine has also been shown to have a faster onset of action (<2 weeks) than TCAs, MAOIs or SSRIs.

Noradrenaline reuptake inhibitors such as reboxetine have therapeutic efficacy in major depression similar to that of imipramine, desipramine and fluoxetine, but not in mild depression. Adverse effects include dry mouth, sweating, constipation, insomnia and blurred vision.

One of the most recent introductions to depression therapeutics is ketamine, which is an antagonist at NMDA glutamate receptors. Ketamine has a rapid onset of action, and a single intravenous infusion of ketamine has been shown to induce alleviation of symptoms within 24 hours after infusion. In 2019, the US Food and Drug Administration approved the use of esketamine (the S-isomer of ketamine) as a nasal spray in conjunction with an oral antidepressant in patients with treatment-resistant depression. Another new drug is agomelatine, which is an agonist at melatonin receptors. Melatonin is a hormone produced in the pineal gland and involved in the regulation of the sleep-wake cycle. The beneficial effects of agomelatine may be due at least in part to an improvement in sleep patterns.

Table 16.5 Selectivity of antidepressants as inhibitors of monoamine reuptake

Drug	Selectivity ratio 5-HT:NA
TCAs	
Desipramine	0.003
Nortriptyline	0.015
Imipramine	0.31
Amitriptyline	0.36
Clomipramine	5.2
SSRIs	
Fluoxetine	23
Paroxetine	33
Fluvoxamine	71
Sertraline	73
Citalopram	4000

5-HT, 5-hydroxytryptamine; NA, noradrenaline; TCA, tricyclic antidepressant; SSRI, selective serotonin reuptake inhibitor.

Electroconvulsive therapy

The first electroconvulsive treatment occurred in 1938 as a treatment for catatonia and depression, and was performed by Cerletti and Bini. This had been preceded by the historical observations of Meduna in 1934 (Box 16.4). Although there was a high risk of significant medical morbidity, the results clearly indicated that electroconvulsive therapy (ECT) was efficacious in severely mentally ill patients. Unfortunately, evidence of its success led to a rather indiscriminate use in its early phase. The use of general anaesthesia and muscle relaxants has made ECT much safer.

ECT is reserved for second-line treatment of patients who fail to respond to antidepressant drugs. It is particularly useful in very disturbed patients who are at high risk for suicide. ECT is administered two or three times a week, over several weeks. Electrodes are placed unilaterally or bilaterally on each side of the head. If cognitive side effects following treatment become significant, electrodes can be placed only unilaterally and the frequency of treatments reduced. Several factors can affect the seizure threshold, either by increasing it (age, anticonvulsants or dehydration) or decreasing it (caffeine or hyperventilation).

Headache and nausea are common side effects of ECT, but the major problems with ECT are its effects on learning and memory, which may be considered unacceptable by some patients. Patients lose the memory of events that preceded the treatment (retrograde amnesia). However, the loss is transient, and the patient usually recovers after a few weeks. Patients who respond to treatment have a better quality of life than before and may consider that the lost memories are an acceptable price to pay. Other patients feel very affected by the loss of memory and feel alienated in both their private life and their work.

ECT can be used only for a short time. However, continuation and maintenance can be used to prevent relapse of depression after a successful first course of ECT. The information available so far suggests that long-term use (>1 year) of ECT is efficacious and relatively well tolerated and reduces hospital use for a population of chronically depressed patients who are refractory to various types of medication.

ECT utilization varies widely worldwide, for example from 1.1 ECT patients per 100,000 people in Poland to 36 and 41 ECT patients per 100,000 people in Australia and Sweden, respectively. More than 22,500 individual ECT sessions were recorded in England in 2015–2016, and since the turn of the century, over a million ECTs are performed worldwide per annum. ECT has been used not only in major depression but also in other psychiatric disorders: mania, schizophreniform psychoses, neuroleptic malignant syndrome and catatonic states. Patients treated with ECT or with a combination of antidepressant drugs and ECT show a better response than patients treated only with drugs. The mechanism of action

underlying the efficacy of ECT in a wide spectrum of disorders is still unclear. It has been shown that seizures upregulate the expression of neurotrophic factors such as nerve growth factor (NGF) and BDNF. They also increase hippocampal neurogenesis (i.e. production of new neurons) and hippocampal synaptic plasticity. The technique is continuously optimized (e.g. novel electrode placements, optimization of electrical stimulus parameters and treatment frequency). New methods for inducing more localized seizures are also under development, such as repetitive transcranial magnetic stimulation.

Box 16.4 Electroconvulsive therapy: still an unsolved therapeutic enigma

It is possible that the first attempt by Meduna to use ECT therapeutically was encouraged by the benefits reported by Wagner-Jauregg, who used induction of fever to treat the dementia associated with neurosyphilis. The underlying idea was that of treating a disease using mechanisms associated with another disease. Interestingly, Meduna tried the idea of inducing the seizure therapeutically in a patient with schizophrenia. What follows is the account of that first attempt (recounted by Fink in 2001).

'At 10.30 on the morning of January 24, 1934, the Hungarian neuropsychiatrist Ladislas Meduna approached the bed of Zoltan, a 30-year-old Budapest labourer who appeared lifeless. Zoltan had hardly spoken or cared for himself for more than 4 years; his mental condition of catatonic schizophrenia was considered hopeless. No remedy was available and none looked for, as the doctors believed the illness to be an immutable genetic fault, laid down at the moment of conception. Meduna injected an oily extract of camphor into the patient's right buttock. Soon the patient's heart raced, sweat rose on his brow, and he became increasingly fearful, and after 45 minutes, his eyes suddenly closed, his jaw clenched, breathing stopped and he lost consciousness. With a deep and noisy sigh, his arms and legs extended, he convulsed, and his bed thumped rhythmically, as the attendants caught him as he was about to roll on the floor. His skin became ashen and he wet the bed. As suddenly as the spasm started, it ended. His eyes opened and a pink colour slowly returned to his cheeks. Zoltan continued to stare and was as speechless as before. He had survived an induced grand-mal epileptic fit. Meduna injected camphor at 3–4 days intervals, and 2 days after the 5th seizure, Zoltan awakened, looked about, got out of bed, asked where he was and requested breakfast. He did not believe that he had been in hospital for 4 years and knew nothing of the intervening history. Later that day, he again relapsed into stupor. After each of the next seizures Zoltan remained alert and interested, for longer and longer periods, until after the 8th injection he left the hospital to return to his home and work. His mental condition was relieved and five years later he was well and working.'

The use of magnetic fields provides more control over the site and extent of stimulation than ECT. This enhanced control is a means of focusing the treatment on target cortical structures that may be critical for the antidepressant response and reducing spread to the medial temporal regions implicated in the unwanted effects of ECT on cognition.

Other stimulation therapies

Other stimulation methods used in depression include vagus nerve stimulation and deep brain stimulation. These techniques are also used in other pathologies, i.e. epilepsy and Parkinson's disease (see Chapters 10 and 13). There is evidence that vagus nerve stimulation leads to an activation of neurons in the locus coeruleus and raphe nuclei, and this may underlie its efficacy. In depressive disorders, the deep brain stimulation procedure may target a variety of sites, for example, the orbitofrontal cortex and subcallosal anterior cingulate cortex. The information collected so far on the efficacy of these interventions in major depression is still limited compared with the vast amount of data on the use of pharmacological interventions, but the observations are encouraging so far, especially in patients with treatment-resistant depression. In addition, non-invasive methods such as repetitive transcranial magnetic stimulation (using an electromagnetic coil placed against the scalp) and transcranial direct current stimulation (using a constant direct current of low intensity passed across the brain via surface electrodes) are also being explored and gradually introduced in specialised clinics.

Psychotherapy

The efficacy of various forms of psychotherapy in the management of depression is well accepted, especially in mild forms of this condition. Cognitive behavioural therapy (CBT) is a form of psychotherapy used in depression. This therapy is based on the premise that behaviour is learned, and that change can be stimulated by the positive experiences resulting from new behaviour. CBT focuses on affect and cognitive regulation skills. It consists of a minimum of six to eight sessions administered over 2–3 months. CBT is also available as a computerised version, that is, it can be provided via a computer-based or web-based programme.

Chronic psychotherapy significantly reduces relapse and recurrence in the highest-risk patients—those with recurrent major depressive disorder. Specific CBT strategies can also be used in the management of anxiety disorders, such as specific phobias, panic disorder and agoraphobia, social phobia, generalized anxiety disorder and obsessive-compulsive and posttraumatic stress disorders.

Other forms of psychotherapy include interpersonal therapy, behavioural activation therapy, couple therapy and short-term psychodynamic therapy. All psychotherapy regimes can be combined with antidepressant drugs. Functional imaging data indicate that psychotherapy interventions, such as CBT or interpersonal therapy, can normalise some of the metabolic changes seen in cortico-limbic circuits in depression.

Bipolar disorder and its treatment

Bipolar disorder is a form of mood disorder consisting of an alternation of manic phases and depressive episodes. The natural course of the disease is characterized by relapse and recurrence. The goal of treatment is to treat both the acute phase (acute depression or mania) and the recurrence of these episodes. The duration of episodes ranges from 2 to 6 weeks, and their frequency varies considerably between patients. Between 5% and 15% of patients have four or more mood episodes (depressive, manic or mixed) within a year, and this rapid cycling is associated with a poor prognosis. The treatment continuation phase continues for up to 6 months after the remission of acute symptoms. Lifelong treatment may be necessary for a significant number of patients. Bipolar disorder is a clinically heterogeneous disease, so treatment varies with disease subtype, within the three subtypes mentioned previously: bipolar I, bipolar II and cyclothymia.

There is clearly a genetic component to this disease. Its heritability is more than 70%. As for other common and complex diseases, such as diabetes and hypertension, the transmission of bipolar disorder is multifactorial rather than the result of simple Mendelian inheritance. Genetic linkage studies have suggested the involvement of chromosomal regions 4p, 6p, 13q, 15q and 18q. A large-scale genome-wide association study published in 2019 identified 30 distinct loci associated with bipolar disorder.

As with major depression, imaging studies and postmortem morphometric observations in bipolar disorder show neuronal atrophy and cell loss in cortical areas. Bipolar disorder can be associated with a larger third ventricle, smaller cerebellum, smaller temporal lobe and larger amygdala. The pathophysiology of the disease has not yet been elucidated. The recently identified new genetic loci are associated with voltage-gated calcium channels and sodium channels, glutamate receptors and synapse components.

The successful treatment of bipolar disorder remains a challenge in psychiatry. It is generally agreed that patients should be maintained on a mood-stabilizing drug. The most commonly prescribed stabilizers are lithium and the anticonvulsants carbamazepine and sodium valproate. Antipsychotic drugs and antidepressant drugs can be added to these to control mania and depression episodes, respectively.

The discovery of the efficacy of lithium in bipolar disorder represents a landmark in the history of 20th century medicine. Lithium was the first drug for which recurrence-preventing action was demonstrated in mood disorders. It may prevent recurrences not only in bipolar disorder but also in recurrent major depression. This monovalent cation continues to be used for both mainstay treatment for the acute manic phase and prophylaxis for recurrent manic and depressive episodes. The beneficial effects consist of reductions in both the number of episodes and their severity. Long-term lithium treatment is also associated with lower mortality and reduced suicidal behaviour. The drug has efficacy, but it also has many side effects that may lead to cessation of treatment. The major side effects include nausea, tremor, fatigue, polyuria and polydipsia. The recommended serum lithium range is 0.4–1.2 mmol/L. The risk of lithium intoxication is a drawback of the treatment. Lithium is eliminated through the kidneys, and it should be used with caution in the case of dehydration, sodium deficiency or kidney disease.

Research on the mechanism of action underlying the efficacy of lithium has focused extensively on the hydrolysis of phosphatidylinositol 4,5-bisphosphate (PIP_2) (see Fig. 2.14, Chapter 2). Inositol phospholipids, such as PIP_2 are involved in receptor-mediated signal transduction pathways. Several receptor subtypes (e.g. 5-HT_2 serotonergic; α_1-noradrenergic; M_1, M_3 and M_5 muscarinic) are coupled to the hydrolysis of inositol phospholipids. The activation of receptors leads to stimulation of phospholipase Cβ. The enzyme catalyses the conversion of PIP_2 to inositol 1,4,5-trisphosphate (IP_3) and diacylglycerol (DAG). IP_3 stimulates the mobilization of intracellular Ca^{2+}, and DAG activates protein kinase C. IP_3 can be phosphorylated and dephosphorylated. Lithium interferes with these processes. At therapeutically relevant concentrations, it inhibits inositol monophosphatase. The effect on protein kinase C may be equally important. Interestingly, it was recently shown that tamoxifen—a drug that has protein kinase C inhibitory activity—could significantly reduce acute mania. However, the story of lithium, which is still an enigma in psychiatry, continues with even more exciting developments (Box 16.5).

Anticonvulsants such as carbamazepine and sodium valproate have comparable efficacy to lithium and may be better tolerated. There is also evidence that combinations of lithium with an anticonvulsant drug can help in atypical cases of bipolar disorder or in patients resistant to treatment. During a depressive episode, it is often necessary to add an antidepressant drug. This, unfortunately, may induce a switch to a manic phase. The antidepressant bupropion and, more recently, lamotrigine, are also useful in the treatment of depressive episodes, especially in comparison with TCAs, as the latter may induce a switch to a manic phase.

General comments on mood disorders

Mood disorders are among the most prevalent, recurrent and disabling of all illnesses. They cover a wide spectrum, from severe intractable depression to the milder forms, such as seasonal affective disorder and postnatal depression (Box 16.6). Drugs that can be used to treat mood disorders with some success were discovered accidentally, not as a result of following a scientific rationale. Drug development has focused heavily on

---

Box 16.5 Lithium: a story of serendipity and surprises!

A new era in psychiatry started in the second half of the 20th century, and one of the key discoveries triggering this change was the introduction of lithium into therapeutics.

In 1949 the Australian John Cade hypothesized that mental illness is caused by intoxication with a xenobiotic, and that this toxic agent could be eliminated in the patient's urine. In order to explore the effects of uric acid, he injected lithium urate into guinea pigs. This choice was made because of the good solubility of this salt. The effects were surprising: the animals were docile and sedated. Cade immediately thought of treating manic patients with lithium. Following administration of lithium urate, the manic patients showed significantly decreased symptoms. The rest is medical history.

The efficacy of this monovalent cation intrigued researchers for years and, for a while, emphasis was placed on its modulatory role in inositol-related biochemical pathways. However, the most recent discoveries suggest that the effects of lithium (and possibly of other mood stabilizers, such as valproate) involve concomitant changes in the expression of numerous genes, for example, through modulation of the activity of transcription factors such as AP-1. Furthermore, at therapeutically relevant concentrations, lithium is an inhibitor of the enzyme glycogen synthase kinase 3. This enzyme plays an important role in cytoskeletal dynamics, as well as in nuclear transcriptional events. Finally, differential analysis of the transcriptome (i.e. cellular pool of transcribed mRNA) after treatment with lithium suggests that the cation upregulates neuroprotective genes such as BCL2. Therefore, the emerging view of the effect of lithium is that of action at multiple levels and significant neuroprotective potential.

---

monoaminergic targets, and there is a need for more mechanistic diversity. Several major challenges remain: the delayed effect of antidepressants, resistance to treatment and, most of all, an understanding of the pathophysiology of the disease and its causes. Our understanding of the circuits responsible for the regulation of mood and affect is still rudimentary. Some of these issues are discussed below.

Treatment resistance in depression

Although new-generation compounds are much better tolerated than the original tricyclic drugs, they are not necessarily more efficacious. Furthermore, many patients are resistant to drugs. It is suggested that up to 50% of patients who receive drugs still experience symptoms and are somewhat functionally impaired. Combinations of drugs (e.g. lithium and antidepressants) can be attempted, but no optimum strategy to address treatment resistance in depression has been defined as yet.

Postnatal depression

Depressive episodes in women after childbirth are relatively common. During the first 6 months after delivery, the prevalence is 12%–13%. Risk factors for postnatal depression include poor marital relationship, past history of psychopathology, low social support, unplanned pregnancy, antenatal parental stress and depression in fathers. Treatment consists of antidepressant medication and/or cognitive behavioural therapy. Postnatal depression must be distinguished from the very transient period of tearfulness or emotional lability that many mothers experience in the first 1–2 weeks after birth ('baby blues'), which resolves naturally.

Seasonal affective disorder

This type of depression received formal recognition only in the early 1980s. Symptoms of depression affect patients regularly during the autumn or winter months, whereas spontaneous remission is seen in spring and summer. This disorder is correlated with the level of light and may be connected with an abnormality in the production/secretion of melatonin, a hormone secreted by the pineal gland. As days become shorter and darker, the production of this hormone increases. Many people affected by this disorder respond to bright light therapy. For example, they can be exposed daily for a limited time to a bank of fluorescent lights shielded with a plastic screen. Antidepressant drugs such as selective serotonin reuptake inhibitors (SSRIs) can also be used successfully to treat this disorder.

One of the major complications of depressive mood disorders is the increased risk for suicide. A common biological marker of suicide is a reduced concentration of the 5-HT metabolite 5-hydroxyindoleacetic acid in the CSF of suicide cases versus controls. Although suicide prevention is ideally primary, before the event, most treatment is in fact secondary or tertiary, after initial unsuccessful suicide attempts. Depending on the individual characteristics of the patient, suicide prevention usually includes a pharmacological cocktail (e.g. one of the SSRIs to raise 5-HT concentrations, perhaps combined with an anxiolytic, mood-stabilizing or antipsychotic agent), supportive psychotherapy and/or ECT. The existence of a significant risk of suicide in a patient necessitates treatment in hospital.

The failure of medication may sometimes be due to the use of inadequate doses. Thus, many patients who receive TCAs are prescribed relatively low doses, and an improvement is seen if doses are increased. At higher doses, plasma monitoring may be required in the case of tricyclic compounds, because of the risk of cardiotoxicity.

Another strategy that can be used is switching to a different class of antidepressant. There is evidence that switching may benefit approximately 50% of the patients initially unresponsive to medication. One of the problems encountered when attempting to switch to a different antidepressant drug is that withdrawal from the first compound is difficult. It may be more appropriate to add a second compound to the first. Patients with depression with psychotic features have low rates of response to TCAs but may improve when an antipsychotic drug is added to the treatment (e.g. amitriptyline with perphenazine, or olanzapine with fluoxetine). There is also evidence that lithium added to TCAs, MAOIs or SSRIs leads to an improved response. Finally, maintenance therapy with antidepressant drugs for a minimum of 6 months after the successful treatment of an episode has been shown to decrease the risk of recurrence.

Delayed onset of antidepressant action: a consequence of autoregulation?

Although drugs such as TCAs and SSRIs block 5-HT reuptake rapidly, their therapeutic action is delayed. A possible explanation for this delay has been suggested, using the SSRIs as an example. It has been suggested that the increase in synaptic 5-HT activates feedback mechanisms mediated by $5\text{-}HT_{1A}$ receptors situated on the cell body and $5\text{-}HT1_B$ receptors situated on the nerve terminals. The activation of these two types of autoreceptor reduces the firing of 5-HT neurons and decreases the amount of 5-HT released. Long-term treatment with SSRIs desensitizes the inhibitory $5\text{-}HT_1$ autoreceptors, and 5-HT neurotransmission is ultimately enhanced. The time course of desensitization is similar to the delay in clinical effect. This explanation is supported by the observation that the addition of pindolol (a drug that blocks $5\text{-}HT1_A$ receptors) to SSRI treatment accelerates and enhances the antidepressant response.

Need for new therapeutic targets

As mentioned earlier, the monoamine theory of depression has certainly served a useful purpose, but the field now needs to move beyond this concept, and it is important to consider, in parallel with monoamines, the other neurotransmitters that are likely to be dysfunctional in depressive disorders. Evidence suggests that it is possible to target glutamatergic systems (e.g. NMDA receptor antagonists or 4-amino-3-hydroxy-5-methyl-4-isoxazole propionic acid [AMPA] receptor potentiators) or peptidergic systems (CRF receptor antagonists) and obtain significant antidepressant effects. It may be possible in the near future to develop drugs that will address the cause of mood disorders and not only treat the symptoms during depressive episodes. The recent success of esketamine opens up new therapeutic avenues.

Comments on case history

The unpredictable evolution of depression is illustrated by the case history. Depression emerged unexpectedly, possibly triggered by the stress intrinsic to a high level of activity. However, a genetic susceptibility is also suggested by the family history. The patient responds to an SNRI and tolerates it well but makes the mistake of stopping the medication immediately after improvement. Relapse occurs, and it is severe, with added anxiety. This leads to the choice of combination therapy (medication and psychotherapy). It cannot be ruled out that this patient will experience periods of remission and relapse throughout his life.

Anxiety disorders

'The mind is its own place, and in itself can make a heaven of hell, a hell of heaven.'

John Milton (1608–1674)

Anxiety is an unpleasant emotional experience characterized by fear disproportionate to the severity of stressful factors in the environment, or fear without a cause. An optimum level of anxiety may improve performance. However, when it is intense and persists for a prolonged period, it is an extremely disabling disorder. Anxiety disorders are the most common of all mental health disorders and can occur at any age. They are more common in women, and their prevalence is highest in midlife. There is a substantial underrecognition and undertreatment of anxiety disorders worldwide. They are associated with a considerable degree of impairment and a significant economic burden for society.

The heritability of anxiety disorders is approximately 30%–50%. These disorders are categorized into different subtypes (Table 16.6). Some of them are phobic disorders, whereas others do not have a phobic component (Table 16.7). Phobias are characterized by irrational fear and avoidance of objects and situations. Specific phobias are the most common forms of anxiety disorder, followed by panic disorder. Although previously included in the class of anxiety disorders, posttraumatic stress disorder is a complex and unique syndrome, which includes clear manifestations of anxiety, and is now classified separately in DSM-5 as a form of trauma and stress-related disorder (Box 16.7). In order to monitor severity and response to treatment, scales such as the Hamilton Anxiety Rating Scale (HAM-A) can be used.

Anxiety and depression are distinct disorders, but mixed disorders combining the two occur frequently; it is estimated that >42% of all depressive disorders are

Table 16.6   Classification of anxiety disorders (DSM-5)

Panic disorder
Agoraphobia
Specific phobia
Social anxiety disorder (social phobia)
Separation anxiety disorder
Selective mutism
Anxiety disorder due to another medical condition
Generalized anxiety disorder
Substance/medication-induced anxiety disorder
Other specified anxiety disorder
Unspecified anxiety disorder

Table 16.7   General characteristics of phobias and of non-phobic anxiety disorders

Phobias		
Agoraphobia	**Social phobias**	**Specific (isolated) phobias**
Anxiety in situations where escape or help is difficult Fear of being alone in public places or in a crowd	Intense fear of embarrassment or humiliation in public or social gatherings Subject feels that other people think them stupid or incompetent	Intense fear provoked by appearance or anticipation of specific situations or objects (e.g. fear of spiders, snakes, heights, water, travelling by plane or train)
Non-phobic anxiety disorders		
Generalized anxiety disorder	**Panic disorder**	**Selective mutism**
Ill-defined apprehension not related to a specific situation/object, lasting for more than 6 months Exaggerated worries about health, personal safety, work or finances	Recurrent unexpected panic attacks (accompanied by dizziness, nausea, palpitations, chest pain, hyperventilation, sweating, tremor and sometimes incontinence)	Anxiety disorder characterized by an adult or a child's inability to speak and communicate effectively in specific social settings, e.g. at school. It can be accompanied by extreme shyness and fear of social embarrassment, and social withdrawal

Box 16.7   Posttraumatic stress disorder

Posttraumatic stress disorder (PTSD) is a syndrome that emerges after one or more traumatic events, and involves a series of anxiety symptoms including emotional numbing, flashbacks and avoidance of reminders of the event. This disorder was associated in the past mainly with the psychological consequences of war, but today it is increasingly recognized as a serious complication after rape, abuse, assault, accidents or natural disasters. It is classified as a trauma and stress-related disorder. In the acute aftermath of a traumatic event, those affected experience hyperarousal, agitation, insomnia and nightmares. These reactions may serve an adaptive role and may remit in a short time. When they do not remit, they evolve into PTSD. The presentation of this syndrome is heterogeneous, with symptoms that vary significantly between patients.

Several brain circuits and neurotransmitters are involved in the pathophysiology of PTSD. Catecholamines, serotonin, the hypothalamic–pituitary–adrenal axis (in particular corticotrophin-releasing factor) and corticolimbic circuits are involved in the modulation of fear, anger, arousal and aggression.

Approaches to treatment of PTSD are both pharmacological and non-pharmacological. Different drugs can be used, sometimes on a semi-empirical basis, to reduce the flashbacks, anxiety, hyperarousal and depression. Interestingly, compounds from the same pharmacological class appear to have effects on different symptoms. For example, imipramine decreases nightmares and flashbacks but has no effect on avoidance behaviour. In contrast, amitriptyline reduces avoidance and anxiety. Monoamine oxidase inhibitors such as phenelzine or moclobemide have been shown to be effective in some patients. Selective serotonin reuptake inhibitors have been shown to be effective in civilian and military trauma victims. Anticonvulsants (carbamazepine and valproate) decrease flashbacks and impulsivity. Overall, approximately 70% of patients get some benefit from pharmacotherapy. Psychotherapy can include cognitive behavioural therapy (CBT) and group therapy. More recently, encouraging results have been reported with eye movement desensitisation and reprocessing therapy (EMDR), during which the patient makes rapid lateral eye movements guided by the therapist, while recalling the traumatic events.

mixed anxiety-depressive syndromes. Depression is often comorbid with conditions such as generalized anxiety disorder, panic disorder and obsessive-compulsive disorder. That many types of depression involve a degree of anxiety is illustrated in the case history, during the second depressive episode of the patient.

Anxiety manifestations have affective, behavioural and somatic components. The affective component is characterized by the feeling of panic and dread when confronted with a perceived threat. Behavioural reactions tend to be aimed at avoiding the source of anxiety.

Somatic reactions reflect a state of autonomic hyperre-activity, including cardiopulmonary, urinary and gastrointestinal symptoms. The neural circuitry underlying anxiety disorders includes the amygdala (both the basolateral amygdala and the central nucleus of the amygdala), lateral septum, bed nucleus of the stria terminalis, insula, hippocampus and prefrontal cortex. These structures are highly interconnected, with multiple reciprocal projections. The amygdala is a key structure for the interpretation of environmental stimuli as potentially threatening. The sensory information flows forwards from the amygdala to the bed nucleus of the stria terminalis (an area important in stress-related behavioural processing), the ventral hippocampus and medial prefrontal cortex, and then to effector nuclei (such as the reticular formation, see Fig. 1.17). The hippocampus has a major role in fear learning and anxiety-related behaviour. The medial prefrontal cortex controls the evaluation of threat and may permit or prevent anxiogenic interpretations of perceived threat situations.

Treatment of anxiety disorders

The management of anxiety disorders can be pharmacological, non-pharmacological (psychological therapies) or a combination of both. Psychological therapies are recommended as first-line treatment especially for milder forms of anxiety disorders. Such interventions include cognitive behavioural therapy, interpersonal therapy, insight-oriented therapy, biofeedback, relaxation therapy and exposure psychotherapy. Support groups and stress-management techniques may also help. Even after psychotherapy has led to improvement, some patients may still have residual symptoms, and they may benefit from psychotherapy combined with pharmacotherapy.

Anxiety symptoms can be managed using a variety of pharmacological treatments. Currently, the first-line recommended treatment is represented by SSRIs such as citalopram or paroxetine. Antidepressant drugs such as imipramine can be used to treat panic and social phobias. Side effects include dry mouth, constipation, tachycardia and blurred vision, as discussed above. SNRIs such as venlafaxine have also shown potential in the treatment of various anxiety disorders. The drug pregabalin can also be used for generalised anxiety disorder.

β-blockers (e.g. propranolol) do not affect the psychological aspects of anxiety but reduce the physical symptoms (e.g. tremor and palpitations). They are used in the treatment of social phobias and also to treat 'stage fright' in performers.

Barbiturate drugs were used in the past and have become obsolete, being replaced by benzodiazepines. Barbiturates have a narrow therapeutic window, and there is a risk of major cardiovascular and respiratory depression resulting from overdose. Furthermore, their induction of liver metabolic enzymes may lead to dangerous drug interactions due to changes in the metabolism of co-administered drugs.

Table 16.8   Pharmacokinetic profiles of commonly used benzodiazepines and non-benzodiazepine drugs

Drug	Onset of action (min)	Elimination half-life (h)	Duration of action	Active metabolites
Diazepam	20–40	20–60	Long	Yes
Flunitrazepam	20–30	11–20	Intermediate	No
Flurazepam	30–60	47–100	Long	Yes
Nitrazepam	20–50	25–35	Long	No
Oxazepam	15–30	8–12	Intermediate	No
Temazepam	45–60	3–25	Intermediate	No
Triazolam	15–30	1.5–5	Short	No
Zaleplon	15–30	1	Short	No
Zolpidem	30	1.5–4.5	Short	No
Zopiclone	15–30	3.5–6.5	Short	Yes

Benzodiazepines represent a major class of drugs that can be used for treating anxiety disorders. They are prescribed for the short-term relief of severe anxiety, but their long-term use should be avoided. They comprise a large class of related compounds with sedative, anxiolytic, muscle relaxant and anticonvulsant activity (see Chapter 13). These compounds bind to the $GABA_A$ receptor—a ligand-gated ion channel associated with a chloride conductance. The $GABA_A$ receptor is a pentamer assembled from several subunits that exist in different isoforms: $\alpha(1–6)$, $\beta(1–3)$, $\gamma(1–3)$, $\varrho(1–3)$, δ, ε, π and θ. Many $GABA_A$ receptor subtypes contain α-, β- and γ-subunits with the composition $2\alpha.2\beta.1\gamma$. The most abundant $GABA_A$ receptor type is composed of $\alpha_1\beta_{2/3}\gamma_2$ subunits. Benzodiazepines enhance the actions of the inhibitory neurotransmitter GABA by binding to a specific recognition site on $GABA_A$ receptors containing α_1, α_2, α_3 and α_5 subunits. Two types of benzodiazepine (BZ) binding sites have been described: BZ1 and BZ2. $GABA_A$ receptors and the BZ sites, which are present on these receptors, have an abundant and heterogeneous distribution in the central nervous system (CNS) (Box 16.9).

Benzodiazepine binding involves the α subunits or the $\alpha–\gamma$ interface, and these drugs act as positive allosteric modulators, that is, they increase the frequency of opening of the ion channel in the presence of the endogenous agonist GABA. Benzodiazepines replaced barbiturates (which can also act as positive allosteric modulators of the receptor) and became the most prescribed drugs in the world in the 1970s. However, apart from being anxiolytic, benzodiazepines also cause acute sedation. Therefore, benzodiazepines can also be used as hypnotics, that is, to induce sleep (see below). Chronically, they have abuse potential and can cause physical dependence. A withdrawal syndrome can emerge upon treatment discontinuation, especially if treatment is stopped without gradual tapering of the dose. Recent estimates suggest that 10%–30% of chronic benzodiazepine users are physically dependent on the drugs and 50% of all users suffer withdrawal symptoms.

Overall, compounds that bind at BZ sites on the $GABA_A$ receptor can have a variety of pharmacological profiles. If they enhance the inhibitory actions of GABA (they act as agonists at the BZ site), they are classified as positive allosteric modulators of the receptor complex. The compounds that induce effects opposite to those induced by benzodiazepines are termed inverse agonists, and those that reverse the effects of benzodiazepines (e.g. flumazenil) are benzodiazepine site antagonists. Between the opposite ends of the spectrum (i.e. full agonist and full inverse agonist action) are a range of compounds with differing degrees of efficacy, such as, partial agonists and partial inverse agonists. Attempts have been made to develop compounds that have the anxiolytic properties of the full agonist benzodiazepines but have reduced sedation and dependence (withdrawal) liabilities. Such compounds may interact with all four (i.e. α_1-, α_2-, α_3- and α_5-containing) $GABA_A$ receptor subtypes and have partial rather than full agonist efficacies. Alternatively, a compound might have comparable binding affinities but different efficacies at the various subtypes, thereby preferentially exerting its effects at subtypes thought to be associated with anxiety (α_2- and/or α_3-containing receptors) rather than the subtype associated with sedation (α_1-containing receptors).

Benzodiazepines differ in terms of pharmacokinetic properties (Table 16.8). These drugs undergo hepatic metabolism. The long half-life benzodiazepines, such as chlordiazepoxide, clorazepate, diazepam and flurazepam, undergo phase I and phase II metabolic transformations, which occur mostly in the liver, and lead to the formation of more polar derivatives and conjugated drug forms, which enable drug elimination from the body. These long half-life compounds are metabolized via phase I reactions (e.g. oxidation) into active compounds with even longer half-lives. Short half-life benzodiazepines, such as lorazepam, oxazepam and temazepam, require only phase II metabolism and are inactivated by hepatic conjugation. Phase II metabolism is less affected by age, so short-acting compounds should be prescribed

Table 16.9	Complications of chronic benzodiazepine use in the elderly

Psychomotor impairment

Risk of falls

Daytime drowsiness

Intoxication

Amnesia

Depression

Respiratory problems

Abuse and dependence

for the elderly. It is important to be aware of these aspects, especially when prescribing for the elderly for the management of either insomnia or anxiety. Chronic administration of benzodiazepines in this patient population can be accompanied by serious complications (Table 16.9).

One of the most prescribed anxiolytics is diazepam. Diazepam can be used intravenously for controlling panic attacks. In acute overdose, benzodiazepines are much safer than older anxiolytic/hypnotic drugs such as barbiturates; this is an important consideration given that anxiolytic compounds may be used in suicide attempts. Overdose, in general, leads to prolonged sleep without depression of respiration or cardiovascular function. However, when benzodiazepines are taken in combination with other CNS depressants, such as alcohol, respiratory depression can become severe. If this occurs, patients can be treated with flumazenil, a benzodiazepine site antagonist.

5-HT$_{1A}$ agonists, such as buspirone, ipsapirone and gepirone, can be used in the treatment of generalized anxiety disorder instead of benzodiazepines. In contrast with the latter, buspirone and related compounds have a delay of action of at least 2 weeks, which makes compliance difficult. Unwanted effects include nausea, headaches and dizziness.

It is important to be aware that patients who have anxiety comorbid with depression tend to discontinue treatment early. It is considered preferable to address the anxiety component first (e.g. using a drug such as venlafaxine, which has a shorter onset of action). Resolution of anxiety improves patients' compliance.

Insomnia

Sleep is an essential physiological process and is controlled by several neuronal pathways that regulate the degree of wakefulness. The Viennese neurologist von Economo was the first to suggest, in 1930, that prolonged sleepiness is due to injury to neurons in the posterior hypothalamus and rostral midbrain. However, a real understanding of the complex circuitry that controls sleep and wakefulness was possible only during the last two decades of the 20th century. It gradually became possible to correlate the activity of neuronal groups with the different sleep phases (Box 16.8). An arousal system ('the ascending reticular activating system') consisting of monoaminergic and cholinergic neurons has been well described (Fig. 16.5). Cholinergic neurons from the pedunculopontine and laterodorsal tegmental nuclei project to several thalamic nuclei and modulate the activity of thalamocortical neurons. During wakefulness, cholinergic neurons fire rapidly. Their activity decreases during the first stages of sleep. In contrast, during rapid eye movement (REM) sleep, their activity increases again as a consequence of decreased monoamine-mediated inhibition. Monoaminergic control originates in the locus coeruleus (noradrenaline), raphe nuclei (5-HT) and tubero-mamillary nucleus (histamine). Neurons in these nuclei fire fast during wakefulness and gradually decrease their activity during sleep. They are almost completely inhibited during REM sleep. Neurons in the ventrolateral preoptic nucleus contain galanin and GABA. In contrast to cholinergic and monoaminergic neurons, they are active during sleep. Reciprocal connections exist between these various nuclei, as well as with other groups of neurons containing neuromodulatory peptides such as orexin (hypocretin). Orexin is a peptide produced in the hypothalamus and has a major role in the maintenance of wakefulness. The balance of activity in these various circuits involving neurotransmitters and neuromodulators is probably a major determining factor in the natural evolution of a sleep–wake cycle. Good quality sleep is essential for the maintenance of health, and in particular, for optimum mental performance. Following a set of simple rules, for example, avoiding prolonged exposure to blue light (such as that emitted by smartphones, tablets, computers, TV screens) at the end of the day, avoiding short naps during the day, reducing the consumption of caffeine late in the day and adhering to regular sleeping habits, can maintain sleep quality.

Sleep disorders are classified into primary sleep disorders and secondary sleep disorders, the latter being associated with other mental health problems, other medical conditions, or medication/substance misuse. Insomnia is defined as a disturbance of normal nocturnal sleep patterns that affects daily activities. Patients may have difficulty in initiating sleep, or difficulty in maintaining sleep (early-morning awakening or frequent nocturnal awakenings). Primary insomnia is diagnosed when present for at least 3 months and not attributable to other causes.

Insomnia can be transient, short-term or chronic. Transient insomnia can be caused by an acute disturbance or environmental stress (e.g. jetlag). Shift work may be associated with transient insomnia. It lasts for less than a week and usually resolves when the cause is eliminated, without intervention, or with only a brief exposure to a short-acting hypnotic drug. Short-term insomnia lasts longer (<3 months) and is often associated with stressors such as illness, or emotional upset caused by bereavement, loss of a job, etc.

Box
16.8   The neurobiology of sleep and wakefulness

Sleep is a necessary activity, as its disturbance leads to a decreased quality of life. However, the fundamental role of sleep remains incompletely understood. The suprachiasmatic nucleus—in the hypothalamus—acts as a master regulator of circadian rhythms and sleep-wake cycles.

During a normal night's sleep, there are usually five consecutive phases of sleep: stages 1, 2, 3 and 4 and rapid eye movement (REM) sleep. These stages progress in a cycle from stage 1 to REM sleep, and then a new cycle starts again with stage 1. A complete cycle lasts 90–120 min on average. The electrical activity of the brain is very different during each stage of this cycle (Fig. 16.4). Almost 50% of the total sleep time is spent in stage 2 sleep, approximately 20% in REM sleep and the remaining 30% in the other stages. Babies spend about half of their sleep time in REM sleep.

Stage 1 is light sleep, from which one can be awakened easily. Muscles are relaxed, but sudden muscle contractions (hypnic myoclonia), similar to a startle reaction while awake, are sometimes experienced. These may be preceded by a sensation of starting to fall. In stage 2 sleep, sudden bursts of rapid waves called sleep spindles start appearing on the electroencephalogram trace, on a background of slower electrical activity. In stage 3, extremely slow brain waves called delta waves begin to appear; these dominate in stage 4. Stages 3 and 4 are called deep sleep. There is no eye movement or muscle activity. People awakened during deep sleep do not adjust immediately and may feel disoriented for several minutes. It is during deep sleep that some children experience bedwetting. Sleepwalking can also occur during this phase.

The first REM sleep period usually occurs 70–90 min after the onset of sleep. During this phase, breathing is rapid, irregular and shallow, and the eyes move rapidly in the orbit. There are increases in heart rate and blood pressure, and males develop penile erections. Limb muscles become temporarily paralysed. When people are woken during REM sleep, they often describe dreams.

The first sleep cycles during the night contain relatively short REM periods and long periods of deep sleep. As the night progresses, REM sleep periods increase in length, and deep sleep periods decrease in length. By the morning, sleep consists almost entirely of stages 1 and 2 and REM sleep.

It is also notable that sleep patterns change as a function of age. Normal ageing is associated with changes in sleep patterns that mirror the neurophysiology of depression: reduced slow-wave sleep, reduced REM sleep latency and decreased continuity of sleep (i.e. more awakenings). These are accompanied by a blunting of body temperature rhythms and circadian cortisol variations.

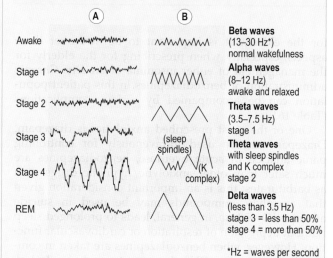

Fig. 16.4 Representation of the profiles of electrical activity of the brain during sleep stages: normal sleep electroencephalogram (A) and diagrammatic representation of types of electrical activity that appear in the various sleep stages (B). The wakeful/alert and relaxed/awake electroencephalogram and the rapid eye movement (REM) sleep electroencephalogram are characterized by desynchronized activity (alpha and beta waves), whereas stage 1 and especially stage 2, are characterised by the appearance of theta waves, which are slower and stronger than beta waves. Stages 3 and 4 are characterized by the gradual emergence of synchronized activity, represented by high altitude delta waves.

Chronic insomnia lasts longer than 3 months. It can be associated with a chronic underlying medical condition, with major psychiatric disease (e.g. depression) or chronic drug abuse. For example, in the case history, the patient suffers from insomnia. When a cause is suspected, it is important to attempt to first identify and treat the possible underlying problem, and then check if the insomnia persists. The first element of management is based on recommendations for improved sleep hygiene (e.g. good sleep environment, regular sleep schedule, avoidance of bright lights and noise or exposure to psychostimulants). Drugs that lead to improved sleep (hypnotics) can be used intermittently and for limited periods only. They should not be prescribed routinely. Non-pharmacological treatment could be attempted (e.g. use of cognitive behavioural therapy or relaxation techniques).

The pharmacological treatment of insomnia can involve the use of benzodiazepines. These drugs have replaced barbiturates for the treatment of this condition. Barbiturates such as pentobarbitone act as positive allosteric modulators at the GABA$_A$ receptor, like benzodiazepines, but they increase the duration of the opening of the chloride channel. At high doses, barbiturates can open the channel in the absence of GABA.

Benzodiazepines have different pharmacokinetic profiles (see Table 16.8); some of them have long half-lives, and they also have active metabolites leading to prolongation of the effect of the parent compound. A typical example is diazepam, whose metabolite N-desmethyldiazepam is active and has a longer half-life than the parent compound. This increases the risks of cumulative effects and a feeling of 'hangover' after use.

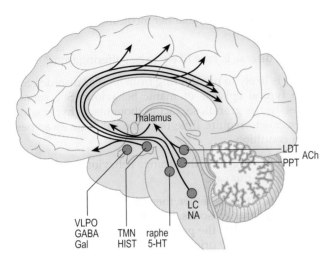

Fig. 16.5 Circuits involved in sleep and wakefulness: the ascending arousal system. Neurons of the laterodorsal tegmental nuclei (LDT) and pedunculopontine tegmental nuclei (PPT) send cholinergic fibres (ACh) to forebrain structures including the thalamus. Neurons of the tuberomamillary nucleus (TMN) contain histamine (HIST). Neurons of the raphe nuclei contain 5-HT, and neurons of the locus coeruleus (LC) contain noradrenaline (NA). Neurons of the ventrolateral preoptic nucleus (VLPO) contain GABA and galanin (Gal). (From Saper CB et al., The sleep switch: hypothalamic control of sleep and wakefulness, (2001), Trends In Neurosciences, 24: 726-731.)

Overall, benzodiazepines are much safer drugs than barbiturates and have larger therapeutic windows. Nevertheless, their use is associated with several unwanted effects:

- Change in sleep patterns: they suppress sleep stages 3 and 4. These stages of sleep are restorative, so benzodiazepine use does not lead to good sleep quality. They also suppress REM sleep. A rebound increase in REM sleep, accompanied by frightening dreams, may occur at the end of a period of treatment with benzodiazepine hypnotics.

- Daytime sedation: the use of benzodiazepines may be associated with sedation and a 'hangover' feeling and impaired psychomotor performance and concentration. This effect is particularly marked with long-acting benzodiazepines.

- Rebound insomnia: this phenomenon may occur at the end of treatment with short-acting or long-acting benzodiazepines. For example, administration of triazolam, for even one night, can lead to rebound insomnia on the night after treatment. This leads to chronic use of the drug and facilitates the development of dependence and the development of a vicious circle.

- Tolerance: the use of benzodiazepines is associated with tolerance, although the rate at which tolerance develops varies (it is faster for short-acting agents). Tolerance leads to the use of increasing doses.

Box 16.9 Benzodiazepine receptors for better sleep

Benzodiazepine 1 (BZ1) binding sites on GABA$_A$ receptors are located in brain areas involved in the control of sleep and wakefulness, whereas BZ2 binding sites on these receptors are present in areas involved in memory and cognition. Most benzodiazepine compounds do not differentiate between these two types, and this may account for their unwanted effects. Several non-benzodiazepine hypnotics are now available that have different selectivity for the subtypes of benzodiazepine binding site, and they offer the promise of being better than the existing drugs. Examples are zopiclone, zolpidem and zaleplon (also known as 'z-drugs'). These are short-acting compounds (pharmacokinetic data in Table 16.8) that act mainly as agonists at the BZ1 sites on the receptor complex.

Zolpidem is comparable in efficacy to short-acting benzodiazepines such as triazolam. However, it disturbs sleep patterns less. It does not depress respiration, which makes it safer in elderly patients or other patients with respiratory problems. It lacks anticonvulsant and muscle-relaxant properties. There is no evidence that zolpidem induces tolerance, rebound insomnia or withdrawal symptoms. Zopiclone binds to a site close to the benzodiazepine site on the GABA$_A$ receptor complex. It induces less sedation and respiratory depression than benzodiazepines. Tolerance is low, and rebound insomnia is more infrequent than with benzodiazepines. Zaleplon is a very short-acting compound, ideally suited for patients who have difficulty in initiating sleep. Because of its short half-life, it can be taken late at night, without having effects on performance and memory the next day. Its tolerance and abuse potential appear to be low. Therefore, in clinical practice, non-benzodiazepine compounds are preferable and safer alternatives to benzodiazepines.

- Physiological dependence: this is a significant problem associated with the long-term use of benzodiazepines. In order to limit this problem, intermittent use of drugs, for short durations, is recommended. Dependence is reflected in the emergence of a withdrawal syndrome (muscle cramps, increased anxiety, nausea and vomiting, sweating, photophobia, tremors and seizures). This syndrome can be minimized by gradual tapering of doses at the end of treatment.

Benzodiazepines can depress respiration and potentiate sleep apnoea. Therefore, in patients with compromised respiratory function, and particularly in elderly patients, benzodiazepines must be used carefully.

More recently, new non-benzodiazepine hypnotics have been developed, and they offer significant clinical advantages over previous drugs in the treatment of insomnia (Box 16.9). Finally, orexin receptor antagonists have recently emerged as interesting new therapeutics for insomnia.

Self-assessment case study

Jane is a young, aspiring actress. After a rather indifferent career start, she recently secured her first major role in a West End theatre production. One afternoon, her sister comes home to find Jane very busy unpacking a series of 40 travel books that she has just bought. Their flat is filled with the books for which there is no shelving or storage space. Her sister is concerned at the money spent by Jane and suggests that they should take some of the books back to the bookshop. Jane disagrees: she is in an ebullient good mood and cannot stop talking about the future and about her great projects. As tactfully as possible, her sister asks her about her medication. Jane dismisses the question and says that 'everything has changed now' and all her problems are part of the past. Her sister is worried, remembering how depressed Jane was only a few months ago, a state in total contrast to her present exuberance.

One late morning, after 4 days during which Jane is barely seen at home, as she seems to share her time between her work in the studio and going out all night, indulging in drink binges, her sister receives a phone call from the police. Jane has been caught stealing from a store. Her response is that 'she could not wait in the queue because it was too slow'. After a discussion with the police and her general practitioner, Jane is brought home and care is taken that her medication is immediately reinstated.

1. What disease is Jane likely to be suffering from?

Jane is likely to be suffering from bipolar disorder. She has a typical episode of manic behaviour. She spends recklessly, has grandiose, racing thoughts, is hyperactive and seems to require little rest. She has little awareness of her condition.

2. What has triggered the strange behaviour of the patient in this case?

It is uncertain whether there are specific triggers for bipolar disorder episodes. The disease evolves in cycles, and it appears that the patient has already experienced a depressive episode prior to this manic attack.

3. What is the best management for this type of case?

Jane is likely to have received a mood stabiliser, such as lithium, carbamazepine or sodium valproate, but she may have stopped taking the medication. Management of her manic phase would consist of immediate reinstatement of lithium treatment or another mood stabiliser and also prescription of an antipsychotic drug (e.g. olanzapine, quetiapine or risperidone). Antidepressant drugs should be discontinued, gradually. There should be close monitoring of her compliance and response to the drugs.

ADDICTION

17

Chapter summary

1. Addiction is a complex medical condition, characterized by compulsive drug seeking and drug use, and intense cravings that are difficult to control. This substance use disorder may involve a variety of compounds, such as alcohol, nicotine, cannabis, opiates, amphetamines and substituted amphetamines. Addictive behavioural patterns may also develop in connection with habits such as compulsive gambling.

2. The addiction cycle is characterized by three phases: (a) binge/intoxication, (b) withdrawal/anhedonia and (c) preoccupation/craving. The reward experienced during misuse of many drugs, in particular in the first exposure/intoxication phase, involves activation of reward pathways such as the mesolimbic dopaminergic projections. Subsequently, there is involvement of additional structures, such as the hippocampus, amygdala and prefrontal cortex, and additional neurotransmitter systems.

3. The development of addiction involves changes in gene transcription programmes and can lead to significant structural and functional changes in the nervous system. The specific targets of drugs of abuse may also undergo up- or down-regulation, leading to behavioural changes that become apparent during the manifestations of drug-withdrawal states. Many misused drugs can induce a combination of psychological and physical dependence.

4. The management of addiction is challenging and there are frequent relapses across all types of addiction. Treatment involves pharmacological and non-pharmacological approaches. Examples of drug therapies include: (a) methadone, buprenorphine and naloxone for opiate addiction, (b) use of disulfiram, acamprosate and naltrexone for alcohol-use disorder, and (c) nicotine-replacement therapy and varenicline for tobacco addiction. Behavioural approaches include cognitive-behavioural therapy and contingency management.

Introduction

The compulsion of humans to repeatedly use specific substances or develop certain persistent habits, with significant negative consequences, in order to obtain a general feeling of well-being and pleasure, to relieve sadness or induce euphoria, and to alter their perception of the world, can be traced back to ancient times and remains a characteristic feature of human society. 'If we could sniff or swallow something that would, for five or six hours each day, abolish our solitude as individuals, atone us with our fellows in a glowing exaltation of affection and make life in all its aspects seem not only worth living, but divinely beautiful and significant, and if this heavenly, world-transfiguring drug were of such a kind that we could wake up next morning with a clear head and an undamaged constitution—then, it seems to me, all our problems (and not merely the one small problem of discovering a novel pleasure) would be wholly solved and earth would become paradise,' said the writer Aldous Huxley. Unfortunately, seeking pleasure or consolation through psychoactive substances or certain repetitive behavioural patterns, is far from safe and the long-lasting consequences can be dramatic. Drug abuse (also called drug misuse or substance use disorder) and the development of addiction to drugs or habits such as gambling is a problem with considerable negative consequences, both for the individual and society. An example of addiction is illustrated in the case history in Box 17.1, and this case also encapsulates some of the misconceptions associated with drug abuse.

Addiction and drug misuse: general comments

'Ecstasy' and cocaine, which are mentioned in the case history, are two examples of drugs that can be misused by people irrespective of age, social background, gender or race. Some drugs are mainly used intermittently, such as 'ecstasy', which is used in a recreational context, whereas the misuse of others becomes part of daily life; especially for the latter, there is an irresistible drive to use them on a regular, permanent basis, and this reflects a state of strong physical and/or psychological dependence. Some of the substances misused can be quite common and widely accessible such as nicotine or alcohol. What is dispiriting is the significant percentage of young people worldwide who use and abuse drugs. Misuse of drugs has acute consequences, reflected in the number of admissions to emergency units. Fig. 17.1A shows that more than half of admissions in several European countries are correlated with three major misused drugs: cannabis, cocaine and heroin. According to data reported in 2020 in the UK, the prevalence of any drug use in the previous year was highest amongst 16–19-year-olds and 20–24-year-olds (21.1% and 21%, respectively). This significant impact of drug misuse on the young is also reflected in Fig. 17.1B. Apart from the acute, immedi-

Box 17.1 Case history

Sarah J., a vivacious 17-year-old, went out with her friend James on a Friday night to meet other friends, drink and dance, and 'have a good time' before the end-of-year examinations. Everything went well until around midnight, when Sarah took two 'ecstasy' pills. A short time after that, she started feeling ill and dizzy. The temperature in the club had been high, and Sarah kept drinking alcoholic drinks and a lot of water to compensate for the dehydration caused by hours of dancing. At about 3 a.m., she felt sick and vomited several times, complaining of a terrible headache. James took her to a friend's house nearby for a rest, but Sarah's state deteriorated rapidly. She kept vomiting and drifted in and out of consciousness. James and his friend took her to hospital around 6 a.m. and phoned her parents. The doctors immediately suspected intoxication with 'ecstasy', and her blood Na^+ level (123 mmol/L) confirmed their suspicion. After a day in hospital, her situation remained critical and the consultant expressed reserved optimism as to her survival. Sarah's state gradually started improving the next day. James is puzzled and explains that she only took some 'ecstasy' pills, as usual, and cannot see the harm in it. He argues that it was only 'a little bit of fun' and that neither he nor Sarah 'have done any hard stuff like cocaine', as some of his older friends do.

This case gives rise to the following questions:

1. What has led to Sarah's critical state after her use of 'ecstasy'?
2. Is 'ecstasy' a safe drug, and what differentiates it from cocaine?
3. What is the incentive that leads to the use of life-threatening drugs?
4. Is it correct to assume that there are 'hard' and unsafe drugs of abuse, in contrast to 'light' and generally safe drugs?
5. What treatment saved Sarah's life after admission to hospital?

ate impact of addictions, there are also life-long consequences, including the heightened risk of developing additional mental health disorders and major medical complications. For example, addicts who use drugs by injectable routes are at high risk of infections with the hepatitis C virus or human immunodeficiency virus (HIV), from the sharing of injection-related material.

As a preamble to the discussion of various substances that are abused, it is useful to define some of the concepts discussed in this chapter. Addiction is defined as a compulsion to take a drug, with loss of control over drug taking, and it is considered a psychiatric disease in the Diagnostic and Statistical Manual of Mental Disorders, fifth edition (DSM-5). This chronic relapsing disorder is characterized by the inability to limit or stop drug intake. Tolerance refers to the necessity to escalate the drug dose in order to obtain the same effects as those obtained initially. Sensitization, in

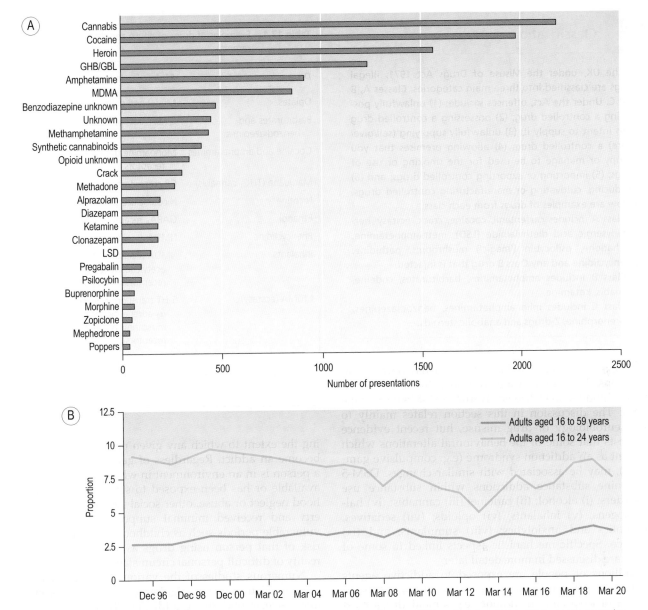

Fig. 17.1 (A) Top 25 drugs associated with admissions to emergency services in a selection of 27 sentinel hospitals in 19 European countries. *GHB/GBL*, γ-hydroxybutyrate/γ-butyrolactone; *LSD*, lysergic acid diethylamide. *MDMA*, methylenedioxymethamphetamine. (B) The proportion of users of Class A drugs in England and Wales as a function of age. (A, From the European Drug Report 2020, European Monitoring Centre for Drugs and Drug Addiction. B, From the Office for National Statistics, Crime Survey for England and Wales, 2020.)

contrast to tolerance, refers to a gradually enhanced effect of drugs that are misused chronically. Dependence refers to drug-induced adaptations in cells and tissues after prolonged use, which leads to the need to continue drug intake. The abrupt cessation of drug intake can lead to a withdrawal syndrome, which has both physical and psychological components. Psychological dependence involves emotional symptoms such as dysphoria, depression, anhedonia and restlessness. Physical dependence involves significant unpleasant physical–somatic symptoms such as fatigue, nausea, seizures, pain and autonomic hyperactivity.

Drugs that are misused are subject to specific regulations defined by national laws (described for the UK in

Box 17.2). Table 17.1 shows examples of drugs that are misused and their main molecular targets. They belong to a wide range of pharmacological classes. Some common mechanisms involved in the development of addiction are discussed and the examples of specific types of misused drugs are reviewed.

Neurobiology of addiction

Addictions are diseases (although some may prefer the term 'conditions' and not 'diseases') of the brain associated with complex and widespread neurobiological

In the UK, under the Misuse of Drugs Act 1971, illegal drugs are classified into three main categories: Classes A, B and C. Under the Act, offences include: (1) unlawfully possessing a controlled drug; (2) possessing a controlled drug with intent to supply it; (3) unlawfully supplying (sell/give/share) a controlled drug; (4) allowing premises that you occupy or manage to be used for the smoking or use of drugs; (5) importing or exporting controlled drugs; and (6) producing, cultivating or manufacturing controlled drugs. Below are examples of drugs from each class.

Class A includes carfentanil, cocaine, crack, ecstasy, heroin, lysergic acid diethylamide (LSD), methamphetamine, methadone, psilocybin ('magic') mushrooms, pethidine, phencyclidine and any Class B drug that is injected.

Class B includes amphetamines, barbiturates, codeine, cannabis, ketamine.

Class C includes mild amphetamines, benzodiazepines, buprenorphine, Z-drugs and anabolic steroids.

Table 17.1 Examples of drugs of abuse and their main cellular targets

Drugs	Molecular targets
Opiates	Mu (μ) and delta (δ) opioid receptors
Barbiturates and benzodiazepines	$GABA_A$ receptors
Cocaine and amphetamines	Monoamine transporters, TAAR1 receptors
Marijuana (THC, cannabis)	CB_1 receptors
Nicotine	Nicotinic acetylcholine receptors
Ethanol	$GABA_A$ receptors, NMDA receptors
Phencyclidine	NMDA receptors
Inhalants	NMDA receptors? Nicotinic acetylcholine receptors? $GABA_A$ receptors? $5\text{-}HT_3$ receptors?
MDMA (ecstasy)	5-HT transporter, $5\text{-}HT_2$ receptors, α_2-adrenergic receptors, M_1 muscarinic receptors, H_1 histamine receptors

5-HT, 5-hydroxytryptamine; CB, cannabinoid; GABA, γ-aminobutyric acid; NMDA, N-methyl-D-aspartate; TAAR1, trace amine-associated receptor 1.

changes and characterized by specific behavioural manifestations. They are considered among the most incompletely understood chronic dysfunctional states of the brain. The discussion in this section relates mainly to the neurobiology of drug misuse, but recent evidence suggests that some of the behavioural alterations which present as an addiction syndrome (e.g. compulsive gambling), may be associated with similar changes. DSM-5 lists nine substance addictions within substance use disorders: (i) alcohol; (ii) caffeine; (iii) cannabis; (iv) hallucinogens; (v) inhalants; (vi) opioids; (vii) sedatives, hypnotics and anxiolytics; (viii) stimulants; and (ix) tobacco. Specific mechanistic aspects linked to some of these are discussed in more detail later.

Millions of people are exposed to addictive agents each year (either in an illegal context or within the period of use of a specific medication, e.g. opioid drugs used for pain-relief) but only a minority develop addictions. Genetic factors play a role both in experimentation with drugs and the transition to addiction. Approximately 50% of the risk of developing addiction is linked to genetic factors; heritability is lower for hallucinogens and highest for cocaine. The genetic risk for addiction is polygenic, and there are genes that have been associated with multiple addictions or addiction to specific substances only. The genes encode a variety of proteins and examples include dopaminergic D_2 receptors, nicotinic cholinergic receptor subunits, the 5-hydroxytryptamine (5-HT) transporter and the noradrenaline transporter, the $5\text{-}HT_3$ receptor, the monoamine-degrading enzymes monoamine oxidase (MAO_A) and catechol-O-methyltransferase (COMT), corticotropin-releasing factor (CRF) receptor 1 and the opioid mu receptor. Evidence suggests that epigenetic mechanisms are also involved in addiction, but it is clear that environmental factors are very important in modulat-

ing the extent to which any given person will ultimately become an addict. Regardless of genetic vulnerability, if a person is in an environment in which drugs are widely available or has been exposed to stresses such as childhood neglect or abuse, other social stressors such as poverty and received minimal support during especially vulnerable periods such as childhood or adolescence, the risk of that person using drugs as a way to escape the reality of difficult personal circumstances becomes high.

Numerous studies of the various types of drug that can be misused have highlighted some common cellular aspects underlying addiction. There is strong evidence that the dopaminergic mesolimbic system, with its origin in the midbrain ventral tegmental area (VTA) and projection to the nucleus accumbens, plays a major role from the very early stage of addiction (Fig. 17.2). The dopaminergic mesolimbic system is associated with both natural rewards and the reward induced by addictive drugs. It has been suggested that the powerful effect of addictive drugs may be due to the inability of the brain to distinguish between activation of reward circuitry by natural stimuli such as food or sex, and activation by drugs. Addictive drugs appear to 'hijack' the body's natural response, and stimulate the reward circuits with an intensity that is overwhelming and superior to that of natural stimuli. Although addictive drugs belong to a variety of pharmacological classes, many of them (psychostimulants in particular) increase the levels of dopamine in the nucleus accumbens. Some of them act directly in the VTA, and others activate endogenous

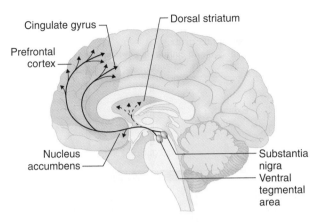

Cingulate gyrus

Dorsal striatum

Prefrontal cortex

Nucleus accumbens

Substantia nigra

Ventral tegmental area

Fig. 17.2 The dopaminergic projections associated with reward and addiction. Projections from the ventral tegmental area to the nucleus accumbens (the mesolimbic pathway), and from the ventral tegmental area to the prefrontal cerebral cortex and cingulate gyrus (mesocortical pathway). Also shown is the projection from the substantia nigra to the dorsal striatum (caudate and putamen) that has a role in habit formation and motor behaviours related to drug use. (From Nestler EJ. Goldman-Cecil Medicine, Published January 1, 2020. pp. 137–9.e2. © 2020. From Hyman SE, Malenka RC, Nestler EJ. (2006) Neural mechanisms of addiction: the role of reward-related learning and memory. Annual Review of Neuroscience 29:565–98.)

opioid pathways that ultimately lead to activation of the VTA dopaminergic neurons (e.g. alcohol and nicotine). Dopaminergic cells have a complex response to rewarding stimuli. When the reward is still novel and unanticipated, the dopamine neurons fire intensely. After a prolonged period of repeated exposure to the reward, dopaminergic neurons fire in anticipation of the reward. If a predicted reward is not presented, the firing of cells is suppressed. If, on the contrary, the reward exceeds expectation, the firing of the cells is amplified. The increased release of dopamine in the nucleus accumbens then leads to an increased activity of nucleus accumbens neurons, which project back to the VTA, releasing γ-aminobutyric acid (GABA) and dynorphin. Evidence suggests that the increased release of dynorphin onto dopaminergic neurons and the associated activation of kappa opioid receptors, which exerts an inhibitory effect, is associated with the dysphoria experienced after cessation of drug intake and during the emergence of withdrawal.

Several other brain structures are also involved in the addiction process as it unfolds through repetition of the three key elements of bingeing, withdrawal and craving/anticipation. For example, the craving for a drug long after withdrawal symptoms have vanished and the relapse upon exposure to certain cues, involves structures such as the amygdala, prefrontal cortex and hippocampus. Experimental evidence shows that drug-associated cues can elicit activation of these areas. Imaging studies in addictive behaviours have identified a key role for the prefrontal cortex, whose dysfunction in addiction is linked to the major changes in executive function seen in addicts: loss of self-control, impaired salience attribution and the lack of awareness

and insight. Concerning the neurotransmitters involved, apart from dopamine, there is evidence of involvement of noradrenaline, glutamate and stress-associated factors such as CRF. A summary of the complex circuitry and various structures involved in maintenance of the addicted state is shown in Fig. 17.3.

Prolonged exposure to drugs triggers complex and long-lasting changes in gene expression and also epigenetic changes. Among the various cellular transcription factors regulated by drugs of abuse, two have received particular attention: the cyclic AMP response-element-binding (CREB) protein and the transcription factor ΔFosB. CREB is a transcription factor that regulates the expression of genes containing a cyclic AMP-responsive element in their regulatory regions. For example, chronic opiate or cocaine exposure leads to a significant increase in the expression of CREB in several brain regions. Interestingly, transgenic animals with a mutated CREB gene show decreased dependence after chronic opiate administration. However, changes in CREB are reversed within a week of drug intake cessation. Therefore, it is likely that they are involved only in the subacute changes induced by abused drugs, and in particular the withdrawal phase. In contrast, ΔFosB is a much stronger candidate for playing a role in long-term changes. As shown in Fig. 17.4, the acute single administration of a drug can induce a transient increase in the expression of the transcription factor c-fos. Administration of a drug of abuse also induces upregulation of members of the Fos-related antigen (Fras) family of proteins in the nucleus accumbens. The upregulation is transient for Fras proteins (although longer than that of c-fos), apart from certain ΔFosB isoforms, which are much more stable. Upon chronic exposure, the modifications in these isoforms, although discrete at the beginning, begin to take on increasing importance and the cumulative effect is significant. As a result, ΔFosB persists in the brain for a long time and may act as a master regulator of sustained transcriptional changes. ΔFosB acts as a heterodimer with Jun family proteins, to form a complex—activator protein 1 (AP1)—which binds to gene regulatory elements.

Epigenetic changes seen after acute and chronic drug exposure include increased histone acetylation, altered DNA methylation and also changes in the levels of specific miRNAs (non-coding RNAs, which can act as repressors of translation, therefore leading to silencing of gene expression). Very interesting recent developments in addiction research show that specific epigenetic inhibitors are able to reduce the rewarding effects of drugs such as heroin, thus opening new therapeutic avenues.

Finally, it has been shown experimentally that drugs of abuse, such as cocaine and amphetamine, can induce significant and long-lasting structural changes, such as increased branching of dendrites and an increased number of dendritic spines on neurons in structures such as the prefrontal cortex and nucleus accumbens. Such structural changes alter synaptic dynamics and can be seen for a very long time after cessation of drug intake.

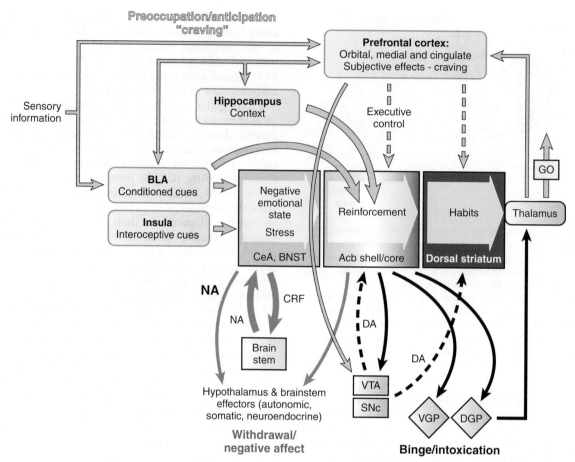

Fig. 17.3 The circuits involved in the three stages of the addiction cycle: binge intoxication, withdrawal and craving. Multiple adaptations occur during the development of addiction as a chronic state. The extended amygdala, nucleus accumbens and dorsal striatum are persistently driven by cues, the prefrontal cortex loses executive control, and there is increased nucleus accumbens to ventral tegmental area output underlying the dysphoria, which drives the addict to maintain drug intake. The dotted lines indicate gradual reduction in activity. *Acb*, Nucleus accumbens; *BLA*, basolateral amygdala; *BNST*, bed nucleus stria terminalis; *CeA*, central amygdala; *CRF*, corticotropin-releasing factor; *DA*, dopamine; *DGP*, dorsal globus pallidus; *NA*, noradrenaline; *SNc*, substantia nigra compacta; *VGP*, ventral globus pallidus; *VTA*, ventral tegmental area. (From Koob GF, Volkow ND. (2010) Neuropsychopharmacology Reviews 35:217–38. Nature Publishing Group.)

Opiates

Opium is the dried juice of the unripe seed capsule of the poppy *Papaver somniferum*. The ancient Greeks and Romans were aware of the sedative and euphoria-inducing properties of opium, as well as its analgesic and anti-diarrhoea effects. In the 19th century opium was a commodity that was freely available. Morphine (or 'morphia') was introduced in the 1820s, and the hypodermic syringe in the 1850s. The German company Bayer produced heroin in 1898 and described it as a 'heroic drug, that has the ability of morphine to relieve pain, yet is safer'. The number of prescriptions soared and the Ebert Prescription Survey in the USA in 1885 showed that the ingredients most used in medicines were quinine and morphine. Doctors became aware of the emergence of dependence and withdrawal symptoms, and addiction became defined as a disease. In 1934 the term 'drug addiction' first appeared in the American Psychiatric Association's diagnostic handbook.

Opiate drugs ('opiate' and 'opioid' are interchangeable terms in this context; 'opiate' refers more to compounds derived from opium) exert their effects by binding to opioid receptors. Of the three opioid receptor types—mu (μ), kappa (κ) and delta (δ)—it is the mu type that is critical for the addictive effects of morphine and heroin. Blockade of this receptor type reduces self-administration of opiates in experimental animals. Agonists at mu receptors activate dopaminergic neurons in the VTA and enhance dopamine release in the nucleus accumbens. This activation is indirect, through inhibition of GABAergic neurons. The mesolimbic dopaminergic pathway, shown in Fig. 17.2, is involved in the reward mechanisms underlying the abuse of several drugs, as discussed in the previous section. Dopamine released from the mesolimbic terminals can modulate the glutamatergic cortical input received by medium-sized spiny output neurons in the nucleus accumbens. After chronic exposure to opiates such as morphine and heroin, functional changes occur in the mesolimbic dopaminergic

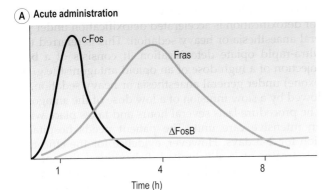

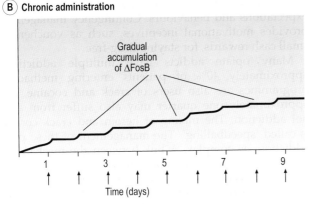

Fig. 17.4 Regulation of genes encoding transcription factors by drugs of abuse. (A) Acute administration of drugs of abuse leads to a marked transient increase in c-Fos, a smaller but more durable increase in certain Fos-related antigens (acute Fras) and a small but very long-lasting increase in ΔFosB. (B) Upon chronic exposure, the effect on ΔFosB becomes cumulative (bottom panel).

neurons. Upon cessation of drug intake, decreased dopaminergic transmission in the mesolimbic dopaminergic pathway (partly triggered by dynorphin input from the nucleus accumbens) may underlie the anhedonia and dysphoria experienced in this phase. It has been suggested that the need to avoid this strongly aversive state leads to the reinstatement of drug use. It is known that stress is one of the main factors in relapse. Stress responsiveness appears to be influenced by the intensity of the previous exposure to the addictive drug; the more prolonged or intense the exposure, the higher the risk of relapse after a stressful experience.

Heroin is the typical opiate drug used by addicts. Heroin is diacetylmorphine; acetylation leads to higher lipid solubility than that of morphine and increased availability to the brain. Heroin can be injected, sniffed, snorted or smoked. An overdose of heroin can induce death through respiratory depression. The intravenous administration of heroin leads to an intense euphoria, described as a 'rush', and a feeling of intense pleasure. This is soon followed by dysphoria. If drug administration is not reinstated, the first symptoms of the withdrawal syndrome emerge. The signs and symptoms of the withdrawal syndrome vary in intensity according to the dosage and duration of opiate exposure.

At approximately 8–12 h after the last dose, the user experiences headaches, irritation and anxiety, muscular aches and pains, and can become agitated and aggressive; there is restlessness and difficulty sleeping, loss of appetite, sweating, rhinorrhoea, tremor and drug craving. After another 1–2 days, nausea, vomiting and gastrointestinal symptoms become intense. In this later phase, heart rate and blood pressure increase, and there are alternating chills and intense sweating, and diarrhoea-linked dehydration. The phrases 'cold turkey' and 'kicking the habit' that are used to describe withdrawal reflect the gooseflesh and muscle spasms that occur in the arms and legs, respectively. Towards the end of the first week, withdrawal starts to subside, and there is fatigue, depressed mood and insomnia. The post-acute withdrawal syndrome can continue for months after the last dose and symptoms may include persistent tiredness, depression, sleep disturbance and drug craving. The withdrawal syndrome may only last for a couple of weeks, but the drug craving may continue for many years and never fully subside. Clonidine and other α_2-adrenergic agonists alleviate symptoms of autonomic hyperactivity during withdrawal, which may be due to excessive release of noradrenaline. Clonidine stimulates presynaptic receptors, leading to reduction in noradrenergic tone, and thus helps to ameliorate some of the more distressing symptoms of heroin withdrawal. A small proportion of patients prescribed clonidine may develop hypotension. Lofexidine is a drug similar to clonidine but with possibly fewer adverse cardiovascular effects. The adrenergic agonists are usually used in combination with several other drugs to provide symptomatic relief. These drugs include paracetamol for bone pain, diphenoxylate or loperamide for control of diarrhoea, and hyoscine to control abdominal cramps. Benzodiazepines such as nitrazepam can be used for the short-term treatment of insomnia during withdrawal.

Opioid misuse affects large numbers of individuals worldwide and there is clear evidence that it can be initiated by the misuse of prescribed opioid drugs. Prescription opioid analgesics such as oxycodone have effects similar to heroin and their misuse may open the door to heroin use. Statistics from 2017 show that 1.7 million individuals in the United States suffered from opiate misuse linked to the abuse of prescribed opioid drugs, and more than 0.6 million were specifically affected by heroin use disorder. Opioids alone account for approximately 50,000 deaths in the United States each year. This is 20,000 more people than those dying from prostate cancer and 10,000 more than those dying from breast cancer. Heroin users are largely intravenous drug users, and they often suffer from and die of diseases associated with their dangerous and promiscuous lifestyles: HIV infection, hepatitis B or C infection, and sexually transmitted diseases. Contrary to the view that opiate addiction occurs only in a limited section of society and affects mainly socially marginalized people, heroin addiction cuts across the social spectrum. Patients enrolled in detoxification programmes include students, lawyers, artists, bankers and doctors. A major hurdle during opioid detoxification remains the intense withdrawal syndrome experienced by individuals.

The treatment of opiate-dependent patients consists of a detoxification phase, during which withdrawal symptoms are managed as described above, and then a regimen of substitution to prevent relapse. One of the most used regimens is methadone substitution. Methadone is an orally active, long-acting opioid drug. It acts preferentially at mu receptors and also has some weak N-methyl-D-aspartate (NMDA) receptor antagonist activity. Its long half-life leads to a constant level of stimulation of the opioid receptors. Taken orally once a day, methadone suppresses withdrawal symptoms for between 24 and 36 h. Because methadone is effective in eliminating withdrawal symptoms, it is the opioid drug of choice for detoxifying addicts. Methadone reduces the cravings associated with heroin use and blocks the 'high' from heroin. For many addicts, 12 months of maintenance is an appropriate duration, whereas other addicts may require maintenance for years. For most patients, optimal results are achieved with a dose of 60–100 mg/day, although careful titration and use of higher doses may be required in other patients. The lack of development of tolerance to methadone may be due to its NMDA receptor antagonist properties, as it has been suggested that NMDA receptors are involved in the development of tolerance.

Methadone produces no serious unwanted effects. Some patients may experience constipation, water retention, drowsiness and skin rashes. In a survey of the National Institute on Drug Abuse, it was reported that the weekly heroin use of addicts decreased by 69% while they were on methadone maintenance. This allows the patient to reintegrate into normal life and even full-time employment, and thus stops the life of crime that was required to sustain the drug habit. Methadone maintenance programmes help to reduce the risk of infection in addicts, resulting from intravenous drug use. Methadone also helps with the management of addiction in convicted addicts. However, the absolute efficacy in terms of relieving opiate addiction remains controversial, as many argue that one addiction is replaced by another and the core problem remains unsolved. Buprenorphine, a partial agonist at mu receptors, can also be used. It has the advantage of being more difficult to overdose, but its efficacy remains lower than that of methadone, even at high doses. Opioid antagonists such as naloxone or naltrexone can also be used in the management of addiction. Naltrexone slow-release preparations can be used in detoxification to provide a constant block of opioid receptors. Overall, it is considered that buprenorphine or buprenorphine–naloxone combinations, may be valuable for the treatment of addiction, especially in the early phase of treatment, with conversion to methadone maintenance only at a later stage. Although all these medications (methadone, buprenorphine, naloxone/naltrexone) significantly improve clinical outcomes and reduce the risk of overdoses, major challenges remain regarding patient compliance and relapse. Another method used for detoxification is accelerated detoxification under general anaesthesia or heavy sedation. This is referred to as ultra-rapid opiate detoxification. It consists of a bolus injection of a high dose of an opioid antagonist (e.g. naloxone) under general anaesthesia or heavy sedation, followed by a slow infusion of a low dose of the antagonist. The procedure lasts several hours and takes place within an intensive care unit. The patient needs hospitalization for 2–3 days. However, evidence for the efficacy of this treatment is still limited. Behavioural therapies for heroin addiction include cognitive behavioural therapy and contingency management. Cognitive behavioural therapy helps to modify the patient's thought patterns, expectations and behaviours. Contingency management provides motivational incentives, such as vouchers or small cash rewards, for staying drug-free.

Many opiate addicts have multiple addictions: approximately 40% of patients entering methadone programmes are also users of crack and cocaine, and approximately one quarter may also suffer from alcohol addiction. The mixing of heroin and crack cocaine is called 'speedballing'. The management of these poly-addictions is complex. A link between the mechanisms involved in various simultaneous addictions is the fact that the percentage of opiate/cocaine addicts who continue to use cocaine after 1 year of methadone maintenance falls to around 30%, highlighting a possible role of an endogenous opioid tone in cocaine addiction.

Cocaine and crack

Cocaine is an alkaloid present in the leaves of the shrub *Erythroxylon coca*. In pre-Columbian history coca leaves were reserved for the royal Incas. Their stimulant properties countered fatigue and hunger and boosted physical endurance, especially at high altitudes. The Spanish conquistadores introduced coca leaves to Europe, and in 1860 cocaine was isolated by Albert Niemann. A coca leaf contains 0.1%–0.8% cocaine. Cocaine use became widespread after its introduction into Europe. Coca Cola was initially sold as a 'brain tonic and cure for all nervous afflictions', and until 1904 contained small amounts of cocaine. There are approximately two million users of cocaine in the United States, and cocaine is the major cause of strokes and heart attacks in people under the age of 35 years. In 2019 approximately 70% of all drug users in the UK were taking cocaine; 91% of cocaine users aged between 19 and 45 years were also found to abuse two or more other substances alongside cocaine.

The cocaine most commonly used is in the form of a salt—cocaine hydrochloride. The drug inhibits the reuptake of dopamine, noradrenaline and serotonin. It also has local anaesthetic effects (as well as being a potent vasoconstrictor, which is useful during surgery). When taken systemically, it leads to an increase in the release of dopamine in the nucleus accumbens, and therefore increased transmission in the mesolimbic pathway. Cocaine can be snorted or injected. Its effects reflect its psychostimulant properties. It induces enhanced mood and self-confidence and increases libido. Crack cocaine is a form of cocaine that can be smoked. When cocaine in its salt form is heated, it is converted to the base and this substance makes a cracking noise when heated (hence its name). It vaporizes at relatively low temperatures, so it can be inhaled through a heated pipe. Crack cocaine induces strong sensations of pleasure, which are described by addicts as a 'whole-body orgasm'. The intense stimulation and euphoria are followed by a 'crash', characterized by depression, anxiety, irritability and paranoid delusions. Regular users of crack may develop hallucinations, such as formication (insects crawling under the skin) and a form of delirium. During crack cocaine binges lasting several days, users can consume a large amount of the drug. The habit becomes expensive and crack users will commit theft or violent crime in order to be able to sustain their consumption of the drug, a pattern of behaviour common in those with 'hard' drug addictions.

Regular ingestion of cocaine by snorting can damage the nasal membranes and smoking of crack may lead to partial loss of voice. As cocaine is a very strong sympathomimetic, high doses and chronic exposure have significant adverse cardiovascular effects: hypertension, tachycardia and risk of myocardial infarction. Seizures or extreme agitation associated with overdose can be treated with anticonvulsants and dopaminergic antagonists. Recent studies have also shown that cocaine can be rapidly cleared from the body after infusion of butyrylcholinesterase.

There is still debate about whether cocaine or crack induce tolerance or withdrawal in a similar manner to heroin. It is well established that regular users experience distressing symptoms if they stop taking the drug. They may feel tired and exhausted but unable to sleep, suffer from diarrhoea and vomiting, and experience intense anxiety. Dependence is not inevitable and may well be determined by individual characteristics.

Treatment for cocaine addiction is notoriously difficult. Cocaine is one of the most potent and addictive psychostimulants known and there are no available pharmacotherapies to treat successfully cocaine addiction. Despite the significant health risks associated with cocaine abuse, >95% of cocaine addicts who try to quit fail. As with treatment for opiate addiction, there is first a detoxification phase, and then an abstinence phase, during which relapse must be prevented. In the acute phase, β-receptor blockers such as propranolol may offer symptomatic relief. For the later phase, several categories of drug have been tried, with limited or no success. These include: (1) dopamine receptor antagonists (e.g. haloperidol, flupenthixol and risperidone); (2) dopamine receptor agonists (e.g. pergolide and bromocriptine); (3) dopamine receptor partial agonists (e.g. terguride); (4) dopamine reuptake inhibitors (e.g. amantadine and methylphenidate); (5) monoamine oxidase (MAO) inhibitors (e.g. selegiline); (6) antidepressant drugs (e.g. imipramine, desipramine, fluoxetine and venlafaxine); (7) Ca^{2+} channel blockers (e.g. nimodipine); (8) β-blockers (e.g. propranolol); and (9) opioid antagonists (e.g. naltrexone). The most promising recent strategies involve the use of long-acting dextroamphetamine and the GABA agonist/glutamate antagonist topiramate. Encouraging results have also been reported in studies of the cholinesterase inhibitor galantamine and modafinil, a mild stimulant that blocks the dopamine transporter. Psychotherapy interventions remain the treatment of choice and include contingency management and cognitive behavioural therapy.

One of the most recently explored, novel strategies to treat cocaine addiction involves the use of a vaccine. A cocaine vaccine works by triggering the formation of antibodies against the drug. These bind the drug and prevent it from accessing the brain. The majority of work in developing vaccines against addiction has been conducted in the field of cocaine and nicotine addiction. Preliminary results are promising and vaccines for cocaine and nicotine are now in clinical trials. However, there are certain aspects of the use of vaccines in addicts that still cause concern: (1) lack of protection against a structurally dissimilar drug (which would not be recognized by antibodies); (2) lack of effect of the vaccine on drug craving, which triggers relapse; and (3) the variability between individuals in antibody formation. The induction of passive immunity, by administering the antibody and not the vaccine, is also under investigation.

Cannabis

Cannabis (marijuana) is the most widely abused drug in the UK, and this has been the case for at least the last 20 years. In 2019/20, approximately 30% of people in England and Wales aged between 16–59 years had used cannabis at least once during their lifetime. There are at present over 250 million cannabis users worldwide, with the highest number of users found in Asia, followed by the Americas and Africa. Cannabis is the dried female flower of *Cannabis sativa*. Pyrolysis leads to the formation of several dozen compounds that are inhaled when a cannabis cigarette is smoked. The plant contains several psychoactive substances, but the most significant is the terpenoid Δ-9-tetrahydrocannabinol (THC). The content of THC in the cannabis flower is between 2% and 5%, whereas the THC content of hashish (resin-soaked flower buds) is closer to 20%. More recently, stronger types of cannabis have become available, such as 'super skunk'. Smoking of cannabis is associated with a THC bioavailability of 18%, whereas the consumption of THC in cakes or teas is associated with a bioavailability of approximately 6%. The effects of cannabis are use- and context-dependent. Overall, cannabis has a mild sedative effect and users describe a feeling of relaxation. First-time users may experience feelings of panic or anxiety. The smoking of cannabis leads to decreased blood pressure and bloodshot eyes, a feeling of dizziness and an increased appetite. Memory and coordination can also be transiently affected (Box 17.3).

A potted history of 'dope'

Cannabis, or the hemp plant *(Cannabis sativa)*, originated in central Asia. The earliest evidence of hemp use comes from the Neolithic age, with pieces of hemp cloth being found in archaeological sites in western China. It is likely that it was cultivated by the Anglo-Saxons from about 400 AD onwards. The economic importance of hemp throughout history as a source of fibre cannot be overstated. Under King Henry VIII of England, a law stipulated that all subjects with arable land should reserve some of it for the cultivation of hemp and flax, which was essential for the rigging of ships. A less fortunate use of hemp was as the fibre that made the hangman's noose! There is evidence, for example, in the earliest Chinese Pharmacopoeia, that very early on there was awareness of its effects on consciousness: 'To take too much makes people see demons and throw themselves about like maniacs.' The ancient Indian text, Artharvarveda, describes it as an herb that will 'release us from anxiety'. Interestingly, in 1848 a text in the British Pharmacopoeia clearly outlined the effects of cannabis, in particular the antispasmodic and analgesic potential: 'Numerous observers have described the Indian hemp as producing in the natives of the East, who familiarly use it instead of intoxicating spirits, sometimes a heavy, lazy state of agreeable reverie, from which the individual may be easily roused to discharge any simple duty—sometimes a cheerful, active state of inebriation causing him to dance, sing and laugh, provoking the venereal appetite, and increasing the desire for food—and sometimes a quarrelsome drunkenness, leading to acts of violence. During this condition pain is assuaged and spasm arrested.' In Southeast Asia, its traditional use is in the form of 'grass'; that is, its leaves, stalks and flowering tops are smoked, sometimes mixed with tobacco.

The mode of action of THC remained poorly understood until the discovery of cannabinoid-sensitive sites in the central nervous system (CNS). The cannabinoid CB_1 and CB_2 receptors were cloned and identified in the 1990s. A search began after their identification to isolate endogenous cannabinoid ligands. The first was a lipid compound that is an amide of arachidonic acid with ethanolamine, and was named anandamide. Other endogenous ligands for cannabinoid receptors were subsequently identified, such as 2-arachidonoylglycerol (2-AG), virodhamine, noladin ether and *N*-arachidonoyl dopamine. The formation of endogenous ligands such as anandamide is Ca^{2+}-dependent. There is evidence that stimulation of neurotransmitter receptors such as the D_2 dopamine receptor can lead to increased availability of anandamide.

Cannabinoid ligands are hydrophobic compounds, and thus tend to remain associated with lipid membranes. Endocannabinoid signalling appears to be modulated by two processes: carrier-mediated transport into cells and intracellular hydrolysis. The transport is not driven by transmembrane Na^+ gradients, as is the case with other transporters, but instead may depend on facilitated diffusion. The hydrolysis involves several enzymes such as fatty acid amide hydrolase and monoacylglycerol lipase.

The CB_1 receptor mediates most of the effects of cannabinoids on the CNS, whereas the CB_2 receptor is found in the periphery (especially on immune cells) and also on microglia. The CB_1 receptor is present in the neocortex, hippocampus, basal ganglia, cerebellum, thalamus, hypothalamus, midbrain (periaqueductal grey [PAG] and superior colliculus), medulla and spinal cord. The CB_1 receptor is the most abundant G-protein-coupled receptor in the mammalian brain. Activation of CB_1 receptors leads to a series of signalling events: inhibition of N- and P/Q-type voltage-activated Ca^{2+} channels, opening of K^+ channels, and inhibition of adenylate cyclase.

Cannabinoids are involved in the phenomenon called 'depolarization-induced suppression of inhibition', seen in structures such as the hippocampus and the cerebellum. Thus, when pyramidal neurons in the CA1 region of the hippocampus are firing, it is likely that they release anandamide or 2-AG. This may activate CB_1 receptors on the terminals of GABAergic neurons situated in the vicinity, thus inhibiting GABA release. The net result may be a facilitation of long-term potentiation in CA1 neurons. This may seem paradoxical, as cannabinoids have amnesic effects. However, the amnesic effects may involve other circuits and/or mechanisms, distinct from the local depolarization-induced suppression of inhibition. A regulatory role of cannabinoids has also been suggested in the striatum, in terms of modulation of glutamatergic signals from corticostriatal fibres (Fig. 17.5). In this model, intense firing of corticospinal neurons leads to release of glutamate, and through the influx of Ca^{2+}, subsequent activation of the synthesis of endocannabinoids in the medium-sized striatal spiny neurons. These could act retrogradely and stimulate CB_1 receptors on corticostriatal fibres, leading to decreased release of glutamate. This mechanism may underlie long-term depression at this synapse. Thus, cannabinoids can exert complex modulatory effects on the CNS, at both inhibitory and excitatory synapses. Some of these may underlie the beneficial effects of cannabinoids, such as the analgesic, antiemetic and antispasmodic effects. It has also been shown that agents that reduce CB_1 receptor function, such as the partial agonist rimonabant, may reduce the potential for relapse in certain addictions such as alcohol, nicotine and heroin addiction.

One of the most disquieting trends in recreational cannabis use is the increasing number of people who are regular users of cannabis. The percentage of adolescents in England reporting the use of cannabis increased from 3.9% to 4.4% during 2014–2018. There is also evidence of a strong link between repeated use of cannabis and the development of depression and psychosis in later life. Someone who starts using cannabis at the age of 15 years has more than four times the risk of developing schizophrenia over the next 11

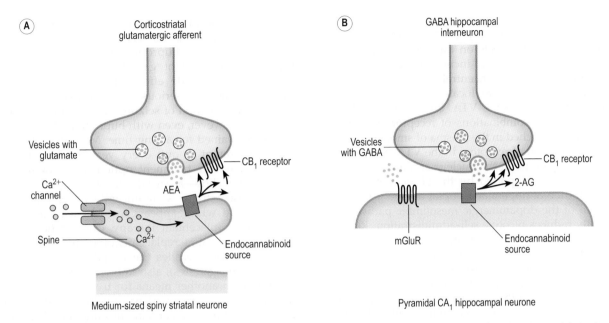

Fig. 17.5 Modulatory effects of cannabinoids. (A) Modulation by anandamide (AEA) of glutamatergic release in the striatum. (B) Modulation by 2-arachidonoylglycerol (2-AG) of GABA release in the hippocampus. *mGluR*, metabotropic glutamate receptor; *GABA*, γ-aminobutyric acid.

years as someone who starts using cannabis at the age of 18 years. After the age of 18 years, those who have used cannabis at least 50 times have a seven-fold risk of developing psychosis over the next 15 years.

There is an increasing call worldwide, from certain groups, to legalize cannabis—a change that has already occurred in many countries. Some addiction specialists' reflection on this is that the data so far clearly show that legalisation of drugs that can induce addiction (e.g. the common use of nicotine and alcohol) increases the number of people who are exposed to them, and the more people who are exposed to a drug, the greater the number who will become addicted, and the subsequent personal consequences and burden of medical care on society will also increase. Evidence also indicates that cannabis may prime the brain for the rewarding effects of other drugs and this increases the risk of spiralling into deeper addiction. However, there is also evidence that controlled use of cannabis in the form of well-regulated formulations would have a clear therapeutic value, for example, in the control of spasticity and chronic pain in multiple sclerosis, and the nausea and vomiting associated with chemotherapy. Furthermore, an interesting development in the field of cannabinoid research in the last decade is the accumulating evidence that cannabidiol, a non-psychoactive component of cannabis, could exert many beneficial effects, for example, in treatment-resistant forms of juvenile epilepsy and also in the management of opioid use disorder.

Nicotine

Nicotine is the main psychoactive component of tobacco. The Spanish conquistadores were the first to discover the widespread use of tobacco—the dried leaves of the plant *Nicotiana tabacum*—by the natives of Cuba. Within less than two centuries, tobacco use was well established throughout Western Europe, some of its success probably being due to its supposed activity as an aphrodisiac! In parallel, opposition to the habit of smoking developed. For example, King James I of England described smoking as 'a custom loathsome to the Eye, hateful to the Nose, harmful to the Brain, dangerous to the Lungs', showing remarkable insight into the characteristics of the abused substance. Most of the tobacco used in the UK is in the form of cigarettes; a smaller amount is consumed in the form of cigars or pipe tobacco. Addiction to nicotine constitutes one of the most serious health problems worldwide. Over 8 million smoking-related deaths are reported annually. Approximately 1.2 million of these deaths are due to passive smoking, that is, exposure to smoke produced by smokers in one's vicinity. Nicotine is the largest killer in the western world, with smoking-related diseases accounting for 20% of all deaths.

Nicotine was first isolated in 1828. It exerts widespread effects on the autonomic nervous system and also complex effects on the CNS. The effects are mediated by agonist action at neuronal nicotinic receptors, which are a particular type of acetylcholine receptor. These have a widespread distribution in the central and peripheral nervous systems. They are ligand-gated ion channels and have a pentameric structure (see Chapter 2), which can result from combinations of 12 different subunits: α_2 to α_{10} and β_2 to β_4. The activation of the receptor leads to an influx of Na^+ and K^+ (and to a lesser extent Ca^{2+}) into the neuron, and subsequent depolarization. Nicotine increases both sympathetic and parasympathetic activity. Furthermore, it increases muscle tone through its effects on nicotinic receptors at the neuromuscular junction. Nicotine also has monoamine oxidase (MAO) inhibitory activity. Overall, its effects on the CNS are reflected in mild arousal, a sensation of increased energy and focus, improved memory and concentration.

Nicotinic receptors are located on GABAergic and dopaminergic cells in the VTA, but the two cell types express different combinations of receptor subunits. At doses that are reached in the plasma of smokers, nicotine leads to activation of receptors in the VTA and increased release of dopamine in the nucleus accumbens. The role of dopamine is supported by the observation that the administration of dopamine receptor antagonists, as well as lesion of the dopaminergic mesolimbic pathway, significantly reduces nicotine self-administration. Repeated exposure leads to desensitization, which may underlie nicotine tolerance. Tolerance to nicotine develops rapidly. It disappears almost as quickly as it develops (6–8 h) and smokers report that the cigarette they enjoy the most is the one they smoke first thing in the morning! Compounds present in cigarette smoke also act as potent inducers of the P450 liver microsomal enzyme system, thus affecting the metabolic transformations of other substances. Therefore, several types of drug may have decreased efficacy in smokers (e.g. opiates, antianginal drugs and benzodiazepines), necessitating a dose increase.

Apart from addiction to nicotine *per se*, smoking is also associated with other health risks. The most well established fact is the significantly increased risk of developing lung cancer. The risk of death is directly related to the number of cigarettes smoked daily and the age when smoking starts. The risk of smokers developing cancers of the mouth, throat and oesophagus is almost 10 times greater than for non-smokers. Other forms of cancer also appear to be more frequent in smokers. Smoking also leads to increased platelet adhesiveness and narrowing of coronary arteries. More than 30% of deaths from coronary heart disease in the UK are attributed to smoking. Smoking also leads to a high-risk of developing chronic obstructive lung disease. Women who smoke give birth to babies that are significantly lighter than those born to women who do not smoke, and these babies are at higher risk of death during the perinatal period. In the last decade the dangers of passive smoking (i.e. exposure to cigarette smoke without being a smoker) have also become clearer. Passive exposure to cigarette smoke may significantly increase the risk of ischaemic heart disease, asthma, chronic obstructive pulmonary disease and lung cancer.

Attempts to stop smoking lead to symptoms such as craving, irritability, headaches, insomnia and weight gain. The most common approach to dealing with nicotine addiction is the use of a nicotine replacement therapy—nicotine transdermal patches, lozenges, inhalers, gums or sprays—which maintain a certain plasma nicotine level. The drug bupropion, developed initially as an antidepressant, is also used as an aid in the treatment of nicotine addiction. Its primary mechanism of action involves an increase in dopaminergic and noradrenergic signalling through inhibition of the reuptake of the amines. Bupropion reduces the withdrawal symptoms and weight gain associated with smoking cessation. Minor side effects include dry mouth and insomnia. The only serious risk with the use of bupropion is the induction of seizures (approximately 0.1% of patients). However, even with bupropion, the abstinence is not maintained for a long time. More than 20 million smokers attempt to quit every year but less than 10% succeed. Another treatment option for smoking cessation is varenicline—a partial $\alpha_4\beta_2$ nicotinic receptor agonist—whose activity is significantly lower than that of nicotine, and which appears to be at least as effective as nicotine replacement therapy. Combinations of varenicline and nicotine replacement therapy are also under study. In recent decades the introduction of electronic cigarettes (e-cigarettes), also known as 'vaping' devices, has provided another means for trying to reduce smoking. E-cigarettes are small hand-held devices that heat a liquid that usually contains nicotine and flavourings. Nicotine is inhaled in a vapour rather than in smoke. Therefore, e-cigarettes do not expose users to the same levels of toxins as those associated with smoking involving conventional cigarettes. There is some evidence that these devices may help more people to stop smoking compared to nicotine replacement therapy.

Alcohol

Alcohol is one of the most commonly used psychoactive substances. Alcohol (ethyl alcohol or ethanol) is a natural product of the fermentation of fruits and cereals. A major portion of the alcohol produced and consumed worldwide is derived from fermentation of grapes from various *Vitis* species, in particular *Vitis vinifera* or grain, and consumption occurs in the form of wine, beer or spirits.

The pharmacokinetics and pharmacodynamics of alcohol are complex. It is absorbed almost completely from the gastrointestinal tract and 95% of this is metabolized, while the rest is eliminated in the urine, sweat and breath. Pure alcohol decreases gastric emptying and mixed alcohol (e.g. as found in alcoholic sweetened carbonated drinks such as 'alcopops') is absorbed faster than pure alcohol. The absorption of alcohol is slowed by the fat content of food. Alcohol is metabolized by alcohol dehydrogenase, an enzyme whose activity is controlled by the availability of the cofactor nicotine adenine dinucleotide. When alcohol dehydrogenase activity is saturated (at approximately 10 mg/100 mL blood) the metabolism of alcohol becomes zero-order, which means that even small increases in ingested alcohol will lead to large increases in plasma concentration. Alcohol dehydrogenase shows genetic polymorphism and this explains the significant variability between individuals in resistance to the intoxicating effects of alcohol. Mild intoxication occurs at a concentration of 30–50 mg of alcohol in 100 mL of blood. When the concentration is higher than 100 mg/100 mL, most individuals suffer significant neurological symptoms, the most common being slurred speech and disturbed, staggering gait. Aggressive behaviour emerges, and vision and movement are impaired. At higher concentrations, alcoholic coma ensues. Chronic ingestion of alcohol induces the P450 microsomal system, which leads to pharmacokinetic changes and increased tolerance to alcohol, but also changes the biotransformation of other drugs (similar to chronic smoking).

Alcohol induces a range of peripheral and central effects. Acute ingestion increases blood pressure and induces peripheral vasodilatation. It reduces secretion of the anti-diuretic hormone and so increases diuresis. It increases the level of blood glucose and inhibits gluconeogenesis. It irritates the gastric mucosa, leading to the development of chronic gastritis in many alcoholics. Heavy drinking sessions ('boozing', or 'binging'), a pattern of drinking common in northern Europe, particularly in the UK, can trigger acute hepatitis. Chronic use of alcohol leads to severe thiamine deficiency, as this compound is used in the metabolism of alcohol, and its absorption is decreased by alcohol itself. This thiamine depletion ultimately leads to Wernicke's encephalopathy and Korsakoff's psychosis (also known as the Wernicke–Korsakoff syndrome). The symptoms include confusion, peripheral neuropathy, ataxia, aphasia, memory loss, confabulation and significant cognitive dysfunction. Fine motor function may also be affected and there are vision changes (nystagmus and ophthalmoplegia). If alcohol consumption stops and supplementation with thiamine is started, recovery is possible. If treatment is not administered, up to 20% of patients with Wernicke–Korsakoff syndrome will die of it. In the majority of patients the loss of memory and cognitive impairment are permanent due to damage of the mammillary bodies, thalamus and periaqueductal grey—structures involved in the Papez circuit.

Alcohol also affects pregnancy; the number of miscarriages is significantly higher among alcoholic women and approximately 10% of babies born to alcoholics present with 'foetal alcohol syndrome'. Symptoms include mental retardation and microcephaly, low body weight and length, poor motor coordination, hypotonia, and a typical facies characterized by a smooth philtrum (due to lack of a nasal bridge), a thin upper lip and small eyeballs with short palpebral fissures (Fig. 17.6). Multiple neurotransmitter systems are involved in the effects of alcohol on the brain. Like other abused drugs, alcohol activates the dopaminergic mesolimbic system and this is likely to be associated with its rewarding effects. Alcohol increases the firing of dopaminergic cells in the VTA and, as a result, increases dopamine release in the nucleus accumbens. Genetic studies have shown a clear association between alcoholism and both the D_2 dopamine receptor and the dopamine plasma membrane transporter. Brain imaging has shown alterations in the expression of the D_2 dopamine receptor and the dopamine transporter in the brain of alcoholics. Recent studies suggest that the increased vul-

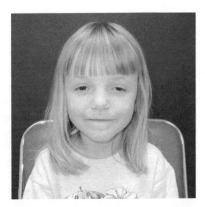

Fig. 17.6 Facial characteristics in foetal alcohol syndrome. Note the bilateral ptosis, short palpebral fissures, smooth philtrum and thin upper lip. (From Seaver LH. (2002) Adverse environmental exposures in pregnancy: teratology in adolescent medicine practice. Adolesc Med State Art Rev 13:269–91.)

nerability to relapse in alcoholic patients is associated with an increased density of D_2 receptors. However, it has been shown that destruction of the dopaminergic mesolimbic pathway does not lead to total cessation of the self-administration of alcohol. Alcohol binds to several neurotransmitter receptors: 5-HT₃, GABA and NMDA receptors. Acutely, it facilitates the inhibitory effects of GABA and decreases the stimulatory effects of glutamate. Chronic exposure to alcohol increases the number of NMDA receptors and L-type Ca^{2+} channels. Alcohol intake is also associated with increased release of endogenous opioids.

Alcoholism is a disorder with high heritability (50%–60%). It is often comorbid with other disorders such as anxiety and depression. Alcoholism can be defined as a chronic and progressive disease characterized by loss of control over the use of alcohol. After chronic use of alcohol, one of the most severe complications of withdrawal is the development of delirium tremens (Box 17.4).

Strategies to treat alcoholism include pharmacological and non-pharmacological approaches. The most common strategies employed to treat alcoholism are psychosocial interventions and self-help groups such as 'Alcoholics Anonymous'. Pharmacological treatment is used to treat three aspects: (1) alleviation of the symptoms of acute withdrawal (e.g. β-blockers and benzodiazepines, which reduce anxiety), (2) anticonvulsant agents for the management of seizures during delirium tremens and (3) aversive drugs such as disulfiram, which irreversibly blocks acetaldehyde dehydrogenase (an intermediate product in the metabolic pathway that leads from alcohol to acetic acid). Taking disulfiram before ingestion of alcohol, disrupts the metabolism of alcohol. Alcohol is metabolized in the liver to acetaldehyde by alcohol dehydrogenase. Acetaldehyde is then oxidized to acetate by acetaldehyde dehydrogenase. Disulfiram reduces the rate of oxidation of acetaldehyde, causing a large increase in the concentration of acetaldehyde. The increased acetaldehyde levels produce unpleasant side

The abrupt cessation of intake of alcohol in chronic alcoholics leads to a complex withdrawal syndrome termed 'delirium tremens'. This often occurs when a person who has developed physical dependence is admitted to hospital, for example, for accidental injury, and they cannot continue drinking alcohol according to their regular pattern. Withdrawal symptoms vary and unfold slowly: some of them may occur as early as 6–8 h after the last drink, others at 48–72 h and yet others after 8–10 days. The syndrome is characterized by nervousness and irritability, anxiety, nausea and vomiting, insomnia, palpitations, tremor, sweating and headaches. Confusion and disorientation and a state of extreme agitation may follow. The patient may become very sensitive to sensory stimulation such as light, sound or touch. Hallucinations (mainly visual) may occur, with the patient complaining of insects crawling under the skin. The delirium may become severe, and some patients may become lethargic or develop seizures of a tonic–clonic type. Associated symptoms include stomach cramps and chest pains and a very irregular heartbeat. Delirium tremens is a medical emergency. First, the blood pressure, fluid and electrolyte balance, and respiration are checked. Seizures require administration of anticonvulsant. Clonidine can be used to decrease anxiety and reduce cardiovascular symptoms. Hallucinations are treated with antipsychotic drugs for as long as necessary. A β-blocker may reduce the symptoms of sympathetic overactivity. It is also important to provide vitamin supplements, in particular thiamine, as alcoholics are usually deficient in thiamine. If the symptoms are severe, the patient may require sedation (e.g. benzodiazepines) for several days. Even after the successful management of a delirium tremens episode, patients may suffer for several months from tiredness, anxiety, depression and fluctuations in mood.

effects: vasodilatation, headaches, hypotension, nausea, vomiting and circulatory collapse.

Naltrexone and acamprosate are two drugs recently introduced for the management of alcohol use disorder. Naltrexone is a long-acting opiate antagonist that appears to improve abstinence rates and reduces relapse. In the United States it is the most commonly used pharmacotherapy for alcoholism. Interestingly, it has been shown that there is a pharmacogenetic aspect in the efficacy of naltrexone for the management of alcoholism: individuals with the 118G polymorphism in the OPMR1 gene encoding the mu opioid receptor are better responders to naltrexone than individuals with the more common 118A allele. Acamprosate (calcium acetylhomotaurine) exerts its effects through interactions with NMDA receptors and also as a positive allosteric modulator of the $GABA_A$ receptor. Like naltrexone, acamprosate can reduce relapse and increase abstinence rates. Patient compliance is better with acamprosate than with naltrexone.

Phencyclidine

Phencyclidine (PCP) was introduced in 1950 as an anaesthetic. It soon became obvious that patients experienced psychotic-like symptoms after a single exposure. PCP was withdrawn from therapeutic use, but remained a popular street drug. One of its street names is 'angel dust' because it is often sprinkled on tobacco or marijuana and then smoked. PCP has a variety of effects on the CNS: anaesthesia, analgesia, psychostimulation, hallucinations, distorted perceptions and other psychotomimetic actions. It induces very little tolerance. Individuals can become addicted and develop both a physical and psychological dependence. Withdrawal symptoms experienced upon abrupt cessation of use include agitation, anxiety, sweating, muscle spasms, psychosis, diarrhoea and hyperthermia. PCP is an NMDA receptor antagonist. It can also block nicotinic cholinergic receptors and block dopamine uptake. Experimental studies have shown that chronic use of PCP leads to degenerative changes in cortical neurons, with vacuolization of cells and increased cell death. It has a complex toxic profile. Males in particular become agitated, belligerent and violent. The individuals present with increased respiration, hypertension and tachycardia, hyperpyrexia, increased secretions, stereotypies and often a blank stare. Blood pressure may fluctuate widely and seizures are common, with possible conversion to status epilepticus. The toxic syndrome induced by PCP may require patient restraint because of the aggressive behaviour. Sedation can be induced with benzodiazepines. Death may occur due to respiratory and cardiovascular complications, and also to rhabdomyolysis and consequent kidney failure, in a manner similar to intoxication with substituted amphetamines (see below).

Amphetamines

Examples include amphetamine, methamphetamine and other related derivatives. These compounds are indirect agonists at noradrenergic, dopaminergic and serotonergic synapses. They inhibit monoamine reuptake, promote monoamine release and can also inhibit MAO activity. Amphetamine is also a potent agonist at the trace amine-associated receptor 1 (TAAR1). Amphetamines and related compounds are second only to cannabis in terms of their widespread use. Administration of amphetamine leads to reduced need for sleep, decreased reaction times, increased motor activity and improved concentration. Amphetamine also increases blood pressure and heart rate and dilates pupils. Methamphetamine is a derivative with a longer duration of action than amphetamine and better bioavailability.

The stimulant effects of amphetamines have been known for a long time. Amphetamine was used extensively during World War II to increase resistance to fatigue. Not only soldiers, but also politicians, were users of amphetamine, including Winston Churchill and Adolf Hitler. Amphetamine was presumed to be safe, although the effects of stopping intake were well known: after the rush of energy and euphoric state, and the decreased need to sleep or eat, the users would experience a 'crash', dominated by tiredness and depression. Typically, this would lead to further drug intake. The only amphetamines currently used for medical purposes are dexamphetamine for narcolepsy and methylphenidate (an amphetamine-related compound) for the treatment of hyperactive children suffering from attention-deficit/hyperactivity disorder.

Amphetamines can be snorted, taken orally or injected. After heroin, amphetamine is the most abused injected drug in the UK. There is particular concern over the use of methamphetamine, which is stronger than amphetamine and causes an intense and longer-lasting 'high'. Its chronic use can lead to strong psychological dependence and bouts of intense depression after the 'high'. In 2020 it was estimated that there were 7.4 million dependent amphetamine users worldwide. Dependence on amphetamine/methamphetamine is associated with depression, psychosis, anxiety and cardiovascular disease.

Amphetamine overdose can lead to cardiac arrhythmia, paranoid ideation, hyperactivity and hyperthermia. Paranoia may be accompanied by hallucinations, and it is known that amphetamine ingestion can precipitate relapse in schizophrenic patients. The combination of hyperthermia and hyperactivity may lead to an acidotic state, convulsions and death. Intense headache and dyskinesias may also occur. The management of amphetamine overdose relies on the use of benzodiazepines and antipsychotics. In the latter category, drugs with an α-adrenergic component are preferred, such as chlorpromazine, in order to counter the increased sympathetic activity. Since amphetamine is a base that is excreted unchanged in the urine, it is possible to acidify urine with ammonium chloride and thus significantly increase the rate of excretion.

At present, there is no satisfactory treatment for addiction to amphetamines. A very wide range of treatments have been explored so far, including antidepressant drugs (e.g. mirtazapine), GABA agonists (e.g. baclofen), partial nicotinic cholinergic agonists (varenicline), different stimulants (dexamphetamine and methylphenidate), glutamatergic agents (riluzole), opiate antagonists (naltrexone) and CRF_1 antagonists. However, the benefits shown are mild and inconsistent across studies. Antipsychotic drugs and short-term benzodiazepines can be used for the management of acute withdrawal symptoms. Psychosocial interventions that have shown some benefits include cognitive behavioural therapy and contingency management.

Methylenedioxymethamphetamine—'Ecstasy'

One of the most abused recreational drugs is a substituted amphetamine: 3,4-methylenedioxymethamphetamine (MDMA), also called 'ecstasy'. MDMA is an amphetamine derivative structurally related to the hallucinogenic compound mescaline. Since the mid-1980s, MDMA has become a very popular recreational drug associated with live music venues, especially 'rave' parties. Ecstasy tablets come in a variety of shapes, sizes and colours. Doses and purity vary widely. A 2012 Dutch study found that the occurrence of significant adverse events after ecstasy use, for example, palpitations, agitation, hyperthermia and seizures, were attributed to the presence of contaminants such as methylenedioxyamphetamine and meta-chlorophenylpiperazine. The effects of the drug occur after a latent period of 20–60 min and may last for 3–6 h. MDMA users report a state of relaxation and euphoria. The drug appears to increase empathy and to sharpen emotions. It decreases inhibitions and heightens the perception of sounds and colours.

The case history illustrates the dangers associated with the use of this drug and the misperception that it is rather mild and innocuous. According to the 2014 United Nations World Drug Report, Australia ranks as the highest per capita consumer of the drug. Most hospital admissions and, ultimately, deaths associated with this drug are the result of hyperthermia, which leads to breakdown of skeletal muscle (rhabdomyolysis), and associated multiple organ failure. Furthermore, ingestion of large volumes of water in an attempt to decrease the effects of hyperthermia and dehydration (due to many hours of dancing, for example) may lead to a typical hyponatraemic syndrome, exacerbated by increased secretion of anti-diuretic hormone. The retention of water leads to dilution of the extracellular medium. The subsequent brain swelling is accompanied by signs of increased intracranial pressure. Death may occur as a result of brain herniation. The case history illustrates a typical toxic ecstasy syndrome, which luckily resolved within 48 h but which may have also ended in the death of the young person involved. Young women are particularly sensitive to the toxic effects of ecstasy. In the case history the restoration of a normal Na^+ level was probably crucial in saving the life of the patient.

There is increasing concern that the use of ecstasy leads to irreversible brain structural changes. The pharmacodynamic profile of this drug is complex. The acute administration of MDMA leads to increased release of 5-HT in the brain. This effect involves an interaction with the 5-HT reuptake system. MDMA also inhibits MAO activity (with a 10-fold higher potency at MAO_A than at MAO_B). The drug can also increase dopamine release but its effects may not involve the dopamine transport system; instead, diffusion into the dopaminergic terminal followed by displacement of dopamine from vesicles. Finally, MDMA can also acutely increase the release of noradrenaline. MDMA binds to a variety of receptors; it shows high affinity for $5-HT_2$, $α_2$-adrenergic, M_1 muscarinic and H_1 histamine receptors, and lower affinity for $5-HT_1$, β-adrenergic and $α_1$-adrenergic receptors.

Research in monkeys has shown that MDMA has a neurotoxic effect on the 5-HT innervation of the forebrain (see Fig. 17.7). The loss of 5-HT fibres may be partly reversible in some brain structures, but it is question-

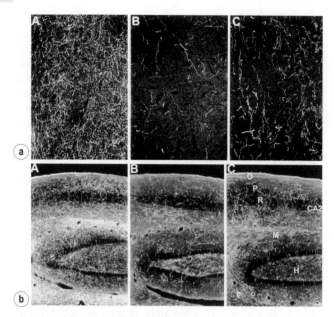

Fig. 17.7 Neurotoxicity of MDMA in monkeys exposed semi-acutely to the drug. (a) Dark-field photomicrograph showing 5-hydroxytryptamine (5-HT) fibres in the caudate nucleus (A) in control animals, (B) 2 weeks after a 3-day exposure to MDMA, and (C) 7 years after a 3-day exposure to MDMA. (b) Dark-field photomicrographs showing 5-HT fibres in the hippocampus (A) in control animals, (B) 2 weeks after a 3-day exposure to MDMA, and (C) 7 years after a 3-day exposure to MDMA. *H*, Hilus; *M*, the molecular layer; *O*, stratum oriens; *P*, stratum pyramidale; *R*, stratum radiatum. (From Hatzidimitriou et al. (1999). Journal of Neuroscience 19:5096–107.)

able whether full recovery ever occurs. As illustrated in Fig. 17.7, the effects are spectacularly long lasting. Thus, after only three administrations of ecstasy, 7 years before their brain tissue was analysed, the monkeys still showed significantly decreased serotonergic innervation of the striatum and of the hippocampus. Positron emission tomography (PET) studies in chronic ecstasy users confirm that serotonin transmission is altered, raising the possibility that the regular use of ecstasy in humans irreversibly affects serotonergic signalling. Furthermore, it has been shown that long-term use of recreational MDMA leads to discrete changes in brain glucose metabolism, which can be correlated with specific verbal memory deficits.

Hallucinogens

Drugs that induce mental changes similar to psychotic states are called hallucinogens or 'psychedelic' drugs. In 1938 the Swiss chemist Albert Hofmann synthesized the compound lysergic acid diethylamide (LSD) and a few years after its synthesis accidentally ingested some powder, subsequently experiencing the 'mind-expanding' properties of this compound. The effects (also known as 'the trip') were described as a 'dream-like state' during which sensory modalities fused. Hallucinations during which sensory modalities are mixed up are called 'syn-

esthetic'. Interestingly, such hallucinations are sometimes encountered in patients with temporal lobe epilepsy. The sense of time is disrupted but memory is unaffected. Feelings of total detachment and depersonalization may occur. Hallucinogens may affect mood, but the type of effect seen is context-dependent and depends on the mindset of the user. Good 'trips' as well as terrifying, bad 'trips' can be experienced by the same user. There is increased sympathetic activity, with increased blood pressure and pulse rate, dilated pupils and increased body temperature.

The structure of LSD and other hallucinogens, such as the compounds extracted from the psilocybe mushroom (i.e. psilocybin) or the peyote cactus (i.e. mescalin), are very similar to that of serotonin. It is now well established that LSD can activate presynaptic 5-HT receptors, and thus decrease the activity of raphe serotonergic neurons. This may underlie, at least partly, the effects of the hallucinogen, but the compound has a complex pharmacology, involving several types of 5-HT receptor. LSD is a very potent compound, with 25 µg being sufficient to induce hallucinations. Death from LSD overdose is rare, as the safety range of this compound is wide. When overdose occurs, it manifests as vomiting, respiratory arrest and coma. There is rapid tolerance to the effects of LSD. Hallucinogens may lead to psychological but not physical dependence. Together with cannabis, ecstasy and amphetamine, LSD is among the most popular drugs with club-goers. Experiencing the effects of psychedelic compounds through ingestion of LSD or 'magic mushrooms' (its street name) is a common temptation among teenagers in particular, and some of the self-reported effects and consequences are quite disturbing. Box 17.5 contains edited fragments of the comments of two people who have eaten 'magic mushrooms'.

An interesting development in the past 2–3 years has been the new recognition of the potential therapeutic value of certain hallucinogens, such as psilocybin, which could have unique therapeutic effects in depression and the management of addictions (e.g. alcohol and tobacco). Like other psychedelic compounds, psilocybin exerts agonist effects at 5-HT$_{2A}$ receptors, which are abundantly expressed on the large cortical pyramidal cells. Magnetoencephalography and electroencephalography show that psilocybin induces an increase in cellular firing and, subsequently, desynchronized cortical activity. This enhanced entropy effect leads to an increase in cerebral connectivity patterns, possibly underlying more insights into feelings, motives, beliefs and actions. Notably, the regimen of treatment with these psychedelic agents is quite different from the usual regimens of drug treatment in these conditions: for example, instead of taking the drug daily, it is administered only on a few occasions over several weeks, and it is used in conjunction with very structured psychotherapy support. Overall, the proponents of this new 'psychedelic psychiatry', such as the scientists and clinicians at the newly created Centre for Psychedelic Research, at Imperial

Going on 'trips'

'I had a terrible experience yesterday on mushrooms. I had eaten them twice before with no problem... This time, when I ate the 8th, I didn't even finish them all. I felt fine at first. We were going to go to the beach to "people watch". I got up to go to the bathroom first and all of a sudden I felt extreme anxiety. I have never been so scared in my life. I felt like I was fighting with myself. I started screaming at my boyfriend. Everything I saw was changing and I didn't know where I was. I was being really mean to him one second and the next second I was apologizing, trying to tell him I didn't mean it. I could not understand anything that was going on. I had no concept of anything. Even time. I kept asking what time it was. Literally, a minute felt like it should have been 2 or 3 hours... He tried to put on some soothing music and I made him take it out. I couldn't even watch commercials with music on television. Now, 24 hours later, I feel extremely sad and not quite myself. I would appreciate it if you could ... tell me what happened. How can I get myself feeling normal again?'

'I took mushrooms at the age of 20 and had a very bad experience. I became suicidal and for about 4 days I was totally wasted. Today at the age of 47 I suffer from severe depression and phobias and have had to have electroshock treatment for a breakdown. Could this be related to that bad experience all those years ago, and if so, what help could I get, if there is a cure available?'

College in London, suggest that these agents trigger a profound and long-lasting beneficial neural plasticity.

Solvents

A wide variety of organic compounds that are used as solvents, e.g. in paint, nail varnish remover and glue, as well as cigarette lighter gas or propellant gas used in aerosols, can be abused through inhalation (and so are termed 'inhalants'). Solvent abuse is commonly called 'glue-sniffing' and is a form of addiction that affects mainly adolescents. It is quite common in the UK, and it particularly affects young people in socially deprived areas. These inhalants are rapidly absorbed and lead to a sensation similar to that of being drunk. Irrespective of their structures (i.e. aliphatic or aromatic hydrocarbons, chlorinated hydrocarbons, acetates, ketones, ether or chloroform), these agents initially produce a stimulating effect, which is followed by depression. The molecular targets activated by solvents to induce these effects are not well defined. They include NMDA glutamate receptors, nicotinic cholinergic receptors, $5\text{-}HT_3$ receptors and $GABA_A$ receptors. The effect is short-lived (usually a few minutes) and repeat doses are required every hour. The user can develop hallucinations and delusions and may slip into a delirious state. Tolerance to solvents can develop very quickly. There is no physical dependence but there is strong psychological dependence. Chronic exposure to solvents is likely to cause not only neurotoxicity but also hepatotoxicity and renal toxicity. Accidental death can also be caused by suffocation or choking on vomit after intense periods of sniffing that may trigger emesis. There is at present no treatment for solvent abuse. Changes in legislation which restricts sales of glues and solvents with high volatile organic compound content are an example of a means of controlling this type of addiction.

Addiction and rehabilitation: general comments

In the treatment of addiction there are three stages at which interventions play an important role: (1) during the active use of the drug, (2) to alleviate the symptoms of withdrawal and (3) to prevent relapse. That addiction is a disease of the brain, with complex physical and emotional aspects, is a relatively recent concept in the history of medicine; some scholars have proposed different theories of addiction and question or reject the brain disease model. For example, an alternative theory is that addiction reflects a distorted deep learning process that can be unlearned. Multiple drug addiction is a common and significant societal problem. Addicts may use, at the same time, varying combinations of alcohol, cocaine, crack, methadone and PCP, and also sniff glue. Each of these drugs, as discussed above, has its own characteristics and sometimes their negative effects can be synergistic. Cocaine and heroin can lead to tolerance. However, under certain conditions, drugs of abuse such as amphetamine can lead to the opposite phenomenon, that of sensitization, that is, an enhancement of the effects of the drug. Ethanol and opiates lead to physical dependence, whereas cocaine and amphetamine much less so. Cues associated with drug taking play a major role in relapse, either a short time after abuse or after a long period of abstinence. Thus, places, people or the paraphernalia associated with drug abuse can trigger relapse. Stress also appears to act as a triggering factor for relapse in many addictions.

In parallel with the main substance use disorders discussed in this chapter, another trend in society is the emergence of new psychoactive substances, that is, drugs designed to replicate the effects of substances like cannabis, cocaine and 'ecstasy' while remaining legal—hence the alternative names: 'legal highs' or 'designer drugs'. They represent a heterogeneous class of substances, known under various brand names, and include synthetic cannabinoids, psychostimulants, compounds with sedative and anti-anxiety effects, and also substances with hallucinogenic properties. These drugs are easily available online and are often adulterated with other compounds. There is increasing evidence that demonstrates their short-term and long-term harm, in particular their strong addictive potential. The Psychoactive Substances Act came into force in the UK in 2016, and it is illegal to produce, supply, or import these new substances for human consumption—including for personal use.

The life of an addict can lead to extreme physical and moral degradation, as described by the autobiographies or diaries of addicts: 'I wake to the feeling of something warm dripping down my chin. I lift my hand to feel my face. My four front teeth are gone. I have a hole in my cheek, my nose is broken and my eyes are swollen nearly shut... I look at my clothes and my clothes are covered with a colourful mixture of spit, snot, urine, vomit and blood'. There are at present very few efficient ways of treating addiction and, in the future, the answer may lie in an approach based on a better understanding of the complex changes induced in the brain by chronic consumption of drugs. Our present understanding of the neurobiology of addiction indicates that, in the brain of an addict, homeostasis has been replaced by 'allostasis', that is, a totally different set point, and efficiently treating addiction will require better characterization of all the neurotransmitter and circuit changes involved in this allostatic transformation. What is also clear is that the life trajectory of addicts and their substance misuse can be very different: persistent use, declining use, cessation followed by relapse or sustained cessation. There is a need for a better understanding of the factors that underlie this heterogeneity and the development of reliable biomarkers of relapse, thus leading to improved management of this significant and life-changing brain condition.

Self-assessment case study

Alex recently graduated in engineering and was offered a choice position to work on an oil platform in Scotland. He has decided to celebrate with friends and go out for a drink. He intends to make it a special occasion and drink more than the usual few pints that he drinks almost every night during the week. Whenever he is out with his friends he has a reputation for 'drinking everybody under the table'. On the night of the celebration they start the evening with a few whiskies and continue with beer. After several hours of drinking, all of them are seriously drunk. As they leave the pub, they attempt to cross the road and Alex is hit by a car that he did not see. He suffers multiple fractures and is taken to the accident and emergency department. The first 24 h in hospital seem to go by in a haze and after the first day Alex starts to feel very unwell, with alternating chills and sweating. During the afternoon of the second day, he becomes aggressive with the nurses and attempts to hit one of them. He also claims that there are bugs in his bed 'that crawl all over him'. The doctor on duty decides to administer diazepam and keep him under observation over the next 2–3 days.

After studying this chapter, you should be able to answer the following questions:

1. What is Alex suffering from?
   The symptoms that Alex is suffering from, taking into account his history of alcohol consumption, correspond to the development of a withdrawal syndrome and a state of 'delirium tremens'.
2. What are the main risks associated with the condition that he develops in hospital?
   A patient who develops symptoms of 'delirium tremens' must be maintained under observation: there may be onset of seizures, increased confusion and psychotic episodes, and also autonomic instability that will require appropriate management before patient discharge.
3. What long-term treatment can you suggest in Alex's case?
   After discharge from hospital, Alex would require an assessment of his habit of consuming regularly large quantities of alcohol. He is likely to have developed alcohol use disorder, which could be managed using a combination of pharmacological and non-pharmacological strategies.

Index